FUNDAMENTAL MECHANISMS
IN HUMAN CANCER IMMUNOLOGY

DEVELOPMENTS IN CANCER RESEARCH

FUNDAMENTAL MECHANISMS IN HUMAN CANCER IMMUNOLOGY

Proceedings of the First International Conference on Fundamental Mechanisms in Human Cancer Immunology, Galveston, Texas, U.S.A., October 27–29, 1980.

Editor:
J. PALMER SAUNDERS, PH.D.
Professor of Pharmacology, Dean of the University of Texas, Graduate School of Biomedical Sciences, Galveston, Texas, U.S.A.

Associate Editors:
JERRY C. DANIELS, M.D., PH.D.
Associate Professor of Internal Medicine and Microbiology, University of Texas Medical Branch, Galveston, Texas, U.S.A.

BERNARD SERROU, M.D.
Center Paul Lamarque, University of Montpellier, Montpellier, France

CLAUDE ROSENFELD, M.D.
Institut de Cancerologie, Villjuif, France

Assistant Editor:
CONSTANCE B. DENNEY, PH.D.
Research Coordinator, Multidisciplinary Research Program on Schizophrenia, Division of Biochemistry, University of Texas Medical Branch, Galveston, Texas, U.S.A.

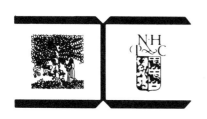

ELSEVIER/NORTH-HOLLAND
NEW YORK • AMSTERDAM • OXFORD

Published by:

Elsevier North Holland, Inc.
52 Vanderbilt Avenue, New York, New York 10017

Sole distributors outside the USA and Canada:

Elsevier Science Publishers B.V.
P.O. Box 211, 1000 AE Amsterdam, The Netherlands

Library of Congress Cataloging in Publication Data

International Conference on Fundamental Mechanisms in
    Human Cancer Immunology (1st : 1980 : Galveston, Tex.)
    Fundamental mechanisms in human cancer immunology.

    (Developments in cancer research, ISSN 0163-6146 ;
v. 5)
    Bibliography: p.
    Includes indexes.
    1. Cancer--Immunological aspects--Congresses.
I. Saunders, J. Palmer. II. Title. III. Series.
[DNLM: 1. Neoplasms--Immunology. W1 DE997WM v.16 / QZ 200
F9815]
RC268.3.I463 1981   616.99'4079   81-9845
ISBN 0-444-00648-6   AACR2

Manufactured in the United States of America

Contents

viii

Preface

J. Palmer Saunders, Ph.D.

Professor of Pharmacology and Toxicology; Executive Director, UTMB Cancer Research Center; Dean, The University of Texas, Graduate School of Biomedical Sciences at Galveston, The University of Texas Medical Branch, Galveston, Texas

Cancer is probably the most feared of human diseases. The very word "cancer" strikes terror in the hearts of most of us. It is not the fear of dying that frightens us. After all, heart disease and strokes kill more people each year than do malignancies. No, it is the frightening prospect of a prolonged, painful illness resulting in isolation from the rest of humanity, and, frequently, dehumanizing disfigurement produced by heroic surgical procedures aimed at rooting out the disease. Death, when it comes, is regarded as a welcome release from a long period of exquisite torture. Cancer then stands as the great challenge to medical science and to the physicians who must bear the burden of treating its sufferers. Cancer is regarded as a universal evil, and no other disease so stirs the emotions. As a consequence, people use such terms as "crusade" and "war" for the constant battle against the disease. No other disease has the ability to loosen the purse strings both of the federal government and of individual citizens. All of us wish to do all we can to stop cancer and each one of us secretly prays that a cure will be discovered before it engulfs us too.

Cancer is not a single disease—there are probably two hundred different cell types. But it is convenient to speak of cancer as if it were a single entity. Cancer affects most living things and it is part of the life process itself. There is no cell which has a greater will to survive and multiply than the cancer cell. Cancer was well-known even to the ancients, and Hippocrates gave it its name because its pattern of cell growth resembles a crab. The Greeks and Romans thought that cancer was caused by an imbalance in the bodily humors. After 2500 years marked by constant research and study, we still cannot improve very much on that description. In fact, we can state with fair confidence that cancer in its many manifestations is not a disease but a symptom of a fundamental disorder in the host organism's defense mechanisms.

In the nineteenth century, the diagnosis of cancer was uniformly considered a sentence of death. Great secrecy surrounded the diagnosis and families went to great lengths to prevent it from being known—not only to persons outside the family, but to the victim. Cancer caused great dread and physicians themselves avoided the diagnosis as long as possible—thus surely aggravating the situation. Many persons felt that cancer was a degrading disease and there was fear of "catching" cancer, as if it were an infectious disease. As a result of these various emotions, the cancer victim was often condemned to a lonely and horrifying death. Surgery was the accepted method of treatment. To isolate the tumor and cut it out seemed the only rational approach. And of course this sometimes worked. When a tumor was localized, surgical removal was quite effective. Unfortunately, the majority of cancer victims were not that lucky. Cancer cells migrating to other parts of the body soon began to grow and the disease returned, this time without much hope of a surgical cure.

At the end of the century, with the discovery of Roentgen rays and their effects on living cells, a new modality of treatment was introduced. At first crude x-rays were effective only on superficial lesions, but as the principles of radiobiology were slowly uncovered, more sophisticated techniques were used. With the introduction of more powerful beams, scientists learned how to control the rays—thus avoiding some of the damage to normal tissue and concentrating on the tumor. At its best, however radiation was another form of surgery. Once a tumor was detected—and this was the crucial step—the decision to use surgery or radiation depended more upon the specialty of the oncologist rather than on any rational protocol.

After World War II, clinical groups in Chicago and New Haven attempted a systematic study of the use of nitrogen mustard as a treatment of cancer. Cancer chemotherapy—or the treatment of cancer with various chemical agents—was born out of chemical warfare, and it was not long before other compounds were introduced. Only the leukemias and lymphomas however seemed to be susceptible to treatment with drugs, and even then little success was obtained. Then, in 1955, the proponents of chemotherapy research persuaded the Congress to appropriate large (for that time) amounts of money. Using the successful search for an antimalarial drug to support their case, prominent advocates of chemical treatment argued that it was almost certain that somewhere—on the laboratory shelves of synthetic chemists or among the many biologically active plants of the country—there existed a "magic bullet" which would cure cancer. "Give us $5 million a year for the search and we'll find a cancer cure in 5 years," they claimed. Congress was convinced and established within the National Cancer Institute a Cancer Chemotherapy Service Center to carry out the search for new agents and to screen them against tumor cells. Provisions were also made for the establishment of special clinical teams to try out the expected new compounds in human cancer therapy.

Unfortunately, the hope for a cure engendered by these words proved naive. The oversimplification broke down and researchers belatedly came to realize that the struggle against cancer was far more complex than finding a "magic bullet." Nevertheless, the screening mechanism of the National Cancer Institute produced several new compounds, each of which gave partial promise of activity against the childhood leukemias and lymphomas. Vincent de Vita and his co-workers pioneered the use of complex mixtures of compounds (the MOPP program) and were able to secure long-term remissions in Hodgkin's disease and some leukemias.

During this time, surgical procedures and more powerful radiation therapy were still being employed against the so-called solid tumors (which remain the major killers), since it appeared that chemotherapy was only partially effective in most cases. The use of all three modalities of treatment (multimodal therapy) was gradually introduced in the late 1960's. Today, the treatment of cancer can involve all three therapies, surgery and/or radiation to reduce the tumor's bulk, and selective and appropriately timed chemotherapy to eradicate metastatic foci throughout the body.

The outlook for cancer today is far brighter than it was a generation ago. There are over 1.5 million people in the United States whose cancers can be said to be "cured," as judged by survival five years beyond first diagnosis. It is estimated that better than 30% of the approximately 650,000 new cases of cancer diagnosed each year will be added to this group. Among patients treated in specialized and comprehensive cancer centers, the rate may even exceed this figure. The key to this success is early diagnosis, since few would disagree that the chances for a favorable outcome depend on early detection and diagnosis, followed by aggressive treatment.

Despite improved prognosis for childhood leukemia, lymphomas, and other limited cancers, the mortality data for the major cancer killers—lung, colon, breast, prostate, and bladder—remain alarmingly stable. In fact, for the first time in 25 years, cancer incidence has begun to rise (Pollack and Horm, 1980). Not all of this increased incidence is due to smoking. Cancer epidemiologists claim that even discounting the increased incidence of smoking-related cancer, the overall cancer rate is still on the upswing. Some scientists feel that the tremendous increase in the synthesis of new chemical compounds since World War II and their almost universal employment in all phases of human activity must be tied in somehow to this cancer increase. Marvin Schneiderman, Associate Director of the National Cancer Institute, has stated categorically that these trends "suggest industrial exposure may be contributing more and could contribute substantially to the cancer burden in the future (Wade, 1980). Even if one does not entirely agree with this point of view, it is clear that the ubiquitous chemical carcinogen is with us to stay—in our food, in our water, and in the air we breathe. In the face of this ever increasing danger and in view of the resistance to treatment of the cancers responsible for the greatest mortality, biomedical science should expect an even tougher battle in the future. New concepts must be devised and new approaches employed.

Immunology is the basic science of how the body copes with foreign invaders. It has always been a mystery how a cancer cell can by transformation become a "foreign substance," and yet escape detection and destruction by host defense mechanisms. There are reasons to suspect that malignant transformation is a common occurrence, and that the host's immune system normally operates continually to seek out and destroy these wild cells. According to this hypothesis, it is only when this system becomes defective that cancer cells can establish themselves and multiply. At later stages in its differentiation, the colony may create its own perimeter defense and thus thwart the body's natural immune defense mechanisms. At this point, the cancer emerges as a frank disease entity.

Efforts to employ immunotherapy against cancer therefore cannot be based purely on the administration of additional amounts of substances normally found in the body, such as interferon, unless one can predict precisely at what period the body's defense mechanism needs augmentation. We need to learn much more about basic immunologic mechanisms of normal and malignant cells before we can mount any large scale program of immunotherapy. The purpose of the Symposium is to facilitate and stimulate an exchange among laboratory and clinical scientists who are leading investigators of those basic mechanisms.

Today, we can look forward to many advances in cancer research which were beyond expectation just a few short years ago. The biological revolution that is now in full swing argues convincingly for an eventual solution to the dreadful problem of cancer. That hope, coupled with the great advances already made, should give new inspiration to all of us and impel us to redouble our efforts to uncover the basic principles of cell biology.

References

Pollack, E.S. and Horm, J.W. (1980) Trends in cancer incidence and mortality in the United States, 1969–76. *J.N.C.I.* 64:1091–1103.

Wade, N. (1980) Government says cancer rate is increasing. *Science* 209:998–1001.

Acknowledgments

This Symposium is the first of a series to be sponsored jointly by The University of Texas Medical Branch, Galveston, Texas and The University of Montpellier, Montpellier, France. The Editor wishes to thank the administration of both universities for their encouragement and support during both the planning of the conference and the meeting itself.

Financial support for the Symposium was provided in part by a Grant from the National Cancer Institute— CA 27958-01A1. The Editor wishes to express his appreciation to the staff of the National Cancer Institute for their support during preparations for the conference. Financial support was also provided through generous gifts from the Harris and Eliza Kempner Fund of Galveston, the American Cyanamid Company, Bristol Laboratories, Eli Lilly and Company, Hoffman LaRoche, Inc., and Stuart Pharmaceuticals. The Editor wishes to convey grateful thanks to these organizations for their additional support, without which it would have been difficult if not impossible to complete arrangements for the meeting.

An international Symposium of this nature is not accomplished without much hard work and dedication from a number of individuals. The Editor would particularly like to express his thanks to the Assistant Editor, Dr. Constance Denney, who worked many long hours in editing and preparing the manuscripts for publication. Thanks are also due to the efforts of the staff of the UTMB Cancer Center—Mr. Fred C. Delaney, Ms. Margie Taylor, Mrs. Karen Lewis, and Mrs. Roxanne Schuster.

If the Symposium has achieved a measure of success, it can be attributed to the excellent presentations by the individuals who participated in the Symposium. The Editor wishes to thank them all for their enthusiasm and vigorous participation in the many fruitful and stimulating discussions which occurred during the conference.

FUNDAMENTAL MECHANISMS
IN HUMAN CANCER IMMUNOLOGY

PART I:

Cell Membranes

Published 1981 by Elsevier North Holland, Inc.
Saunders, Daniels, Serrou, Rosenfeld, and Denney, eds.
FUNDAMENTAL MECHANISMS IN HUMAN CANCER IMMUNOLOGY

CHAPTER 1

Modulation of C3b Receptor Synthesis on a Human B Lymphoblastoid Cell Line (Raji)[1]

R. Frade,[2] M. Barel,[3] and C. Charriaut

Institut de Cancérologie et d'Immunogénétique, Département de Culture et de Production de Cellules Humaines, 16 Avenue Paul-Vaillant Couturier, 94800 Villejuif, France

Summary

It has been reported by Hampar et al. (1972) and Gerber (1972) that treatment of Raji cells, an Epstein Barr Virus (EBV)[4] negative cell line, by 5-bromodeoxyuridine (BrdU) resulted in activation of infectious virus synthesis. In the present report, using a FACS II, we have shown that treatment of Raji cells by BrdU results in an enhancement of C3b receptor synthesis on the cell surface. The mechanism of BrdU action on the regulation of C3b receptor synthesis on Raji cells is discussed.

Introduction

The presence of receptors for the third component of complement, C3, has been extensively described on a variety of mammalian cells (Lay et al., 1968; Philipps-Quagliata et al., 1971). The exact role of C3 receptors on the cell surface is not yet understood, but the most recent results suggest that C3 receptors could be involved in: (a) cell-cell cooperation (Pepys, 1976), (b) the maturation state of cells (Ross et al., 1978), or (c) an association with other

[1] This research was supported by the University Pierre et Marie Curie (Paris) and by research grants from the Délégation Générale à la Recherche Scientifique et Technique (DGRST 79-7-0794) and from Unité d'enseignement et de Recherche de Kremlin-Bicêtre (n° 782).
[2] To whom correspondence should be addressed.
[3] M.B. is a fellow of la Ligue Nationale Française contre le Cancer.
[4] Abbreviations used: EBV: Epstein Barr Virus; FITC: Fluorescein Isothiocyanate; HMBA: Hexamethylenebisacetamide; BrdU: 5-Bromodeoxyuridine; Me$_2$SO: Dimethylsulfoxide; db cAMP: Dibutyryl cyclic AMP; Raji (BrdU) cells: Raji cells rendered resistant to BrdU.

membrane antigens as histocompatibility antigens (Ferreira et al., 1976; Curry et al., 1976) or EBV receptors (Jondal et al., 1976; Rosenthal et al., 1978). Little is yet known about the biochemistry of C3b receptors. Lay et al. (1968) first described its trypsin sensitivity, and recently, Fearon (1980) identified a membrane glycoprotein, gp 205, as the C3b receptor on human peripheral blood cells. In biochemical studies of C3b receptors on human B lympho-blastoid cells (Raji), we have shown (Frade et al., 1980) that C3b receptors interact with purified and ^{125}I labeled C3b as low affinity receptors with a dissociation constant of 10^{-6} M, and that binding sites numbered 5×10^4 per cell. We have mentioned that only 60% to 70% of the Raji cells react with particle bound C3b. On analyzing the data from other laboratories, we have found that Raji cells were described as either 100% or 60% C3b receptor positive, and no explanation for these discrepancies has been offered. To study the regulation of C3b receptor synthesis on human B lymphoblastoid cells, we thought it necessary to elucidate the exact expression of C3b receptors on the Raji cell line and to establish the conditions under which the largest number of C3b receptors could be induced. In the present report, we have attacked this problem by measuring C3b receptor synthesis on human B lymphoblastoid cells (Raji) grown in the presence of several cell differentiation effectors.

Methods

Cells

Raji wild type, a B cell line derived from a Burkitt's lymphoma, Molt 4, a T cell line derived from a T acute lymphoblastoid leukemia, and Reh 6, a "non T-non B" cell leukemia, were grown in RPMI 1640 (Gibco), supplemented with 10% heat inactivated fetal calf serum (Gibco) at 37°C in a 5% CO_2 incubator.

Purification of Human C3

Human C3 was purified following the method described by Tack et al. (1976) to homogeneity as assessed by polyacrylamide gel electrophoresis in the presence of sodium dodecyl sulfate and by immunoelectrophoresis using goat anti-human C3 (Cordis, Flo). C3b was freshly prepared from the purified C3 trypsin cleavage under the conditions described by Bokish et al. (1969).

Detection of C3b Receptor on Human Lymphoblastoid Cells

5×10^6 cells were incubated with 1 ml purified human C3b at a saturating dose of 0.5 mg per ml for 30 min at 37°C. After two washes with dextrose gelatin veronal buffer, cells were incubated with 100 μl fluorescein isothiocyanate (FITC) anti-human C3 (Cappel) at a saturating dose dilution of 1 : 50, for 1 hour at 4°C. After two washes, cells were analyzed for fluorescence with the Fluorescence Activated Cell Sorter (FACS II) from Beckton Dickinson. Under conditions of growth with or without drugs and during FITC anti-C3 labeling of cells, the number of dead cells never exceeded 5-8%. The percent of C3b reporter positive cells was calculated from the number of fluorescent cells per 50,000 living cells, counted after selection of channels on the FACS to avoid dead cells. Negative controls were obtained by incubating cells with buffer in place of C3b and then with FITC anti-human C3 serum. Preliminary experiments using either the FITC labeled IgG fraction of the anti-human C3 serum of the F (ab')$_2$ fragment purified from these IgG fractions have shown that the binding of anti C3 antibody on cell surfaces preincubated with purified C3 does not occur through its Fc fragment. These results discount the possibility of interference with the Fc receptor in the conditions of incubation used.

Results

Human lymphoblastoid cells were incubated at 5×10^5 per ml in culture medium at 37°C for 72 hr and then chemical compounds were added. Cell growth and the percentage of C3b receptor positive cells were measured over 72 hr, the time needed for the culture to reach the stationary phase. Drug treatment had no effect on the measure of fluorescence; cells incubated with a drug and tested immediately showed no change in fluorescence intensity.

When Raji wild type cells were grown without cell differentiation compounds, the percentage of C3b receptor positive cells was 60% at t=0 and 70% at t=72 hr (Figure 1.1) with a low fluorescence intensity which indicated a low density of C3b receptors on each positive cell (see Figure 1.4A). Two other cell lines were used as controls: Molt 4, a T cell leukemia line, whose cells are consistently 25% C3b receptor positive, and Reh 6, a "non T-non B" cell leukemia line whose cells are consistently 100% C3b receptor negative (Figure 1.1).

Effect of Polar Compounds on C3b Receptor Expression on Raji Cell Surface

Polar compounds such as dimethylsulfoxide (Me$_2$SO) and hexamethylenebis-acetamide (HMBA) have been reported to be highly efficient inducers of cell differentiation. Studying the differentiation of the murine erythroleukemia cells incubated in the presence of Me$_2$SO, Yeoh and Morgan (1979) have shown an increase in transferrin receptor levels, whereas Parker and Hopper (1979) have described a loss of Fc receptors at the cell surface. Nudel et al. (1977) have demonstrated that after these cells are grown for 4 days with HMBA or Me$_2$SO, the B^{maj} containing hemoglobin (Hb^{maj}) predominates.

When the human lymphoblastoid cell line, Raji (wild type), was incubated with these polar compounds, the expression of C3b receptors on the cell surface was modulated as follows: (a) HMBA (2 mM) had no effect during the first 48 hours and a slight decrease from 65% to 55% was observed only at 72 hours (Figure 1.1), whereas cell growth was substantially increased from 2.2×10^6 to 2.9×10^6 cells per ml (Figure 1.2). (b) In the presence of Me$_2$SO (2%), an increase was detected at 36 hours which reached a maximum of 80%

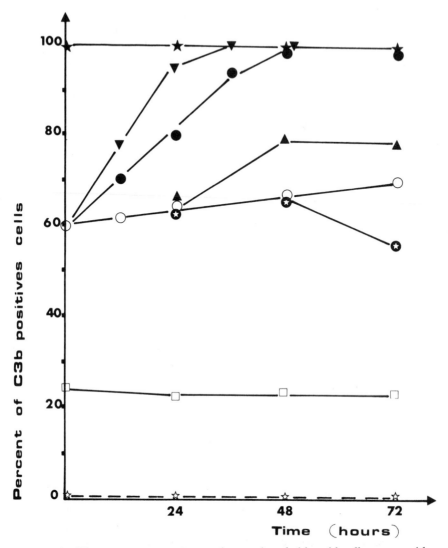

Figure 1.1. C3b receptor expression on human lymphoblastoid cells grown with or without cell differentiation effectors: (○—○) Raji wild type grown without compounds; Raji wild type grown in presence of: (✪—✪) HMBA (2 mM); (▲—▲) Me$_2$SO (2%); (▼—▼) dbcAMP (5×10^{-4} M); (●—●) BrdU (30 μM). (□—□) Molt 4; (☆—☆) Reh 6; and (★—★) Raji (BrdU) grown with or without BrdU).

at 48 hours (Figure 1.1), whereas cell growth was significantly diminished from 2.2×10^6 to 1.2×10^6 cells per ml (Figure 1.2).

Lower concentrations of these polar compounds had no effect on C3b receptor expression or on cell growth; higher concentrations were toxic. At no concentrations did they affect C3b receptor expression of Molt 4 and Reh 6 cells.

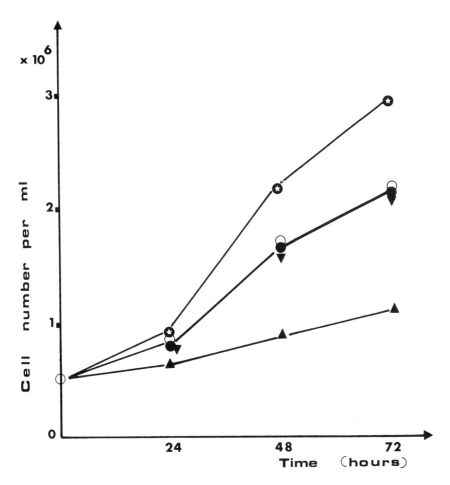

Figure 1.2. Growth curve of Raji wild type, incubated with or without cell differentiation effectors. (○—○) control; (✪—✪)+HMBA (2 mM); (▲—▲)+Me$_2$SO (2%); (▼—▼)+dbcAMP (5×10^{-4} M); (●—●)+BrdU (30 μM).

Effect of BrdU on C3b Receptor Synthesis on Raji Cell Surfaces

5-Bromodeoxyuridine (BrdU), an analogue of thymidine (TdR), was described by Coleman et al. (1970) as a promising tool to manipulate experimentally the determination of cell type. These compounds have been extensively described as activators or inhibitors of cell differentiation, depending on the type of cells and the cell differentiation marker studied.

When Raji cells (wild type) were incubated in the presence of an optimal concentration of BrdU (30 μM), a tremendous increase in C3b receptor expression on the cell surface was measured (Figure 1.1) without any change in cell growth (Figure 1.2). This increase was detected at as early as 6 hr, and by

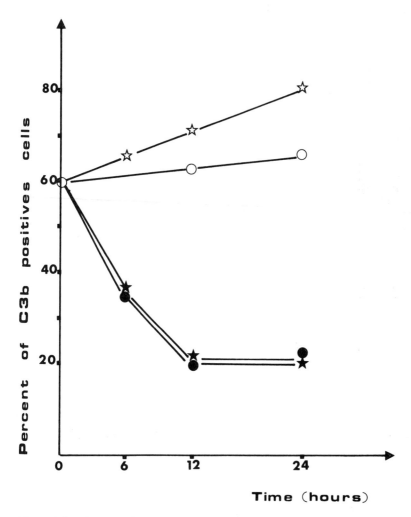

Figure 1.3. Effect of inhibition of protein synthesis on C3b receptor expression on Raji wild type. Cells were grown without: (O—O) or with: (☆—☆). BrdU (30 μM) in absence (white symbols) or in presence (black symbols) of cycloheximide (200 μg/ml).

48 hr, 100% of the cells were C3b receptor positive. This increase was related to "de novo" protein synthesis, since the increase was abolished in the presence of cycloheximide (200 μg/ml) (Figure 1.3). BrdU (30 μM) had no effect on the C3b receptor expression of the Molt 4 and the Reh 6 cell lines.

The increase of C3b receptor synthesis on Raji (wild type) by BrdU (30 μM) was analyzed using the FACS II. Whereas Raji (wild type) cells grown without BrdU showed a low fluorescence intensity over 72 hours (Figure 1.4A), which indicates a low density of C3b receptors on cell surface, the same cells grown

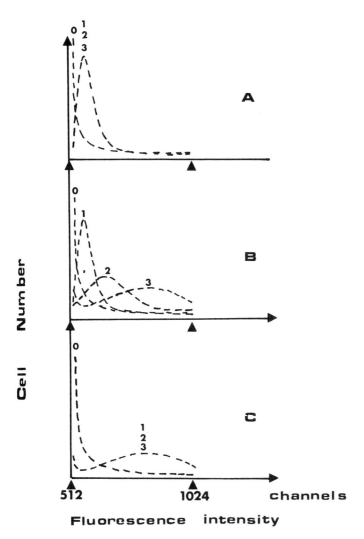

Figure 1.4. Fluorescence Activated Cell Sorter (FACS) analysis of C3b receptor expression on Raji cell surface. (A) Raji wild type grown in absence of BrdU (30 μM). (B) Raji wild type grown in presence of BrdU (30 μM). (C) Raji (BrdU) grown in absence or in presence of BrdU (30 μM). (O) Corresponds to the negative control, i.e., Raji cells incubated without C3b but with FITC anti-C3. (1), (2), and (3) correspond respectively to t=0, t=24 hours, and t=48 hours of growth.

for 72 hr in the presence of BrdU showed fluorescence profiles which changed from a low to a high fluorescence intensity (Figure 1.4B). These results indicate that the increase in the number of C3b receptor positive cells from 60% to 100% was accompanied by an increase in the density of C3b receptors on the cell surface. This phenotype is conserved for several weeks in presence of BrdU and at least for 2 weeks after removing BrdU and growing cells in drug free medium. It appears from these data that a Raji strain, Raji (BrdU), with a high density of C3b receptors on the cell surface could be selected in the presence of BrdU (30 μM). Hampar et al. (1972) have shown that Raji (BrdU) have thymidine kinase at about 1% of the enzyme levels expressed by Raji (wild type) cells.

Effect of Exogeneous Dibutyryl Cyclic AMP on C3b Receptor Synthesis on Raji Cell Surfaces

Exogeneous cyclic AMP or its analogue, dibutyryl cyclic AMP (db cAMP) have been described as inducers of cell differentiation *in vitro* (Scheid et al., 1973). When Raji (wild type) was grown in the presence of db cAMP (5×10^4 M), 100% of cells expressed C3b receptor at their surface with a high density of receptors per cell within 24 hours (Figure 1.5).

Discussion

The present study was undertaken to quantitate the expression of C3b receptors on a human B lymphoblastoid cell Raji (wild type) and determine the

Figure 1.5. Fluorescence Activated Cell Sorter (FACS) analysis of C3b receptor expression on Raji wild type cell surface, grown in presence of db cAMP (5.10^{-4} M) for 36 hours. (O) corresponds to the negative control, i.e., Raji cells incubated without C3b but with FITC anti-C3.

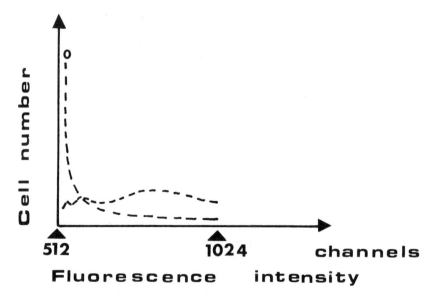

growth conditions required to increase C3b receptor synthesis on the cell surface in the presence of cell differentiation effectors.

When Raji (wild type) cells were grown in the absence of cell differentiation compounds, 60 to 70% of the cells expressed the C3b receptor on their surface, with a low density of receptors per cell.

When Raji (wild type) cells were grown in the presence of polar compounds such as HMBA (2 mM) or Me₂SO (2%), the percentage of C3b receptor positive cells was 55% or 80% respectively, at 72 hours, with alterations in the rate of cell growth.

When Raji (wild type) cells were grown in presence of BrdU (30 μM) C3b receptor synthesis was increased tremendously; in 48 hours, 100% of the cells expressed a high density of C3b receptors, with no change in the rate of cell growth. The high density of C3b receptors on Raji (BrdU) cells was unchanged during a continuous treatment of 4 weeks and after the removal of BrdU for a period of at least 2 weeks. From these data, it can be concluded that:

1. Two strains of cells, Raji (wild type) and Raji (BrdU), could be selected, each showing different C3b receptor expression. Use of either one of these strains without any specification could explain the discrepancy in C3b receptor expression reported by other investigators.
2. Using Raji (BrdU) or Raji (wild type) cells grown in the presence of BrdU, it is possible to obtain a population of 100% C3b receptor positive cells, with a high density of C3b receptors on each cell, which will be helpful for further C3b biochemical analysis.
3. On the basis of their C3b receptor expression on the cell surface, Raji (BrdU) and Raji (wild type) appear to represent two different blocks in the differentiation of the same lymphoblastoid cell whose differences can be abolished by incubating the cells with BrdU.

The mechanism of BrdU action in regulating C3b receptor synthesis on Raji cells remains to be determined. However, two mechanisms are usually reported: a DNA linked mechanism and a non-DNA linked mechanism.

Inhibition of BrdU activation of C3b receptor synthesis by thymidine (50 μg/ml) in our experiments (not shown) suggests that incorporation of the analog into DNA may be an essential step in the induction process. Moreover, Hampar et al. (1972) have shown that Raji (wild type) cells incorporate BrdU into DNA, whereas Raji (BrdU) does not. This result was confirmed by Billard (personal communication).

However, a non-DNA linked mechanism cannot be ruled out, since db cAMP (5.10^{-4} M) can enhance C3b receptor synthesis in 24 hours, and it has been mentioned by Rutter et al. (1973) that BrdU influences cyclic AMP levels. Schubert et al. (1970) have suggested that the halogenated pyrimidine need not be incorporated into DNA to alter the phenotype of the cell.

Finally, the BrdU activation of Raji cells is not restricted to the C3b receptor synthesis. Gerber (1972) and Hampar et al. (1972) have shown that treatment of Raji cells and E. B. virus negative cells by BrdU results in activation of infectious virus synthesis, and Tovey et al. (1977) have described the enhancement of interferon production in BrdU-treated Raji cells. BrdU could be an interesting tool to study the possible relationship between E. B. virus synthesis, E. B. virus receptor synthesis, and C3b receptor synthesis.

ACKNOWLEDGMENTS
We are grateful to Dr. C. Rosenfeld for access to the FACS II and to Mr. Z. Mishal for skillful technical assistance with it.

References

Bokish, V.A., Muller-Eberhard, H.J., and Cochrane, C.G. (1969) Isolation of a fragment (C3a) of the third component of human complement containing anaphylatoxin and chemotactic activity and description of an anaphylatoxin inactivator of human serum, *J. Exp. Med.* 129:1109–1130.

Coleman, A.W., Coleman, J.R., Kankel, D., and Werner, I. (1970) The reversible control of animal cell differentiation by the thymidine analog 5 bromodeoxyuridine. *Exp. Cell Res.* 59:319–328.

Curry, A.R., Dierich, M.P., Pellegrino, M.A., and Hoch, J.A. (1976) Evidence for linkage between HLA antigens and receptors complement components C3b and C3d in human mouse hybrids. *Immunogenetics* 3:465–471.

Eisen, H., Nasi, S., Georgopoulos, G.P., Ardnt-Jovin D., and Ostertag, W. (1977) Surface changes in differentiating Friend erythroleukemia cells in culture. *Cell* 10:689–695.

Fearon, D.T. (1980) Identification of the membrane glycoprotein that is the C3b receptor of the human erythrocyte, polymorphonuclear leukocyte, B lymphocyte, and monocyte. *J. Exp. Med.* 152:20–30.

Ferreira, A., Fotino, M., and Nussenzweig, V. (1976) Relationship between 4a and 4b HLA determined specifications and C3 receptors of leukocytes membrane. *Eur. J. Immunol.* 6:832–833.

Frade, R. and Strominger, J. (1980) Binding of soluble ^{125}I human C3b—the third component of complement, to specific receptors in human cultured B lymphoblastoid cells. *J. Immunol.* 125:1332–1339.

Gerber, P. (1972) Activation of Epstein-Barr Virus by 5 Bromodeoxyuridine in "virus-free" human cells. *Proc. Natl. Acad. Sc. U.S.A.* 69:83–85.

Hampar, S., Derge, G.J., Martos, L.M., and Walker, J.L. (1972) Synthesis of Epstein-Barr virus after activation of the viral genome in a "virus negative" human lymphoblastoid cell (Raji) made resistant to 5 Bromodeoxyuridine. *Proc. Natl. Acad. Sc. U.S.A.* 69:78–82.

Jondal, M., Klein, G., Oldstone, M.B.A., Bokish, V., and Yefenof, E. (1976) Surface markers on human B and T lymphocytes. VIII. Association between complement and Epstein-Barr Virus (EBV) receptors on human lymphoid cells. *Scand. J. Immunol.* 5:401–410.

Lage-Davila, A., Krust, B., Hofman-Clerc, F., Torpier, G., and Montagnier, L. (1979) Bromodeoxyuridine induced reversion of transformed characteristics in BHK 21 cells: changes at the plasma membrane level. *J. Cell. Physiol.* 100:95–108.

Lay, W.H. and Nussenzweig, V. (1968) Receptors for complement in leukocytes. *J. Exp. Med.* 128:991–1009.

Nudel, U., Salmon, J.E., Terada, M., Bank, A., Rifkind, R.A., and Marks, P.A. (1977) Differential effects of chemical inducers on expression of B globin genes in murine erythroleukemia cells. *Proc. Natl. Acad. Sc. U.S.A.* 74:1100–1104.

Parker, C.L. and Hooper, W.C. (1979) The loss of Fc surface receptors by erythroleukemia cells following stimulation to differentiate. *Cell Differentiation* 8:365–373.

Pepys, M.B. (1976) Role of complement in the induction of immunological responses. *Transplant Rev.* 32:93–120.

Philipps-Quagliata J.M., Levine B.B., Quagliata, F., and Uhr, J.W. (1971) Mechanisms underlying binding of immune complexes to macrophages. *J. Exp. Med.* 133:589–601.

Prasad, K.N. and Sinha, P.K. (1976) Effect of sodium butyrate on mammalian cells in culture: a review. *In Vitro* 12:125–132.

Rosenthal, K.S., Yanovitch, S., Inbar, M., and Strominger, J. (1978) Translocation of a hydrocarbon fluorescent probe between Epstein-Barr Virus and lymphoid cells: an assay for early events in viral infection. *Proc. Natl. Acad. Sc. U.S.A.* 75:5076–5080.

Ross, G. D., Jarowski, C.I., Rabellino, E.M., and Winchester R.J. (1978) The sequential appearance of Ia like antigens and two different complement receptors during the maturation of human neutrophils. *J. Exp. Med.* 147:730–744.

Rutter, W.J., Pictet, R.L., and Morris, P.W. (1973) Toward molecular mechanisms of developmental processes. *Ann. Rev. Biochem.* 42:601–646.

Scheid, M.P., Goldstein, G., Hammerling, U., and Boyse, E.A. (1975) Lymphocyte differentiation from precursor cells *in vitro. Annals N.Y. Acad. Sci.* 249:531–540.

Schubert, D. and Jacob, F. (1970) 5 Bromodeoxyuridine-induced differentiation of a neuroblastoma. *Proc. Natl. Acad. Sc. U.S.A.* 67: 247–254.

Tack, B.B. and Prahl, J.W. (1976) Third component of human complement: purification from plasma and physicochemical characterization. *Biochemistry* 15:4513–4521.

Tovey, M.G., Begon-Lours, J., Gresser, I., and Morris, A.G. (1977) Marked enhancement of interferon production in 5 Bromodeoxyuridine treated human lymphoblastoid cells. *Nature* 267:455–457.

Published 1981 by Elsevier North Holland, Inc.
Saunders, Daniels, Serrou, Rosenfeld, and Denney, eds.
FUNDAMENTAL MECHANISMS IN HUMAN CANCER IMMUNOLOGY

CHAPTER 2

Membrane Lipids and Cellular Functions of Normal and Malignant Lymphocytes

Michael Inbar, Ph.D.

Head, Department of Cell Biology, Miles-Yeda Ltd. and Department of Membrane Research, Weizmann Institute of Science, Rehovot, Israel

Introduction

During the last decade, technological innovations have allowed extensive study of the involvement of different membrane components in reactions regulating normal and abnormal cell growth and differentiation (Gitler, 1972; Signer and Nicolson, 1972; Edidin, 1974). Out of these studies has emerged the hypothesis that the cell surface membrane plays a major role in biological control mechanisms associated with malignant transformation of normal cells (Inbar and Sachs, 1969; Inbar et al., 1971). The membrane changes associated with transformation are complex, and involve different properties of the membrane, including (a) changes in the relative composition of membrane components, and (b) changes in the dynamic and structural organization of membrane constituents (Inbar et al., 1973; Shinitzky and Inbar, 1974). These two major types of membrane alterations, which are partially interrelated, are now believed to determine to a large extent the functional activities of the membrane (Shinitzky and Inbar, 1974).

Recent studies attempting to elucidate the molecular basis of membrane changes in normal and malignant transformed cells suggest that the composition and the distribution pattern of membrane components in an intact cell are controlled by several alternate mechanisms: (a) lateral and rotational mobilities of membrane protein receptors, (b) lateral diffusion of membrane phospholipids, (c) modulation of membrane antigens, (d) exchange of membrane cholesterol, and (e) exfoliation and shedding of lipoprotein complexes. It is now widely accepted and in some cases well documented that these processes which differ in normal and tumor cells primarily determine functional properties of their respective surface membranes (Inbar and Shinitzky, 1974). However, although several hypotheses have recently been advanced which propose a direct relationship between surface interactions and malignant transformation events, experimental evidence has generally demonstrated only indirect correlations.

Although direct evidence that membrane changes are required for malignant transformation of normal cells is not yet available, studies of membrane differences between normal and tumor cells have illuminated general biological problems such as the molecular mechanisms of cell differentiation and growth regulation (Inbar and Shinitzky, 1974). Moreover, quantitative tools for the early detection of malignant cells by analysis of membrane changes will prove valuable for both the study and treatment of cancer (Yanovich et al., 1978; Rosenfeld et al., 1979).

Since biological processes such as cellular differentiation, growth regulation, and malignant transformation are interrelated in lymphoid cells, and since all these processes involve changes in the structure and function of membrane components, we have undertaken a systematic study of the membranes of normal and leukemic lymphocytes. Our studies during the last 5 years were carried out with lymphoid cells and membranes obtained from both experimental model systems and humans.

Membranes of Intact Cells

In 1974, we introduced a new method for monitoring dynamic parameters of membranes in lymphoid cells (Shinitzky and Inbar, 1974). This method is based on fluorescence polarization (P) properties of the fluorescent hydrocarbon probe, 1,6-diphenyl 1,3,5-hexatriene (DPH) when embedded in hydrophobic regions of cellular membrane. For labeling, lymphoid cells are incubated in an aqueous dispersion of DPH at the concentration of 2×10^{-6} M which is practically void of fluorescence. The penetration of the DPH molecules into cellular membranes is indicated by a rapid increase in the fluorescent intensity of the system which levels off after about 30 min of incubation at $25°C$ (Shinitzky and Inbar, 1974). The labeled cells are then immediately submitted to fluorescence polarization analysis with a Microviscosimeter (Elscint Ltd., Haifa, Israel). The DPH-labeled cells are excited with polarized U.V. light and emitted fluorescence is detected in two independent, cross-polarized channels. Fluorescence polarization (P) is measured by simultaneous intensities polarized vertically (Iv) and horizontally (Ih) to the direction of polarization of the excitation beam. The values obtained related to the degree of fluorescence polarization (P), to the fluorescence anisotropy (r), and to the total fluorescence intensity (F) according to the following equations:

$$P = \frac{Iv - Ih}{Iv + Ih} \tag{2.1}$$

$$r = \frac{Iv - Ih}{Iv + 2Ih} \tag{2.2}$$

$$F = Ih(Iv/Ih + 2) \tag{2.3}$$

These measurements are rapid and the Microviscosimeter directly records the P value within 30 sec per sample. The sample temperature is controlled by a built-in thermoelectric system which minimizes variability in the recorded temperature to less than 0.3°C. Under these conditions of constant temperature, the accuracy of the obtained P value was found to be P = ±0.005.

By measuring the degree of fluorescence polarization, which is determined by the degree of rotation of the excited DPH molecules, the dynamics of the region where the probe molecules are embedded can be calculated. Our studies employed two independent methods for quantitative evaluation of the dynamic state of cellular membranes: (a) the degree of microviscosity, $\bar{\eta}$ (Shinitzky and Inbar, 1974) and (b) the degree of lipid fluidity, LFU (Yanovich et al., 1978).

Our method for evaluating membrane microviscosities ($\bar{\eta}$) is based on the fluorescence polarization properties of a fluorescent probe as described by the Perrin equation for rotational depolarization of a non-spherical fluorophore:

$$\frac{r_0}{r} = 1 + C_{(r)} \frac{T \cdot \tau}{\bar{\eta}} \tag{2.4}$$

where r and r_0 are the measured and the limiting fluorescence amisotropies (respectively), T is the absolute temperature, τ is the excited state life time of DPH, $C_{(r)}$ is a parameter that relates to the molecular shape of the fluorophore, and $\bar{\eta}$ is the membrane microviscosity (Shinitzky and Inbar, 1974).

The method employed for the qualitative evaluation of the degree of membrane fluidity (LFU) is a simple treatment in which the recorded P is related to a constant P value which is the theoretical upper limit of P:

$$LFU = \frac{\frac{P_{(max)}}{P_{(r)}} - 1}{P_{(r)}} = \left[\frac{P_{(r)}}{\frac{P_{(max)}}{P_{(r)}} - 1} \right]^{-1} \tag{2.5}$$

where $P_{(r)}$ and $P_{(max)}$ are the measured and limiting values of fluorescence polarization, respectively. The theoretical lower and upper limits of fluorescence polarization are 0 and 0.5 respectively, and therefore $P_{(max)} = 0.5$ (Yanovich et al., 1978). In general, the relation between P and LFU extends between the upper limit value of LFU which reaches ∞ value when $P_{(r)} = 0$ and the lower limit value of LFU which is 0 when $P_{(r)} = P_{(max)} = 0.5$. It is important to note that the P values are recorded directly from the Microviscosimeter, whereas $\bar{\eta}$ and LFU are calculated values obtained by Equations 2.4 and 2.5 respectively. The microviscosity treatment represents the dynamic nature of the membrane in absolute viscosity units (poise), whereas the LFU represents only a relative value.

Our method allowed characterization of dynamic parameters of cellular membranes in intact normal and leukemic lymphocytes obtained from 3 independent mouse systems. The leukemic lymphocytes used in these experiments were obtained from (a) a spontaneous thymus-derived lymphoma, (b) a Moloney virus-induced lymphoma, and (c) a methylcholantrene-induced lymphoma. Normal lymphocytes used as control cells were (a) mouse lymphnode lymphocytes, (b) mouse thymocytes, and (c) peritoneal exudate, cytotoxic T lymphocytes. A higher degree of fluorescence polarization (P) was obtained with DPH-labeled normal lymphocytes as compared to the P values obtained with DPH-labeled leukemic lymphocytes, indicating a lower degree of microviscosity and a higher degree of fluidity (LFU) in leukemic cells. This result was obtained in all of the large spectrum of normal and leukemic cells tested (Inbar, 1980). In order to provide direct evidence that leukemic cells show a lower P as compared to normal lymphocytes, a special fluorescence polarization instrument was constructed in our laboratory in collaboration with Elscint Ltd., Haifa, Israel. Experiments with this instrument demonstrated that on the single-cell level, most of the leukemic cells showed lower P values than the P value distribution in a normal lymphocyte population (Inbar, 1976; Van-Blitterswijk et al., 1977). It was therefore concluded that these differences represent differences between normal and leukemic cells and not differences between normal and leukemic cell populations.

Our demonstration of increased fluidity in the membranes of mouse leukemic lymphocytes led us to initiate a parallel study in humans. Our first objective was to search for possible differences in the membrane viscosity of lymphocytes obtained from normal donors and leukemic lymphocytes obtained from patients with leukemia. Our results indicated that the mean P value of lymphocytes isolated from peripheral blood of 131 normal donors and non-malignant patients is $P_{25}o = 0.294$. T, B, and Null, normal lymphocytes showed similar dynamic characteristics (Yanovich et al., 1978). Parallel experiments carried out with lymphocytes isolated from peripheral blood of patients with malignant lymphoma, chronic lymphatic leukemia, and acute lymphoblastic leukemia are 0.280, 0.273, and 0.245, respectively (Yanovich et al., 1978), indicating a marked decrease in cellular membrane microviscosity and a significant increase in membrane fluidity as compared to the same properties in normal lymphocytes. Similar results were obtained with leukemic lymphocytes isolated from both peripheral blood or bone marrow (Inbar, 1980).

In order to assess the possibility that these membrane differences between normal and leukemic lymphocytes are related to the disease state, lymphocytes isolated from leukemic patients during their illness and during remission were compared. Our results demonstrated a marked increase in the P value during remission in both peripheral blood and bone marrow lymphocytes (Rosenfeld et al., 1979). These results suggest that lymphocytes isolated from leukemic patients in remission show membrane characteristics similar to those of normal lymphocytes. Such a change from disease to remission was only obtained in patients with a long duration of remission. The decrease in the obtained P value in the different types of the leukemia disease correlates with prognosis. Chronic lymphatic leukemia shows a higher P value as compared to acute lymphoblastic leukemia, and T cell acute lymphoblastic leukemia shows a lower P value as compared to Null cell acute lymphoblastic leukemia.

In order to confirm our correlation of fluidity changes in cellular membranes of lymphocytes with clinical manifestation of acute lymphatic leukemia, lymphocytes isolated from 139 samples of peripheral blood obtained from 52 acute lymphatic leukemic patients in complete hematological remission were subjected to fluorescence polarization analysis with the aid of DPH. From the recorded P value the degree of microviscosity was calculated, and according to these values the 52 patients were divided into two groups: Group A, including 20 patients with a mean $\bar{\eta}$ value of 2.95 ± 0.38 and an upper limit value lower than 3.44, and group B, including 23 patients with a mean $\bar{\eta}$ value of 4.22 ± 0.38 and a lower limit value higher than 3.76. Nine patients showed an intermediate value between groups A and B. By correlating microviscosity of cells during remission and the clinical manifestation of the disease, we found that systematic relapse and neurological localization of tumor cells were 2.85 and 3.84-fold higher in group A as compared to group B. Data accumulated over a period of 3 years suggest that an abnormality low microviscosity of membranes of peripheral blood lymphocytes in leukemic patients in complete hematological remission may indicate a poor prognosis of the disease months in advance of the re-appearance of lymphoblasts in the circulation (Rosenfeld et al., 1979). This test is now being incorporated into follow-up protocols for the treatment of patients with acute lymphatic leukemia, since a very early prediction of relapse can be obtained. Our recent observations, indicating that leukemic patients in remission contained a large population of lymphocytes that show abnormal microviscosity and fluidity under conditions where no leukemic lymphoblasts can be detected, suggest that these cells may exist in a premalignant state which cannot be monitored by standard hematological nor immunological parameters. Indirect support for this hypothesis was obtained from our finding that such cells are only present in the peripheral blood of acute lymphatic leukemic patients with a short duration of remission (Rosenfeld et al., 1979; Inbar, 1980).

In order to explore the hypothesis that the low microviscosity and high fluidity of lymphoid cell membranes is characteristic of malignant cells, cellular membranes were studied in human lymphoblastoid cell lines established from patients with hematopoietic disorders. Twenty-five human hematopoietic cell lines established from patients with malignant and non-malignant diseases were studied for membrane fluidity. Our results show that cells derived from malignant diseases have a lower microviscosity and a higher fluidity than cells derived from non-malignant disorders (Inbar and Ben-Bassat, 1976). It was concluded that the malignant origin of a cell line grown *in vitro* can be related to low microviscosity and high fluidity, the characteristic parameters of freshly isolated leukemic cells.

Since the introduction of fluorescence polarization analysis of DPH-labeled intact cells in 1974, several investigators have questioned the validity of such measurement as a direct indicator of membrane fluidity in the cell surface membrane in intact cells. These reports have suggested that part of the DPH molecules are internalized from the cell surface into cytoplasmic membranes. At present we cannot discount the possibility that, with DPH-labeled intact cells, some of the fluorescent signals originate from inner membranes, but the measurements obtained by fluorescence polarization analysis may still be a valid biological and clinical tool in the study of human leukemia, assuming the clinical studies just described can be confirmed. Recent studies have also questioned the validity of microviscosity data obtained from steady state fluorescence polarization measurements. The term microviscosity is derived from the Perrin's equation for rotational depolarization of a non-spherical fluorphore, which is only valid where both emission anisotropy and total emission exhibit exponential decay. Nanosecond time-dependent fluorescence depolarization measurements of DPH embedded in artificial liposomes or dissolved in oils have indicated that decays are non-exponential. Thus, the relation between steady state fluorescence polarization and microviscosity may be more complex than anticipated. Nevertheless, microviscosity data of cellular membranes may be valid for a qualitative comparison between different populations of lymphoid cells. Therefore, although no reliance should be placed upon the absolute values of microviscosity, different $\bar{\eta}$ values of different cell types or different stages of the same cell type are valid. Moreover, similar clinical conclusions will be reached, if the data is presented in terms of fluorescence polarization, which is the value directly recorded from the Micro-viscosimeter. Due to these limitations in the method used in all our recent studies, results are given in P, $\bar{\eta}$, and LFU values, and significance should be only attached to relative values but not to absolute units (Inbar, 1980).

Isolated Plasma Membranes

During the last few years, since the introduction of the DPH fluorescence polarization method, dynamic parameters of lipid layers have been studied extensively, mostly with liposomes as membrane model systems (Shinitzky and Inbar, 1974). These studies have established that three main characteristics determine the physical state of a lipid region in the membrane. The most important of these is the molar ratio of cholesterol to phospholipids, the two major classes of lipids in the cell surface membrane of mammalian cells. Under physiological conditions, with a constant composition of phospholipids and at a constant temperature, an increase in the molar ratio of cholesterol to phospholipids will cause an increase in the rigidity of the system. The physical state of the lipid layer is also influenced by the relative composition of the different phospholipids in the membrane, more specifically, the molar ratio of sphingomyeline to phosphatidylcholine, and by the degree of saturation of the phospholipid acyl chains or the presence or absence of saturated and un-saturated free fatty acids in the systems. An increase in the ratio of sphingomyeline to phosphatidylcholine will cause an increase in the rigidity of the membrane, whereas an increase in the degree of unsaturation will cause an increase in the fluidity of the complex (Inbar, 1980).

To follow up our studies of lipid structures in intact cells and in membrane model systems, we attempted to directly determine the lipid composition of plasma membranes isolated form normal and leukemic lymphocytes. Plasma membranes were isolated from both cell types and analyzed for lipid composition and dynamic parameters. Our results confirmed those of our studies of intact cells: plasma membranes isolated from leukemic cells showed a lower degree of microviscosity and a higher degree of fluidity than plasma membranes isolated from normal lymphocytes. The molar ratio of cholesterol to phospholipids in isolated membranes was shown by direct biochemical analysis to be markedly reduced in leukemic cells as compared to normal lymphocytes. This reduction appears to explain in large part the significant increase in membrane fluidity in leukemic cells. Direct evidence to support this conclusion was obtained from the following experiments (Shinitzky and Inbar, 1974; Van-Blitterswijk et al., 1977; Petitou et al., 1978):

1. Plasma membranes of both normal and leukemic lymphocytes were subjected to a total lipid extraction. From the lipid extracts, liposomes were prepared and the degree of DPH fluorescence polarization of such liposomes was compared to the P values obtained with the intact membranes. The results have shown that the P values were 0.306 and 0.305, respectively, for membranes and liposomes of total lipids in membranes of normal lymphocytes, and 0.269 and 0.256 in intact membranes and liposomes of total lipids in leukemic membranes (Van-Blitterswijk et al., 1977). These results indicate that in lymphoid membranes, the obtained P value is determined only by the lipid composition of the membrane, without direct effect of membrane proteins.
2. Additional evidence was obtained from the dynamic behavior of liposomes prepared only from membrane phospholipids. Phospholipids were isolated from the total lipid extract of the two types of membranes by thin-layer chromatography. From the isolated phospholipids, liposomes were prepared and labeled with DPH. The results show a marked decrease in the P value where total lipid liposomes were compared to phospholipid liposomes, indicating as expected, the major effect of cholesterol. Phospholipid lipo-

somes extracted from both normal and leukemic membranes showed similar dynamic characteristics, indicating a similar composition of phospholipids in the two types of membranes. This conclusion was confirmed directly by a complete phospholipid analysis, which showed that the only difference in membrane phospholipids between normal and leukemic cells is a very slight decrease in sphingomyeline in leukemic cells. This decrease may account for the slight difference in P of 0.209 and 0.193, respectively, between phospholipid liposomes of normal and leukemic membranes (Van-Blitterswijk et al., 1977).

These observations support two conclusions: (a) Plasma membranes isolated from leukemic cells, like those on intact cells, are more fluid than plasma membranes isolated from normal lymphocytes, and therefore the observed differences between intact normal and leukemic cells may have a direct relation to differences in lipid composition of the cell surface membrane. (b) The major biochemical parameter that determines these dynamic differences is a significant change in the molar ratio of cholesterol to phospholipids in the cell surface membrane.

Exchange of Cholesterol

Previous studies have shown that introduction of exogeneous cholesterol into membranes of leukemic cells can be performed by an *in vitro* incubation of cells with phosphatidylcholine/cholesterol liposomes at mole per mole concentrations. This translocation of cholesterol in mouse leukemic cells resulted in an increase in membrane microviscosity until it equalled that of normal lymphocytes (Shinitzky and Inbar, 1976). Inversely, extraction of native cholesterol from normal mouse lymphocytes can be performed by an *in vitro* incubation of cells with phosphatidylcholine liposomes. This treatment resulted in a decrease in the membrane microviscosity of normal lymphocytes to a value similar to that found in mouse leukemic cells. These induced *in vitro* changes in cholesterol content and corresponding microviscosity are practically reversible for both cell types in both directions, and in principle, can be varied in both cell types within the upper and lower limits prescribed by untreated normal and leukemic cells respectively (Inbar and Shinitzky, 1974). The facile *in vitro* exchange of cholesterol between liposomes and intact lymphoid cells suggests that similar translocation of cholesterol can also occur *in vivo* between lymphoid cells and serum lipoproteins (Inbar et al., 1977a; Petitou et al., 1978). To explore this hypothesis, peripheral blood lymphocytes and serum were collected from normal human donors and from chronic lymphatic leukemic patients. Isolated normal lymphocytes were incubated *in vitro* with leukemic serum, whereas leukemic cells were incubated in normal serum. The results show that with incubation of leukemic cells in normal serum, the degree of microviscosity of the incubated cells increased to a level that is characteristic of untreated normal lymphocytes, and that incubation of normal cells in serum of leukemic patients resulted in a decrease in the degree of microviscosity of the incubated cells to a level that is characteristic of untreated leukemic cells. No changes in P, $\bar{\eta}$, or LFU could be observed when normal or leukemic cells were incubated *in vitro* in their own serum or buffer (Inbar et al., 1977a). These results indicate that changes in dynamic parameters of lymphoid cells induced by incubation in different sera are fully reversible in both directions for both human cell types, as they were for mouse lymphocytes incubated with artificial liposomes (Shinitzky and Inbar, 1974).

To follow up these studies, attempts were made to obtain more direct information regarding the interrelation between cellular membranes and serum lipoproteins, and to determine which fraction in serum is responsible for the changes in dynamic parameters of lymphoid cells and the translocation of cholesterol. Lymphocytes isolated from acute lymphatic leukemic patients in relapse were incubated *in vitro* with pure fractions of low-density lipoproteins and high-density lipoproteins isolated from serum of human normal donors. The results show a marked increase in the degree of cellular microviscosity of leukemic lymphocytes upon *in vitro* incubation with normal low-density lipo- proteins, while under the same conditions, no effects were observed with normal high-density lipoproteins. No changes in microviscosity were observed when normal lymphocytes were incubated under the same conditions as normal low- or high-density lipoproteins (Petitou et al., 1978; Rosenfeld et al., 1979).

Experiments involving both translocation of cholesterol between lymphoid cells and artificial liposomes and translocation of cholesterol between lymphoid cells and serum lipoproteins indicate that the leukemic cell membrane can absorb cholesterol up to the upper limit represented by the cholesterol content of normal lymphocytes, once this lipid is available. This conclusion led to the hypothesis that the composition of serum lipids in leukemic patients is abnormal, compared to that of normal donors. To test this hypothesis, dy- namic parameters of serum lipids obtained from normal donors and acute lymphatic leukemic patients both in relapse and remission were studied. Our results show a marked reduction in microviscosity of serum lipids obtained from leukemic patients in relapse as compared to that of lipids in sera obtained from normal donors or leukemic patients in remission. This reduction of microviscosity of serum lipids in leukemic patients in relapse indicates a dramatic alteration of the composition of serum lipids. A complete analysis of serum lipids has shown that the decreased microviscosity of serum lipids in leukemic patients in relapse is associated with a marked decrease in the ratio of cholesterol to triglycerides and phospholipids. Moreover, these changes in the composition of serum lipids are associated with two major alterations in the composition of serum lipoproteins (Rosenfeld et al., 1979): (a) a significant increase in very low-density lipoprotein triglycerides and (b) a marked decrease in low-density lipoprotein cholesterol.

Analysis of microviscosity and lipid content both in lymphoid cells and serum lipoproteins suggests that in human acute lymphatic leukemia, the decrease in the molar ratio of cholesterol to phospholipids in the cell surface membrane of lymphoid cells isolated from patients in relapse is associated with a concomitant decrease in the ratio of cholesterol to phospholipids and triglycerides in serum lipoproteins. However, this correlation is not so simple as it appears, for studies have shown that erythrocytes isolated from serum of leukemic patients have the same cholesterol content as erythrocytes isolated from serum of normal donors (Inbar, unpublished data). Therefore, it is possible that exchange of cholesterol between lymphoid cells and serum lipoproteins and between erythrocytes and serum lipoproteins is determined by different biological mechanisms. Another possibility is that the structural organization of membrane cholesterol is different in lymphocytes and erythrocytes. Indirect evidence for this alternative was obtained from the following experiment. Incubation of normal lymphocytes with lecithin liposomes for 4 hr at 4°C resulted in the extraction of up to 50% of the membrane cholesterol. However, incubation of erythrocytes with the same concentration of lecithin liposomes for 24 hr at 37°C resulted in the extraction of only 15% of the membrane cholesterol (Inbar, unpublished data). Lymphocytes may therefore be more susceptible to lipid exchange with serum than are erythrocytes. To understand more fully the mechanism for cholesterol exchange in leukemia, it will be necessary to study the structural organization of the apoprotein in leukemic low-density lipoprotein and the functional activities of cellular receptors for binding of low-density lipoproteins on the surface membrane of leukemic cells.

Exfoliation of Membrane Vesicles

Immune reactions to tumors in experimental animals immunized by inoculation of non-viable tumor cells are well established and provide evidence for the presence of tumor specific antigens on the cell surface of tumor cells (Alexander et al., 1966; Baldwin and Barker, 1967). However, the fact that a tumor can grow in the face of the host immune response has suggested the existence of mechanisms that enable the escape of tumor cells from host immune effector processes (Currie, 1973). Recent studies attempting to elucidate the nature of escape mechanisms and to assess the possibility that these mechanisms are related to specific dynamic processes on the cell surface of leukemic cells have suggested the possibility of an active mechanism for shedding off plasma membrane vesicles with a specific lipid and protein composition from the cell surface of leukemic cells (Raz et al., 1978b) Such membrane vesicles have been isolated from ascites fluid and blood serum of both experimental animals and human leukemia patients in several independent studies (Van-Blitterswijk et al., 1977; Raz et al., 1978a; Petitou et al., 1978).

Biochemical and biophysical studies of isolated membrane vesicles have indicated that they have a specific lipid and protein composition (Van-Blitterswijk et al., 1977; Raz et al., 1978a). These vesicles are characterized by a high molar ratio of cholesterol to phospholipids and a high content of membrane sphingomyeline, and therefore they show a high degree of microviscosity and a low degree of membrane fluidity. Moreover, they demonstrate a marked increase in the specific activity of membrane proteins such as 5′-nucleotidase, receptors for plant lectins, and specific tumor antigens in comparison with membranes of intact cells (Van-Blitterswijk et al., 1977; Raz et al., 1978a,b; Petitou et al., 1978).

These studies suggest that such membrane vesicles are generated *in vivo* both in experimental and human leukemia by actively growing leukemic cells, and originate mainly from the cell surface of leukemic cells, presumably by a shedding-off mechanism (Petitou et al., 1978; Raz et al., 1978a). They express a very high specific activity of plasma membrane enzyme markers such as 5′-nucleotidase, but only a low specific activity of cytoplasmic enzyme markers such as glucose-6-phosphatase or acid phosphatase (Raz et al., 1978a). Moreover, the ratio of specific activity of 5′-nucleotidase (plasma membrane marker) to acid phosphatase (cytoplasmic marker) in mouse leukemia has indicated a 3–5-fold enrichment in plasma membrane components in the ascites fluid vesicles as compared to leukemic cell homogenate obtained from the same tumor. Similar results were obtained with human acute lymphatic leukemia: the ratio of specific activity of 5′-nucleotidase to glucose-6-phosphatase indicated a 3–5-fold enrichment in plasma membrane components in membrane vesicles isolated from pleural effusion as compared to a homogenate of leukemic cells of the same patient (Petitou et al., 1978). Along with this enrichment in plasma enzyme markers, vesicles isolated from a Moloney-induced lymphoma also showed an enrichment of 3–5-fold in the number of their receptors for Concanavalin A.

In order to study the extent to which such vesicles also have a specific lipid composition, the molar ratio of cholesterol to phospholipids was determined to be 1.19 and 1.08, respectively, in membrane vesicles isolated from mouse GRSL leukemia and blood serum of human acute lymphatic leukemia (Van-Blitterswijk et al., 1977; Petitou et al., 1978). This ratio, which is 3–4-fold higher than that found in membranes isolated *in vitro* from leukemic cells was, as expected, associated with a high degree of microviscosity and a low degree of lipid fluidity (Van-Blitterswijk et al., 1977; Petitou et al., 1978). The formation of such vesicles, like cholesterol exchange, may be a mechanism by which leukemic cells decrease their cholesterol content and increase their membrane fluidity (Inbar, 1980).

Since these membrane vesicles contain specific plasma membrane proteins, such as 5′-nucleotidase, other cell membrane antigens that might also be embedded in these membranes were looked for (Raz et al., 1978a). Membranes from plasma membrane vesicles isolated from cell-free ascites fluid of Moloney virus-induced lymphoma-bearing mice were found to contain a high specific activity of the MLV-P-30 antigen (Raz et al., 1978a). A specific radioimmunoassay for the P-30 antigen indicates that the specific activity of this antigen is 20-fold higher in the ascites membrane vesicles than in cell homogenate of leukemic cells obtained from the same tumor (Raz et al., 1978a). Similar results were obtained with the MLr antigen in the GRSL mouse leukemia. In a recent study, antisera were raised against leukemic lymphoblasts isolated from the peripheral blood of an Ia positive acute lymphatic leukemic patient as well as against membrane vesicles isolated from cell-free peripheral blood of the same patient. Both antisera were obtained from rabbits and adsorbed with human red blood cells, human platelets, and with a T leukemic cell line. Studies using the Fluorescence Activated Cell Sorter (FACS-I) have shown that both antisera specifically bind to Null cell acute lymphatic leukemic cells, chronic lymphatic leukemic cells, normal B lymphocytes, and B lymphoblastoid cell lines. Neither antiserum reacts with T cell acute lymphatic leukemia cells, T leukemic cell lines nor with normal T lymphocytes (Yanovich and Inbar, in preparation). These findings show that peripheral blood of leukemic patients in relapse contain a subcellular membrane fraction that carries the same immunological determinants as the circulating intact leukemic lymphoblasts.

Results of studies of both experimental and human leukemia suggest that the presence of membrane vesicles that contain a high specific activity of tumor antigens in the circulation may have a direct effect on host immune reactions against the intact tumor cells (Raz et al., 1978b). To test this hypothesis, several biological experiments were carried out. In vitro studies have demonstrated that plasma membranes isolated from cell-free ascites fluid of a Moloney virus-induced lymphoma in A/J mice can specifically inhibit the association of normal macrophages and leukemic cells, if the macrophage monolayers are incubated for a short period of time with membrane vesicles prior to the addition of the leukemic cells. In vivo studies have shown that these membrane vesicles can immunize against intact leukemic cells if injected intramuscularly or subcutaneously into adult mice (Raz et al., 1978b).

The shedding off mechanism of plasma membrane vesicles from the cell surface of leukemic cells may take part in determining the composition of membrane components. A controlled reduction of specific and non-specific membrane proteins at different stages of cell differentiation may determine different physiological functions of leukemic cells. Supporting this hypothesis are the results of experiments on the dynamic structural organization of the plasma membrane enzyme marker 5'-nucleotidase in normal and leukemic lymphocytes. The specific activity of 5'-nucleotidase was reduced in intact human chronic lymphatic leukemic cells as compared to intact human normal lymphocytes. Similar results were also obtained in human acute lymphatic leukemia cells. A marked reduction was found in the specific activity of 5'-nucleotidase in leukemia, both on an intact cell level and on an isolated plasma membrane level (Inbar, 1980). This significant reduction in the specific activity of 5'-nucleotidase in leukemic lymphoblasts can be related to the high specific activity of 5'-nucleotidase found in plasma membrane vesicles isolated from the blood serum of leukemic patients (Inbar, 1980). It is plausible to conclude that the specific activity of membrane proteins on the intact cell surface is controlled by the degree of membrane shedding.

The experiments just summarized reveal a provocative correlation between high specific activity of specific proteins such as the P-30 antigen and non-specific proteins such as Concanavalin A receptors or 5'-nucleotidase, the high molar ratio of cholesterol to phospholipids, and the corresponding high degree of membrane microviscosity in the membrane vesicles exfoliated from the cell surface of leukemic cells. This correlation may represent direct experimental evidence for the dynamic redistribution of both membrane proteins and membrane lipids in the cell surface of leukemic lymphocytes. It will be of interest to determine to what extent membrane antigens or membrane enzymes in normal and leukemic cells have a specific lipid requirement for their optimal activity. More interesting is the possibility that membrane vesicles generated *in vivo* by one type of cell are transported via the body fluids to a different organ and by a fusion mechanism interact with a different type of cells. Such a mechanism may provide an *in vivo* control for communication of membrane signals between cells without a requirement for cell-cell interaction.

Although at present the mechanism of *in vivo* formation of membrane vesicles is not yet fully understood, it is of interest to note that both exfoliated cellular plasma membranes and virus envelopes contain a specific lipid composition (Petitou et al., 1978; Moore et al., 1976) which is characterized by a high membrane rigidity, presumably due to an increase in the ratio of cholesterol to phospholipids in the bilayer lipid core (Rosenthal et al., 1979). Although this similarity between cellular plasma membrane vesicles and enveloped viruses is not necessarily related, it is possible that membrane vesicles and viruses are formed in conjunction with the same mechanism on the cell surface membrane.

The behavior of leukemia cells may be to a large extent determined by the two associated events examined here: the fluidization of cellular membrane lipids via a decrease in the ratio of cholesterol to phospholipids, which may be directly related to an increase in cell proliferation (Collard et al., 1977; Inbar et al., 1977b), and the formation of extracellular plasma membrane vesicles with a high specific activity of membrane antigens, which may be directly related to an increase in immunosuppression (Raz et al., 1978a,b; Inbar, 1980).

Conclusions

1. The molar ratio of cholesterol to phospholipids in the lipid core of the cell surface membrane of leukemic cells obtained from both experimental and human leukemia is significantly lower as compared to the molar ratio of

cholesterol to phospholipids in plasma membranes isolated from normal lymphocytes.

2. This structural difference in the lipid composition of membranes from normal and leukemic lymphocytes determines to a large extent dynamic differences between the two types of cells, resulting in an increase in the fluidity of the leukemic cell membranes.

3. Two possible mechanisms are suggested for these structural and dynamic differences between normal and leukemic cells: (a) Translocation of cholesterol between cellular membranes and serum low-density lipoproteins and (b) exfoliation of plasma membrane vesicles from the surface membrane of leukemic cells.

4. The behavior of leukemic cells may be to a large extent determined by the two associated events observed in their membranes: (a) The fluidization of the cell surface via the decrease in the molar ratio of cholesterol to phospholipids, which has a direct relation to increases in cell proliferation and cell migration and (b) the formation, via the exfoliation mechanism, of extracellular plasma membrane vesicles with a high specific activity of surface antigens, which have a direct relation to the increase in immunosuppression.

References

Alexander, P., Connel, D.I., and Mikulska, Z.S. (1966) Treatment of murine leukemia with spleen cells or sera from allogeneic mice immunized against the tumor, *Cancer Res.* 26:1508–1513.

Baldwin, R.W. and Barker, C.R. (1967) Tumor specific antigenicity of aminoazo-dye induced rat hepatomas. *Int. J. Cancer* 2:355–361.

Collard, J.G., De-Wildt, A., Oomen-Meulemans, E.P.M., Smeekens, J., Emmelot, P., and Inbar, M. (1977) Increase in fluidity of membrane lipids in lymphocytes, fibroblasts, and liver cells stimulated for growth. *FEBS Letters* 77:173–178.

Currie, G. (1973) The rule of circulating antigen as an inhibitor of tumor immunity in man. *Brit. J. Cancer* (Suppl. 1): 153–155.

Edidin, M. (1974) Rotational and translational diffusion in membranes. *Ann. Rev. Biophys. Bioeng.* 3:179–201.

Gitler, C. (1972) Plasticity of biological membranes. *Ann. Rev. Biophys. Bioeng.* 1:51–102.

Inbar, M. (1976) Fluidity of membrane lipids: a single cell analysis of mouse normal lymphocytes and malignant lymphoma cells. *FEBS Letters* 67:180–184.

Inbar, M. (1980) Membrane fluidity and cell transformation: membranes of normal and leukemic lymphocytes. In *Biology of Cancer Cell*. Letnansky, K., (ed.), Amsterdam: Kugler Publications, pp. 269–294.

Inbar, M. and Ben-Bassat, H. (1976) Fluidity difference in the surface membrane lipid core of human lymphoblastoid and lymphoma cell lines. *Int. J. Cancer* 18:293–297.

Inbar, M. and Sachs, L. (1969) Interaction of the carbohydrate-binding protein concanavalin A with normal and transformed cells. *Proc. Natl. Acad. Sci. U.S.A.* 63:1418–1422.

Inbar M. and Schinitzky, M. (1974) Cholesterol as a bioregulator in the development and inhibition of leukemia. *Proc. Natl. Acad. Sci. U.S.A.*, 71:4229–4231.

Inbar, M., Ben-Bassat, H., and Sachs, L. (1971) A specific metabolic activity on the surface membrane in malignant cell transformation. *Proc. Natl. Acad. Sci. U.S.A.* 68:2784–2788.

Inbar, M., Shinitzky, M., and Sachs, L. (1973) Rotational relaxation time of Concanavalin A bound to the surface membrane of normal and malignant transformed cells. *J. Mol. Biol.* 81:245–253.

Inbar, M., Goldman, R., Inbar, L., Bursuker, I., Goldman, B., Akstein, E., Segal, P., Ipp, E., and Ben-Bassat, I. (1977a) Fluidity difference of membrane lipids in human normal and leukemic lymphocytes as controlled by serum components. *Cancer Res.* 37:3037–3041.

Inbar, M., Yuli, I., and Raz, A. (1977b) Contact-mediated changes in the fluidity of membrane lipids in normal and malignant transformed mammalian fibroblasts. *Exptl. Cell. Res.* 105:325–335.

Moore, N.F., Barenholz, Y., and Wagner, R.R. (1976) Microviscosity of toga-virus studied by fluorescence depolarization: influence of envelope proteins and the host cell. *J. Virol.* 49:126–135.

Petitou, M., Tuy, F., Rosenfeld, C., Mishal, Z., Paintrand, M., Jasmin, C., Mathe, G., and Inbar, M (1978) Decreased microviscosity of membrane lipids in leukemic cells: two possible mechanisms. *Proc. Natl. Acad. Sci. U.S.A.* 75:2306–2310.

Raz, A., Barzilai, R., Spira, G., and Inbar, M. (1978a) Oncogenicity and immunogenicity associated with membranes isolated from cell-free ascites fluid of lymphoma-bearing mice. *Cancer Res.* 38:2480–2485.

Raz, A., Goldman, R., Yuli, I., and Inbar, M. (1978b) Isolation of plasma membrane fragments and vesicles from ascites fluid of lymphoma-bearing mice and their possible role in the escape mechanism of tumors from host immune rejection. *Cancer Immunol. Immunother.* 4:53–59.

Rosenfeld, C., Jasmin, C., Mathe, G., and Inbar, M. (1979) Dynamic and composition of cellular membranes and serum lipids in malignant disorders. In *Recent Results in Cancer Research*, Vol. 67. Bonadonna, G., Mathe, G., and Salmon, S.E. (eds.), Berlin-Heidelberg-New York: Springer-Verlag.

Rosenthal, K.S., Yanovich, S., Inbar, M., and Strominger, J.L. (1979) Translocation of a hydrocarbon fluorescent probe between Epstein-Barr virus and lymphoid cells: an assay for early events in viral infection. *Proc. Natl. Acad. Sci. U.S.A.* 75:5076–5080.

Shinitzky, M. and Inbar, M. (1974) Difference in microviscosity induced by different cholesterol levels in the surface membrane lipid layer of normal lymphocytes and malignant lymphoma cells. *J. Mol. Biol.* 85:603–615.

Signer, S.J. and Nicolson, G.L. (1972) The fluid mosaic model of the structure of cell membranes. *Science* 175:720–731.

Van-Blitterswijk, W.J., Emmelot, P., Hilkmann, H.A.M., Oomen-Meulemans, E.P.M., and Inbar, M. (1977). Differences in lipid fluidity among isolated plasma membranes of normal and leukemic lymphocytes and membranes exfoliated from their cell surfaces. *Biochim. Biophys. Acta* 467:309–320.

Yanovich, S., Harris, K. Sallan, S.E., Schlossman, S.F., and Inbar, M. (1978) Dynamic parameters of membrane lipids in normal and leukemic human lymphocytes isolated from peripheral blood and bone marrow. *Cancer Res.* 38:4654–4661.

Published 1981 by Elsevier North Holland, Inc.
Saunders, Daniels, Serrou, Rosenfeld, and Denney, eds.
FUNDAMENTAL MECHANISMS IN HUMAN CANCER IMMUNOLOGY

CHAPTER 3

Tumor Cell Heterogeneity and Blood-Borne Metastasis

Garth L. Nicolson,[a,b] Karen M. Miner[b] and Christopher L. Reading[a,b]

[a]Department of Tumor Biology, University of Texas System Cancer Center,
M.D. Anderson Hospital and Tumor Institute, Houston, Texas 77030 and
[b]Department of Developmental and Cell Biology, University of California,
Irvine, California

Introduction

Successful blood-borne metastasis or colonization of distant organ sites appears to be dependent on unique host and tumor cell properties (Poste and Fidler, 1980; Fidler and Nicolson, 1980). Tumor cell characteristics important in hematogenous metastatic colonization include the ability to invade surrounding tissues and penetrate blood vessel walls, detach and circulate as viable cells, implant successfully in the microcirculation, invade at the site of arrest, and survive to grow into gross metastatic colonies (Zeidman, 1957; Fidler et al., 1978). Clinical observations (reviews: Sugarbaker, 1952; del Regato, 1977) and information obtained from experimental metastatic systems (reviews: Nicolson, 1978; Poste and Fidler, 1980) indicate that there is a tendency for metastatic colonization of particular organ sites.

In order to study tumor cell properties important in metastasis, we have developed animal tumor models in syngeneic hosts that show distinctive metastatic behavior, according to the principles of variant selection used by Fidler (1973). Several of these models have been developed by sequential selection for enhanced blood-borne arrest, survival, and growth, or for spontaneous metastasis to specific organs. Sublines of murine B16 melanoma have been sequentially selected for their abilities to preferentially colonize lungs (Fidler, 1973), brain (Brunson et al., 1978), liver (Tao et al., 1979), or ovary (Brunson and Nicolson, 1979). Similarly, we have selected *in vivo* murine RAW117 lymphosarcoma sublines that show enhanced liver (Brunson and Nicolson, 1978) or lung (Belloni and Nicolson, unpublished results) colonization. Selection for spontaneous subcutaneous metastasis to regional lymph nodes or lungs has been achieved with a rat 13762 mammary carcinoma line

(Neri et al., 1979). It has also been possible to select tumor cell sublines with altered properties such as resistance to lymphocyte killing (Fidler et al., 1976), attachment to immobilized lectins (Reading et al., 1980a), or enhanced invasion of isolated tissues (Hart, 1979) or veins (Poste et al., 1980). The success of these selection methods is thought to indicate the presence of distinct tumor cell subpopulations in the initial tumor (Prehn, 1970), although these variants could also have arisen by a process of sequential adaptation to a particular organ environment during the process of selection.

Materials and Methods

Cell Lines

Murine B16-F1 melanoma which shows some preference for lung, but also colonizes a variety of extrapulmonary sites (Fidler and Nicolson, 1976, 1977), was obtained from Dr. I.J. Fidler (Frederick Cancer Research Center, Frederick, Maryland) and was used to select sublines that preferentially colonize brain or ovary (see Brunson and Nicolson, 1979, for details). Murine RAW117 lymphosarcoma line was selected sequentially for liver colonization according to the method of Brunson and Nicolson (1978). All lines were grown in Dulbecco-modified Eagle's medium (DME) containing 5 or 10% fetal bovine serum (Flow Laboratories).

Biologic Assays

B16 melanoma cells were grown to subconfluency and were detached with 2 mM calcium- and magnesium-free, phosphate buffered saline and suspended in serum-free DME. Viable single cells (2×10^4) were injected (0.2 ml) intravenously into groups of C57BL/6 mice, and experimental metastases were located after 3–4 weeks. RAW117 lymphosarcoma cells grown in suspension in DME containing 10% fetal bovine serum were washed three times in serum-free media and injected intravenously (5×10^3 cells in 0.2 ml) into groups of BALB/c mice. After 10–14 days, the locations of metastases were determined. Cell lines were cloned by limiting dilution techniques (Reading et al., 1980b).

In Vitro Selection of RAW117 Lines

RAW117 lymphosarcoma lines were sequentially selected in vitro for non-adherence to polystyrene-immobilized concanavalin A (Con A) or wheat germ agglutinin (WGA), according to the method of Reading et al. (1980a).

Results

Antigen Determination of RAW117 Lines

Viral antigens gp70, p12 and p20 were determined by competition radioimmune assay according to Reading et al. (1980). Brunson et al. (1978) selected a pigmented variant B16 subline by harvesting small pigmented tumor colonies from rhinal fissure regions of brain and selectively growing the melanoma cells in culture to yield the first selected subline. After ten sequential selections, a subline (B16-B10N) was obtained which formed small pigmented tumors in brain rhinal and longitudinal fissures, but failed to form large numbers of tumor colonies in other organs (Brunson et al., 1978; Brunson and Nicolson, 1980). We have selected another brain-preferring variant subline from B16-F1 by similar methods, except that small tumor colonies were sequentially harvested from brain cerebral meninges and cultured *in vitro* (Nicolson et al., 1978). This latter selection for meningeal metastasis proved to be less specific with respect to organ preference of colonization. Organs other than brain were involved at autopsy in experimental metastasis assays using sublines selected ten (B16-B10B) to thirteen (B16-B13B) times *in vivo* (Table 3.1). In addition, many animals (26% in this assay for B16B) displayed neurologic symptoms indicative of brain tumor presence. These results were not obtained when a lung-selected B16-F10 subline was assayed (Table 3.1).

Increased or altered organ preference of tumor cell colonization has also been noted during selection of murine RAW117 lymphosarcoma sublines for liver colonization (Table 3.2). With each sequential selection for liver colonization, the number of visible lymphosarcoma tumors increased, so that by selection ten, subline RAW117-H10 formed an average of greater than 200 liver tumor colonies (Table 3.2). Although the potential for liver colonization increased with each selection cycle from one (RAW117-H1) to ten (RAW117-H10), the number of lung tumor colonies formed after tail vein injection of tumor cells was not altered significantly (Table 3.2).

Malignant variant sublines were also obtained by a completely *in vitro* route in which lymphosarcoma lines were sequentially selected for lack of binding to immobilized lectins. *In vitro* selection of RAW117-parental cells for lack of

Table 3.1. Selection and Assay of B16 Melanoma Variant Sublines.

| Subline | Colonization of organ sites | | | |
	Lung	Ovary	Brain	Other sites
B16-F1	15/15	0/15	2/15[a]	4/15 adrenal; 4/15 thoracic; 2/15 liver; 5/15 skin
B16-F10	10/10	3/15	1/15[a]	2/15 thoracic; 2/15 skin
B16-B13B	19/19	15/19	16/19[b,c]	1/15 adipose

Note: Animals were injected intravenously with 2×10^4 viable, single tumor cells and experimental metastases were determined after 2-4 weeks.

[a]Rhinal fissure cell colony pigmentation indicative of melanoma.

[b]Meningeal cell colony pigmentation indicative of melanoma.

[c]5/19 animals possessed neurological symptoms such as irregular head twisting or turning, loss of equilibrium, turning to one direction only or uncoordinated movements.

Table 3.2. Selection and Assay of RAW117 Lymphosarcoma
Variant Sublines.

RAW117 subline	Average no. visible liver colonies (range)	Average no. visible lung colonies (range)
Parental	0.6 (0-4)	0.4 (0-1)
H1	2.7 (1-7)	0.4 (0-1)
H5	25.1 (9-39)	0.6 (0-2)
H10	237.0 (200-250)	1.0 (1-4)

Note: Lymphosarcoma cells (5×10^3) were injected intravenously into groups of
ten BALB/c mice, and the locations and numbers of visible tumor colonies were
determined after ten days.

(Source: Brunson and Nicholson, 1978.)

binding to immobilized-Con A yielded after ten such selections a subline
(RAW117-P Con A^{a10}) which was distinctly more malignant compared to the
original unselected parental line, while ten selections *in vitro* of the highly
malignant RAW117-H10 subline resulted in a subline (RAW117-H10 WGA^{a10})
which was less malignant (Reading et al., 1980a). These results suggested that
tumor cell subpopulations exist in the initial cell line used for selection, and the
selections yield cell populations enriched in more metastatic cells.

In both the B16 melanoma (Fidler and Kripke, 1977) and RAW117
lymphosarcoma (Reading et al., 1980b) metastatic systems, cell clones have
been obtained from both the unselected and selected tumor cell lines that show
variations in metastatic potential compared to the lines from which they were
cloned. In order to explain the metastatic behavior of unselected and selected
tumor cell lines in terms of their polyclonal properties, we compared the
experimental metastatic properties of uncloned cell lines with the pooled data
obtained from several clones. Our results (Table 3.3) indicated that the
metastatic properties of uncloned, unselected or uncloned, selected RAW117
cell lines can be mimicked by pooling data obtained from several individual
clones. Furthermore, sequential selection *in vivo* (or *in vitro*) for variant cell
sublines appeared to enrich the cell population for clones with variant phenotypes.

Cell surface analysis of RAW117 parental line, *in vivo* and *in vitro* selected
RAW117 sublines, as well as cloned cell populations derived from the parental
line and selected sublines indicates that a major cell surface modification exists
which correlates with enhanced metastasis. Lactoperioxidase-catalyzed cell
surface iodination reveals the presence of a prominant iodinable cell surface
component of approximate molecular weight 70,000 in the RAW117 parental
line and certain clones of low metastatic potential. In RAW117 cell sublines
and clones of high metastatic potential, this component is reduced or missing
(Table 3.4). Similar results have been obtained by labeling slab gels with

Table 3.3. Analysis of RAW117 Sublines and Clones with Respect to Heterogeneity of Liver Colonization.

Subline or clone (no.)	Percent of animals with number (N) visible liver tumor colonies				
	N=0	$1 \leqslant N \leqslant 10$	$10 < N \leqslant 100$	$100 < N \leqslant 200$	$N > 200$
Parental line	30	60	0	10	0
Parental clones (20)	35	50	15	0	0
H10 subline	0	0	10	0	90
H10 clones (12)	0	0	17	0	83
P Con A[a]10 subline	20	40	20	0	20
P Con A[a]10 clones (41)	37	27	32	0	5
H10 WGA[a]10 subline	9	10	10	40	40
H10 WGA[a]10 clones (14)	0	7	7	50	36

[125]I-lectins (Reading et al., 1980a, b). When the quantities of RNA tumor virus envelope glycoprotein gp70 were analyzed by competition radioimmune assay, the parental RAW117 line and sublines and clones of low metastatic potential possessed high amounts of gp70, while the *in vivo* and *in vitro* selected sublines and clones of high metastatic potential had low quantities of gp70 (Table 3.4).

Table 3.4. Cell Surface Properties of RAW117 Lymphosarcoma Sublines and Clones.

RAW117 subline or clone	Median liver tumor colonies (range)	70,000 mol. wt. component[a]	gp70 content ng/10^6 cells (±SE)[b]
Parental line	1 (0–5)	++	407 ± 9.9
P clone 13	0 (0–1)	++	1074 ± 236
P clone 21	13 (7–>200)	+	158 ± 6.6
H10 subline	>200 (>200)	−	65 ± 12.7
H10 clone 3	28 (0–>200)	+	354 ± 3.7
H10 clone 101	>200 (>200)	−	71 ± 8.6
P Con A[a]10 subline	95 (9–>200)	+	309 ± 4.6
P Con A[a]10 clone 40	200 (>200)	−	60 ± 7.2
P Con A[a]10 clone 63	0 (0–5)	++	1088 ± 19.8
H10 WGA[a]10 subline	85 (0–>200)	+	575 ± 25.6
H10 WGA[a]10 clone 11	>200 (49–>200)		437 ± 34.9
H10 WGA[a]10 clone 15	0 (0–1)	++	870 ± 27.3

[a]Presence of 70,000 mol. wt. component identified by lactoperoxidase-catalyzed iodination-SDS polyacrylamide gel electrophoresis.

[b]Data from Reading et al. (1980b).

Discussion

The existence of clonal variability in unselected lines of B16 melanoma (Fidler and Kripke, 1977), RAW117 lymphosarcoma (Reading et al., 1980b) and other metastatic models (Kripke et al., 1978; Nicolson, 1978; Suzuki et al., 1978) suggested that tumors are heterogeneous with respect to the metastatic pheno-types of individual tumor cells and that the selected tumor cell lines represent particular subpopulations derived from originally heterogenous tumor cell populations. The data for B16 melanoma and RAW117 lymphosarcoma clones agreed with this hypothesis and further suggested that sequential adaptation in particular organ environments is not as important as selective processes. Indeed, metastatic variants of RAW117 lymphosarcoma can be obtained by an *in vitro* selection scheme based entirely upon lack of binding to immobilized lectins such as Con A or WGA. In Table 3.3, the biologic properties of sublines selected ten times from the parental line (or from the liver-selected H10 line) for lack of binding to immobilized-Con A or -WGA indicated that after selection *in vitro*, the metastatic properties of these sublines are shifted compared to the unselected parental or selected H10 lines. When the data for several RAW117 clones were pooled, there was essentially no difference between the pooled data for RAW117 clones compared to the sublines from which they were derived, suggesting that the *in vivo* selection process resulted in an enrichment of stable, highly metastatic clones.

In addition, experiments aimed at adapting B16 melanoma lines to survive in particular organ environments such as brain have failed to enhance meta-static properties. Brunson and Nicolson (1980) attempted to adapt B16-F1 cells sequentially during ten *in vivo* adaptation cycles in brain. Each cycle involved direct inoculation into brain, growth in that organ, and recovery of brain tumor lesions for culture *in vitro*. After ten sequential cycles of brain survival, adaptation, and growth, a ten-times adapted melanoma line was tested for its ability to form experimental metastases in syngeneic mice. In contrast to two different B16 sublines selected for blood-borne implantation, survival, and growth in brain (Table 3.1 and Brunson et al., 1978), the ten-times-adapted melanoma line was no more effective in forming experimen-tal brain metastases than the parental B16 line (Brunson and Nicolson, 1980).

These experiments suggest that adaptation to organ environment per se is insufficient for generating a highly metastatic phenotype. Consistent with these observations are other experiments in which cell sublines have been obtained that possess widely different metastatic properties by selection *in vitro* (Fidler et al., 1976; Hart, 1979; Poste et al., 1980). In each case, variant sublines with quite different metastatic properties were obtained during a completely *in vitro* selection process where site adaptation was eliminated.

Environmental factors also play an important role in metastasis. For exam-ple, endocrine state appears to be important in human and experimental animal metastasis. Proctor et al. (1976) found that B16 melanoma, like malignant melanoma in humans (Cochran, 1973), grew more slowly and metastasized less often in female compared to male mice, and these differences in metastatic properties were eliminated by oblation of female hormonal systems. The development of metastatic lesions at sites of trauma or tissue damage is well known (Fisher et al., 1967), and it has been proposed that local anti-tumor host immunity may be important in determining the distribution of metastatic colonies *in vivo* (Fidler and Kripke, 1980).

In the B16 melanoma and RAW117 lymphosarcoma systems, host immunity appears to be an important factor in metastasis (Fidler and Nicolson, 1978, 1980; Reading et al., 1980b). Although recognizable cell surface immunological determinants related to metastatic phenotype have not yet been found in the B16 melanoma variant system (Fidler and Nicolson, 1980), RAW117 lymphosarcoma malignancy and metastasis to liver has been related to specific cell surface properties including: quantities of lectin-binding sites and RNA tumor virus antigens, exposure of specific cell surface glycoproteins, and quantities of certain cell surface glycoproteins visualized in gels with ^{125}I-labeled lectins or antibodies. Specifically, the amounts or exposures of cell surface RNA tumor virus envelope glycoprotein gp70 in cell sublines and clones correlated with metastasis; enhanced malignancy and metastasis to liver was accompanied by decreases in gp70 cell surface expression. This may be similar to the results of Mora et al. (1977), who found that tumor forming SV40-transformed fibrosarcoma lines lose SV40 cell surface antigens, possibly by immunological selection. In the RAW117 lymphosarcoma system, the host immune system may also eliminate individual pre-existent cells with strong viral antigens, allowing survival only of subpopulations of cells that have lowered contents or expression of gp70. In other tumor systems, different, unique cell surface antigens may be involved in determining metastasis. For example, Shearman et al. (1980) found that the presence of a unique antigen recognizable on a Marek's disease virus-transformed, non-producer, lymphoma subline (Shearman and Longenecker, 1980) correlated with metastasis to liver. The antigen could be identified by indirect cell rosette formation and complement-dependent cytotoxicity using a particular monoclonal antibody preparation. These monoclonal antibodies also inhibited *in vivo* metastasis to liver but not *in vitro* invasion of the chorioallantoic membrane, suggesting that these events are mediated by different, unique properties of the tumor cells. These studies and our own on target organ cell recognition and adhesion by metastatic tumor cells (Nicolson and Winkelahke, 1975; Nicolson et al., 1976; Nicolson and Fidler, 1978) indicate that unique cell surface determinants may determine both the site and degree of metastatic spread.

References

Brunson, K.W. and Nicolson, G.L. (1978) Selection and biologic properties of malignant variants of a murine lymphosarcoma. *J. Natl. Cancer Inst.* 61:1499–1503.

38

Brunson, K.W. and Nicolson, G.L. (1979) Selection of malignant melanoma variant cell lines for ovary colonization. *J. Supramol. Struct.* 11:517–528.

Brunson, K.W. and Nicolson, G.L. (1980) Experimental brain metastasis. In *Brain Metastasis.* Weiss, L., Gilbert, H. and Posner, J.B. (eds.), Boston: G.K. Hall & Co., pp. 50–65.

Brunson, K.W., Beattie, G., and Nicolson, G.L. (1978) Selection and altered tumor cell properties of brain-colonizing metastatic melanoma. *Nature* 272:543–545.

Cochran, A.J. (1973) Malignant melanoma. A review of ten years experience in Glasgow, Scotland. *Cancer* 23:1190–1199.

del Regato, J.A. (1977) Pathways of metastatic spread of malignant tumors. *Sem. Oncol.* 4:33–38.

Fidler, I.J. (1973) Selection of successive tumor lines for metastasis. *Nature New Biol.* 242:148–149.

Fidler, I.J. and Kripke, M.L. (1977) Metastasis results from pre-existing variant cells within a malignant tumor. *Science* 197:893–895.

Fidler, I.J. and Kripke, M. (1980) Tumor cell antigenicity, host immunity, and cancer metastasis. *Cancer Immunol. Immunother.* 7:201–205.

Fidler, I.J. and Nicolson, G.L. (1976) Organ selectivity for implantation, survival, and growth of B16 melanoma variant tumor lines. *J. Natl. Cancer Inst.* 57:1199–1202.

Fidler, I.J. and Nicolson, G.L. (1977) Fate of recirculating B16 melanoma metastatic variant cells in parabiotic syngeneic recipients. *J. Natl. Cancer Inst.* 58:1867–1872.

Fidler, I.J. and Nicolson, G.L. (1978) Tumor cell and host properties affecting the implantation and survival of blood-borne metastatic variants of B16 melanoma. *Israel J. Med. Sci.* 14:38–50.

Fidler, I.J. and Nicolson, G.L. (1980) The immunobiology of experimental metastatic melanoma. *Cancer Biol. Rev.* (in press).

Fidler, I.J., Gersten, D.M., and Budmen, M.B. (1976) Characterization *in vivo* and *in vitro* of tumor cells selected for resistance to syngeneic lymphocyte-mediated cytotoxicity. *Cancer Res.* 36:3160–3165.

Fidler, I.J., Gersten, D.M., and Hart, I.R. (1978) The biology of cancer invasion and metastasis. *Adv. Cancer Res.* 28:149–250.

Fisher, B., Fisher, E.R., and Feduska, N. (1967) Trauma and the localization of tumor cells. *Cancer* 20:23–30.

Hart, I.R. (1979) The selection and characterization of an invasive variant of B16 melanoma. *Am. J. Pathol.* 97:587–600.

Kripke, M.L., Gruys, E., and Fidler, I.J. (1978) Metastatic heterogeneity of cells from an ultraviolet light-induced murine fibrosarcoma of recent origin. *Cancer Res.* 38:2962–2967.

Mora, P.T., Chang, C., Couvillion, L., Kuster, J.M., and McFarland, V.W. (1977) Immunological selection of tumor cells which have lost SV40 antigen expression. *Nature* 269:36–40.

Neri, A., Ruoslahti, E., and Nicolson, G.L. (1979) Relationship of fibronectin to the metastatic behavior of rat mammary adenocarcinoma cell lines and clones. *J. Supramol. Struct.* [Suppl. 3]:181.

Nicolson, G.L. (1978) Experimental tumor metastasis: characteristics and organ specificity. *BioScience* 28:441–447.

Nicolson, G.L. and Winkelhake, J.L. (1975) Organ specificity of blood-borne tumor metastasis determined by cell adhesion? *Nature* 255:230–232.

Nicolson, G.L., Winkelhake, J.L., and Nussey, A.C. (1976) An approach to studying the cellular properties associated with metastasis: some *in vitro* properties of tumor variants selected *in vivo* for enhanced metastasis. In *Fundamental Aspects of Metastasis.* Weiss, L. (ed.), Amsterdam: North-Holland Publishing Co., pp. 291–303.

Nicolson, G.L., Brunson, K.W., and Fidler, I.J. (1978) Specificity of arrest, survival, and growth of selected metastatic variant cell lines. *Cancer Res.* 38:4105–4111.

Poste, G. and Fidler, I.J. (1980) The pathogenesis of cancer metastasis. *Nature* 283:139–146.

Poste, G., Doll, J., Hart, I.R., and Fidler, I.J. (1980) *In vitro* selection of murine B16 melanoma variants with enhanced tissue invasive properties. *Cancer Res.* 40:1636–1644.

Prehn, R.T. (1970) Analysis of antigenic heterogeneity within individual 3-methyl-cholanthrene-induced mouse sarcomas. *J. Natl. Cancer Inst.* 45:1039–1045.

Proctor, J.W., Auclair, B.G., and Stokowski, L. (1976) Endocrine factors and the growth and spread of B16 melanoma. *J. Natl. Cancer Inst.* 57:1197–1198.

Reading, C.L., Belloni, P.N., and Nicolson, G.L. (1980a) Selection and *in vivo* properties of lectin-attachment variants of malignant murine lymphosarcoma cell lines. *J. Natl. Cancer Inst.* 64:1241–1249.

Reading, C.L., Brunson, K.W., Torrianni, M., and Nicolson, G.L. (1980b) Malignancies of metastatic murine lymphosarcoma cells lines and clones correlate with decreased cell surface display of RNA rumor virus envelope glycoprotein gp70. *Proc. Natl. Acad. Sci. U.S.A.* (in press).

Shearman, P.J. and Longenecker, B.M. (1980) Selection for virulence and organ-specific metastasis of herpesvirus-transformed lymphoma cells. *Int. J. Cancer* 25:363–369.

Shearman, P.J., Gallatin, W.M., and Longenecker, B.M. (1980) Detection of a cell-surface antigen correlated with organ-specific metastasis. *Nature* 286:267–269.

Sugarbaker, E.V. (1952) The organ selectivity of experimentally induced metastasis in rats. *Cancer* 5:606–612.

Suzuki, H., Withers, H.R., and Koehler, M.W. (1978) Heterogeneity and variability of artificial lung colony-forming ability among clones from a mouse fibrosarcoma. *Cancer Res.* 38:3349–3351.

Tao, T-W., Matter, A., Vogel, K., and Burger, M.M. (1979) Liver-colonizing melanoma cells selected from B16 melanoma. *Int. J. Cancer* 23:854–857.

Zeidman, I. (1957) Metastasis: a review of recent advances. *Cancer Res.* 17:157–162.

Published 1981 by Elsevier North Holland, Inc.
Saunders, Daniels, Serrou, Rosenfeld, and Denney, eds.
FUNDAMENTAL MECHANISMS IN HUMAN CANCER IMMUNOLOGY

CHAPTER 4

Relationship Between Cell Surface Thrombin Receptors and Cytoplasmic Microtubules: Potential Involvement in Regulation of Normal and Neoplastic Cell Proliferation[1, 2]

Darrell H. Carney and Kathryn L. Crossin

Department of Human Biological Chemistry and Genetics, The University of Texas Medical Branch, Galveston, Texas

Introduction

A number of differences between the cell surface molecules of normal and transformed cells have been found. Some of these differences are now being used to develop specific antibodies directed against tumor cells for possible use in tumor immunotherapy. (Several examples of this approach are described in Part III of this book). The correlations between alteration of specific cell surface molecules and transformation, however, have not held up in all systems, making the therapeutic value of this approach somewhat uncertain. A more basic approach has been first to identify the molecular events which initiate normal cell proliferation and then to determine whether transformation alters these events. This report will focus on the initiation of cell division by thrombin and the molecular events which appear to be involved in this initiation. Our hope is that through a more basic understanding of normal growth control we might begin to understand the lesions which lead to abnormal proliferation of neoplastic cells.

We will first review data from several laboratories which led to the discovery of a thrombin receptor on the surface of fibroblasts and showed the role of this receptor in initiation of cell division by thrombin. Next, we will review recent

[1]Research was supported by Grant AM 25807 from the National Institute of Arthritis, Metabolism, and Digestive Diseases. KLC is supported by a University of Texas Graduate Assistantship.
[2]Please address correspondence to: Darrell H. Carney, Ph.D., Division of Biochemistry, The University of Texas Medical Branch, Galveston, Texas 77550, Phone (713) 765-3210.

studies which indicate that following transformation of various cells, the thrombin receptor is no longer available to bind thrombin. Since we know that thrombin binding to this receptor can trigger initiation of cell division, the alteration or occupancy of this receptor by transformation products may be related to uncontrolled proliferation in neoplastic cells. Finally, we will present recent experiments from our laboratory which indicate that microtubule depolymerization may be involved in initiation of cell division by thrombin and that disruption of cytoplasmic microtubules by various agents is itself sufficient to initiate DNA synthesis and events leading to cell division. These studies have broad implications for the control of normal and neoplastic cell proliferation—especially since many transformed cells have altered cytoskeletons, some but not all with grossly depolymerized microtubules (Brinkley et al., 1975; Edelman and Yahara, 1976; Fuller and Brinkley, 1976; Miller et al., 1977; Osborn and Weber, 1977). Throughout this review we have taken the liberty to speculate and have proposed several working models which explain our results to date. We hope these models will provoke further experimentation and lead to a better understanding of this important process.

Initiation of Cell Division by Thrombin

Early studies with both chick embryo fibroblasts and mouse 3T3 cells indicated that trypsin could initiate cell division in otherwise nonproliferating cultures (Sefton and Rubin, 1970; Burger, 1970; Noonan and Burger, 1973). Because trypsin treatment of these cells mimicked several morphological and biochemical effects of transformation, this system was widely studied as a potential model for transformation (for review, see Noonan, 1978). Trypsin-induced changes in cell morphology and cell surface properties which cause increased agglutinability, however, did not correlate with initiation of cell proliferation (Cunningham and Ho, 1975; Zetter et al., 1976). Studies also showed that trypsin was not able to initiate division of various types of mammalian cells (Glynn et al., 1973; Holley and Kiernan, 1974; Carney et al., 1978). In contrast, highly purified human thrombin could initiate division of both chick embryo fibroblasts and various mammalian cells in culture without generating many of the unrelated surface changes associated with trypsin (Chen and Buchanan, 1975; Teng and Chen, 1975; Zetter et al., 1976; Pohjanpelto, 1977; Carney et al., 1978). Thus it appeared that initiation of cell division by thrombin might provide a much more reliable model system for studying the specific molecular events that lead to cell division. In addition, since thrombin is a pivotal enzyme in the blood clotting process, its involvement in initiating fibroblast cell proliferation could play an important role in the wound healing process.

Other features of the thrombin system have also facilitated molecular studies of initiation events. First, highly purified thrombin initiates cell division in serum-free cultures, permitting studies under chemically defined conditions

(Chen and Buchanan, 1975; Carney et al., 1978). Second, as will be discussed, proteolytic activity of thrombin is required for its mitogenic action. Thus, it has been possible to label cell surface proteins and look for a primary cleavage which relates to initiation (Glenn and Cunningham, 1979). Finally, proteolytically inhibited thrombin binds to its receptor but does not initiate cell division (Glenn et al., 1980). Thus by comparing thrombin and proteolytically inhibited thrombin, we can begin to identify events following thrombin binding which might be causally involved in initiation.

Initiation by Cell Surface Interaction with Specific Receptors

To elucidate the molecular events by which thrombin initiates cell division, one of the first questions raised was whether thrombin can initiate proliferative events by action at the cell surface or whether internalization is necessary (Carney and Cunningham, 1978a,b). Indeed, there is uncertainty about this question for polypeptide hormones and growth factors in general. For these studies, ^{125}I-thrombin was covalently linked to carboxylate-modified polystyrene beads using a carbodiimide condensation. When added to nonproliferating cultures of chick embryo cells, these thrombin beads caused a 25% to 50% increase in DNA synthesis and cell number over cultures incubated with control beads. By monitoring radioactivity released from the beads into the medium or directly into the cells, it was possible to demonstrate that the amount of thrombin released from the beads was 10- to 30-fold less than the amount of active intact soluble thrombin required to initiate an equivalent amount of cell division. Thus these studies indicated that initiation of cell division was the result of thrombin attached to the beads, and that the cell surface action of thrombin is sufficient to initiate division of chick cells (Carney and Cunningham, 1978a,b).

We next attempted to determine whether there was a specific receptor for thrombin on the surface of fibroblasts which might be involved in initiation of cell division. Our studies revealed that a large portion of the total binding of ^{125}I-thrombin to mouse fibroblasts was specific (about 80% at a concentration of up to 50 μg/ml), since it was saturable and could be displaced by non-labeled thrombin (Carney and Cunningham, 1978c). Scatchard analysis of this binding data suggested a single affinity class of receptors with a dissociation constant of about 10^{-9} M. The existence of a single class of binding sites for thrombin was further indicated by photoaffinity labeling experiments, which demonstrated that up to 70% of the specifically bound thrombin cross-linked to a single molecule on mouse embryo cells of about 50,000 daltons (Carney et al., 1979).

Several lines of evidence from these studies suggested that this binding was physiologically important to thrombin initiation of cell division. First, neither insulin, epidermal growth factor, nor prothrombin (which does not initiate cell division) significantly competed for binding to this receptor. Second, approximately half of the thrombin receptors were occupied at thrombin concentrations which were half maximal for initiation of cell division. Third, low concentrations of serum inhibited both the binding of thrombin to its receptors and its mitogenesis without affecting either the proteolytic activity of thrombin or its non-specific associations with the cells. Together these observations indicated that thrombin binding to its receptor was the critical interaction with the cell surface which was necessary for thrombin to initiate cell division.

Effects of Transformation on the Thrombin Receptor

Early studies on thrombin initiation of cell division in normal and Rous sarcoma virus transformed chick embryo cells revealed that transformed cells were relatively unresponsive to thrombin and that binding and internalization of ^{125}I-thrombin was significantly decreased in these cells (Zetter et al., 1977). Recently, it was discovered that this defect in transformed cells is associated with an apparent loss of the thrombin receptor (Perdue et al., 1981). In these studies, chick, rat, and mouse cells appeared to lose most, if not all, of their high affinity binding sites for thrombin following spontaneous transformation or transformation induced by viruses or methylcholanthrene.

Several molecular models can be proposed to explain this apparent loss of high affinity thrombin binding by transformed cells. Some of these models are presented in Figure 4.1. First, it is possible that following transformation, the cell produces an abnormal thrombin receptor either by a stable mutation or through a general effect of transformation on receptor or glycoprotein processing (Figure 4.1a). Indeed, it appears that many cell surface proteins are altered by transformation. Second, one might imagine that the receptor molecules are no longer present on the surface of the membranes (Figure 4.1b). If, for example, the thrombin receptor required cytoskeletal anchorage for proper insertion in the membrane, then in transformed cells, where many changes occur in microtubules and microfilaments, these receptors might be released from the cells. Third, it is possible that normal thrombin receptors are inserted into the membrane but that these receptors are occupied by products produced by the transformed cells (Figure 4.1c). For example, urokinase and other plasminogen activators compete with ^{125}I-thrombin for binding to both chick and human fibroblasts (D.D. Cunningham and J.F. Perdue, personal communications). The fourth model (Figure 4.1d) simply indicates that, either through production of an abnormal receptor (model a) or through proteolytic cleavage following binding of a transformation product (model c), the cleaved or altered thrombin receptor no longer binds thrombin. Since protolytic cleavage of the receptor appears to be involved in thrombin initiation of cell division (Glenn et al., 1980; Glenn and Cunningham, 1979), this type of model would explain how the defect in the thrombin receptor might be causally involved in the uncontrolled proliferation of transformed cells.

Proteolytic Cleavage of the Thrombin Receptor is Necessary for Initiation

To determine whether proteolytic cleavage of the thrombin receptor was necessary for thrombin to initiate cell division, several proteolytically inhibited thrombin derivatives were prepared and examined for their ability to bind to thrombin receptors and initiate division of chick, mouse, human, and Chinese hamster fibroblasts (Glenn et al., 1980). Two of these derivatives with active site inhibitors were able to bind as well as unmodified thrombin to receptors on mouse and Chinese hamster cells. However, none of the derivatives initiated cell division. These experiments indicated that receptor binding alone is not sufficient for initiation of cell division and that proteolytic cleavage is a necessary step subsequent to receptor binding.

That proteolytic cleavage by thrombin of the thrombin receptor itself is involved in initiation was suggested by the recent studies of Glenn and Cunningham (1979). Thrombin cleavage and disappearance of an iodinated surface protein corresponding in size to the thrombin receptor correlated with initiation of cell division by thrombin. This iodinated protein was present on the surface of both responsive and non-responsive chick cells (as was the receptor; Carney and Glenn, unpublished), but was only cleaved and removed from the surface of responsive cells after treatment with mitogenic concentra-

Figure 4.1. Models for the apparent loss of high affinity thrombin binding following transformation. See text for detailed description.

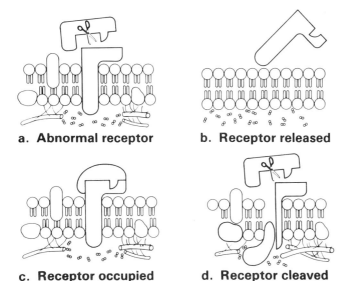

a. **Abnormal receptor**   b. **Receptor released**

c. **Receptor occupied**   d. **Receptor cleaved**

tions of thrombin. Thus, it appears that proteolytic cleavage of the thrombin receptor is necessary to initiate cell division.

As shown in Figure 4.2, such cleavage could generate a mitogenic signal in several different ways. First, it could release a peptide fragment which either interacted with other membrane bound molecules or was itself released intracellularly to generate a mitogenic signal (Figure 4.2a). This type of model is similar to the model suggested by Das and Fox (1978) to explain mitogenic action of epidermal growth factor through receptor cleavage. Second, receptor cleavage could alter the conformation of the receptors or release them from anchorage, which then would allow receptor aggregation (Figure 4.2b). Once receptors are aggregated, a mitogenic signal might be produced through an influx in cationic molecules or by other means. For example, aggregation of receptors could create ionic channels in the lipid bilayer through which calcium ions or other molecules might enter to initiate various events. A final possibility is that by proteolytic cleavage, a conformational change in the receptor activates the receptor itself or an adjacent molecule, which then generates a signal (Figure 4.2c). In this model, the concept of protease activation of other enzymes is carried over to membrane receptor activation by thrombin, which is itself both a product and an activator in the cascade of events leading to blood coagulation.

Visualization of Thrombin Binding and the Question of Aggregation

To determine whether thrombin receptors aggregate following thrombin binding, we prepared a highly fluorescent thrombin by linking 4-(N-6-aminohexyl

Figure 4.2. Models depicting possible roles of proteolytic cleavage of the thrombin receptor in generating the transmembrane signal that initiates cell division.

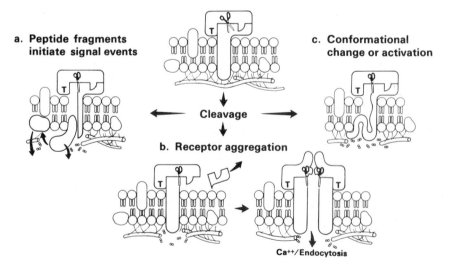

a. **Peptide fragments initiate signal events**

c. **Conformational change or activation**

← Cleavage →

b. **Receptor aggregation**

Ca++/Endocytosis

thioureal)-fluorescein to the carbohydrate moiety of the thrombin molecule. This thrombin preparation had about four fluoresceins per thrombin molecule and still retained its affinity for the thrombin receptor and its mitogenic activity (Carney, 1981). As shown in Figure 4.3a, incubating mouse embryo cells with a mitogenic concentration of fluorescein amine labeled thrombin (250 ng/ml) at 4°C for 6 hr produced a diffuse fluorescent pattern. This pattern was specific in that it was not observed when a 50-fold excess of unlabeled thrombin was included in the incubation (Figure 4.3b). Thus, the thrombin receptors appear to be randomly distributed over the surface of the cells when thrombin binds at 4°C.

Increasing the temperature to 37°C following 4°C binding resulted in a rapid unexpected disappearance of the fluorescent pattern from the cells, leaving only a pattern equivalent to that which could be observed in cells never exposed to fluorescent thrombin (Figure 4.3c). Thus with this approach we have been unable to establish whether there is aggregation of receptors following thrombin binding.

Several interpretations of these fluorescent experiments are possible and have been described in detail (Carney, 1981). One possible explanation is that incubating the cells at 4°C altered a cytoskeletal anchorage of the receptors

Figure 4.3. Specificity and pattern of aminohexyl fluorescein thrombin binding to mouse embryo cells at 4°C. Aminohexyl fluorescein labeled thrombin (250 ng/ml) was incubated with nonproliferating cultures of mouse embryo cells plated on glass coverslips at 4°C for 5 hours in the presence or absence of unlabeled thrombin (5 μg/ml). These coverslip cultures and ones incubated without fluorescent thrombin were then rinsed 4 times with PBS at 4°C, fixed with 3% formaldehyde and photographed using identical exposure through a fluorescent microscope (4250X). (A) Aminohexyl fluorescein thrombin alone. (B) Aminohexyl fluorescein plus 5 μg/ml unlabeled thrombin. (C) Autofluorescence of cells incubated without fluorescent thrombin.

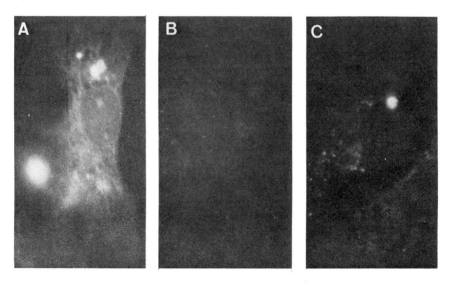

48

and accelerated the release of thrombin or the thrombin receptor complex as the temperature was increased. This possibility has now been further examined to determine whether in fact thrombin receptors are anchored in the cytoskeleton and whether this type of interaction is involved in generation of a mitogenic signal.

Interaction of Microtubules with the Thrombin Receptor

To determine whether the thrombin receptor was anchored by cytoskeletal elements, we examined the effects of colchicine and other agents which disrupt microtubules and microfilaments on binding and mitogenic action of thrombin. As shown in Figure 4.4, treating mouse embryo cells with 10^{-6} M colchicine for 2 hours prior to incubation with ^{125}I-thrombin appears to result in a concentration dependent release of thrombin receptors from the cells. That

Figure 4.4. Effect of microtubule depolymerization on specific binding of ^{125}I-thrombin to mouse embryo cells. Secondary cultures of mouse embryo cells were incubated with the indicated concentrations of ^{125}I-thrombin for 1 hr at 37°C. Each point was corrected for non-specific binding in the presence of excess unlabeled thrombin as described previously (Carney and Cunningham, 1978c). Cells treated for 2 hr with 10^{-6} M colchicine prior to thrombin binding (●—●); control cells, no drug treatment (○—○).

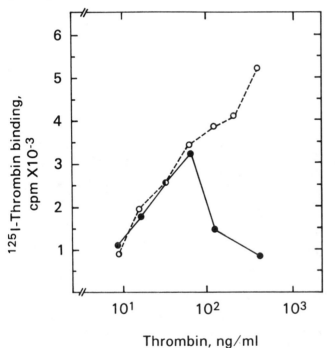

is, at low concentrations of ^{125}I-thrombin, there was no difference in binding between colchicine treated and untreated cells, but at concentrations above 125 ng/ml, in the presence of colchicine, there is a decrease in ^{125}I-thrombin binding as the concentration of thrombin increases. Such a decrease could represent either shedding of the thrombin receptor complex or a conformational change in the receptor which prevents binding. Interestingly, the concentration at which the receptors appear to be lost corresponds to the concentration of thrombin required for half maximal binding and the threshold concentration of thrombin for initiating cell division (Carney and Cunningham, 1978c). These observations suggest that thrombin receptors are in some way anchored to microtubules and that perhaps the concentration dependent event which leads to initiation of cell division involves interaction with microtubules.

Role of Microtubule Depolymerization in Initiation of Proliferative Events

Since the thrombin receptor appeared to be anchored to microtubules, we decided to determine whether microtubule depolymerization could affect initiation of DNA synthesis by thrombin (for complete description of these studies, see Crossin and Carney, 1981). As shown in Figure 4.5, a 2-hour incubation with colchicine completely disrupts the cytoplasmic microtubules of

Figure 4.5. Effects of colchicine and taxol on the cytoplasmic microtubules of mouse embryo fibroblasts. Secondary cultures of mouse embryo cells were plated on glass coverslips and examined with immunofluorescent techniques as described previously (Crossin and Carney, 1981), using monospecific tubulin antibody provided by Dr. Gerald M. Fuller (Fuller et al., 1975). *Panel A.* Control cells. *Panel B.* Cells treated with 10^{-6} M colchicine for 2 hr prior to fixation. *Panel C.* Cells treated for 1 hr with taxol (5 μg/ml), followed by 2-hr treatment with 10^{-6} M colchicine.

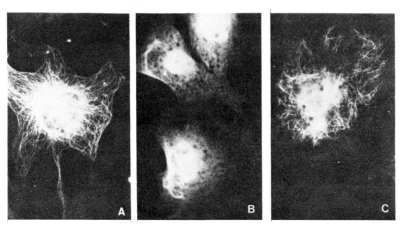

mouse embryo cells cultured in serum-free medium. This treatment did not cause an appreciable decrease in thrombin initiation of DNA synthesis in these cells, nor was there a concentration of colchicine which enhanced thrombin stimulated DNA synthesis above that of the maximal stimulation by thrombin alone. Interestingly, however, in all cases colchicine itself stimulated DNA synthesis in controls to levels 60 to 75% as high as the maximal stimulation by thrombin. Thus, colchicine treatment alone appeared sufficient to initiate DNA synthesis in these cultures. Similar results were obtained with serum-free cultures of chick and human primary fibroblasts and with other drugs which depolymerized microtubules. Lumicolchicine and cytochalasin did not initiate DNA synthesis. Interestingly, we found that initiation of DNA synthesis could be achieved by a brief 2-hr exposure to colchicine or colcemid and that, if colcemid was removed from cultures, the initiated cells continued through the cell cycle with up to a 50% increase in cell number over control cultures within 48 hours. Thus it appeared that a transient depolymerization of the microtubules early in the cell cycle could initiate both DNA synthesis and events leading to cell division.

Even more convincing evidence for the causal involvement of microtubule depolymerization in initiation emerged from experiments in which microtubule stabilization prevented initiation of DNA synthesis. For these experiments, cells were treated with taxol (5 μg/ml) for one hour prior to addition of colchicine or other microtubule disrupting drugs. As shown in Figure 4.5c, this taxol pretreatment alters the normal appearance of the microtubules as described earlier (Crossin and Carney, 1981), but prevents their depolymerization by a 2-hour colchicine treatment. In the same type of experiment, taxol completely inhibited 10^{-6} M colchicine initiation of DNA synthesis in cultures of mouse embryo cells. Thus, these experiments indicate that microtubule depolymerization is necessary for colchicine to initiate DNA synthesis.

To determine whether microtubule depolymerization might be necessary for normal growth factors to initiate DNA synthesis, we have recently examined the effect of taxol on initiation of DNA synthesis by thrombin (Crossin and Carney, 1981 and manuscript in preparation). As shown in Figure 4.6, a one-hour pretreatment of mouse embryo cell cultures with taxol inhibits up to 50% of the DNA synthesis stimulated by thrombin. Preliminary control experiments indicate that this inhibition cannot simply be explained by taxol's effects on thymidine transport or binding or thrombin to the cells. Thus it is tempting to speculate that microtubule depolymerization may be required for thrombin and other growth factors to initiate proliferative events.

Potential Involvement of Microtubules and the Thrombin Receptor in Regulation of Normal and Neoplastic Cell Proliferation

In the preceding sections, we have summarized evidence which allows us to speculate on the interaction between thrombin receptors and microtubules and

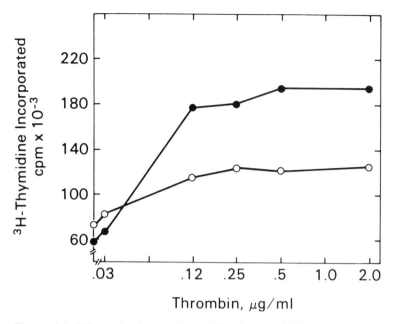

Figure 4.6. Effect of microtubule stabilization on initiation of DNA synthesis by thrombin. Nonproliferating cultures of mouse embryo cells were incubated for 1 hr with or without taxol (10 μg/ml), prior to addition of the indicated concentrations of thrombin. Acid precipitable thymidine incorporation was determined after 28 hr of incubation with 3H-thymidine (1 μCi/ml). Taxol treated cells (O—O); control cells with no taxol (●—●).

their possible involvement in regulating cell proliferation. Several points should be reiterated:

1. Interaction of thrombin with its specific receptor is necessary for thrombin to initiate cell division. Thus this molecule is causally involved in generating a signal for cell division.
2. Transformed cells lose their ability to bind thrombin—perhaps because they make a thrombin-like molecule, because they produce an altered receptor, or because the receptor is released. Regardless of the exact mechanism involved, this finding raises the possibility that transformed cells utilize the thrombin receptor system to initiate uncontrolled proliferation.
3. Colchicine and other drugs which cause microtubule depolymerization appear to release the thrombin receptor from the surface of cells at mitogenic thrombin concentrations. This result indicates that the thrombin receptors are in some way anchored to microtubules and that the concentration dependent event which leads to initiation of cell division involves interaction with microtubules.
4. Microtubule depolymerization itself is sufficient to initiate DNA synthesis and cell division. This observation is especially interesting because many

52

transformed fibroblasts have been shown to lose their microtubule integrity (Brinkley et al., 1975; Edelman and Yahara, 1976; Fuller and Brinkley, 1976; Miller et al., 1977; Osborn and Weber, 1977). If microtubule depolymerization is sufficient to initiate events leading to cell division, then the depolymerization of microtubules in transformed cells may be causally involved in neoplastic proliferation of these cells.

5. Thrombin initiation of DNA synthesis is inhibited by taxol stabilization of microtubules, indicating that microtubule depolymerization may be a necessary event in initiation of cell division by normal growth factors.

The speculative cartoon presented in Figure 4.7 represents a further attempt to summarize these findings and unify our concept of how they might relate to control of normal and neoplastic cell proliferation. We now know that thrombin binding to its receptor and proteolytic cleavage of this receptor are necessary to initiate proliferative events. The molecular signal could be generated through the released peptide fragment, a conformational change in the receptor, or receptor aggregation. In any event, it now appears that microtubule depolymerization may be necessary for thrombin to initiate proliferative events. The observations that colchicine treatment releases thrombin receptors at mitogenic thrombin concentrations further suggests the anchorage of

Figure 4.7. Possible interrelationships between thrombin receptors and microtubules in initiating cell proliferation in normal and transformed cells.

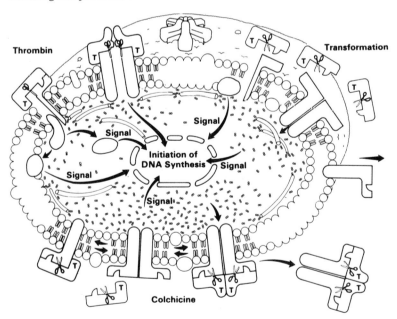

thrombin receptors to microtubules and the interaction with microtubules as part of the signal generating event. That a transient microtubule depolymerization alone is sufficient to initiate DNA synthesis and cell division suggests that the equilibrium between microtubules and free tubulin may be extremely important as a regulator of proliferative events as well as in maintenance of cell shape. It should be noted, however, that the actual mitogenic signal could arise following microtubule depolymerization by resulting changes in calcium ions or nucleotides or by the spontaneous aggregation or activation of membrane enzymes following cytoskeletal disruption.

In transformed fibroblasts, there is a loss of high affinity thrombin binding (Perdue et al., 1981). This observation could be explained by a number of models, including abnormal receptor synthesis, receptor occupancy, or release of receptors from the membrane. It is tempting to speculate that the loss of high affinity thrombin binding indicates that transformed cells utilize this receptor system to potentiate uncontrolled proliferation. Several previous studies have shown that there is a loss of microtubule integrity following transformation; however, microtubule depolymerization has not been observed in all types of transformed cells (Osborn and Weber, 1977). Thus if microtubule depolymerization is causally involved in neoplastic proliferation, only local depolymerization at or around mitogenic receptors may be involved.

The exact mechanism of initiation of proliferative events by growth factors, microtubules, and transformation remain to be elucidated. It should be remembered that the models presented are still speculative and that many of the described observations have only been made in cultured primary fibroblasts. Thus it is presently impossible to generalize these findings to other systems. For example, lymphocytes do not have extensive cytoplasmic microtubule complexes. Hence, the ability of microtubule depolymerization to initiate proliferative events may be limited to fibroblast-like cells. Moreover, thrombin receptors have only been demonstrated on a limited number of cell types. It is hoped, however, that as we begin to understand how these interrelated events initiate fibroblast proliferation, a more fundamental understanding of normal and neoplastic control of cell division will be achieved.

References

Baker, J.B., Low, D.A., Simmer, R.L., and Cunningham, D.D. (1980) Protease-nexin: a cellular component that links thrombin and plasminogen activator and mediates their binding to cells. *Cell* 21:37–45.

Brinkley, B.R., Fuller, G.M., and Highfield, D.P. (1975) Cytoplasmic microtubules in normal and transformed cells in culture: analysis by tubulin antibody immunofluorescence. *Proc. Natl. Acad. Sci. U.S.A.* 73:4981–4985.

Burger, M.M. (1970) Proteolytic enzymes initiating cell division and escape from contact inhibition of growth. *Nature* 227:170–171.

Carney, D.H. (1981) Visualization of thrombin receptors on mouse embryo fibroblasts using fluorescein-amine conjugated human α-thrombin. *J. Supramol. Struct.* 13:467–478.

Carney, D.H. and Cunningham, D.D. (1978a) Cell surface action of thrombin is sufficient to initiate division of chick cells. *Cell* 14:811–823.

Carney, D.H. and Cunningham, D.D. (1978b) Transmembrane action of thrombin initiates chick cell division. *J. Supramol. Struct.* 9:337–350.

Carney, D.H. and Cunningham, D.D. (1978c) Role of specific cell surface receptors in thrombin-stimulated cell division. *Cell* 15:1341–1349.

Carney, D.H., Glenn, K.C., and Cunningham, D.D. (1978) Conditions which affect initiation of animal cell division by trypsin and thrombin. *J. Cell Physiol.* 95:13–22.

Carney, D.H., Glenn, K.C., Cunningham, D.D., Das, M., Fox, C.F., and Fenton, J.W. II. (1979) Photoaffinity labeling of a single receptor for α-thrombin on mouse embryo cells. *J. Biol. Chem.* 254:6244–6247.

Chen, L.B. and Buchanan, J.M. (1975) Mitogenic activity of blood components. I. Thrombin and prothrombin. *Proc. Natl. Acad. Sci. U.S.A.* 72:131–135.

Crossin, K.L. and Carney, D.H. (1981) Evidence that microtubule depolymerization early in the cell cycle is sufficient to initiate DNA synthesis. *Cell* 23:61–71.

Cunningham, D.D. and Ho, T.-S. (1975) Effect of added proteases on concanavalin A-specific agglutinability and proliferation of quiescent fibroblasts. In *Proteases and Biological Control.* Reich, E. Rifkin, D.B., and Shaw, E. (eds.), New York: Cold Spring Harbor Laboratory, pp. 795–803.

Edelman, G.M. and Yahara, I. (1976) Temperature-sensitive changes in surface modulating assemblies of fibroblasts transformed by mutants of Rous sarcoma virus. *Proc. Natl. Acad. Sci. U.S.A.* 73:2047–2051.

Fuller, G.M. and Brinkley, B.R. (1976) Structure and control of assembly of cytoplasmic microtubules in normal and transformed cells. *J. Supramol. Struct.* 5:497–514.

Fuller, G.M., Brinkley, B.R., and Boughter, J.M. (1975) Immunofluorescence of mitotic spindles by using monospecific antibody against bovine brain tubulin. *Science* 187:948–950.

Glenn, K.C. and Cunningham, D.D. (1979) Thrombin-stimulated cell division involves proteolysis of its cell surface receptor. *Nature* 278:711–714.

Glenn, K.C., Carney, D.H., Fenton, J.W. II, and Cunningham, D.D. (1980) Thrombin active site regions required for fibroblasts receptor binding and initiation of cell division. *J. Biol. Chem.* 255:6609–6616.

Glynn, R.D., Thrash, C.R., and Cunningham, D.D. (1973) Maximal concanavalin A-specific agglutinability without loss of density-dependent growth control. *Proc. Natl. Acad. Sci. U.S.A.* 70:2676–2677.

Holley, R.W. and Kiernan, J.A. (1974) Control of the initiation of DNA synthesis in 3T3 cells: serum factors. *Proc. Natl. Acad. Sci. U.S.A.* 71:2908–2911.

Miller, C.L., Fuseler, J.W., and Brinkley, B.R. (1977) Cytoplasmic microtubules in transformed mouse x nontransformed human cell hybrids: correlation with *in vitro* growth. *Cell* 12:319–331.

Noonan, K.D. (1978) Proteolytic modification of cell surface macromolecules: mode of action in stimulating cell growth. In *Current Topics in Membranes and Transport.* Bronner, F. and Kleinzeller, A. (eds.), *New York: Academic Press,* 11:397–461.

Noonan, K.D. and Burger, M.M. (1973) Induction of 3T3 cell division at the monolayer stage. *Exp. Cell Res.* 80:405–414.

Osborn, M. and Weber, K. (1977) The display of microtubules in transformed cells. *Cell* 12:561–571.

Perdue, J.F., Lubenskyi, W., and Kivity, E. (1981) Loss of α-thrombin binding sites in spontaneously, virally or chemically transformed chick and rat embryo fibroblasts and C3H 10T$\frac{1}{2}$ mouse embryo cells. Submitted to *Natl. Acad. Sci. U.S.A.*

Pohjanpelto, P. (1977) Proteases stimulate proliferation of human fibroblasts. *J. Cell Physiol.* 91:387–392.

Sefton, B.M. and Rubin, H. (1970) Release from density dependent inhibition by proteolytic enzymes. *Nature* 227:843–845.

Teng. N.N.H. and Chen, L.B. (1975) The role of surface proteins in cell proliferation as studied with thrombin and other proteases. *Proc. Natl. Acad. Sci. U.S.A.* 72:413–417.

Zetter, B.R., Chen, L.B., and Buchanan, J.M. (1976) Effects of protease treatment on growth, morphology, adhesion, and cell surface proteins of secondary chick embryo fibroblasts. *Cell* 7:407–412.

Zetter, B.R., Chen, L.B., and Buchanan, J.M. (1977) Binding and internalization of thrombin by normal and transformed chick cells. *Proc. Natl. Acad. Sci. U.S.A.* 74:596–600.

Published 1981 by Elsevier North Holland, Inc.
Saunders, Daniels, Serrou, Rosenfeld, and Denney, eds.
FUNDAMENTAL MECHANISMS IN HUMAN CANCER IMMUNOLOGY

CHAPTER 5

Electrical Potentials and Related Membrane Properties of Human and Murine Mononuclear Cells[1]

Richard C. Niemtzow, A. Michael Frace,
Douglas C. Eaton, Steven N. Becker,
Cynthia H. Robbins, J. Regino Perez-Polo,
and Jerry C. Daniels

Divisions of Radiotherapy and Immunology; Departments of Physiology and Biophysics, Pathology, Human Biological Chemistry and Genetics, University of Texas Medical Branch, Galveston, Texas

Introduction

Cells of the immune system are unique among the various classes of mammalian cells in their ability to respond to immunological stimulation. Even though they possess extraordinary immunologic properties, they nonetheless share many characteristics with other mammalian cells. In particular, the cells of the immune system have small electrical potentials across their cellular boundary membranes that are similar to the potentials found in all cells (Suckling, 1961; Niemtzow et al., 1978; Dumont, 1974; Cone et al., 1973). These membrane potentials can be correlated directly with the state of the boundary membrane and events that are affecting the membrane (Suckling, 1961; Cone, 1974; Niemtzow et al., 1979b; Poste and Nicolson, 1977).

In cells of the immune system, measurement of the membrane potential may be particularly important in revealing events related to the immune response for two reasons: first, the initial event in a variety of immune mechanisms involves interaction of immunogenic agents with surface membrane receptors which may change the state of the surface membrane, and second, several of the final events in the transduction process involve alteration in the character-

[1]This research was supported in part by Career Development Award AM00432 to Douglas C. Eaton, National Institutes of Health Grant AM20068 to Douglas C. Eaton, and Grants from the Dora Roberts and Lola Wright Foundations to J. Regino Perez-Polo.

istics of the surface membrane of immune cells (Niemtzow et al., 1978; Goldstine et al., 1974).

Besides the fact that measurement of membrane potential may give us insight into the fundamental membrane processes associated with the immune response, the potentials may also be of practical use. In many cells, membrane properties such as the membrane potential provide a "fingerprint" of the cell (Niemtzow et al., 1978). Among various cells of the immune system, whose membrane characteristics are quite different, one would expect this membrane potential "fingerprint" to allow positive identification of different cell types (Niemtzow et al., 1978; Dumont, 1974; Becker et al., 1980; Wioland and Mehrishi, 1979). This approach is particularly promising because cell surface charge directly affects membrane potential, and differences in surface charge, as determined electrophoretically, are already used to identify various cell types (Andersen et al., 1973; Goldstine et al., 1974; Hanning, 1971; Wioland et al., 1972).

Because of these arguments, we decided to examine the membrane potentials and some related cellular properties in a variety of different cell types of the immune system.

Materials and Methods

In Vivo Experiments

Animals

Male C57 B1/6J mice, aged 6 to 8 weeks, were obtained from the Jackson Laboratory, Bar Harbor, Maine. B-16 malignant melanoma was obtained from the same source and maintained by serial subcutaneous transplants in the right thigh of the experimental mice (Niemtzow et al., 1979b).

Tumor Cell Suspensions

Tumor cell suspensions were prepared after removal of the subcutaneous transplant by aseptic technique. The tumor was pressed through a sterile stainless steel screen and suspended in RPMI 1640 tissue culture media (Grand Island Biological Company) with glutamine (0.3 mg/ml) (Niemtzow et al., 1979b).

Tumor Implantation

On day zero, 10 mice were chosen at random and injected with 0.2 ml of a tumor cell suspension containing 10^6 cells/ml, i.e., a total of 2×10^5 cells per mouse. Subsequently, at approximately two-day intervals, one mouse was randomly selected for examination and sacrifice. The entire area of the injection site was dissected and removed for pathological examination. If there was a visible tumor mass, the size of the tumor at its maximum dimension was measured with calipers (Niemtzow et al., 1979b).

Macrophage Collection

The peritoneum was washed with a small volume of RPMI 1640 and the cells were centrifuged to a pellet at 150 g for 10 minutes. The pellet was then resuspended in 0.5 ml of RPMI-1640 containing 2% agarose (Seaplaque, Marine Colloids, Rockland, Maine) to immobilize the cells. The approximate ionic composition of this solution was Ca $(NO_3)_2$ (0.4 mM), KCl (5.4 mM), Mg SO_4 (0.4 mM), NaCl (103 mM), $NaHCO_3$ (24 mM), and Na_2HPO_4 (5.6 mM) (Niemtzow et al., 1979b).

Similar peritoneal wash specimens were prepared for cytologic evaluation. They were centrifuged to form a film of evenly dispersed cells, fixed in ethanol, and stained by the Papanicolaou method (Clark, 1973). Macrophages were several times larger, having more abundant and irregular cytoplasm than lymphocytes or other cells present.

Intracellular Electrical Potentials

Using these criteria, macrophages were identified when the cell suspension was placed on the stage of an inverted phase contrast microscope (Unitron) (Niemtzow et al., 1979a,b; Becker et al., 1980). They were then impaled with glass microelectrodes whose resistance was in excess of 75 megohms. This resistance implied a tip diameter of less than 0.5 microns. Tip potentials of these electrodes were less than 3 mV. The potentials detected with these electrodes were measured with a high input impedance electrometer (Fredrich Haer Co.) and monitored on an oscilloscope (Phillips) (Suckling, 1961; Niemtzow et al., 1977, 1978).

Statistical Evaluation

The relationships between palpable tumor size, time of tumor growth, and membrane potential were plotted as lines of best fit to which linear regression analysis was applied (Figures 5.1, 5.2, r = coefficient of correlation from the fit of the equation: $y = mx + b$). Mean membrane potentials and standard deviation for Table 5.1 were calculated by the unpaired t test (Niemtzow et al., 1979b).

In Vitro Measurements

Membrane Potential Measurements

A classical electrophysiological system was adapted so that cell membranes penetrated by a microelectrode could be visualized simultaneously as potential differences were recorded at the microelectrode tip. Single cells were penetrated with a glass microelectrode whose resistance was in excess of 75 megohms, implying a tip diameter of less than 0.5 microns. The potentials detected with these electrodes were connected to a bridge amplifier (CBA-1. Frederick, Haer & Co., Brunswick, Maine) modified to include a high cutoff filter adjusted to 1 hz. This filter eliminated line interference, thus permitting measurements

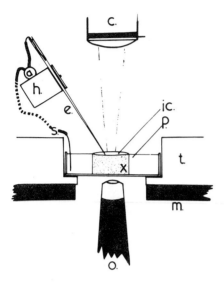

Figure 5.1. Schematic of recording methods. a: electrometer to record membrane potentials. c: condenser of inverted microscope. e: microelectrode. h: motor drive for microelectrode. m: inverted microscope stage. o: inverted microscope objective lens. p: agarose torus without cells. s: Ag-AgCl reference electrode. t: lucite holder for Petri plates. x: agarose containing cells. ic: overlying saline for checking electrode.

without Faraday shielding. An audio-analyzer signalled electrode penetration and variations in electrical potential at the electrode tip. A silver chloride wire electrode completed the electrode circuit by connecting the cell-free agarose in the Petri dish to the pre-amplifier. Measurement of the impedance before and after cell penetration with an impedance check module (Frederick, Haer & Co.) allowed the monitoring of microelectrode integrity (Suckling, 1961; Niemtzow et al., 1978, 1979).

Preparation of Agarose Cell Suspension

In order to achieve reliable and consistent microelectrode penetration, non-adherent cells had to be immobilized in an environment that avoided micro-electrode fracture. This was accomplished by suspending the cells in a highly purified agarose (Seaplaque, Marine Colloids, Rockland, Maine or Indubiose: Industrie Biologique Francaise S.A.) which solidified at 37°C. The agarose was made up to a 2% solution (w/v) in RPM1 1640 plus glutamine prior to use and kept at 38°C. The agarose was mixed with the cells to a final concentration of $5-10 \times 10^6$ cells/ml, then immediately transferred to a 2 cm well cut into a layer of identically constituted agarose in a 3.5 cm Petri dish. Over this well was placed a thin layer of cell-free agarose, which served as an impedance-check layer (Figure 5.1). When the agarose had cooled to 21°C, the measurement of

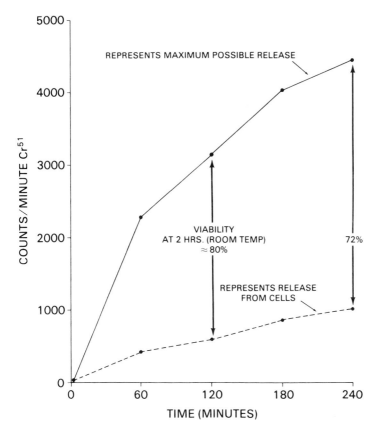

Figure 5.2. Viability of cultured macrophage. Cells were incubated in ^{51}Cr containing saline to load the cells with isotope. Samples of cells were then placed in cold saline and cells were withdrawn at 60-minute intervals. Half the sample was centrifuged and the supernatant counted. This represented ^{51}Cr release from damaged or dead cells. The remainder of the aliquot was sonicated to disrupt the cells, and the sample was counted. The cumulative counts from the two procedures are plotted to demonstrate the percentage of viable cells.

membrane potentials was begun. Between 150–250 individual cells were recorded for each sample during a period of 2–4 hours. Osmolarity measurements of the agarose cell suspension was determined by the freezing-point depression method with the aid of a Fiske osmometer. The 2% agarose RPMI 1640 plus glutamine suspension had a value of 340 ± 5 mOsmol/Kg (Niemtzow et al., 1978, 1979). In experiments where the composition of the external bathing media was altered, the agarose was prepared in the altered saline. The composition of the various salines is given in Table 5.1.

Table 5.1. Solution Composition.[a]

Name	Na^+	K^+	Cl^-	$MeSo_3^-$	$Chol^+$	HCO_3^-	$HPO_4^=$
A. Normal Saline	138.2	5.4	108.4	–	–	24	5.6
B. High K^+	35.2	108.4	108.4	–	–	24	5.6
C. Low K^+	143.6	–	108.4	–	–	24	5.6
D. Na, K free	–	–	108.4	–	143.6	24	5.6
E. Na, K, Cl free	–	–	–	108.4	143.6	24	5.6
F. Na, Cl free	–	143.6	–	108.4	–	24	5.6
G. K, Cl free	143.6	–	–	108.4	–	24	5.6

[a]Besides the ions listed in the table, each of the salines contained 0.4 mM $Ca(NO_3)_2$, 0.4 mM $MgSO_4$, and 1 mM glucose. The solutions were adjusted to pH 7.0 by addition of phosphoric acid.

Techniques of Peripheral Blood Separation, Surface Markers, and Macrophage Separation

Subpopulations of human leukocytes were prepared from heparinized peripheral blood donated by healthy adults. The separation techniques and membrane markers used have been described in detail elsewhere (Niemtzow et al., 1978). Peripheral blood monocytes were prepared by culturing the buoyant mononuclear band separated on ficoll-triosil. These cells were grown overnight in RPMI 1640 plus glutamine and 20% heat-inactivated fetal calf serum at 37°C in a humid atmosphere of 5% CO_2/air mixture. Subsequently, the culture vessels were vigorously washed with RPMI 1640 and the adherent cells either examined while attached to the culture vessel or removed from the surface by a rubber instrument and suspended in agarose as previously described. Over 95% of these cells were phagocytic, as judged by their capacity to ingest particles of colloidal carbon (Niemtzow et al., 1978).

Cell Viability

Prior to agarose inclusion, the viability of cell samples was $95 \pm 2\%$ as judged by Trypan blue dye exclusion. Following incorporation of cells into agarose, the viability was checked by measuring the release of ^{51}Cr into the normal saline supernatant overlying the agarose in the Petri dish from prelabeled cells (Figure 5.2). This was counterchecked by taking trocar biopsies of the cell-containing gel, disaggregating, and exposing to trypan blue (Niemtzow et al., 1978).

^{51}Cr released into the supernatant from prelabeled cells treated with HCl was compared with that released by non-HCl treated cells suspended in agarose. After 2-hr incubation at 21°C, the viability was 81%, and after 4 hr it was 71%. The trypan blue exclusion studies gave similar results: 85% viable at 2 hr and 70% viable at 4 hr (Niemtzow et al., 1978).

Morphologic Methods

Thioglycollate was injected into the peritoneal cavities of the C57 B1/6J mice. Macrophages were obtained from injected mice and control (non-injected) mice at different time intervals, particularly after 72 hours, by intra-peritoneal washing with a small volume of RPMI 1640 tissue culture media containing glutamine (0.3 mg/ml) (Grand Island Biological Co., Long Island, New York). Washings from eight to ten mice were pooled and then divided for various studies (Becker et al., 1980).

Light Microscopy for Nucleoli Counts

Peritoneal exudate washings were centrifuged in a Cyto-Spin centrifuge (Shandon Co.) on non-frosted glass slides providing a uniform cell film. The slides were fixed immediately in 95% ethyl alcohol and stained by the Papanicolaou method, which is used in routine diagnostic cytology for the detection of malignant cells. Nucleoli were counted in 100 nuclei of cells identified as macrophages (Becker et al., 1980).

Scanning Electron Microscopy

Peritoneal exudate washings were centrifuged in a Cyto-Spin centrifuge (Shandon Co.) on non-frosted glass slides previously coated with poly-L-lysine. The slides were fixed immediately with 2.5% glutaraldehyde in 0.1 M cacodylate buffer, pH 7.2. After dehydration in absolute ethyl alcohol, the slide was cut down to a one-square-cm containing the sediment; that volume of tissue could be accommodated as an electron microscope specimen. This piece was dried by the critical point method, mounted on SEM specimen mounts using silver conducting paint, and coated with gold-palladium alloy. Observations were made with the International Scientific Instruments Super III Scanning Electron Microscope operated at 15 KV. Photomicrographs were taken at the desired magnifications with the attached Polaroid camera (Becker et al., 1980).

Results

Response of Macrophage to Immunological Stimulus In Vivo

We were initially concerned that, despite our rationale, there might be no *in vivo* variation after immunologic stimulus in the electrical properties of cells of the immune system. This would make subsequent investigations of immune cells *in vitro* substantially less interesting and relevant. To evaluate this possibility, we examined a murine model in which peritoneal macrophages were immunogenetically challenged with injected neoplastic tissue (Niemtzow et al., 1979b).

Ten mice were examined over a period of 21 days. Our observations are summarized in Table 5.2. As expected, with increasing time after injection of tumor cells, we observed tumor masses of increasing diameter (Figure 5.3). No tumor growth was detected in biopsies of the injection site of the first two mice. Tumor was present in the third mouse and was associated with a few chronic inflammatory cells identified as macrophages, but no necrosis was present. Only a minute focus of tumor cells was present in the fourth mouse. The fifth mouse had a much larger tumor nodule with extensive central necrosis and a slightly increased number of chronic inflammatory cells identified as macrophages at the periphery. In all the mice where it was present, the tumor was characteristic of amelanotic melanoma, having atypical nuclei with massive nucleoli and little apparent melanin in the cytoplasm (Niemtzow et al., 1979b).

When the membrane potentials of the macrophages from these mice were measured, we found a distribution of potentials in any given mouse, but there was a tendency for the potentials to become significantly more electronegative as time after injection increased (Table 5.2). Figure 5.4 shows the mean values of the membrane potential after injection. The increase in electronegativity from control level on day 1 becomes significant between days 3 and 4 ($p = 0.01$). The difference in the potentials remain significant ($p < 0.01$) on all subsequent days (Niemtzow et al., 1979b).

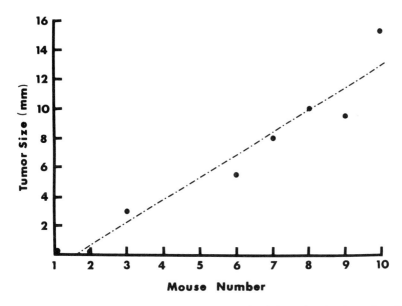

Figure 5.3. Relationship of tumor size to length of time after implantation. The dashed line is the best least-squares linear fit to the data points.

When the membrane potentials of the macrophages are plotted versus the size of the tumor, there is an essentially linear correlation ($r = 0.93$) for all values except that associated with the last mouse sampled (Figure 5.5) (Niemtzow et al., 1979b).

Table 5.2. Variation of Membrane Potential in Peritoneal Macrophage and Tumor Size at Various Times After Tumor Implantation.

Mouse #	Mean mV	± SD mV[a]	Number of cells sampled	Tumor size (mm)	Histology[b]	Weight of mouse (g)
1	−0.29	2.58	31	0	0	17
2	−0.98	2.95	49	0	0	20.5
3	−0.95	3.68	39	3	+	19.5
4	−3.04	3.00	47	−	+	17.5
5	−3.39	3.27	28	−	+	18
6.	−3.81	3.06	32	5.5	+	17.7
7	−3.77	5.36	13	8	+	17
8	−2.11	4.20	37	10	+	12
9	−8.00	3.48	37	15.3	+	25
10	−4.75	3.72	24	27	+	21

[a] $\overline{X}$ ± SD Statistical differences in the means were calculated by the unpaired t test.

[b] By microscopic histology (0 = not present; + = tumor present).

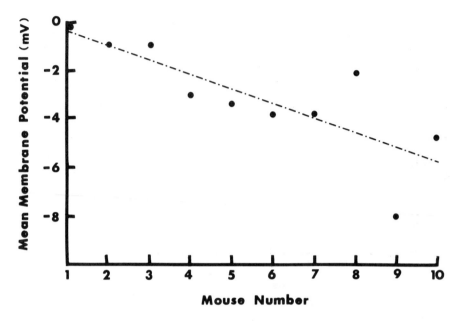

Figure 5.4. Mean value of peritoneal macrophage membrane potential vs time after implantation of tumor.

In Vitro Measurements of Membrane Properties of Immune Cells

The previous experiment showed us that there was a substantial *in vivo* change of membrane potential in macrophage when they were presented with an immunologic challenge (Niemtzow et al., 1979b). Because of this finding, we decided to investigate more thoroughly the source and characteristics of the membrane potential and other related membrane properties in macrophage and other cells of the immune system (Niemtzow, 1979b).

Macrophage

Measurements of intracellular ion concentrations. Although the external environment of the macrophage can be controlled by the experimenter, the internal ion composition cannot be. Under many conditions the membrane properties of cells depend upon the internal ion concentrations; therefore, we measured the intracellular Na^+ and K^+ concentrations of peritoneal macrophage by flame spectrophotometry. The results from eight samples of macrophage prior to any antigenic stimulation were: intracellular $K^+ = 53 \pm 12$ mM and intracellular $Na^+ = 44 \pm 13$ mM. The ratio of intracellular Na^+ to K^+ was 0.91 ± 0.24. These results are similar to those found by Castranova et al. (1979) in rat alveolar macrophage. We also examined macrophage subsequent to their activation by intraperitoneal injection of thioglycollate. Seventy-two hours after the injection, the macrophage obtained by peritoneal washout had

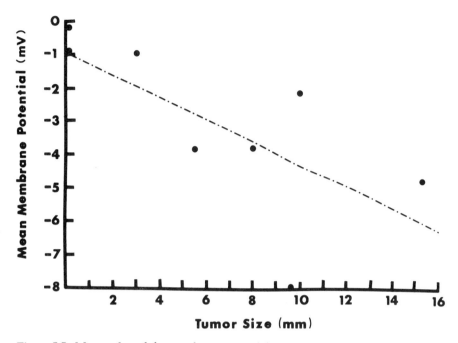

Figure 5.5. Mean value of the membrane potentials of peritoneal macrophage vs tumor size.

dramatically changed their intracellular ion compositions. In six samples, the intracellular K^+ had risen to 84 ± 17 mM while the Na^+ concentration had fallen to 15 ± 8 mM. The new Na^+ to K^+ ratio was now 0.18 ± 0.08.

Selectivity to K^+, Na^+, and Cl^-. Most cell membranes develop potentials through a mechanism of selective permeability. The permeability to K^+ is usually high, while permeabilities to Na^+ and Cl^- are low. These ion gradients are usually maintained by a Na^+-K^+ transport system driven by ATP cleavage. The result of the selective permeability to K^+ is generally a membrane potential that has the inside negative with respect to the outside. One manner of assessing the permeability to various ions is to vary the external ionic environment and note any changes in membrane potential. The relative permeabilities can then be calculated from the equation (Goldman, 1943; Hodgkin and Katz, 1949):

$$V_M = \frac{RT}{F} \ln\left(\frac{P_K(K^+)_o + P_{Na}(Na)_o + P_{Cl}(Cl)_i}{P_K(K^+)_i + P_{Na}(Na)_i + P_{Cl}(Cl)_o} \right)$$

where V_m is the membrane potential; P_x is the permeability of a specific ion, x; $(x)_o$ is the concentration of an ion outside the cell; and $(x)_i$ is the concentration inside, T is the absolute temperature, R is the universal gas constant and F is

Faraday's constant. This equation implies very specific properties of a selective membrane (Hodgkin and Horowicz, 1959). If a membrane is only permeable to potassium, for example, the membrane potential is directly related to the $\log_{10}$ of the potassium concentration with the potential varying 58 mV per ten-fold change in potassium concentration. If the membrane is permeable to other ions, the variation in potential will be less than 58 mV. In fact, given information about the variation in potential and intracellular ion concentrations, one can calculate the relative permeabilities to various ions (Hagiwara et al., 1972; Eaton et al., 1975). Since information of this sort might be useful in understanding the properties of immune cells, we applied solutions of varying potassium concentration to both normal and activated macrophage. In Figure 5.6, the variation of membrane potential of normal macrophage is plotted versus the log of the K^+ concentration. K^+ is varied by equimolar replacement of Na^+ in normal saline (Table 5.1). In this case, the variation in potential as K^+ is varied is only 6.4 millivolts per ten-fold change in K^+ concentration. This implies a membrane very permeable to many of the ions in

Figure 5.6. Membrane potential of non-activated macrophage as a function of potassium concentration in the bathing medium. The potassium in normal saline (solution A, Table 1) is varied by equimolar substitution for Na^+. Chloride ion is kept constant. The dotted line represents a 6.4 millivolt change per 10-fold change in K^+ concentration.

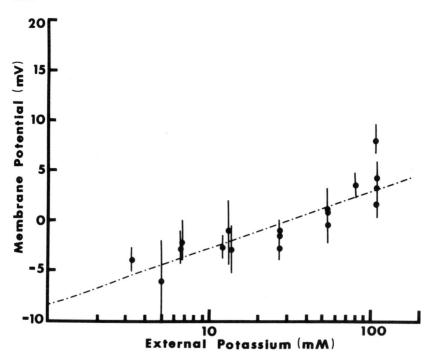

the solution (Eaton et al., 1975). To decide which other ions are permeable besides K^+, we must remove from the external solution by turns the various likely candidates for permeable ions. In the experiments summarized in Figures 5.7 and 5.8, we have removed first Cl^- and then both Na^+ and Cl^- from the external solution. After the removal of each of these ions, there is a substantial increase in the magnitude of the change in potential for changes of K^+. In the absence of Cl^-, the slope becomes 10.5 millivolts per decade change. In the absence of Cl^- and Na^+, the slope becomes 24 millivolts per decade change of K^+. These three figures taken together give us several quantitative measures of the permeability of the membranes of non-activated macrophage (Hodgkin and Horowicz, 1959; Eaton et al., 1975). Potassium ion is 1.85 times more permeable than sodium ion. Chloride ion is 1.15 times more permeable than potassium. The intracellular chloride concentration is 68 ± 6 mM. In addition, the cationic replacement ion, choline, is 0.25 times the permeability of K^+, the anionic replacement ion, methane sulfonate, is 0.65 times as permeable as chloride ion. That so many different ions show substantial permeability is quite unusual for most cells (Hagiwara et al., 1972). The unusual permeability properties of the non-activated macrophage contrasted sharply with those of the activated cells. In Figure 5.9, the effect on the membrane potential of varying the K^+ concentration shows that in the absence of Cl^- the potential changes 31 millivolts per decade change of K^+.

Figure 5.7. The variation of membrane potential with potassium concentration when the product of K^+ concentration and Cl^- concentration is kept constant. This method effectively reduces the contribution of Cl^- to the measured changes in membrane potential. The slope of the dotted line represents a 10.5 millivolt change per 10-fold change in K^+ concentration.

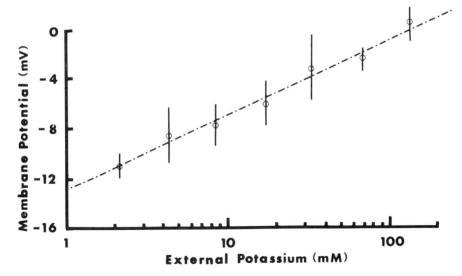

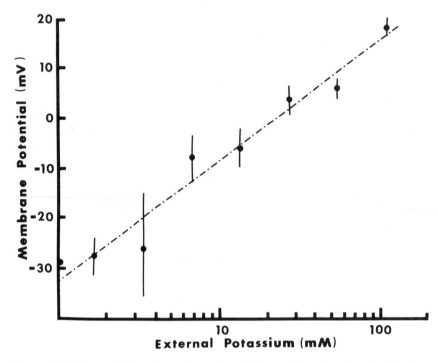

Figure 5.8. The variation of membrane potential as a function of external potassium concentration in the absence of sodium and chloride ions. Na^+ has been replaced with choline while Cl^- ion has been replaced with methane sulfonate. The slope of the dotted line represents a 24 millivolt change per 10-fold change in K^+ concentration.

This implies that K^+ is 5.9 times more permeable than Na^+ through the membrane of the activated cells. The intercept of the line on the potential axis implies an intracellular K^+ concentration of 89 mM. This confirms the observation made by flame photometry that upon activation the intracellular K^+ increases dramatically.

Current-voltage relations of macrophage. Although membrane selectivity can be a strong indicator of membrane state, another traditional way of examining membrane properties is to apply a current across the membrane and measure the resultant voltage. The current acts as a driving force for ions and careful measurement of current and voltage can give information about magnitude of movement and species of ion moving across the membrane. In Figure 5.10, the results of an experiment are depicted in which the current-voltage relationships of several macrophage are depicted. One plot shows the results obtained from a typical cell obtained from a sample of activated cells, while the other plots show the I-V relationship for a non-activated cell and the same cell after addition of the calcium ionophore, A23187. The ionophore causes an alteration

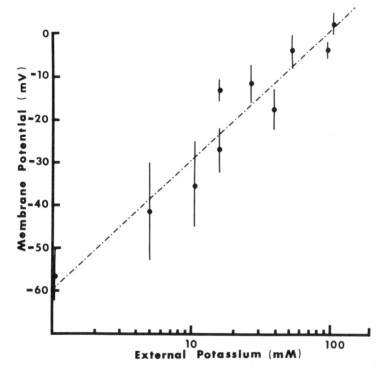

Figure 5.9. The variation of membrane potential as a function of external potassium concentration for thioglycollate activated macrophage. The measurements were made in the absence of chloride. The slope of the dotted line represents a 31 millivolt change per 10-fold change in K^+ concentration. This implies a substantial increase in K^+ permeability over that observed in non-activated macrophage.

of the relationship in a manner suggestive of activation. If Ca^{++} entry is a necessary prerequisite for activation, then other changes associated with activation should be associated with application of Ca^{++} ionophore (Gallin et al., 1975).

Effects of exogenous agents on membrane potentials and respiration. The effect of the calcium ionophore, A23187, on the current voltage relationship caused us to speculate that entry of Ca^{++} into the non-activated macrophage might be an important initial step in the process of activation with a subsequent possible step, the inhibition of phosphodiesterase with consequent increase of intracellular cyclic AMP (Rasmussen and Goodman, 1977).

To test this idea, we decided to compare the effects of application of the ionophore to the natural changes that take place when the macrophages are activated by antigenic stimulation. We also examined the effects of cholera toxin which is an activator of cyclic nucleotide production in some prepara-

72

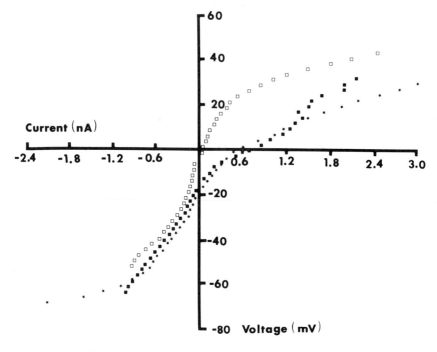

Current (nA)

Voltage (mV)

Figure 5.10. The relationship between voltage response and injected current for activated macrophage (stars), non-activated macrophage (open squares) and non-activated macrophage treated with the calcium ionophore, A23187 (filled squares).

tions (Mertens et al., 1974). The effects are shown of the two agents on activated and non-activated macrophage is given in Table 5.3. The alternative criteria we used to test the effect of the two agents was to examine changes in respiration. Activated macrophage have characteristically higher respiration rates than macrophage measured prior to antigenic stimulation. In Figures 5.11 and 5.12, we compare the respiration of activated macrophage with the respiration of non-activated cells before and after the application of A23187 and cholera toxin. In both cases, there is a substantial increase in respiration of the non-activated cells. For A23187, the respiration of activated and non-activated cells becomes virtually identical.

Effect of lymphokines on the membrane potentials of macrophage. Although the effects of calcium ionophore and cholera toxin are interesting in themselves, the possible importance of these interactions is emphasized by the effect on membrane potential of naturally occurring lymphokines. The effects of the addition of lymphokine to non-activated macrophage are given in Table 5.3. This agent, just like calcium ionophore and cholera toxin, induces a negative change in macrophage membrane potential that appears to mimic the normal activation process (Niemtzow et al., 1979a; Becker et al., 1980).

Table 5.3. Effects of Exogenous Agents on Activated and
Non-Activated Macrophage.

		Agent		
		A23187	Cholera toxin	Lymphokine
Non-activated cells	Control	−0.98 ± 2.95 n = 39	−1.31 ± 3.40 n = 18	−2.48 ± 1.51 n = 48
	Treated	−15.4 ± 3.87 n = 22	−12.8 ± 4.2 n = 12	−11.2 ± 2.04 n = 37
Activated cells	Control	−20.5 ± 1.74 n = 25	−18.9 ± 3.74 n = 13	−11.2 ± 2.04
	Treated	−24.2 ± 2.86 n = 14	−21.3 ± 3.24 n = 9	

Morphological Discriminators of Activation

Can we correlate the dramatic changes in membrane potential, membrane
selectivity, intracellular ion concentrations, cellular respiration, and sensitivity
to exogenous agents that take place as a macrophage is activated with any
morphologic events at the cellular level? To investigate the possibility, we
examined normal and activated macrophage in several ways (Becker et al.,
1980).

Figure 5.11. The effect of calcium ionophore on the respiration of non-activated
macrophage compared with the respiration of activated macrophage.

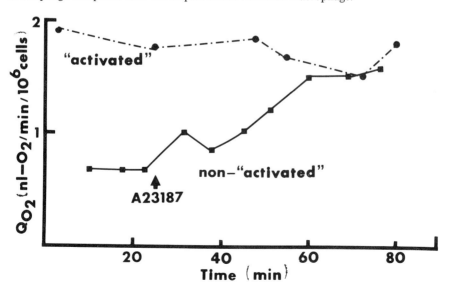

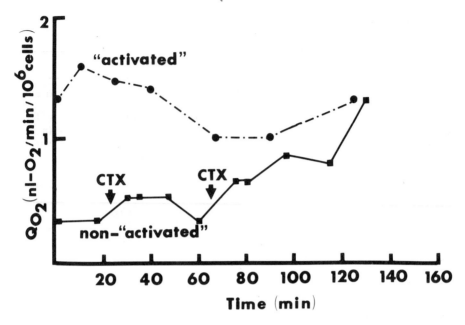

Figure 5.12. The effect of cholera toxin on the respiration of non-activated macrophage compared with the respiration of activated macrophage.

Activated macrophages collected 72 hours after injection of thioglycollate had increased numbers of nucleoli averaging 1.95 ± 0.18 nucleoli/nucleus compared to control macrophages which averaged only 1.01 ± 0.31 nucleoli/nucleus ($p < 0.0001$) (Becker et al., 1980). In addition activated macrophages were much larger with more abundant foamy vacuolated cytoplasm (Figure 5.13). Scanning electron microscopy revealed that activated macrophages had a pronounced, ruffled surface topography compared to the smoother surface with irregular projections observed on the unactivated control cells (Figure 5.14) (Becker et al., 1980; Nabarra et al., 1978).

Protein Synthesis in Macrophage

The 72-hour activated and control macrophages showed no difference in the level of protein synthesis as measured by incorporation of ^{3}H-amino acids into acid-precipitable fractions. Rather, protein synthesis was markedly increased (up to 35-fold) within 24 hours of activation when transmembrane potential and average nucleoli/nucleus differences in activated and control cells were minimal (Becker et al., 1980; Figure 5.15).

Measurements of Membrane Electrical Potentials of Human Peripheral Blood Mononuclear Cells

Results obtained from five donors demonstrated that the membrane potential of the majority of cells fell in the $+4$ mV to -6 mV range. The membrane

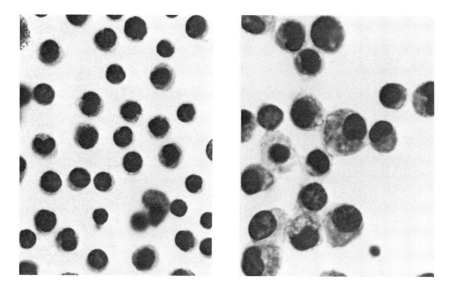

Figure 5.13. Light micrographs of non-activated and activated murine macrophage. On the left are murine peritoneal macrophage prior to activation with thioglycollate. On the right are macrophage 72 hours after the animal was peritoneally injected with thioglycollate.

Figure 5.14. Scanning electron micrographs of non-activated and activated murine macrophage. On the left is a peritoneal macrophage prior to activation. On the right is a similar macrophage 72 hours after injection of the mouse with thioglycollate.

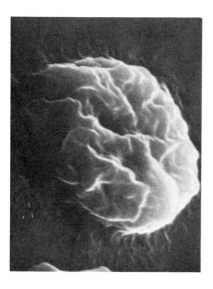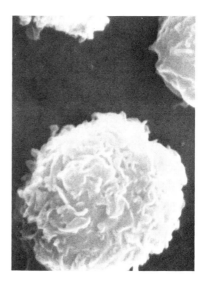

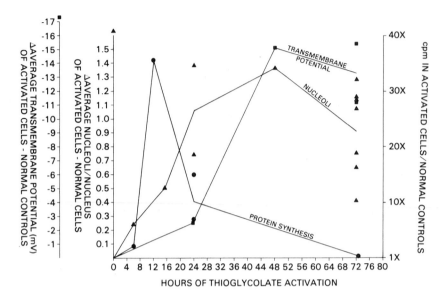

Figure 5.15. Correlates of activation in macrophage. On the horizontal axis, we have plotted the hours after injection of the mice with thioglycollate. On the vertical axis, the average number of nucleoli per cell, the mean membrane potential and magnitude of protein synthesis (as measured by ^{3}H-leucine incorporation) is plotted.

potential frequency distribution for these donors is shown in Figure 5.16. The mean membrane potential was -2.4 ± 8.4 mV. The observations that some cells had a positive rather than a negative potential and that some voltage peaks had more amplitude than others were the first indications that particular cell types might have distinctive electrical potentials (Niemtzow et al., 1978; Dumont, 1974).

Membrane Electrical Potentials of Peripheral Monocytes

The vast majority of cultured monocytes had positive membrane potentials: 89.2% had potentials in the $+2$ to $+20$ mV range, and 10.8% had negative membrane potentials in the -2 to -6 mV range (Figure 5.16). The mean membrane potential and standard deviation for this cell type were 4.0 ± 3.95 mV. These cells were defined as monocytes because they were phagocytic adherent mononuclear cells (Niemtzow et al., 1978; Dumont, 1974).

Membrane Electrical Potentials of T Lymphocytes

96% of the T cell population had membrane potentials in the -2 to -20 mV range with a mean of -4.8 ± 3.2 mV (Figure 5.17). Only 6.4% had positive membrane potentials, in the $+2$ to $+3$ mV range. This population was not completely homogeneous: 78% formed E-rosettes and 15% EA-rosettes, and 3.57% had surface immunoglobulin (Niemtzow et al., 1978; Dumont, 1974).

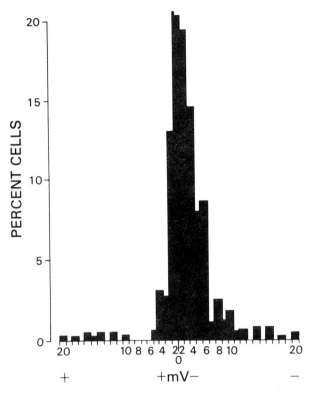

Figure 5.16. Variation of potential in human mononuclear cells. On the abscissa is the percentage of total cells. On the ordinate are the membrane potentials of all measured cells divided into 1 mV bins. The cells were the mononuclear fraction of human peripheral blood cells separated on ficoll-triosil. Erythrocyte and polymorph contamination as 5±3%. The measurements represent 1000 cells obtained from 5 healthy donors. Mean membrane potential is −2.4±8.4 mV.

Membrane Electrical Potentials of B Lymphocytes

The majority of these cells had positive potentials, 61.3% having a potential in the −2 to −7 mV range (Figure 5.17). The mean potential and standard deviation for this cell type were +2.7±6.9 mV. This population of cells was not completely homogeneous; 73% had surface immunoglobulins, 20% formed EA-rosettes, and 2% formed E-rosettes (Niemtzow et al., 1978; Dumont, 1974).

Membrane Electrical Potentials of Null Cells

All of these cells had negative potentials in the −2 to −20 mV range, with a mean potential of −7.39±4.44 mV. Surface markers showed that 5% formed E-rosettes, 29% formed EA-rosettes, and 6.9% had surface immunoglobulin. This implies that 89.9% of these cells did not possess classic T and B lymphocyte surface markers (Niemtzow et al., 1978; Dumont, 1974).

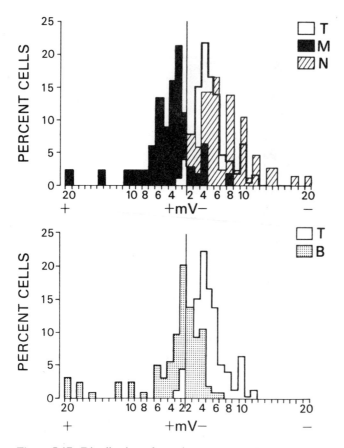

Figure 5.17. Distribution of membrane potentials in various mononuclear cells. On the abscissa is the percent cells. In the upper panel, we have plotted the potentials of T lymphocytes, monocytes, and null cells (non-E-rosette-forming, non-immunoglobulin-bearing). The monocyte population was prepared from total mononuclear fraction, described above, by culturing in plastic Petri dishes for 18 hr at 37°C in a humid atmosphere of 5% CO_2/air in RPMI 1640 with glutamine and 10% decomplemented fetal calf serum. Antibiotics and anti-fungal agents were not added. Dishes were vigorously washed with the remaining adherent cells recovered by scraping with a rubber spatula. This population of cells was 95% phagocytic. The null-cell-enriched population was prepared from carbonyl-treated buoyant ficoll-triosil cells incubated on a nylon wool column for 1 hr at 37°C. Effluent non-adherent cells were separated into two fractions by E-rosetting sedimentation, the non-rosette-forming cells being rich in null cells. The T lymphocyte-enriched population was prepared after removal of phagocytic cells from the total "floating band" of ficoll-triosil-separated peripheral blood by treatment with carbonyl iron; remaining cells incubated twice with sheep erythrocytes in 24 hr, sedimenting rosette-forming cells in ficoll-triosil and recovering them after 60 s exposure to 0.83% NH_4Cl. Below, we have plotted the potentials of a B lymphocyte enriched population with the T lymphocyte population for comparison. The B-lymphocyte-enriched population was prepared from monocyte-depleted ficoll-triosil mononuclear cells incubated on nylon wool in absence of serum for 1 hr at

Membrane Electrical Potentials of Cultured and Mitogen-Stimulated Cells

When the total mononuclear cell preparation was incubated in RPMI 1640 and 20% human AB serum for 72 hr, an increase in the number of cells with positive potentials were noted, with a compensating decrease in the number of cells with negative voltage. The predominantly negative potential mononuclear cell population became increasingly positive when cultured *in vitro*, but this effect occurred more rapidly and was more marked when lymphoblastogenic doses of phytohemagglutinin (PHA) and concanavalin A (Con A) were added to the culture medium (Niemtzow et al., 1978; Dumont, 1974).

The total mononuclear cell population membrane potential was -2.4 ± 8.4 mV, the T-lymphocytes -4.8 ± 3.2 mV, the B-lymphocytes $+2.7 \pm 6.9$ mV, the null cells -7.39 ± 4.4 mV and the monocytes $+4 \pm 3.95$ mV. After polyclonal stimulation by either phytohemagglutinin (PHA) or concanavalin A (Con A), the membrane potentials became less negative, and after 72 hours, a substantial percentage of the population had achieved a positive membrane potential contrarily (Figures 5.18 and 5.19). The monocytes became increasingly negative after phagocytosing colloidal carbon or mineral oil (Niemtzow et al., 1978; Niemtzow et al., 1979a).

Discussion

Our primary objectives in examining the electrophysiological properties of cells in the immune system were three-fold:

1. Are there substantial differences in membrane potential or other membrane properties between the various cell types of the immune system or even between the same cell type when presented with varying immunologic stimuli?
2. If there are differences that we can observe *in vitro*, do they correspond to events which occur during normal *in vivo* immunologic activation by antigenic stimuli?
3. And if the answer to both of these questions is positive, can we gain any insight into the underlying membrane events from the observable changes in the properties of the cellular membranes?

We feel that the answer to each of these questions is a qualified "yes." The qualification is probably attributable to the fact that we have not been able to devote as intensive an effort to some cellular components of the immune

---

37°C; non-adherent cells were then washed through and adherent (B lymphocyte) cells recovered by vigorous washing. Mean membrane potentials for these separated populations: T lymphocytes -4.8 ± 3.2 mV; B lymphocytes $+2.7 \pm 6.9$ mV; Monocytes $+4 \pm 3.95$; Null cells -7.39 ± 4.44 mV.

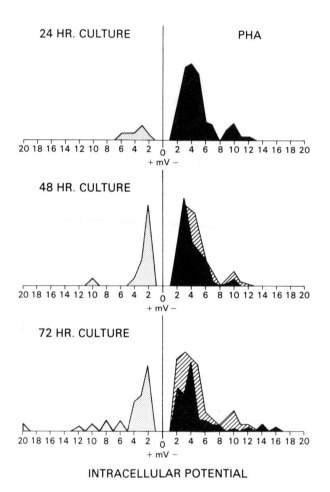

Figure 5.18. *In vitro* stimulation with phytohemagglutinin (PHA). After 72 hours in culture, there is a substantial negative shift of membrane potentials of the cultured cells.

system as we have to others, such as the macrophage. Nonetheless, we feel the methods of electrophysiology offer a unique opportunity to support more conventional approaches to study of the immune system.

Membrane Potentials as an Analytic Tool for Identification of Immune Cell Types

Our results strongly suggest that, under certain circumstances, membrane potential measurements may be used as a correlative measure of cell type along with other identifying characteristics. It has been suggested that some null cells

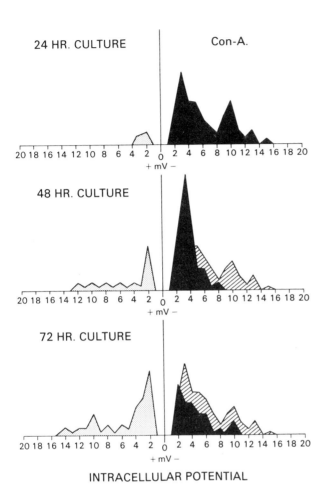

Figure 5.19. *In vitro* stimulation with concanavalin A (Con A). After 72 hours in culture, there is a substantial negative shift of the membrane potentials of the cultured cells.

are T lymphocyte precursors (Ballet and Daguillard, 1977). Our studies have shown that null cells invariably have negative intracellular potentials and the population as a whole is more electronegative than T lymphocytes (-4.8 ± 3.2 mV as compared to -7.39 ± 4.44 mV). Clearly there is an overlap in the intracellular potentials, which may in part be related to the lack of complete homogeneity in the two subpopulations separated (11% of the null cell population had T or B lymphocyte markers and 22% of the T lymphocyte preparation did not form E-rosettes). However, we can postulate that in cells destined to become mature T lymphocytes, there is a progressive change in the intracellular potential towards the less negative end of the spectrum, with an overt change to positivity during blastogenic stimulation (Niemtzow et al., 1978; Dumont, 1974; Stillwell et al., 1973; Cone, 1971).

The hypothesis that the membrane potentials of different populations of cells vary in specific ways is supported by the observation that membrane potentials of a mixed cell population alter systematically in response to antigenic stimuli. A variety of membrane changes besides alterations of membrane potential have been observed in lymphocytes exposed to lectins such as phytohemagglutinin (PHA) and concanavalin A (Con A). Some of the effects described include: increased membrane transport of K^+ (Quastel and Kaplan, 1970; Averdunk, 1972), Ca^{2+} (Allwood et al., 1971; Whitney and Sutherland, 1972), and amino acids (Mendelsohn et al., 1971; Van den Berg and Betel, 1971). Kinetic studies have shown that there is a unidirectional K^+ flux resulting in an increase in the intracellular potassium concentration in rat thymocytes exposed to concanavalin A (Con A) (Inversen, 1976).

The relationship between the external membrane charge and the intracellular potential is not yet clear. Differences in the electrophoretic mobility appear to be related to differences in membrane ionic groups (Mehrishi, 1972; Mehrishi and Zeiller, 1974a,b), and it has been shown that human T and B lymphocytes have different mobilities in an electrical field (Wioland et al., 1972). Depletion experiments strongly suggest that B and T lymphocytes have different intracellular potentials, a hypothesis which has been confirmed by studies on isolated, enriched subpopulations. Similarly, depletion experiments indicate that peripheral blood monocytes have positive intracellular potentials, and although this observation has been confirmed in the purified, isolated population, it is probable that the latter was to some extent activated by in vitro culture and mechanical procedures. Despite these experimental limitations, the evidence argues that distinct subpopulations of human peripheral blood mononuclear cells have different intracellular potentials which are altered by a variety of in vitro factors such as mitogenic stimulation and duration of culture. The maturity of a cell may also play a role in deciding the membrane potential at any given stage. A more precise understanding of this fundamental aspect of cellular physiology may in fact help to explain a number of immunological phenomena that have hitherto been unknown or obscured in complexity.

We must, however, exercise a certain amount of caution in extending our results to an in vivo system. The methods available for the in vitro isolation of monocytes are known to induce variable degrees of non-specific activation. The removal of nylon wool-adherent B lymphocytes could conceivably induce activation or stimulation. Hence the interpretation of the intracellular potentials of in vitro isolated cells must take into account the possible induction of changes that may not necessarily be related to in vivo resting potentials.

Maturation of a cell may also be accompanied by changes in intracellular potential. Electrokinetic studies of mouse thymocytes indicate that subpopulations with different electrophoretic mobilities appear as the animal matures (Dumont, 1974).

The separation procedures involved in deriving distinct subpopulations of mammalian cells have such marked effects on membrane physiology that the use of the intracellular potential alone as a means of determining the specific histogenic or functional nature of that cell appears to us to be fraught with many difficulties, making it by itself an unsuitable method. But employed as an additional identifying marker for cell identification, it may have substantial utility. Moreover, the examination of these potentials may, as in the case of macrophage, give us important insights into fundamental membrane mechanisms involved in the immune response.

Membrane Responses to In Vivo Antigenic Stimuli

Although membrane properties of immune cells may be useful as identifiers of specific cell types or as a method for gaining insight into the normal functioning of these cells, the investigation of the membrane properties would be much more significant if it were clear that, under *in vivo* conditions, there were changes in the membrane properties associated with events in the immune system.

We feel that to a certain extent our observations of the human monocyte population suggests that changes in membrane potential do take place. Our work with tumor induced macrophage addresses this point directly, since tumor cells, but not normal cells, can be killed by activated, but not by normal macrophage (Basic et al., 1974; Chapman and Hibbs, 1977; Cleveland et al., 1974; Den Otter et al., 1972; Hibbs et al., 1972; Hibbs, 1973, 1974a,b; Holtermann et al., 1973; Niemtzow et al., 1978; Piessans et al., 1975).

The activation process involves numerous steps, expressed as morphological, biochemical, and physiological changes (Adams et al., 1973; Hammond and Dvorak, 1972; Joseph et al., 1977; Mackaness, 1970; Nelson, 1979; Stubbs et al., 1973). As macrophages become more activated, they exhibit enhanced bactericidal and tumoricidal activity (Biroum-Noerjasin, 1977; McLeod and Remington, 1977; Keller, 1973; Nelson, 1979). Thus, measurement of a parameter which correlates with tumor-stimulatory activity implies that such a parameter may be a direct reflection of the degree of macrophage activation. The direct correlation of tumor size in the B-16 murine melanoma model with peritoneal macrophage membrane electronegativity suggests that membrane potential may be related to the activation process, as has been supported by other observations using lymphokine treatment of macrophages *in vitro* (Niemtzow et al., 1979a). We offer the hypothesis that progressive macrophage membrane electronegativity may reflect increasing activation, triggered by immunologic reactivity to the tumor.

Macrophage Activation

Since *in vivo* activation of macrophage appears to be correlated with membrane potential changes, we felt that an examination of membrane properties *in vitro* could help to illuminate the response by macrophage to antigenic stimulation.

A number of membrane or cellular events occur when a macrophage is activated (see summary in Table 5.4). By themselves, the various events are not very informative about the underlying processes that lead to activation. However, examination of some treatments which may participate in activation naturally or whose application mimics normal activation give a strong suggestion about these mechanisms.

The calcium ionophore, A23187, when applied to normal macrophage, produces a respiratory response and an alteration of the current-voltage relationship that causes the cells to appear very similar to activated cells (Gallin et al., 1975). In addition, cholera toxin, a potent cyclic nucleotide stimulator (Mertens et al., 1974), also produces events similar to activation. This is particularly interesting, since intracellular Ca^{++} is also known to inhibit phosphodiesterase, the enzyme responsible for hydrolysis of cyclic AMP. It is attractive to speculate that the initial events in activation are a Ca^{++} permeability increase followed by an increase in intracellular cyclic AMP. The work of several other investigators lends support to this hypothesis. The activation of lymphocytes is directly dependent upon external Ca^{++} (Alford, 1970; Whitney and Sutherland, 1972a). There is also increased uptake of ^{45}Ca upon activation (Allwood et al., 1971; Whitney and Sutherland, 1972b; Goldberg et al., 1974). The activation of lymphocytes is thus associated with an increase in the intracellular level of Ca^{++}. Increased intracellular Ca^{++} has been shown to lead to substantial potassium permeability increases in a variety of cells (Meech, 1974). Concomitant with the increase in intracellular Ca^{++} in activated lymphocytes, the cyclic AMP has also been shown to increase (Smith et al., 1971). Cyclic AMP has also been associated with increased Na-K-ATPase activity, the so-called "Na^+ pump" (Hays et al., 1977). These changes, taken together, could easily account for the changes of intracellular ion concentrations, the reduction in membrane resistance, and the alteration of membrane potential observed at the time of activation. Finally, cyclic AMP production has also been associated with increased protein synthesis (Avener et al., 1972; Terasaki et al., 1978).

Table 5.4. Summary of Differences Between Activated and Non-Activated Peritoneal Macrophage.

Membrane or cellular parameter	Non-activated cells	Activated cells
1. Cellular respiration	0.7 nl-O_2/min/10^6 cells	2.0 nl-O_2/min/10^6 cells
2. Membrane resistance	> 100 Mohms	5-20 Mohms
3. Intracellular Na^+	44 mM	15 mM
4. Intracellular K^+	55 mM	84 mM
5. Membrane potential	> −5 mV	< −20 mV
6. Ratio of sodium to potassium permeability	0.54	0.17
7. Permeability to large ions (choline, sulfate)	high	low
8. Morphologic changes	$\simeq$ 1 nucleoli/nucleus	$\simeq$ 2 nucleoli/nucleus
9. Protein synthesis	low	initially high

Are there any other cell preparations which appear to resemble the macrophage? Egg cells, in making the transition between unfertilized to fertilized, display each of the properties listed in Table 5.4 (Hagiwara and Jaffe, 1979). Moreover, a Ca^{++} permeability increase is associated with fertilization and this change leads to increased cyclic AMP activity. The analogy between the two initially quiescent cells is quite striking, and further comparisons may allow testing of a specific hypothesis about the initial membrane events associated with macrophage activation.

Conclusion

We have examined the membrane and cellular characteristics of several cell types in the immune system. On the basis of this examination, we have determined that different cell types have different membrane properties which may be used as criteria for identifying cell types. Our measurements have also given us a suggestive hypothesis about the initial cellular events which occur in immunologic activation of cells.

References

Adams, D.O., Biesecker, J.L., and Koss, L.G. (1973) The activation of mononuclear phagocytes *in vitro*: immunologically mediated enhancement. *J. Reticuloendoth. Soc.* 14:550.

Alford, R.H. (1970) Metal cation requirements for phytohemagglutinin-induced transformation of human peripheral blood lymphocytes. *J. Immunology* 104:698.

Allwood, G., Asherson, G.L., Davey, M.J., and Goodford, P.J. (1971) The early uptake of radioactive calcium by human lymphocytes treated with phytohaemagglutinin. *Immunol.* 21:509.

Andersen, L.C., Nordling, S., and Hayri, P. (1973) Fractionation of mouse T and B lymphocytes by preparative cell electrophoresis. Efficiency of the method. *Cell. Immunol.* 8:235.

Averdunk, R. (1972) Uber die Wirkung von Phytohaemagglutinin und Antilymphozytenserum auf den Kalcium-, Glucose- und Aminsaure-Transport der menschlichen Lymphozyten. *Hoppe-Seylers Z. Physiol. Chem.* 353:79.

Averner, M.J., Brock. M.L., and Jost, J.P. (1972) Stimulation of ribonucleic acid synthesis in horse lymphocytes by exogenous cyclic AMP. *J. Biol. Chem.* 247:413.

Ballet, J.J. and Daguillard, F. (1977) Carcteres membranaires et fonctionnels de lymphocytes precurseurs T du sang et de l'amygdale humaine. *Ann. Immunol. Inst. Pasteur.* 128:C6.

Basic, I., Milas, L., Grdina, D.J., and Withers, H.R. (1974) Destruction of hamster ovarian cell cultures by peritoneal macrophages from mice treated with corynebacterium granulosum. *J. Nat. Cancer Inst.* (USA) 52:1839.

Becker, S.N., Niemtzow, R.C., Eaton, D.C., Olson, M.H., Perez-Polo, R., Robbins, C., and Daniels, J.C. (1980) Morphologic changes in thioglycollate-activated macrophages correlated with protein synthesis and changes in transmembrane potential. *Laboratory Investigation* 42:101.

Biroum-Noerjasin (1977) Listericidal activity of nonstimulated and stimulated human macrophages *in vitro*. *Clin. Exp. Immunol.* 28:138.

Castranova, V., Bowman, L., and Miles, L.P. (1979) Transmembrane potential and ionic content of rat alveolar macrophages. *J. Cell. Physiol.* 101:471.

Chapman, H.A., Jr. and Hibbs, J.B., Jr. (1977) Macrophage tumor killing: influence of the local environment. *Science* 197:279.

Clark, G. (1973) *Staining Procedures Used by the Biological Stain Commission*. Baltimore: Williams and Wilkins.

Cleveland, R.P., Melzer, M.S., and Zbar, B. (1974) Tumor cytotoxicity *in vitro* by macrophages from mice injected with bacterium bovis strain BCG. *J. Nat. Cancer Inst.* 52:1887.

Cone, C.D., Jr. (1974) The role of the surface electrical transmembrane potential in normal and malignant mitogenesis. *Annals of the New York Academy of Sciences* 238:420–435.

Cone, C.D., Jr. and Tongier, M., Jr. (1973) Contact inhibition of division: involvement of the electrical transmembrane potential. *J. Cell. Physiol.* 83(3):373–386.

Cone, C.D., Jr. (1971) Maintenance of mitotic homeostasis in somatic cell populations. *J. Theor. Biol.* 30:183–194.

Den Otter, W., Evans, R., and Alexander, P. (1972) Cytotoxicity of murine peritoneal macrophages in tumor allograft immunity. *Transplantation* 14:220.

Dumont, F. (1974) Electrophoretic analysis of cell population changes in the mouse thymus as a function of age. *Immunol.* 26:1051.

Eaton, D.C., Russell, J.M., and Brown, A.M. (1975) Ionic permeabilities of an *Aplysia* giant neuron. *J. Membrane Biol.* 21:353.

Gallin, E.K., Wiederhold, M.L., Lipsky, P.E., and Rosenthal, A.S. (1975) Spontaneous and induced hyperpolarizations in macrophage. *Cell Physiol.* 86:653.

Goldberg, N.D., Haddox, M.K., Dunham, E., Lopez, C., and Hadden, J.W. (1974) The Yin-Yang hypothesis of biological control: opposing influences of cyclic GMP and cyclic AMP in the regulation of cell proliferation and other biological processes. In *Control of Proliferation in Animal Cells*. Clarkson, B. and Baserga, R. (eds.), Cold Spring Harbor Laboratory, pp. 609–625.

Goldman, D.E. (1943) Potential, impedance, and rectification in membranes. *J. Gen. Physiol.* 27:37–60.

Goldstine, A.H., Urbaniak, S.J., and Irvine, W.J. (1974) Electrophoresis of lymphocytes from normal human subjects and patients with chronic lymphatic leukaemia. *Clin. Exp. Immunol.* 17:113.

Hagiwara, S. and Jaffe, L.A. (1979) Electrical properties of egg cell membranes. *Ann. Rev. Biophys. Bioengineering* 8:385.

Hagiwara, S., Eaton, D.C., Stuart, A.E., and Rosenthal, N.P. (1972) Cation selectivity of the resting membrane of squid axon. *J. Membrane Biol.* 9:373.

Hammond, M.E. and Dvorak, H.F. (1972) Antigen-induced stimulation of glucosamine incorporation by guinea pig peritoneal macrophages in delayed hypersensitivity. *J. Exp. Med.* 136:1518.

Hanning, K. (1971) Free flow electrophoresis. A technique for continuous preparative, and analytical separation. *Methods in Microbiology* 5B:513–542.

Hays, E.T., Horowicz, P., and Swift, J.G. (197) Theophylline action on sodium fluxes in frog striated muscle. *J. Pharm. Exp. Therapeutics* 202:388.

Hibbs, J.B., Jr. (1974a) Discrimination between neoplastic and non-neoplastic cells *in vitro* by activated macrophages. *J. Nat. Cancer Inst. (USA)* 53:1487.

Hibbs, J.B., Jr. (1974b) Heterocytolysis by macrophages activated by Bacillus Calmette-Guerin: lysosome exocytosis into tumor cells. *Science* 184:468.

Hibbs, J.B., Jr. (1973) Macrophage non-immunologic recognition of target cell factors related to contact inhibition. *Science* 180:868.

Hibbs, J.B., Jr., Lambert, L.H., and Remington, J.S. (1972) Possible role of macrophage mediated non-specific cytotoxicity in tumor resistance. *Nature (London)*, New Biol. 2:48.

Hodgkin, A. and Katz, B. (1949) The effect of sodium ions on the electrical activity of the giant axon of the squid. *J. Physiol.* 108:37.

Hodgkin, A.L. and Horowicz, P. (1959) The influence of potassium and chloride ions on the membrane potential of single muscle fibers. *J. Physiol.* 148:127.

Holtermann, O.A., Klein, E., and Casale, G.P. (1973) Selective cytotoxicity of peritoneal leukocytes for neoplastic cells. *Cell Immunol.* 9:339.

Inversen, J.G. (1976) Unidirectional K^+ fluxes in rat thymocytes. *J. Cell. Physiol.* 89:267.

Joseph, M., Dessaint, J.P., and Capron, A. (1977) Characteristics of macrophage cytotoxicity induced by IgE immune complexes. *Cell Immunol.* 34:247.

Keller, R. (1973) Cytostatic elimination of syngeneic rat tumor cells *in vitro* by non-specifically activated macrophages. *J. Exp. Med.* 138:625.

Mackaness, G.B. (1970) The mechanism of macrophage activation. In *Infectious Agents and Host Resistance*. S. Mudd (ed.), Philadelphia: W.B. Saunders Co., p. 61.

McLeod, R. and Remington, J.S. (1977) Studies on the specificity of killing of intracellular pathogens by macrophages. *Cell. Immunol.* 34:156.

Meech, R.W. (1974) The sensitivity of *Helix aspersa* neurons to injected calcium ions. *J. Physiol.* 237:257.

Mehrishi, J.N. (1972) Molecular aspects of the mammalian cell surface. In *Progress in Biophysic and Molecular Biology*, Vol. 25. Butler, J.A.U. and Nole, I. (eds.), Oxford: Pergamon Press, pp. 3–68.

Mehrishi, J.N. and Zeiller, K. (1974a) T and B lymphocytes: striking differences in surface membranes. *Brit. Med. J.* 1:360.

Mehrishi, J.N. and Zeiller, K. (1974b) Surface molecular components of T and B lymphocytes. *Europ. J. Immunol.* 4:474.

Mendelsohn, J., Skinner, A., and Kornfeld, S. (1971) The rapid induction by phytohaemagglutinin of increased α-aminoisobutyric acid uptake by lymphocytes. *J. Clin. Invest.* 50:818.

Mertens, R.B., Wheeler, H.O., and Meyer, S.E. (1974) Effects of cholera toxin and phosphodiesterase inhibitors on fluid transport and cyclic AMP concentrations in rabbit gallbladder. *Gastroenterology* 67:898.

Nabarra, B., Cavelier, J.F., Dy, M., and Dimitri, A. (1978) Scanning electron microscopic studies of activated macrophages in the mouse. *Journal of the Reticulo Endothelial Society.* 24(5):489.

Nelson, D.S. (1979) Macrophages as effectors of cell-mediated immunity. In *Phagocytes and Cellular Immunity*. H.H. Gadebusch (ed.), Boca Raton, Florida: CRT Press, Inc., p. 57.

Niemtzow, R.C., Klein, C., Gauci, C.L., Rabischong, R., and Serrou, B. (1977) Techniques for measurements of intracellular potentials in non-excitable cells. *J. Electrophysiol. Tech.* 5:30.

Niemtzow, R., Gauci, C.L., and Serrou, B. (1978) Variations in the intracellular potentials of subpopulations of human peripheral blood mononuclear cells. *Cancer Immunol. Immunoth.* 4:121–127.

Niemtzow, R.C., Olson, M.H., Rossio, J.L., Serrou, B., Gauci, L., and Daniels, J.C. (1979a) Lymphokine-induced changes in macrophage intracellular electrical potentials. *Biomedicine* 31:264–267.

Niemtzow, R.C., Eaton, D.C., Kunze, D.L., Becker, S.N., Wong, J.Y., Olson, M.H., McBee, J., Moulton, R.G., Gauci, L., Viallet, P., Serrou, B., and Daniels, J.C. (1979b) Correlation between macrophage intracellular electrical potentials and malignant melanoma growth in a murine model. *Biomedicine* 31:257–260.

Piessens, W.F., Churchill, W.H., Jr., and David, J.R. (1975) Macrophages activated *in vitro* with lymphocyte mediators kill neoplastic but not normal cells. *J. Immunol.* 114:293.

Poste, G. and Nicolson, G.L. (1977) Preface. In *Dynamic Aspects of Cell Surface Organization. Cell Surface Reviews, Volume 3*. Poste, G. and Nicolson, G.L. (eds.), Amsterdam: North-Holland Publishing Co., p. 1.

Quastel, S. and Kaplan, J.G. (1970) Early stimulation of potassium uptake in lymphocytes treated with PHA. *Exp. Cell Res.* 63:230.

Rasmussen, H. and Goodman, D.B. (1977) Relationships between Ca^{++} and cyclic nucleotides in cell activation. *Physiol. Rev.* 57:421.

Smith, J.W., Steiner, A.L., Newberry, W.M., and Parker, C.W. (1971) Cyclic AMP in human lymphocyte. Alterations after phytohemagglutinin stimulation. *J. Clin. Investigation* 50:432.

Stillwell, E.F., Cone, C.M., and Cone, C.D. (1973) Stimulation of DNA synthesis in CNS neurons by sustained depolarization. *Nature New Biol.* 246(152):110–111.

Stubbs, M., Kuhner, A.V., Glass, E.A., David, J.R., and Karnovsky, M.L. 1973. Metabolic and functional studies on activated mouse macrophages. *J. Exp. Med.* 137:537.

Suckling, E.E. (1961) *Bioelectricity*. New York: McGraw-Hill Book Co., p. 119.

Terasaki, W.L., Brooker, G., de Vellis, J., Inglish, D., Hsu, C., and Moylan, R.D. (1978) Involvement of cyclic AMP and protein synthesis in catecholamine refractoriness. *Adv. Cyclic Nuc. Res.* 9:33.

Van den Berg, K.J. and Betel, I. (1971) Early increase of amino acid transport in stimulated lymphocytes. *Exp. Cell Res.* 66:257.

Whitney, R.B. and Sutherland, R.M. (1972a) Requirement for Ca^{++} in lymphocyte transformation stimulated by phytohemagglutinin. *J. Cell. Physiol.* 80:329.

Whitney, R.B. and Sutherland, R.M. (1972b) Enhanced uptake of calcium by transforming lymphocytes. *Cell. Immunol.* 5:137.

Wioland, M. and Mehrishi, J.N. (1979) Age-dependent changes in the electrophoretic mobilities of human blood lymphocytes. *Scand. J. Immunol.* 10:453–463.

Wioland, M., Sabolovic, D., and Burg, C. (1972) Electrophoretic mobilities of T and B cells. *Nature (London), New Biol.* 237:274.

Published 1981 by Elsevier North Holland, Inc.
Saunders, Daniels, Serrou, Rosenfeld, and Denney, eds.
FUNDAMENTAL MECHANISMS IN HUMAN CANCER IMMUNOLOGY

CHAPTER 6

The Role of Ia Antigens in T Cell Activation

Ethan M. Shevach, M.D. and Robert B. Clark, M.D.

Laboratory of Immunology, National Institute of Allergy and Infectious Diseases, National Institutes of Health, Bethesda, Maryland

Introduction

The I region of the major histocompatibility complex (MHC) mediates a number of functions that are critical in the regulation of the immune response (Katz and Benacerraf, 1976). The I region encodes a series of antigens, the I region associated (Ia) antigens, that are expressed primarily on B lymphocytes, some T lymphocytes, and on a subpopulation of macrophages (Shevach, 1978). In most cases, the Ia antigens are two-chain molecules consisting of a 33,000 and a 28,000 dalton component. I region products play important roles in regulating immunocompetent interactions between macrophages and T lymphocytes (Rosenthal and Shevach, 1973) and between T lymphocytes and B lymphocytes (Katz et al., 1973). In addition, it is likely that the Ia antigens are identical to the products of the immune response (*Ir*) genes, a set of genes which regulate the capacity of individual animals to make T lymphocyte dependent immune responses to specific antigens. This report will deal with the results of our studies on the function of macrophage Ia antigens in the regulation of T cell activation. Three separate, but related, experimental models will be examined in detail—antigen induced T cell proliferation, the autologous or syngeneic-mixed leukocyte reaction (SMLR), and T cell activation produced by aldehyde determinants on macrophage surfaces.

Antigen Induced T Cell Proliferation

We have previously shown that the proliferative response of guinea pig T lymphocytes which had been primed *in vivo* could only be induced with antigen-pulsed syngeneic macrophages (Rosenthal and Shevach, 1973). A detailed genetic analysis, using combinations of macrophages and T lymphocytes that differed by either B region antigens (the guinea pig homologue of the mouse H-2 K/D antigens) or Ia antigens, demonstrated that the Ia antigens or the products of closely linked genes played the critical role in macrophage-T lymphocyte interaction, and that the B antigens played no role in this collaboration (Shevach, 1976).

The model originally proposed to explain the histocompatibility restriction on macrophage-T cell interaction was termed the "cellular interaction structure model" (Shevach and Rosenthal, 1973; Katz et al., 1973). It stated that the Ia antigens function as specific cellular interaction structures, and homology between these structures was necessary for effective cellular interactions. A second model which we have termed the "complex antigenic determinant model" (Thomas and Shevach, 1976) was also consistent with the data. According to this theory, T cells do not recognize antigens per se, but can only be sensitized to antigen modified membrane components or to complexes of antigen combined with certain membrane molecules. Since all of our previous studies had used T cells primed *in vivo*, the failure of allogeneic macrophage associated antigen to activate immune T cells would be secondary to the fact that the T cells had been primed *in vivo* only to antigen associated with syngeneic macrophages.

In order to test the complex antigenic determinant hypothesis, we developed an assay for the generation of an *in vitro* primary response in which non-immune guinea pig T lymphocytes could be primed and challenged in tissue culture with antigen-pulsed macrophages (Thomas and Shevach, 1976). We found that T cells primed with syngeneic macrophages *in vitro* could be restimulated only with syngeneic, but not allogeneic, antigen-pulsed macrophages, thus confirming our previous findings obtained with T cells primed *in vivo*. Furthermore, we found that F_1 T cells primed with antigen-pulsed macrophages of one parent could be restimulated only with the parental macrophage used for initial stimulation, and not with those of the other parent (Table 6.1, Group A).

If some $(2 \times 13)F_1$ T cells are able to be sensitized to the antigenic complex containing strain 2 I region products, while other T cells are sensitized to the immunogenic complex containing strain 13 I region products, then one might predict that in an immunized F_1 animal, separate T cell subpopulations would exist which have been sensitized to antigen associated with either strain 2 or 13 I region products presented by the $(2 \times 13)F_1$ macrophage. Paul et al. (1977) demonstrated that this was indeed the case with the use of positive and negative selection procedures. T lymphocytes from ovalbumin (OVA)-primed $(2 \times 13)F_1$ donors were selected by culture with strain 2 or 13 OVA-pulsed macrophages for 1 week (Table 6.1, Group B). Cells selected with OVA-pulsed strain 2 macrophages responded well to OVA-pulsed strain 2 macrophages in the second culture and poorly to OVA-pulsed strain 13 macrophages. The opposite result was seen with F_1 T cells selected with OVA-pulsed strain 13 macrophages. In negative selection experiments, the proliferating cells were

Table 6.1. Independent Populations of F_1 Lymphocytes Respond to Antigen-Pulsed Parental Macrophages.

Group	T cell source	First culture		Second culture ΔCPM ^{3}H-TdR incorporation	
				2-OVA	13-OVA
A	Unprimed (2 × 13)F_1	Prime	2-OVA	7,280	1,150
			13-OVA	0	8,382
B	OVA-primed (2 × 13)F_1	Positive selection	2-OVA	85,100	890
			13-OVA	23,200	81,457
C	OVA-primed (2 × 13)F_1	Negative selection	2-OVA	2,000	25,000
			13-OVA	102,750	4,890

Note: T lymphocytes from unprimed or primed F_1 animals were cultured with OVA-pulsed parental macrophages for 7 days (priming and positive selection) or 3 days (negative selection with BUdR and light), washed, and then restimulated for 3 days in the second culture with OVA-pulsed parental macrophages.

killed by treatment of the cultures with bromodeoxyuridine (BUdR) and light (Table 6.1, Group C). F_1 T cells negatively selected with OVA-pulsed strain 2 macrophages responded well to OVA-pulsed strain 13 macrophages, but very poorly to OVA-pulsed strain 2 macrophages.

All of the experimental approaches described above have yielded data which is compatible with the complex antigenic determinant model of T cell antigen recognition. According to this model, T cells from an F_1 animal which had been primed *in vivo* should have been sensitized to antigen in association with the Ia antigens of both parental haplotypes. However, one important exception to this rule was noted in our early studies. Thus, for antigens, the response to which is under the control of specific *Ir* genes, immune (responder×non-responder) F_1 T cells could only be activated by antigen associated with macrophages of the responder parent and not by antigen associated with macrophages of the non-responder parent (Shevach and Rosenthal, 1973). In order to make this result consistent with the complex antigenic determinant model, one must propose that the Ia antigens themselves are the *Ir* gene products and function as antigen recognition structures on macrophages. Macrophages from a non-responder animal would lack the appropriate Ia antigen necessary to process or present the antigen, the response to which is controlled by a specific *Ir* gene.

The Autologous or Syngeneic Mixed Lymphocyte Reaction

The studies described above suggest that the Ia antigen molecule on macrophages plays a highly specific role in the regulation of the immune response—the ability to interact with some antigens, but not others, in the formation of a complex which is then seen by the antigen-specific T cell. Another approach to determine the function of Ia antigens in cell interaction and T cell activation is to examine an antigen-independent system of T cell activation. Studies performed primarily with human cells have demonstrated that a highly significant proliferative response can be observed when T cells are cultured with irradiated non-T cells (Opelz et al., 1975; Kuntz et al., 1976). This reaction, which has been termed the "autologous mixed leukocyte reaction" (AMLR), exhibits both memory and specificity (Weksler and Kozak, 1977), and the products of the HLA-D region of the human MHC are the likely target antigens (Hausman and Stobo, 1979; Thorsby and Nousiainen, 1979).

We have attempted to define the role of Ia antigens in the AMLR by using well-characterized cell populations from inbred strain 2 and 13 guinea pigs whose MHC differ only in the I region (Yamashita and Shevach, 1980). The reactivity of guinea pig T cells with syngeneic non-T cells resembled in many respects what has been described in the human AMLR. A peak proliferative response was seen at 8 days of primary culture and an enhanced secondary response was seen on day 4. Specificity in the response was apparent, in that T cells cultured with syngeneic macrophages responded well to syngeneic macrophages in the secondary cultures, but displayed an absent or diminished response to allogeneic stimulation. The responding cell in the guinea pig was shown to be of T cell origin, while the stimulator belonged to the Ia positive subpopulation of peritoneal exudate macrophages (Yamashita and Shevach, 1977).

Direct proof of the importance of Ia antigens was obtained from studies of the reactivity of F_1 T cells with parental stimulator cells. When $(2 \times 13)F_1$ T cells were cultured with parental macrophages for 14 days and then restimulated with F_1 or parental macrophages, they demonstrated an enhanced proliferative response to the macrophages of the same strain used in the first culture (Table 6.2). These results are identical to those seen in the studies of antigen-induced T cell proliferation and demonstrate that two populations of $(2 \times 13)F_1$ T cells, responsive to one or the other parental macrophage, also exist in the SMLR. When the F_1 T cells which had been positively selected with macrophages of one parent were stimulated with F_1 macrophages in the second culture, the response was specifically inhibited by anti-Ia sera directed to the Ia antigens of the macrophage strain used in the first culture. For example, F_1 T cells positively selected with strain 2 macrophages responded to strain 2 or F_1 macrophages, but not strain 13, in the second culture in the presence of normal guinea pig serum (NGPS); the response of these cells to either strain 2 of F_1 macrophages was markedly inhibited in the presence of anti-2 serum, while anti-13 serum had no effect on the response (Table 6.2). These results strongly favor the view that the Ia antigens are the proliferative stimuli in the syngeneic mixed leukocyte reaction (SMLR).

Table 6.2. Ia Antigens Are the Proliferative Stimuli in the SMLR.

First culture			Second culture		
Responder	Stimulator	Serum	2	13	F_1
$(2 \times 13)F_1$	2	NGPS	110	8	55
		Anti-2	19	7	8
		Anti-13	93	9	48
$(2 \times 13)F_1$	13	NGPS	12	35	80
		Anti-2	10	36	68
		Anti-13	12	8	9

Note: $(2 \times 13)F_1$ T cells were cultured with parental macrophage for 14 days, washed, and then restimulated with parental or F_1 macrophage in the presence of NGPS or anti-Ia serum. The incorporation of ^{3}H-TdR was determined on day 4 of the second culture and is expressed as CPM $\times$ 10^{-3}.

Studies of several immunologic diseases suggest that the reactive cell in the SMLR plays an important role in immunoregulation *in vivo*. Sakane et al. (1978) and Kuntz et al. (1979) have noted an absence of an AMLR in patients with systemic lupus erythematosis. Smith and Pasternak (1978) have shown a similar defect in New Zealand black mice. Glimcher et al. (1980) have analyzed the SMLR in three strains of mice with autoimmune disease and demonstrated that the SMLR is present in young mice of these three strains, but is greatly reduced in their older counterparts; reciprocal mixing experiments demonstrated that the defect in the older mice resides in the responder cell population. Conflicting results have been obtained from other studies of the functional role of the human T cell which is reactive in the AMLR. One study demonstrated that the reactive cell may exhibit T-helper function (Hausman and Stobo, 1979), whereas others have demonstrated that the responding cell has properties of a T-suppressor cell (Sakane and Green, 1979).

Our observations that the genetic requirements for the activation of the SMLR resemble the requirements for antigen-specific T cell activation have suggested a number of different roles for the reactive cell in the SMLR (Figure 6.1). First, one must consider that the proliferative response observed *in vitro* represents a primary or secondary response to an unknown foreign antigen, such as a viral antigen. This explanation is very difficult to definitively rule out although, in our studies, great care was taken to avoid exposure of the cells to a source of foreign serum proteins. A second possibility is that the SMLR represents sensitization to a non-T cell or macrophage specific antigen to which tolerance is maintained *in vivo* but not *in vitro*. An antigen of this type need not necessarily by polymorphic, because the genetic restriction of the

94

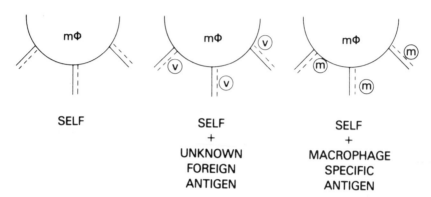

Figure 6.1. Models for the target antigen on the macrophage surface which is the actual stimulator determinant in the SMLR. See text for details. The two-chain Ia molecule is depicted as the two lines on the macrophage surface.

response of the F_1 T cell would be generated because the antigen was seen in association with self-Ia. The third possibility is that T cells do indeed express a receptor for a self-Ia and the SMLR actually represents T cell activation *in vitro*, mediated through this low affinity anti-self receptor. Such a population of T cells might exhibit important immunoregulatory functions, both positive and negative, *in vivo*.

Aldehyde Induced T Cell Activation

Chemical alteration of cell membranes by sodium periodate ($NaIO_4$) or sequential neuraminidase-galactose oxidase (NG) induces extensive proliferation of T lymphocytes from all species studied (Novogrodsky and Katchalski, 1973; Greineder and Rosenthal, 1975). The importance of the aldehyde (CHO) determinant in $NaIO_4$ or NG induced blastogenesis is emphasized by the reversal of activation observed when the treated lymphocytes are reacted with reagents such as sodium borohydrate, which are known to interact with aldehydes. CHO induced T cell proliferation is strictly dependent on the presence of macrophages, although either the T cell or the macrophage may bear the active aldehyde. However, CHO bearing T cells are not able to induce proliferation in untreated T cells even in the presence of macrophages (Greineder and Rosenthal, 1975). CHO induced T cell activation, like the SMLR, offers an opportunity to study T cell recognition of macrophage Ia determinants in the absence of any identifiable antigen. Indeed, it has previously been shown that CHO induced T cell activation resembles both antigen induced T cell activation and the SMLR, in that it can be specifically inhibited by antisera directed toward Ia determinants on macrophages (Greineder et al., 1976).

A logical extension of the comparison of CHO with antigen and SMLR induced T cell activation was to ask whether two independent populations of F_1 T cells could be identified which responded to CHO modified parental macrophages. Initially, we investigated whether we could generate an enhanced secondary response to CHO treated macrophages. $(2 \times 13)F_1$ T cells were stimulated with parental CHO modified macrophages. After 48 hours of culture, the cells were washed and then recultured with untreated macrophages or CHO modified parental macrophages. If the first cultures were stimulated with CHO macrophages of either parental strain, a resultant enhanced secondary response to CHO modified parental macrophages was noted (Table 6.3; compare lines 1 and 2). However, in contrast to the results observed in either antigen or SMLR induced T cell activation, this enhanced secondary response demonstrated no genetic restriction. Thus, $(2 \times 13)F_1$ T cells stimulated with CHO modified strain 13 macrophages in the first culture responded vigorously in the second culture to either strain 2 or 13 CHO modified macrophages (Table 6.3, line 2). The critical role of Ia antigens in this response was demonstrated by the fact that the secondary response of $(2 \times 13)F_1$ T cells to either parental CHO modified macrophage was not generated when the first culture was performed in the presence of anti-Ia serum directed to the Ia antigens of the parental CHO modified macrophage used to stimulate the first culture (Table 6.3, line 3).

The results of these positive selection experiments which suggested that all $(2 \times 13)F_1$ T cells could be activated by either strain of CHO modified parental macrophage were confirmed in negative selection studies. $(2 \times 13)F_1$ T cells were cultured with parental CHO modified macrophages and treated after 24

Table 6.3. The Role of IA Antigens in CHO-Induced T Cell Activation.

Serum	First culture		Second culture	
	Responder	Stimulator	2-NaIO$_4$	13-NaIO$_4$
NGPS	$(2 \times 13)F_1$	13	14	12
NGPS	$(2 \times 13)F_1$	13-NaIO$_4$	86	47
Anti-13	$(2 \times 13)F_1$	13-NaIO$_4$	23	25

Note: $(2 \times 13)F_1$ T lymphocytes were cultured for 2 days with unmodified or sodium periodate (NaIO$_4$) modified strain 13 macrophages in the presence of NGPS or anti-13 serum, washed, and then restimulated with strain 2 or 13 NaIO$_4$-modified macrophages in the presence of NGPS. [3] H-TdR incorporation was determined on day 3 of the second culture and is expressed as CPM $\times 10^{-3}$.

hours with BUdR and light. When these negatively selected cells were restimulated with CHO modified parental macrophages, a significant reduction of the secondary response to either strain of CHO modified macrophages was observed (results not shown). The CHO induced system is therefore unique, in that two populations of responding $(2 \times 13)F_1$ T cells cannot be delineated, in spite of the fact that Ia antigens appear to play a critical role in this response because the generation of the secondary response, as well as the secondary response itself, could be blocked by antisera directed toward Ia determinants on the stimulatory macrophage.

Conclusions

We have described in this report three distinct systems in which macrophage Ia antigens play a critical role in T cell activation. It is appropriate at this point to ask whether any relationship exists between these three *in vitro* models. The activation of T cells by antigen-pulsed macrophage is the most complex of the three but, in some respects, the easiest to understand. Although we have made a strong case for the existence of a complex of nominal antigen and Ia on the macrophage surface, little progress has as yet been made in the biochemical isolation and characterization of this complex. However, recent studies in our laboratory offer further evidence for a very precise function of Ia molecules on the macrophage surface (Burger and Shevach, 1980). We have identified a monoclonal anti-Ia antibody which inhibits the proliferative response of some, but not all antigens, in spite of the fact that our biochemical studies have demonstrated that it reacted with a determinant present on all guinea pig Ia molecules. This result suggests that the monoclonal antibody might react with different parts of the Ia molecule that have different functional roles; certain parts of an Ia molecule might participate in the presentation of certain antigens or antigenic fragments but not others.

Both the SMLR and CHO induced T cell activation are independent of antigen. What then is the stimulus in each case for T cell activation? We have proposed (Figure 6.1) that the polymorphic determinants of the Ia molecule are the target antigens in the SMLR. Indeed, the same portions of the Ia molecule that are capable of binding nominal antigens would be the stimulatory structures in the SMLR. The genetic regulation of the SMLR and antigen induced activation are identical and both are inhibited in a highly specific manner by anti-Ia sera directed towards macrophage Ia determinants.

The results of the studies of CHO induced T cell activation suggest a different role for the Ia molecule in T cell activation. The finding of an Ia requirement without a concomitant genetic restriction was unexpected. We hypothesize that CHO induced T cell activation is a two-step process (Figure 6.2). The initial step is a physical interaction between macrophage and T cell, perhaps mediated by Schiff base formation between CHO modified macrophage and T cell membranes. The second step would involve T cell recognition

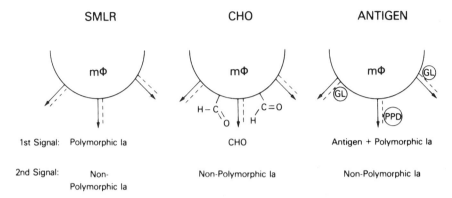

Figure 6.2. Does T cell activation by macrophages require a second signal mediated by the Ia molecule? The polymorphic portion of the Ia molecule is drawn as the hatched line, while the arrow indicates the nonpolymorphic Ia chain.

of, or activation by, a nonpolymorphic portion of macrophage Ia molecules. This would account for the lack of genetic restriction in the positive and negative selection studies. Anti-Ia sera which are directed against polymorphic determinants on the Ia molecule would inhibit the function of the nonpolymorphic portion by steric mechanisms. It is also likely that this two-step mechanism of T cell activation is operative in antigen induced T cell triggering, as well as the SMLR. In the former, recognition of the complex of nominal antigen and polymorphic Ia would constitute the first signal, while in the latter, recognition of polymorphic Ia alone would be the first signal (Figure 6.2). In all cases, the second signal would be mediated by a nonpolymorphic, perhaps species specific, portion of the Ia molecule.

References

Burger, R. and Shevach, E.M. (1980) Monoclonal antibodies to guinea pig Ia antigens. II. Effect on alloantigen-, antigen-, and mitogen-induced T lymphocyte proliferation *in vitro*. J. Exp. Med. 152:1011–1023.

Glimcher, L.H., Steinberg, A.D., House, S.B., and Green, I. (1980) The autologous mixed lymphocyte reaction in strains of mice with autoimmune disease. *J. Immunol.* 125:1832–1838.

Greineder, D.K. and Rosenthal, A.S. (1975) The requirement for macrophage-lymphocyte interaction in T lymphocyte proliferation induced by generation of aldehydes on cell membranes. *J. Immunol.* 115:932–938.

Greineder, D.K., Shevach, E.M., and Rosenthal, A.S. (1976) Macrophage-lymphocyte interaction. III. Site of alloantiserum inhibition of T lymphocyte proliferation induced by allogeneic or aldehyde-bearing cells. *J. Immunol.* 117:1261–1266.

Hausman, P.B. and Stobo, J.D. (1979) Specificity and function of a human autologous reactive T cell. *J. Exp. Med.* 149:1537–1542.

Katz, D.H. and Benacerraf, B. (1976) *The Role of Products of the Histocompatibility Gene Complex in Immune Responses.* New York: Academic Press, Inc.

Katz, D.H., Hamaoka, T., Dorf, M.E., and Benacerraf, B. (1973) Cell interactions between histoincompatible T and B lymphocytes. II. Failure of physiologic cooperative interactions between T and B lymphocytes from allogeneic donor strains in humoral response to hapten protein conjugates. *J. Exp. Med.* 137:1405–1418.

Kuntz, M.M., Innes, J.B., and Weksler, M.E. (1976) Lymphocyte transformation induced by autologous cells. IV. Human T lymphocyte proliferation induced by autologous or allogeneic non-T lymphocytes. *J. Exp. Med.* 143:1042–1054.

Kuntz, M.M., Innes, J.B., and Weksler, M.E. (1979) The cellular basis of the impaired autologous mixed lymphocyte reaction in patients with systemic lupus erythematosis. *J. Clin. Invest.* 63:151–153.

Novogrodsky, A. and Katchalski, E. (1973) Induction of lymphocyte transformation by sequential treatment with neuraminidase and galactose oxidase. *Proc. Natl. Acad. Sci. U.S.A.* 70:1824–1827.

Opelz, G.M., Kiuchi, M., Takasugi, M., and Terasaki, P.I. (1975) Autologous stimulators of human lymphocyte subpopulations. *J. Exp. Med.* 142:1327–1333.

Paul, W.E., Shevach, E.M., Pickeral, S. Thomas, D.W., and Rosenthal, A.S. (1977) Independent populations of primed F_1 guinea pig T lymphocytes respond to antigen-pulsed parental peritoneal exudate cells. *J. Exp. Med.* 145:618–630.

Rosenthal, A.S. and Shevach, E.M. (1973) Function of macrophages in antigen recognition by guinea pig T lymphocytes. I. Requirement for histocompatible macrophages and lymphocytes. *J. Exp. Med.* 138:1194–1212.

Sakane, T. and Green, I. (1979) Specificity and suppressor function of human T cells responsive to autologous non-T cells. *J. Immunol.* 123:584–589.

Sakane, T., Steinberg, A.D., and Green, I. (1978) Failure of autologous mixed lymphocyte reactions between T and non-T cells in patients with systemic lupus erythematosis. *Proc. Natl. Acad. Sci. U.S.A.* 75:3464–3468.

Shevach, E.M. (1976) The function of macrophages in antigen recognition by guinea pig T lymphocytes. III. Genetic analysis of the antigens mediating macrophage-T lymphocyte interaction. *J. Immunol.* 116:1482–1489.

Shevach, E.M. (1978) The guinea pig I-region. A functional analysis of Ia-Ir associations. *Springer Semin. Immunopathol.* 1:207–234.

Shevach, E.M. and Rosenthal, A.S. (1973) Function of macrophages in antigen recognition of guinea pig T lymphocytes. II. Role of the macrophage in the regulation of genetic control of the immune response. *J. Exp. Med.* 138:1213–1229.

Smith, J.B. and Pasternak, R.D. (1978) Syngeneic mixed leukocyte reaction in mice: strain distribution, kinetics, participating cells, and absence in NZB mice. *J. Immunol.* 121:1889–1892.

Thomas, D.W. and Shevach, E.M. (1976) Nature of the antigenic complex recognized by T lymphocytes. I. Analysis with an *in vitro* primary response to soluble protein antigens. *J. Exp. Med.* 144:1263–1273.

Thorsby, E. and Nousiainen, H. (1979) *In vitro* sensitization of human T lymphocytes to hapten (TNP)-conjugated and non-treated autologous cells is restricted by self-HLA-D. *Scand. J. Immunol.* 9:183–192.

Weksler, M.E. and Kozak, R. (1977) Lymphocyte transformation by autologous cells. V. Generation of immunologic memory and specificity during the autologous mixed lymphocyte reaction. *J. Exp. Med.* 146:1833–1838.

Yamashita, U. and Shevach, E.M. (1977) The expression of Ia antigens on immunocompetent cells in the guinea pig. II. Ia antigens on macrophages. *J. Immunol.* 119:1584–1588.

Yamashita, U. and Shevach, E.M. (1980) The syngeneic mixed leukocyte reaction: the genetic requirements for the recognition of self resemble the requirements for the recognition of antigen in association with self. *J. Immunol.* 124:1773–1778.

Published 1981 by Elsevier North Holland, Inc.
Saunders, Daniels, Serrou, Rosenfeld, and Denney, eds.
FUNDAMENTAL MECHANISMS IN HUMAN CANCER IMMUNOLOGY

CHAPTER 7

The Function of Protein-Bound Carbohydrates in Normal and Pathological Cells[1]

Leonard Warren, M.D., Ph.D.

Professor, The Wistar Institute, Philadelphia, Pennsylvania

Introduction

Glycoproteins are being implicated in an ever-increasing number of biological processes, as virologists, immunologists, physiologists, and others learn more about their systems of interest. Glycoproteins differ from other proteins in that they bear covalently-bound carbohydrate polymers. Most workers feel that the carbohydrates must be there because they have special characteristics, and indeed it has been shown that bound carbohydrates are involved in a number of specific cellular processes, including recognition and homing. We and others have shown that the carbohydrate groups in glycoproteins of malignant cells differ from those of normal cells in ways that will be briefly discussed. Despite the widespread occurrence of this change in malignant cells, however, its significance cannot yet be evaluated because the essential role of bound carbohydrate in nature is not known. In this chapter, I will briefly summarize the work of our group and others on the bound carbohydrates of malignant cells, and examine certain properties of protein-bound carbohydrates upon which a new hypothesis of their function is based. Glycolipids will not be discussed because it is felt, though by no means demonstrated, that the non-covalent association of glycolipids with a protein in effect constitutes a glycoprotein.

Glycoproteins in Malignancy

We and others have shown that when cells become malignant, changes take

[1] This work was supported by Grants ACS BC 275 and ACS PRP 28 from the American Cancer Society and Grant CA 19130 from the United States Public Health Service.

place in some of the protein-bound carbohydrate groups of M_r 4000–5000 (see Buck et al., 1970; Van Beek et al., 1973; Warren et al., 1978). These changes have been demonstrated by experiments using the double-label method in which control and malignant cells are grown in the presence of either ^{14}C or ^{3}H-labeled sugars such as L-fucose, D-glucosamine, D-galactose, or D-mannose. Labeled cellular material is treated with pronase to remove as much amino acid as possible, while leaving the labeled carbohydrate structures intact. ^{14}C and ^{3}H-labeled carbohydrate polymers are mixed and chromatographed on a column of Sephadex G50. Figure 7.1 shows that there is an enrichment of carbohydrates in the "group A" region of material derived from transformed (malignant) cells (M_r 4000–5500). The following is a brief summary of our knowledge of this phenomenon.

Figure 7.1. Sephadex G50 chromatography of glycopeptides. Control hamster cells (BHK21/C13) grown in the presence of ^{3}H-D-glucosamine and their virus-transformed, tumorigenic counterpart C13/B4 labeled in culture with ^{14}C-D-glucosamine were treated with trypsin. Both lines of cells grew with approximately the same doubling time (21 hr). The labeled material removed from the surfaces of the cells were mixed and further digested with pronase. The digests with approximately equal numbers of ^{3}H and ^{14}C counts, were applied to a column of Sephadex G50 (1×100 cm) and eluted (Blithe et al., 1980b). The ^{3}H and ^{14}C in the eluted material in each tube was counted and the data was processed and plotted by computer. The material in tubes 1–5 is largely glycosaminoglycan. Note the relatively large amount of group A glycopeptide material derived from malignant C13/B4 cells.

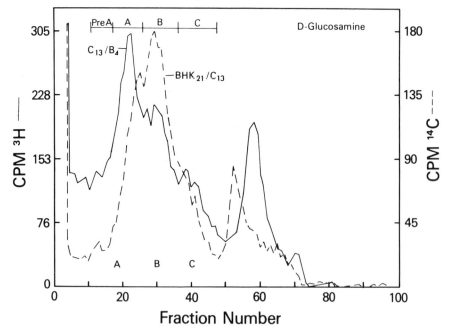

1. The differences seen in the carbohydrate groups of normal and malignant cells appears to be quantitative rather than qualitative. In the past few years, we have devised further fractionation procedures for glycopeptides that separate these structures into approximately 35–40 groups, and we have found no clear-cut, reproducible evidence that new carbohydrate structures appear or others disappear in the malignant cell (Blithe et al., 1980a).

2. The group A carbohydrate groups that increase in number in the malignant cells seem to be those that are particularly growth-sensitive (Buck et al., 1971; Muramatsu et al., 1973; Hakomori, 1975; Ceccarini et al., 1975; Ogata et al., 1976). Many fewer groups are found in non-dividing cells. Thus in our comparative studies, it is imperative that the doubling time of normal and malignant cells be approximately similar. It is under these conditions, at all stages of the growth cycle, that we find considerably more group A glycopeptides in the glycoproteins from malignant cells than in those from control cells.

3. The change in protein-bound carbohydrate of malignant cells takes place in over 80% of the glycoproteins (Van Nest and Grimes, 1977; Tuszynski et al., 1979), in all the membrane systems of the cell (surface, smooth and rough endoplasmic reticular, nuclear, mitochondrial, and Golgi), (Buck et al., 1974; Glick and Buck, 1973). Similar changes are seen in the glycoproteins of viruses grown in transformed cells as compared to those grown in control cells (Lai and Duesberg, 1972). Thus, transformation and malignancy appears to induce a generalized change in the glycosylation mechanism of the cell.

4. Glick et al. (1973; 1974) and Van Nest and Grimes (1977) have shown that the observed carbohydrate increase is more closely linked to the cell's capacity for form tumors *in vivo* than it is to various *in vitro* criteria of transformation.

5. The change takes place virtually without exception in a wide variety of transformed, malignant cells derived from 5 species. (See Warren et al., 1978, for summary). It is seen in cells in culture that are transformed spontaneously, by viruses, or by chemicals. It is also seen in cells transformed by temperature-sensitive viruses when grown at permissive temperatures. It takes place in both solid tumors and leukemia cells, and in cells of the fibroblastic, epithelial, and lymphocytic series (Van Beek et al., 1973, 1975).

In summary, in the malignant as compared to the normal cell, most of the glycoproteins bear larger carbohydrate groups of the "A" type. The cell appears to be capable of shifting the specific forms of the carbohydrate groups covalently bound to its polypeptide chains. Probably a normal cell carries out these alterations in the course of events through the cell cycle, while this activity is exaggerated and/or more persistent in the malignant cell. Since glycoproteins carry on many important cellular functions, and glycoprotein structure is clearly altered in malignant cells, it is possible that function is also altered. The change may slightly affect many processes, such as intercellular adhesiveness and metabolite transport, which involve glycoproteins. Changes of the carbohydrate of some glycoproteins may help the malignent cell to survive and spread. Although the life of the cell may not be threatened by these structural alterations, out of the myriad changes may arise a persistence of cell division, the hallmark of the malignant cell.

The Role of Bound Carbohydrates as Modulators

Hypotheses about the role of bound carbohydrates in malignancy remain largely speculative because we do not yet fully understand the actual function of bound carbohydrates. It is known in a general way that they are extensively hydrated structures situated in exposed positions at the surfaces of molecules. The carbohydrate component of glycoproteins protects them from proteolytic degradation (Olden et al., 1979) and affects their solubility, precipitability, and viscosity in solution (Tarentino et al., 1970; Leavitt et al., 1977; Cheng et al., 1979), their association with other molecules, and their ability to depress the freezing point (Kömatsu et al., 1970). If sialic acid residues are removed from serum glycoproteins, D-galactose residues become exposed and the glycoproteins are readily taken up by liver cells (Ashwell and Morell, 1974).

There are several additional examples of processes which are dependent on specific sugars in glycoprotein effectors (see Hughes, 1976; Rosenberg and Schengrund, 1976), but despite this considerable list we suspect that bound carbohydrates do far more than has been described to date.

At this point, I would like to introduce the notion that a major role of bound carbohydrates resides in their capacity to exert *small* modulating effects on the activities of glycoproteins. When a glycoprotein is involved in a biological process and its sugar structure is altered experimentally, more often than not an investigator reports that "no change is seen," when he might more accurately state that "small changes (perhaps 5–10%) may be seen." Changes of 10% are ignored. The effects are usually observed only under one set of conditions (optimal) and not under a variety of conditions where the effects may vary. Further, small effects cannot be reliably assessed because their magnitude falls within the range of error of the assays employed. In the absence of a theoretical framework within which to evaluate a 10% effect, experimentalists are usually not willing to devote time or attention to it. To provide such a heuristic construct, we would like to offer two hypotheses and explore their consequences. These are (1) that bound carbohydrate groups of glycoproteins are multiple, covalently bound allosteric effectors which exert their relatively small effects indirectly, perhaps by influencing conformation and mobility of polypeptide chains, and (2) that different carbohydrate groups or combinations of them have slightly different modulating activities.

The phenomenon of microheterogeneity of the carbohydrate groups of glycoproteins is a critical element in the construction of our theory of the function of these structures. This phenomenon has been recognized for many years (see Montgomery, 1972; Spiro, 1973) and it is probably the rule rather than the exception. Investigators have chosen to ignore it or dismiss it as the end result of trivial, random degradation. Few, if any, analyses of "pure," isolated glycopeptides derived from glycoproteins yield integral values. The absence of integral numbers in the ratios of one sugar to another in a glycopeptide is probably evidence for heterogeneity. Heterogeneity can usually be found if it is sought. It signifies that during synthesis of a particular glycoprotein, the glycosylation mechanism of the cell ends up by making more than one form of carbohydrate oligomer on each site capable of bearing such groups, and the heterogeneity appears to involve more than terminal sugars. Our recent work on the protein-bound carbohydrate groups suggests that cells in tissue culture bear, in total, perhaps 75 such groups. Work in progress leads us to feel that there are great similarities, though some quantitative and qualitative differences, in glycopeptide material derived from higher animals— specifically, fish, chicken, mouse, hamster, and man (Blithe et al., unpublished data). These results suggest that the library of carbohydrate groups available to all of these cells, although very complex, has been quite stable during evolution. On the other hand, bound carbohydrates of lower animals such as sea urchin seem to be quite different, and those of the insect are totally different.

Given the documented phenomenon of microheterogeneity, and accepting the hypothesis that bound carbohydrates have modulating activities, we would argue that whatever the activity of a glycoprotein (enzyme, hormone, combining or receptor site, structural or clotting factor, etc.) that function is carried out by many forms of the glycoprotein, all differing slightly in their carbohydrate structure. Regardless of the conditions under which the glycoprotein must act, there are always some polypeptides bearing certain carbohydrate groups or combinations of them that are the most effective modifiers for the particular environment. These give the organism a preadaptive, selective advantage. We would argue that the bound carbohydrates broaden the range of conditions in which an organism and its polypeptides can operate, with increased possibility of survival. While a 5–10% difference in activity may be of statistical insignificance to an experimentalist, it could be critical within the evolutionary time scale.

If our hypothesis is correct, we might predict that bound carbohydrates should exist in greater abundance where the cell is least able to control the environment. Sixty to 70% of the bound carbohydrate of a cell is at its surface, outside the lipid barrier, facing the outside world. The smallest quantities are, in fact, found in the nucleus, separated from the outside by three membranes. The enzymes of the cell are almost always proteins rather than glycoproteins, except for the lysozomal enzymes that operate outside the cell or on variable, interiorized bits of the extracellular world. The strictly extracellular compartment of the multicellular organism is exceedingly rich in bound carbohydrate polymers. An inverse relationship exists between the glycoprotein concentration at a given location in a cell and its proximity to the outside world. A plausible explanation of this relationship is that the cell compensates for its inability to control the environment by employing glycosylated polypeptides.

Glycosylation and the Environment

We have proposed that bound carbohydrates enable the organism to cope with a broader range of environmental conditions. In this section, we will discuss the impact of the environment on the glycosylation process, and its possible consequences. The biosynthesis of protein-bound carbohydrate polymers does not proceed under the direction of a template. Construction of the polymer depends on the specificity of many enzymes, the availability of activated sugars and the metabolic state of the cell, the oxidation-reduction state and cation and proton concentrations within the cell and probably many other environmentally influenced factors. The membranes of the cell, which are, in essence, composed of lipid units that are not covalently bound, may also be considered non-template determined polymers. Thus the polymeric elements of the cell can be divided into two categories—those which are template determined (DNA, RNA, and protein) and manifest relatively little polymorphism compared to the non-template determined carbohydrate and lipid polymers. The latter not only manifest extensive polymorphism, but their very structure can, to a significant extent, be determined by the environment at the time of their biosynthesis. Environment as a determinant of structure may also influence any type of post-translational modification (phosphorylation, methylation, acetylation, etc.) of template-determined polymer.

Previous work has shown that the protein-bound carbohydrates can, without obvious damage to the cell, vary with growth, the cell cycle, and the malignant state. A variety of drugs and agents can alter their structure: ethidium bromide (Soslau et al., 1975), cAMP (Van Veen et al., 1976), butyrate (Simmons et al., 1975) and vitamin A (Wolf et al., 1979). Shifts in bound carbohydrate populations are found in mutant cells (Blithe et al., 1980b; Li & Kornfeld, 1978; Via et al., 1980) and in cells grown in culture at different temperatures or pH (unpublished). The patterns of bound carbohydrates appear to vary with the substrate of the cells in culture, i.e., plastic or glass (unpublished). Megaw and Johnson (1979) have shown marked variation in the bound carbohydrates of an epithelial basement membrane glycoprotein of murine carcinoma cells, depending upon the conditions of culture. Differences were seen when the type of buffer or the percentage of serum in the medium were varied. Lipid membranes also vary in composition with the state of the cell (Cheng and Levy, 1979).

It would appear that the environment can influence the final form of the carbohydrate. It is possible that microheterogeneity of the carbohydrates of glycoproteins exists because glycosylation of polypeptides takes place when the cell is subjected to different and varying environmental conditions. It is suggested here that the induced changes that take place in the bound carbo-hydrates are not random and meaningless, but could be of a homeostatic nature, i.e., they could help the organism survive and operate more efficiently in the new environment. The system is now complete, for according to our hypothesis, the bound carbohydrates exist to handle the environment, and in turn their synthesis and their final array is influenced to a significant degree by the environment. Template-determined macromolecules are kept under close control of genetic instructions, while the non-template determined elements are the environmental probes — sensors and buffers. Obviously, carbohydrate and lipid polymers are, despite the special characteristics and functions hypothe-sized here, still largely under genetic control.

Bound Carbohydrates and Pathology

A key to understanding the role of carbohydrates in evolution is that they have small effects that are permitted to act over long periods of time. Is it possible that in chronic, long-term diseases such as arteriosclerosis, diabetes, various metabolic diseases, and even aging, the array of bound carbohydrates is different because the environment is different? The changes from the normal array might be tolerated by the host and would be relatively silent, but ultimately some form of breakdown might follow.

In acute diseases, the environment also changes, and these alterations might be reflected in the protein-bound carbohydrates. Are the bound carbohydrates of a specific serum glycoprotein of a patient with fever different from those of the same individual when healthy? Are the glycoproteins produced by normal cells close to a localized infection or a tumor the same as those produced in the absence of pathology? If so, what are the consequences to the organisms of living with the altered structure?

As discussed before, the protein-bound carbohydrate groups of many types of malignant cells are different from the normal. The origin and the conse-quences of the extensive changes are unknown. The changes, which involve many carbohydrate groups of many glycoproteins, could reflect an altered metabolic state of the malignant cell, and they might be the basis for a cascade of deviate functions, none of which are serious enough to kill the cell. The changes might, however, create a defect in the growth regulatory mechanism that would be responsible for persistent cell division. The structural changes in the carbohydrates might also produce a host of changes of no particular relevance to the malignant process, although some changes, such as in trans-port or intercellular adhesiveness which involve glycoproteins, might promote malignancy.

Conclusions

An attempt has been made to resolve the confusing, anomalous characteristics of protein-bound carbohydrates. Carbohydrates are ancient and ubiquitous. They exist in very complex arrays that appear to be relatively stable over a vast period of time. On the other hand, they are heterogeneous and can vary with shifts in the environmental state, and this polymorphism appears to be central to their cellular functions. It is our impression that despite the striking examples of specific function documented for the oligosaccharides of some glycoproteins, these functions alone are insufficient to justify the elaborate array of glycosylated molecules. There are large areas of ignorance and misconception which prevent us from properly evaluating the complete role of bound carbohydrates in nature.

Our speculations rest primarily on well established evidence for the heterogeneity of carbohydrates in glycoproteins, and on a growing body of evidence suggesting that the glycosylation process is susceptible to environmental influences. There is least hard data to support our argument that bound carbohydrates have only small, modulating effects and that different individual or combinations of carbohydrate groups modulate the activity of the polypeptide differently in different environments. This hypothesis could help us appreciate data that might otherwise be improperly evaluated and discarded. Perhaps differences and changes of small magnitude may be highly significant!

It is possible that the proposed environment handling and responding activities of bound carbohydrates represent their original functions, while the well-known, all-or-none, critical functions of carbohydrates are the result of late, fortuitous events in evolution in which bound carbohydrates happened to become components of specific, structurally-sensitive mechanisms. The original modulating role however may persist—influencing the conformation, mobility, and associations of polypeptide chains.

The hypothesis presented resolves certain confusing and paradoxical elements in the explication of bound carbohydrates. It is logical, and it is in several ways testable. While simplicity, logic, and testability do not make the story true, the notions presented form a rational and useful construct for future experimentation that may enable us to better understand the role of bound carbohydrates in nature.

References

Ashwell, G. and Morell, A.G. (1974) In *Advances in Enzymology*, Vol. 41. Meister, A. and Wiley, J. (eds.) New York: Academic Press, pp. 99–128.

Blithe, D.L., Buck, C.A., and Warren, L. (1980a) Comparison of glycopeptides from control and virus-transformed BHK fibroblasts. *Biochem.* 19:3386–3395.

Blithe, D.L., Pastan, I., Buck, C.A., and Warren, L. (1980b) Carbohydrate groups of glycoproteins in a glycosylation-defective low adherent mutant mouse cell. *Biochem. International* 1:71–76.

Buck, C.A., Fuhrer, J.P., Soslau, G., and Warren, L. (1974) Membrane glycopeptides from subcellular fractions of control and virus-transformed cells. *J. Biol. Chem.* 249:1541–1550.

Buck, C.A., Glick, M.C., and Warren, L. (1970) A comparative study of glycoproteins from the surface of control and Rous sarcoma virus-transformed hamster cells. *Biochem.* 9:4567–4576.

Buck, C.A., Glick, M.C., and Warren, L. (1971) Effect of growth on the glycoproteins from the surface of control and Rous sarcoma virus-transformed hamster cells. *Biochem.* 10:2176–2180.

Ceccarini, C., Muramatsu, T., Tsang, J., and Atkinson, P.H. (1975) Growth-dependent alterations in oligomannosyl cores of glycoproteins. *Proc. Natl. Acad. Sci. U.S.A.* 72:3139–3143.

Cheng, S. and Levy, D. (1979) The effect of cell proliferation on the lipid composition and fluidity of hepatocyte plasma membranes. *Arch. Biochem. Biophys.* 196:424–429.

Cheng, S., Morrone, S., and Robbins, J. (1979) Effect of deglycosylation on the binding and immunoreactivity of human thyroxine-binding globulin. *J. Biol. Chem.* 254:8830.

Glick, M.C. and Buck, C.A. (1973) Glycoproteins from the surface of metaphase cells. *Biochem.* 12:85–90.

Glick, M.C., Rabinowitz, Z., and Sachs, L. (1973) Surface membrane glycopeptides correlated with tumorigenesis. *Biochem.* 12:4864–4869.

Glick, M.C., Rabinowitz, Z., and Sachs, L. (1974) Surface membrane glycopeptides which coincide with virus transformation and tumorigenesis. *J. Virol.* 13:967–974.

Hakomori, S. (1975) Structures and organization of cell surface glycolipid dependency on cell growth and malignant transformation. *Biochim. Biophys. Acta* 417:55–89.

Hughes, R.C. (1976) *Membrane Glycoproteins.* London: Butterworths.

Kōmatsu, S.K., De Vries, A.L., and Feeney, R.E. (1970) Studies of the structure of freezing point-depressing glycoproteins from an Antarctic fish. *J. Biol. Chem.* 245:2909–2913.

Lai, M.M.C. and Duesberg, P.H. (1972) Differences between the envelope glycoproteins and glycopeptides of avian tumor viruses released from transformed and from normal cells. *Virology* 50:259–272.

Leavitt, R., Schlesinger, S., and Kornfeld, S. (1977) Impaired intra-cellular migration and altered solubility of nonglycosylated glycoproteins of vesicular stomatitis virus and Sindblis virus. *J. Biol. Chem.* 252:9018–9023.

Li, E. and Kornfeld, S. (1978) Structure of the altered oligosaccharides present in glycoproteins from a clone of Chinese hamster ovary cells deficient in N-acetyl-glucosaminyltransferase activity. *J. Biol. Chem.* 253:6426–6431.

Megaw, J.M. and Johnson, L.D. (1979) Glycoprotein synthesized by cultured cells: effects of serum concentrations and buffers on sugar content. *Proc. Soc. Exp. Biol. Med.* 161:60–65.

Montgomery, R. (1972) Heterogeneity of the carbohydrate groups of glycoproteins. In *Glycoproteins.* Gottschalk, A. (ed.), Amsterdam: Elsevier Press, Part A, pp. 518–527.

Muramatsu, T., Atkinson, P.H., Nathenson, S.G., and Ceccarini, G. (1973) Cell surface glycopeptides: growth dependent changes in the carbohydrate-peptide linkage region. *J. Mol. Biol.* 80:781–799.

Ogata, S.I., Muramatsu, T., and Kobata, A. (1976) New structural characteristics of the large glycopeptides from transformed cells. *Nature* 259:580–582.

Olden, K., Pratt, R.M., and Yamada, K.M. (1979) Role of carbohydrate in biological function of the adhesive glycoprotein fibronectin. *Proc. Natl. Acad. Sci. U.S.A.* 76:3343–3347.

Rosenberg, H. and Schengrund, C.L. (eds.) (1976) *Biological Roles of Sialic Acid.* New York: Plenum Press.

Simmons, J.F., Fishman, P.H., Friese, L., and Brady, O. (1975) Morphological alterations and ganglioside sialyltransferase activity induced by small fatty acids in Hela cells. *J. Cell Biol.* 66:414–424.

Soslau, G., Fuhrer, J.P., Nass, M.M.K., and Warren, L. (1975) The effect of ethidium bromide on the membrane glycopeptides in control and virus-transformed cells. *J. Biol. Chem.* 249:3014–3020.

Spiro, R.G. (1973) Glycoproteins. In *Advances in Protein Chemistry.* New York: Academic Press, pp. 349–467.

Tarentino, A., Plummer, T.H. Jr., and Maley, F. (1970) Studies on the oligo-saccharide sequence of ribonuclease B. *J. Biol. Chem.* 245:4150–4157.

Tuszynski, G.P., Baker, S.R., Fuhrer, J.P., Buck, C.A., and Warren, L. (1979) Glycopeptides derived form individual membrane glycoproteins from control and Rous sarcoma virus-transformed hamster fibroblasts. *J. Biol. Chem.* 253:6092–6099.

Van Beek, W.P., Smets, L.A., and Emmelot, P. (1973) Increased sialic acid density in surface glycoproteins of transformed and malignant cells. A general phenomenon? *Cancer Res.* 33: 2913–2922.

Van Beek, W.P., Smets, L.A., and Emmelot, P. (1975) Changed surface glycoprotein as a marker of malignancy in human leukemic cells. *Nature* 253:457–460.

Van Nest, G.A. and Grimes, W.J. (1977) A comparison of membrane components of normal and transformed BALB/c cells. *Biochem.* 16:2902–2908.

Van Veen, J., Noonan, K.D., and Roberts, R.M. (1976) A correlation between membrane glycopeptides composition and losses in concanavalin A agglutinability induced by db-cAMP in Chinese hamster ovary cells. *Exper. Cell Res.* 103:405–413.

Via, D.P., Sramek, S., Larriba, G., and Steiner, S. (1980) Effect of sodium butyrate on the membrane glycoconjugates of murine sarcoma virus-transformed rat cells. *J. Cell Biol.* 84:225–234.

Warren, L., Buck, C.A., and Tuszynski, G.P. (1978) Glycopeptide changes and malignant transformation. A possible role for carbohydrate in malignant behavior. *Biochim. Biophys. Acta* 516:97–127.

Wolf, G., Kiorpes, T.S., Masushige, S., Schrieber, J.B., Smith, M.J., and Anderson, R.S. (1979) Recent evidence for the participation of vitamin A in glycoprotein biosynthesis. *Fed. Proc.* 38:2540–2543.

Published 1981 by Elsevier North Holland, Inc.
Saunders, Daniels, Serrou, Rosenfeld, and Denney, eds.
FUNDAMENTAL MECHANISMS IN HUMAN CANCER IMMUNOLOGY

CHAPTER 8

Reduced Metastasizing Potential in Surface Carbohydrate Mutants: The Importance of a Multifaceted Analysis[1]

Max M. Burger, Tien Wen Tao, Jukka Finne, and James Jumblatt

Dept. of Biochemistry, Biocenter of the University of Basel, CH 4056 Basel/Switzerland

Approach and Initial Studies

So far there is no evidence that a specific alteration of biological behavior, let alone a specific macromolecule of a tumor cell, is the cause of its particular metastasizing potential. All the approaches to this question have so far been and most likely will remain correlative. From a wide range of different tumor cells, generally those that have been selected have either a high or a low metastasizing potential, and various morphological, biological, and biochemical characteristics have been compared. The problem with this type of experiment has always been to distinguish differences seemingly correlatable with the metastasizing potential from simple cell strain differences, since the cells generally were not of identical parentage.

Fidler (1973) tried to circumvent this problem by selecting from a melanoma line a cell which had a higher potential for producing lung tumors after injection into the tail vein of mice. No relevant and reproducible biochemical differences were found between these cells and others of the same line. We therefore decided to approach the problem from a different vantage point. Instead of selecting cells for biological changes in the animal and then looking for possible biochemical changes, we began, a few years ago, to select cells with stable changes in their cell surface biochemistry and then search for alterations in their metastasizing behavior. This is still a correlative approach, like every other approach so far taken.

[1]The work described was generously supported by the Swiss National Science Foundation (Grant No. 3.513.79) and the Ministry of Education of Basel.

Since the cell surface may play a role not only in rupture of the metastasizing cell from the primary tumor, but also in cell encounter on the way to and at the place of new metastatic development, we felt that a surface mutant in the cell's outermost molecular layer, i.e., the carbohydrates, may most likely influence invasive behavior. We decided to use lectins which were known to kill tumor cells at high concentrations, and selected resistant cells, among them some that were missing just the carbohydrate to which the particular lectins tend to bind. Initially, we used wheat germ agglutinin (WGA) only and at doses which killed between $10^5 - 10^6$ cells. Such harsh conditions made it more likely that a stable mutant rather than only a variant cell would be selected. Starting with an uncloned B-16 mouse melanoma line, we obtained after about 4 passages a WGA resistant line. This line was cloned (Wa4-bl) and was found to be missing the high affinity binding sites for WGA, while the low affinity sites seemed to remain unaltered.

Metastasizing and tumorigenicity can be measured in a number of ways. It is generally not sufficiently emphasized that these different assays do not necessarily measure the same thing. Each should be independently evaluated, which can sometimes lead to different conclusions. We first chose the most direct assay for metastasis, namely a gross analysis of tumor nodules in other organs like the lung after intraperitoneal administration of the tumor cells. The analysis was usually made prior to death, when the animals became apathic, in order to ensure the largest possible growth time for metastases. The WGA resistant cells did not produce any metastases under these conditions (Table 8.1).

Tumorigenicity was assessed in the most direct way possible, namely by scoring the animals with tumor masses alive or dead after a fixed observation period starting with the intraperitoneal application of a paraoptimal dose of cells. A certain decrease in tumorigenicity (less than 30%) was noted (Table 8.1.) in the Wa4-bl cells, as compared to the parent cell type.

Table 8.1. Metastasizing Capacity and Tumorigenicity of a Lectin Resistant Melanoma Variant.

Cell line	Metastases[a]	Tumorigenicity[b]
F_1	48/50	50/50
Wa4-bl	0/16	23/32

Note: F_1 = an uncloned line of B-16 melanoma cells obtained from Dr. I.J. Fidler, to whom we are very grateful for supplying the stock cells. Wa4-bl = A cloned wheat germ agglutinin resistant F_1 cell variant (see Tao and Burger, 1977).

[a]Number of animals per total number of animals showing metastases in mediastinal or mesenteric lymph nodes or in other organs (liver, adrenal glands, kidneys, and lungs) two to three weeks after i.p. injection of 5×10^4 cells.

[b]Number of animals per total number of animals showing tumors two to three weeks after injection of 2×10^5 cells into the tail vein.

One may ask whether the decrease in tumorigenicity observed in the WGA resistant cells causes the decrease in metastatic potential. Although in the final analysis this interpretation cannot be ruled out, there are reasons which speak against it. A mere reduction in the rate of growth could lead to decreased tumorigenicity, since fewer cells are available to spread elsewhere. However, a reduction of growth rates *in vitro* was not observed in earlier experiments (Tao and Burger, 1977). We also evaluated growth *in vivo* by measuring the volumetric increase of a tumor grown intradermally (Figure 8.1). Although a certain lag in the onset of measurable growth could be detected, no relevant difference in actual growth rate was registered for the WGA resistant cells alone. In order to evaluate this and another possible explanation, namely that the number of potent tumorigenic cells has decreased, reducing simultaneously the number of potentially metastasizing cells, we increased the total dose of cells applied i.p. and detected only an earlier death rate, but no measurable increase in metastases anywhere in these animals.

An extensive search for biological aberrations in these cells which may cause or contribute to their reduced metastasizing potential was initiated some 4 years ago. The most interesting parameters observed were adhesion and the degree of bundling of microfilaments. In general, self-adhesion was somewhat increased in the poorly metastasizing WGA resistant clones. This characteristics was established with three different assays, assessing the size of aggregates

Figure 8.1. *In vivo* growth curve. Comparison of growth curves of tumor nodules developed after intradermal injections of 1×10^6 B-16 (F_1, panel on the left) and WGA resistant variant cells (Wa4-bl, panel on the right) respectively (Tao and Burger, in preparation).

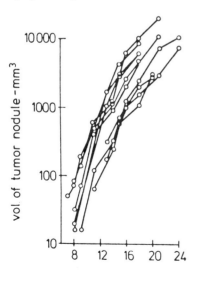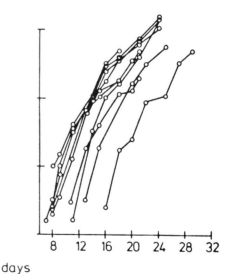

at equilibrium, the rates of aggregation measured by single cell disappearance, and monolayer adhesion. Since the changes were not exactly proportional on a quantitative scale with the changes in metastasizing potential, some caution will have to be used, when interpreting the qualitative correlations which were found.

Preliminary studies on heterotypic adhesion between these mouse melanoma cells and human umbilical cord endothelial cells did not reveal any detectable differences between melanoma parent cells and WGA resistant mutants.

So far, a fairly consistent increase of actin cable expression has been observed in the WGA resistant, poorly metastasizing clones. Whether this phenomenon increases overall cellular rigidity and results in a reduced capability to deform and thus invade other tissues remains speculative.

Biochemical Alterations

Scatchard plots of WGA binding (Burger, 1980) revealed a loss of the high affinity lectin binding sites. Evidence for molecular surface changes first came from the reduction of 5 protein bands in WGA resistant cells after surface labeling with ^{125}I and lactoperoxidase (MW: 144 K, 122 K, 102 K, 94 K, 82 K). Labeling of sialic acid containing surface glycoproteins demonstrated that these 5 reduced proteins were of the glycoprotein type and contained some sialic acid (Finne et al., 1980). Since all of them moved somewhat faster in SDS polyacrylamide gel electrophoresis, a slight reduction in molecular weight could be predicted. That the reduced molecular weight was due to a decrease in peripheral sialic acid, one of the two hapten sugars of the lectin WGA, was strongly suggested by the results obtained from neuraminidase treatment of the cells and labeling of peripheral galactose with $NaB\,^3H_4$ and galactose oxidase. Such a neuraminidase treatment abolished any significant differences between the two types of glycoproteins on SDS-polyacrylamide gel electrophoresis.

The autoradiograms of gel electrophoresis preparations were incubated with labeled lectins, and these confirmed the decrease of total cellular WGA receptors but not of concanavalin A receptors (Jumblatt et al., 1980). A more detailed oligosaccharide analysis of glycopeptides was then initiated. No differences could be observed in the non-sulfated cetylpyridinium chloride precipitable fraction nor in the alkaline cleavable, so called o-glycosidic, glycopeptide fraction.

Separation on a Concanavalin A-Sepharose column produced three principle peaks (Figure 8.2). They were individually fractionated on Sephadex G50 (Figure 8.3), where the neutral mannose-rich N-glycosidically linked glycopeptides (Figure 8.3C) as well as the o-glycosidic glycopeptides (Figure 8.3A:O) revealed no differences between WGA resistant mutants and parent melanoma line. The tetra-antennary sialoglycopetides, i.e., bearing 4 side arms (Figure 8.3A:A) and the biantennary sialoglycopeptides (Figure 8.3B) eluted later, i.e., they seemed to be smaller in the poorly metastasizing cells as compared to their melanoma parent cells.

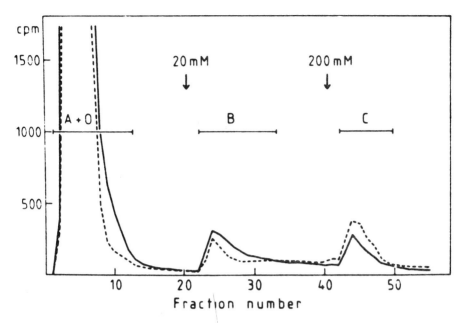

Figure 8.2. Chromatography of [³H] glucosamine-labeled glycopeptides on a column of Concanavalin A Sepharose. The unbound material (Fraction A+O) was obtained by elution with 5 mM sodium acetate buffer (pH 5.2) containing 0.1 M NaCl and CaCl₂, MgCl₂ (1 mM each), and Fractions B and C by including 20 and 200 mM α-methyl-D-glucoside, respectively, in the elution buffers. —, F₁; ---, Wa4-bl glycopeptides. Recovery of radioactivity was 71% for F₁ and 64% for Wa4-bl. The fractions were pooled as indicated by the bars, desalted, and subjected to gel filtration as shown in Figure 8.3.

SOURCE: *Finne et al., 1980.*

A carbohydrate composition analysis of fraction A (Table 8.2) not only reveals a 45% content of sialic acid for the mutant cell, but also (quite unexpectedly) a considerable increase in fucose, and no other significant changes. Methylation and mass fragmentography suggest that two of the four terminal sialic acids are missing in the tetra-antennary oligosaccharide and that two side chains, presumably the same ones, are carrying an additional fucose on the sidearm N-acetylglucosamines (Figure 8.4).

Such a double defect, never before described for any lectin mutant, may provide strong selective advantage for WGA resistance, since not only is one receptor carbohydrate (sialic) missing, but the other one (N-acetylglucosamine), which now would be more accessible to the lectin, is being shielded by the newly attached fucose. In cooperation with Dr. Prieels, we are presently analyzing the enzymatic mechanism that leads to the surface carbohydrate defect, and it seems that only one of the two possible sugar transferases is affected.

114

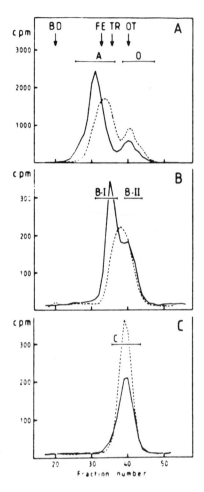

Figure 8.3. Gel filtration of glycopeptides on a column (2×75 cm) of Sephadex G50 of [³H] glucosamine-labeled glycopeptide fractions. (a) Fraction A+O after mild alkaline borohydride treatment; (B) Fraction B glycopeptides; (C) Fraction C glycopeptides. The elution volumes of Blue Dextran (BD), fetuin glycopeptide (FE), transferrin glycopeptide (TR), and the O-glycosidic brain tetrasaccharide (OT) are indicated. Molecular weights are given in text. —, F₁; ---, Wa4-bl. The fractions were pooled as indicated by the bars.

SOURCE: *Finne et al., 1980.*

For a Balanced Assessment of Tumorigenicity and Metastasis, Several Assays Should be Used

The large standard mean errors of whole animal assays indicate that tumor biology is a difficult field for drawing conclusions based on statistical correlations. One should therefore always use different test systems to assay similar parameters.

Table 8.2. Carbohydrate Composition of Fraction A and O Glycopeptides and Oligosaccharides from F₁ and Wa4-bl Cells.

	mol/mol			
	Fraction A		Fraction O	
Sugar	F₁	Wa4-bl	F₁	Wa4-bl
Neuraminic acid	3.8	2.0	1.6	1.5
Fucose	0.8	2.4	0	0
Galactose	4.2	3.8	1.4	1.3
Mannose	2.6	2.4	0.4	0.4
N-Acetylglucosamine	4.9	4.6	0.5	0.5
N-Acetylgalactosaminitol	0	0	1.0	1.0

Note: Sugar determinations were carried out by gas-liquid chromatography after methanolysis. In calculating the data, molecular weights of 3320 and 2870 were used for the Fraction A glycopeptides from F₁ and Wa4-bl cell lines, respectively. The data for Fraction O are expressed relative to N-acetylgalactosaminitol. The values are the average of 2 determinations.

(Source: Finne et al., 1980.)

In the case of tumorigenicity, we could confirm, with two additional assays, the earlier conclusion that the WGA resistant cells lost some but by far not all tumorigenicity. Intradermal injections showed that when we reduced the number of WGA resistant cells injected, the number of "takes" began to drop

Figure 8.4. Altered oligosaccharide portion of glycoprotein in the poorly metastasizing WGA-resistant melanoma cell. The exact location of the N-acetylglucosamine-bound fucose cannot yet be given. Most likely they are located in the two arms of the tetra-antennary oligosaccharide which are missing the sialic acid (AcNeu). The corresponding oligosaccharide in the wild type, i.e., WGA sensitive F₁ cell line, has all four antennae terminating with sialic acid (AcNeu), and does not carry the two fucose residues indicated.

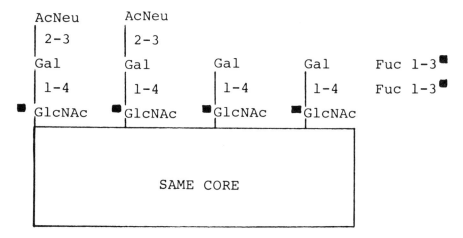

at higher cell doses per injection, as compared with the parental melanoma cells (Figure 8.5).

Further support for the same conclusion comes from survival studies. After intraperitoneal applications of the cells, animals given WGA resistant cells lived longer than those given parental cells. This effect was seen at high and low cell doses (Figure 8.6).

Portions of the metastasizing process can be tested separately (Liotta et al., 1974). Thus the release of tumor cells from a primary tumor can be monitored in the circulation in general only in the draining vessel (Roos & Dingemans, 1979). We have not yet carried out this assay. The establishment of tumors in the next capillary bed (usually the lung) can be monitored after intravenous application of the test cell. However, this procedure monitors only one leg of the metastatic route and since it is an assay where "takes" are measured, it really measures tumorigenicity rather than metastasizing, even though the cells are not directly injected into the tissue of observation. We have had extremely variable results with i.v. applications and have given up this approach for the time being. We decided therefore to measure metastasizing potential in its

Figure 8.5. Intradermal titration of tumorigenicity. Titration assay for tumorigenicity of B-16 and lectin resistant variant cells after intradermal injections of cells in doses of 1×10^3, 1×10^4, 1×10^5, and 1×10^6 per animal: 10–15 animals were used for each variable. Animals were examined for tumor "take" up to 2 months after injection. P: Parental B-16 cells; C: Con A resistant cells, R: Ricin resistant cells; W: WGA resistant cells.

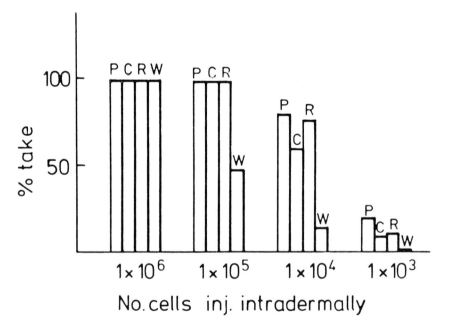

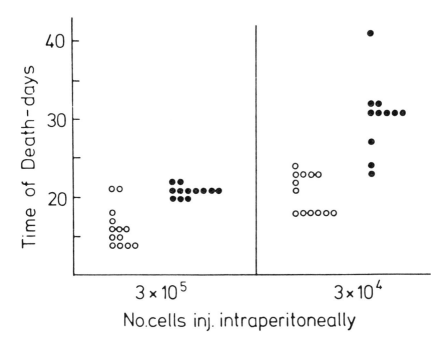

Figure 8.6. Time to death after intraperitoneal application. Each point represents one animal. Note the delayed killing of Wa4-bl cells at the lower cell dose. ○: B-16 or F_1 cells; ●: WGA resistant or Wa4-bl cells.

truest sense by injecting cells intramuscularly in the leg and amputating the leg when the primary tumor reached a specific size. This prevents the animal from being killed by the primary tumor and allows any microscopic metastases to grow up to a size that can be recorded in the assessment. Removal of the primary tumor is not possible with the intraperitoneal assay used earlier (Table 8.1). Using this method, we observed that the WGA resistant clone did give rise to a reduced number of lumbar lymph node metastases, and even to some lung metastases as well. No other organs displayed any metastases. This observation does not invalidate the correlative studies indicating a predominant loss of metastasizing capacity in these WGA resistant cells with a carbohydrate alteration in a specific oligosaccharide, but it indicates that the change is relative rather than absolute.

If a wide variety of assay systems is necessary to construct a complete picture of tumorigenicity and metastasizing capacities, it stands to reason that a wide variety of different cell lines with different surface changes should provide a clearer picture of the relevance of the cell surface to metastasis.

We are following two approaches to the study of such cell surface functions. First, we have begun to isolate other lectin resistant cells, lately also from B-16 melanoma lines that are cloned. As can be seen from Figure 8.5, the Concanavalin A resistant cell showed about the same tumorigenicity as parental cells and in other experiments demonstrated, if anything, an even greater metastasizing potential than parental melanoma cells. The most interesting cell line so far is the Ricin resistant line, which comes very close to providing the ideal test system we are looking for, since it shows a distinctly decreased metastasizing potential but no change in tumorigenicity. If this conclusion holds up in all assay systems, then this line may provide some interesting clues about the distinction between metastatic and tumorigenic phenomena.

Our other approach has been to begin to isolate biochemical revertants. Preliminary experiments with Ricin yielded a revertant with surface labeling patterns detected by iodination similar to those of B-16 melanoma cells (T.W. Tao, unpublished). Using an independent approach that selects for a reversal of the fucose alteration with another lectin, surface labeling patterns similar to those of the original B-16 melanoma line were again observed (J. Finne, unpublished). No reliable data on a reversion of the metatasizing potential are yet available, since we have to test a series of revertant clones before a conclusive statement can be made. The approach however appears quite promising.

Effects of Amputation of the Primary Tumor on Metastasis

Our experience with analyses of amputated mice left over the years the impression that these animals sometimes had more or larger metastases in the lungs than unamputated mice. This unexpected observation was subjected to further examination.

Amputation of the right hind leg was carried out at the time the primary B-16 melanoma reached a standard size (about 300 mg). The mice were sacrified one week thereafter and compared with animals that were not amputated. As can be seen from Table 8.3, the number of animals carrying metastases was increased among the amputated animals (M.M. Burger, unpublished). This unexpected observation could on pure theoretical grounds be attributed to the reduced tumor load after amputation, although realistic explanations for such an interpretation would not be easy to find. However, removal of the healthy leg instead of the one carrying the primary tumor also clearly increased the metastases found in the lungs, as compared to the burden of unamputated animals (Table 8.3). Reduced tumor load can therefore not explain the amputation effect. Animals subjected only to narcosis for a similar duration of time had a slightly increased number of lung metastases, but the difference was statistically barely significant (data not shown).

These unexpected observations, with their possible clinical implications, suggest a series of potential explanations. Unintended manipulation of the primary tumor during the operation (pressure, massage) could for instance increase metastases, as indeed was shown when we tested the effects of tumor massage (data not shown). Manipulation was therefore reduced to a minimum

Table 8.3. Effect of Amputation of the Primary Tumor upon Metastasis.

Treatment	Number of animals with metastases			
	In lungs		In lumbar ln.	
No amputation	8/42	19%	26/42	62%
Tumor bearing hind leg amputated	17/38	45%	31/38	82%
Contralateral hind leg amputated	9/31	29%	21/31	68%

Note: 2 × 10⁵ B-16 melanoma cells (subline of F_1) were injected in 30 μl PBS intramuscularly into the right hind leg. After 14 days, either of the two hind legs was amputated and after another week the animals were sacrificed and lung and lumbar lymphnodes carefully examined for tumor growth.

without significantly decreasing the increased metastases after amputation. We do not believe that this explanation accounts for our results, although it cannot yet be ruled out entirely. Narcosis alone still remains to be ruled out. Loss of blood, minor infections after the operation, hemodynamic changes, blood clots with emboli in the lungs, and many other operative and postoperative causes could contribute, not the least being an effect upon the immune system. Some of the possible causes can and will be tested. Similar results were reported to us by Dr. Keller (Zurich) after the galleys were received.

Some Thoughts on an Organ Distribution Model System: Liver Oriented Variant Cells

In an effort to search for surface changes which promote the settling of tumor metastases in certain organs, we began to select for liver specific B-16 cells (Tao et al., 1979). Nicolson and collaborators (1977) had already looked for brain-oriented variant cells. We chose the liver years ago, since it is the organ where cells other than lymphocytes do "home." Erythrocytes seem to end up in this organ, and Ashwell showed years ago that soluble glycoproteins which had altered sialic acid contents were also rerouted and trapped in the liver.

Injection of B-16 melanoma cells into the portal vein led to an increased number of liver tumors, as expected when capillary system trapping is a major contributory factor in distribution. Regrowth of liver tumors in culture and reinjection led to an increase in liver affinity when the cells were tested by delivery into the tail vein (Figure 8.7).

Three points may be stressed which arise from this work. First, we could not find an obvious change in the cell surface biochemistry of these cell clones. Lactoperoxidase did not reveal an obvious reduction in molecular weight, as was found for the WGA resistant cells, which had several glycoproteins with measurable sialic acid decreases. This observation does not rule out minor carbohydrate changes, (e.g., alterations of minor proteins), but gross changes were clearly absent.

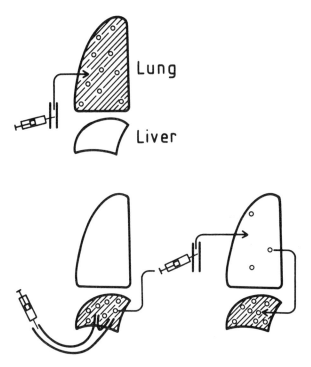

Figure 8.7. Selection of melanoma cells with a tendency to metastasize into the liver. The parent B-16 melanoma cells (F_1) produce almost exclusively lung tumors if injected into the tail vein (see upper part of figure). If they are injected into the portal vein system, primarily liver tumors will be found. If these cells are grown in tissue culture for one passage (not shown) and then injected into the vein, a few liver tumors can be found besides the lung tumors. Repetition of such liver cycles leads to cells with a clearly detectable tendency to colonize the liver if administered intravenously.

Second, the selection process was self-limiting, i.e., the liver specificity of the settled mutants could hardly be improved past the sixth selection cycle. This observation must mean that a ceiling of affinity can be reached early, an unexpected and interesting finding which calls for an explanation.

Third, these liver-specific cells were not going exclusively into the liver after i.v. application. They still went to the lung, although with much lower efficiency, and they certainly seemed to go into some other organs also, although to a minor degree only. We therefore asked whether the increase in liver tumors after i.v. application may be due primarily to a decrease in their affinity to the lung. Perhaps only when these cells escape from the lungs do we detect an increase in the liver and other organs. Intraarterial injections (into the left heart ventricle) clearly showed that this criticism does not apply, since the liver affinity, although not all complete, was clearly better expressed under these conditions, than after i.v. application.

Summary

1. Metastasis is certainly a multistep phenomenon, and therefore more than one biological parameter will be altered to contribute to fast and efficient metastasis. We are most likely going to witness in the future many biochemical changes in metastasizing tumor cells. Over the years to come, some of them will not withstand serious scrutiny for causal relevance. Some of them, representing different single steps of the multistep process, will turn out to be relevant, however.
2. Should the sialic decrease in some very specific oligosaccharides found here be among the relevant causes of metastatic activity, it would certainly not be the only one. We would have to evaluate whether it is a necessary and, if so, a sufficient change for the alteration in the metastatic phenotype.
3. Metastasis and tumorigenicity should always be evaluated with more than one assay. For a given cell line, the particular assay used may not be sufficiently sensitive or not adapted to the growth and organ distribution pattern of the tumor cell line tested.
4. Preliminary observations raise the possibility that amputation of the primary tumor may promote metastatic spread.

ACKNOWLEDGMENTS

Former collaborators who contributed were, in chronological order, Drs. A. Matter, M. Sayare, C. Haskovec, B. Jockusch, K. Vosbeck, and Mr. K. Tullberg. Excellent technical help was provided by Mrs. J. Jenkins, Mr. K. Vogel, and Mrs. H. Haidvogl.

References

Burger, M.M. (1980) The cell surface and metastasis. In *Biology of the Cancer Cell.* Proceedings of the Fifth Meeting of the European Association for Cancer Research, Vienna 9–12 September 1979. Amsterdam: Kugler Publications, pp. 193–208.

Fidler, I.J. (1973) Selection of successive tumor lines for metastasis. *Nature New Biol.* 242:148–149.

Finne, J., Tao, T.W., and Burger, M.M. (1980) Carbohydrate changes in glycoproteins of a poorly metastasizing wheat germ agglutinin-resistant melanoma clone. *Cancer Res.* 40:2580–2587.

Jumblatt, J.E., Tao, T.W., Schlup, V., Finne, J., and Burger, M.M. (1980) Altered surface glycoproteins in melanoma cell variants with reduced metastasizing capacity selected for resistance to wheat germ agglutinin. *Biochem. Biophys. Res. Com.* 95:111–117.

Liotta, L.A., Kleinerman, J., and Saidel, G.M. (1974) Quantitative relationships of intravascular tumor cells, tumor vesicles, and pulmonary metastases following tumor implantations. *Cancer Res.* 34:997–1004.

Nicolson, G.L., Birdwell, C.R., Brunson, K.W., Robbins, J.C., Beattie, G., and Fidler, I.J. (1977) Cell interactions in the metastatic process: some cell surface properties associated with successful blood-borne tumor spread. In *Cell and Tissue Interactions.* Lash, J.W. and Burger, M.M. (eds.), New York: Raven Press.

Roos, E. and Dingemans, K.P. (1979) Mechanisms of metastasis. *Biochim. Biophys. Acta* 560:135–166.

Tao, T.W. and Burger, M.M. (1977) Non-metastasizing variants selected from metastasizing melanoma cells. *Nature* 270:437–438.

Tao, T.W., Matter, A., Vogel, K., and Burger M.M. (1979) Liver colonizing melanoma cells selected from B-16 melanoma. *Int. J. Cancer* 23:854–857.

PART II:

Modulation of Immune Reactions

Published 1981 by Elsevier North Holland, Inc.
Saunders, Daniels, Serrou, Rosenfeld, and Denney, eds.
FUNDAMENTAL MECHANISMS IN HUMAN CANCER IMMUNOLOGY

CHAPTER 9

Interferons: Anti-tumor and Immunoregulatory Activities[1]

Samuel Baron

Department of Microbiology, University of Texas Medical Branch, Galveston, Texas

Introduction

The interferon system was discovered by Isaacs and Lindenmann in 1957 (Isaacs, 1963), during studies of the intriguing phenomenon by which infection by one virus renders hosts and their cells highly resistant to other superinfecting viruses (termed interference). The most widely occurring cause of interference in nature is the production of a new protein, interferon, by host cells themselves (Taylor, 1964). Interferon can react with normal, uninfected cells to render them resistant to most types of viruses.

We will consider some of the physiological and biological aspects of interferon. The interferon system is an inducible genetic function of all somatic cells. It can initiate several pathways which in turn can affect not only viral replication, but also the immune response, cell growth, and other cell functions. There are a number of reviews available—some of which are listed to provide additional information (Baron, 1963; Isaacs, 1963; Grossberg, 1972; Finter, 1973; Johnson and Baron, 1976; Baron and Dianzani, 1977; Gresser, 1977; Baron et al., 1979; Hill et al., 1979; Stewart, 1979). The original studies can be found through these references and the other general references that are included in the text.

Induction of Interferon

The interferon system generally does not function in the absence of viral infection or stimulation by foreign materials. When it is activated, the system

[1]Supported in part by National Eye Institute research Grant EY01715 and Grant 1-515 from the March of Dimes Birth Defects Foundation.

consists of two major mechanisms: first, the induction of interferon and second, the induction of its antiviral, immunoregulatory, anti-tumor, and other activities.

One type of the 3 known types of interferon, IFNβ, can be produced by most body cells (e.g., epithelial and fibroblast) when they become infected by viruses. As shown in Figure 9.1a, during the early stages of viral infection of the cell, some event (probably the presence of foreign viral nucleic acid) derepresses a cellular gene which contains the stored genetic information for the interferon protein. The virus-induced interferon gene appears to be located on specific chromosomes (Chany et al., 1975; Tan et al., 1977).

Figure 9.1. Cellular events of virus-induction and action of interferon (IF). Virus comes in contact with cell (1) and penetrates to the cell membrane. The virus then releases its genetic material and replication of the virus occurs (2). The new virus leaves the cell (3) and enters the fluid around the first cell, and some of the replicated virus infects a second cell (4) where the release of the genetic material again takes place (5). During the early stages of infection of the first cell, some event (viral nucleic acid?) stimulates a gene in the DNA which contains the stored genetic information for interferon (A). This leads to the production of mRNA for interferon (IF), which leaves (B) the nucleus and is translated by the cell's ribosomes (C) into the interferon protein. Several events now occur more or less simultaneously. Some interferon is secreted by the first cell (D) and enters the surrounding fluid where it comes into contact with and stimulates the second cell (E). The second cell is thereby induced to produce a new mRNA (F), which is translated to a new protein(s) (G), the antiviral protein (AVP). This in turn modifies the cell's protein-synthesizing machinery, such that cell mRNA can be translated into protein, but viral RNA is poorly bound or translated or both. In the first cell, processes E, F, and G may also operate to form AVP and thereby reduce the virus yield in the first cell. Shortly after interferon is synthesized in the first cell, another mRNA (H) is believed to be synthesized from the cell's DNA and is translated (I) into a regulatory protein (RP) (hypothesized). This RP combines with the mRNA for IF, thereby preventing further synthesis of more IF (J). There is recent evidence that the antiviral state may be directly transferred between adjacent cells (from second to third cell at right) by the passage of an unknown (?) inducer of the AVP.

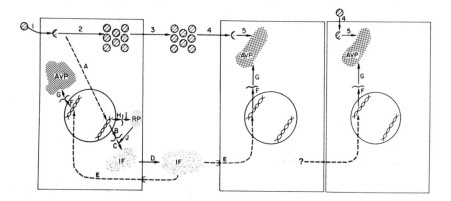

Production of Virus-Induced Interferon

Production of this interferon occurs by cellular protein synthesis from the newly transcribed mRNA (Figure 9.1a). An additional regulatory protein is also produced and is thought to control interferon's production (Vilcek and Kohase, 1977). The interferon molecule, with a small amount of associated carbohydrate, is actively secreted by the cell into the extracellular fluid. Production of this glycoprotein can start as early as 1 hour after stimulation. The synthesis of the interferon molecule is only the first part of the interferon system, since to act, interferon must induce a second process in cells. This activation of cells will be considered below in our discussion of the mechanism of interferon's antiviral action.

Types of the Interferon Molecule

Three clearly distinct types of interferon (IFN) have been identified in humans and probably occur in mouse systems (Epstein, 1977; Paucker, 1977; Youngner, 1977; Osborne et al., 1980) (Table 9.1). These are IFN-α (leukocyte interferon), IFNβ (fibroepithelial interferon) and IFNγ (immune or type II interferon). They may differ (a) antigenically; (b) by producer cell; (c) by stimulus for induction; (d) in major action; (e) in stability; (f) in phylogenetic specificity; and (g) in mechanisms of cell activation. Three distinct gene sites for the three interferons are strongly implied. The most common type, IFNβ, is produced by fibroblasts and epithelial cells during viral infection and it may function mainly as a defense against viruses. Another type, IFNα (Svet-Moldavsky et al., 1974; Trinchieri and Santoli, 1978; Blalock et al., 1979), is produced by lymphoid cells and macrophages when induced by certain viruses and foreign or tumor cells.

Table 9.1. Production of the Three Types of Interferon.

Interferon type	Producer cell	Stimulus
α (Leukocyte)	Null lymphocyte B lymphocyte Macrophage (Other?)	Foreign or transformed cells Bacteria Viruses B mitogens
β (Fibro-epithelial)	Fibroblast Epithelial Macrophage (Other?)	Foreign nucleic acids Viruses Nucleic acids
γ (Immune, Type II)	T (and B?) lymphocyte	Foreign antigens T mitogens

A third type, IFNγ, is produced mostly by T lymphocytes following antigenic or mitogenic stimulation. Recent studies indicate that the mechanism of cellular activation by IFNγ is different from that of the 2 preceding types of interferon (Dianzani et al., 1980). The first antibody to mouse interferon γ has been produced (Osborne et al., 1980). Use of this antibody has shown that interferon γ is antigenically distinct from the other interferons. Furthermore, antigenically indistinguishable IFNγ were induced by various T lymphocyte mitogens *in vitro* and by antigen injected into sensitized mice (Osborne et al., 1980). Purification (10,000-fold) of lymphokine preparations containing IFNγ demonstrated that it could be separated from migration inhibitory factor and lymphotoxin (Georgiades et al., 1979).

Much slower activation of the antiviral state occurs in cells reacting with IFNγ than with the other 2 interferons (Dianzani et al., 1978). The possibility that this slow action is due to a different mechanism of cell activation was raised by studies using sequential inhibition of cellular RNA and protein syntheses (Dianzani et al., 1980). The most probable interpretation of the findings is that IFNγ, unlike interferons α and β, induces cells to synthesize an intermediary protein which then induces antiviral proteins.

Potentiation of the antiviral and anti-tumor action of other interferons may also be an important function of IFNγ. This is indicated by the recent finding that partially purified IFNγ can potentiate the antiviral and anti-tumor action of IFN, α and β, by a factor of approximately ten (Fleischmann, 1979; Fleischmann et al., 1980). IFNγ may also be more potent than IFNα and β as an anti-tumor and immunoregulatory agent (Sonnenfeld et al., 1977; Youngner, 1977).

Antiviral Action

Interferon does not directly inactivate virus. Instead it acts by reacting with membranes of cells surrounding the producer cells to derepress a second gene site, the site encoded for intracellular antiviral protein(s) which must be synthesized before inhibition of virus replication can occur (Figure 9.1b) (Taylor, 1964; Joklik, 1977). The duration of activation of the interferon system during viral infection lasts only 0.5 to 3 weeks during acute infection *in vivo*, depending on the duration of virus replication. The biochemical mechanisms of the viral inhibition by the antiviral protein (Baron and Dianzani, 1977; Riley and Levy, 1977; Ohtsuki et al., 1977, 1980; Joklik, 1977; Jungwirth et al., 1977; Sen et al., 1977; Revel, 1979) are complex and incompletely understood. Interferon effects on cellular protein kinases, initiation factor, ribosomes, various RNAs, oligonucleotide synthesis, endonuclease, elongation, transcription, and induction of new proteins have been reported. Correlation of these biochemical effects with the antiviral or other actions of interferon remains to be accomplished definitively.

Cell-to-Cell Transfer of the Antiviral State

Transfer of antiviral activity from interferon-treated cells to adjacent, untreated cells without the continued presence of interferon can occur as shown in Figure 9.1c (Blalock and Baron, 1977, 1978). The transfer can occur between homologous or heterologous cells, but appears to be most efficient between the homologous cells. Leukocytes may transfer the activation of interferon (Stanton et al., 1980). This transfer mechanism may be an additional means of amplifying the interferon system for antiviral, anticellular, and immunoregulatory activities. For example, a rapid response to interferon occurs in a mixed population of rapid and slowly responding cells because the rapidly responding cells quickly transfer their response to the slowly responding cells. Noradrenaline and follicle stimulating hormone were subsequently found similarly to transfer their cell-specific activities between cells, perhaps by common cyclic AMP-dependent mechanisms (see Blalock and Baron, 1977). The mechanism of antiviral transfer is under study.

Effects on the Immune Response by Interferon

The specifically sensitized lymphocyte may be a unique cell type in its ability to produce IFNγ, along with other lymphokines, in response to reaction with its specific antigen (Green et al., 1969; Salvin et al., 1973; Johnson and Baron, 1976; Epstein, 1977; Johnson, 1977; Youngner, 1977). This finding has raised the possibility that antigen-induced interferon (INFγ) might serve another role. All interferons affect (generally suppress) the antibody response (Braun and Levy, 1972) and preparations (unpurified) of IFNγ have been reported to be the most effective (Sonnenfeld et al., 1977). The suppressive action of interferon on antibody production may be mediated by an interferon-induced suppressor substance (Johnson, 1977). Also, under many conditions, interferon can inhibit induction and expression of cellular immunity (DeMaeyer and DeMaeyer-Guignard, 1977). The sites of interferon action on the immune response are presented as a working model in Figure 9.2. Evidence for a natural role comes from the finding that the concentrations of interferon required for immunosuppression are compatible with those that occur *in vivo*. Also, the timing of production of antigen-stimulated interferon is consistent with a natural regulatory role. Recent evidence indicates that a regulator (inhibitor) of the action of interferon can be produced by stimulated spleen cells (Fleischmann et al., 1978). This inhibitor may be a lymphokine. The several interactions of the interferon and immune systems are listed in Table 9.2.

Anticellular and Anti-tumor Action

There is increasing evidence that interferon and inducers of interferon may

130

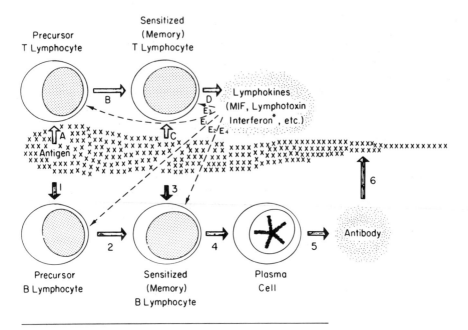

Time ➤

Figure 9.2. Cellular events in the induction and immunosuppressive action of immune interferons. Antigen comes into contact with a precursor T lymphocyte (A), which undergoes differentiation to a sensitized T lymphocyte (B). This cell, driven by antigen (C), may become a memory cell or it may release mediators known as lymphokines (D). Among the mediator produced by the T lymphocyte is antigen-type interferon. Antigen also reacts with a precursor B lymphocyte (1), which undergoes differentiation to a sensitized B lymphocyte (and memory B cell) (2). The sensitized B cell is further driven by antigen (3) to become a plasma cell (4), which is responsible for most of the antibody (5) that is produced. This antibody reacts with the specific antigen (6). Both antigen- and virus-induced interferons are capable of suppressing precursor and sensitized T lymphocytes (E_1) and B lymphocytes (E_2). As differentiation progresses, in part as a result of continued antigen presence, it becomes progressively more difficult to inhibit lymphocyte function by interferons. Plasma cell production of antibody is resistant to inhibition by interferon. The macrophage is not included in the figure, but interferons may exert their immunosuppressive effects via a required macrophage function in the immune response. The diagrammatic scheme does not necessarily imply, therefore, a direct effect of the interferons on the lymphocytes.

function to inhibit the growth of some animal tumors. The mechanisms are not fully understood (Gresser, 1977). Possible anti-tumor effects include direct inhibition of tumor cells, activation of immunocompetent cells, and alteration of the immune response to the tumor (Table 9.3). A new mechanism for anti-tumor action comes from the findings that (a) nonsensitized NK and B lymphocytes can recognize "foreignness" in tumor cells by producing leukocyte

Table 9.2. Interaction of the Interferon and Immune System.

Function	Interaction
IFNγ (lymphokine) production	T lymphocytes + specific antigen or T mitogen
IFNα production	B and NK lymphocytes + foreign or tumor cells or B mitogens
Regulator of IFNγ production	T lymphocyte hyporesponsiveness to repeated induction
Regulation of sensitization to antigen	B and T lymphocytes regulated by IFN
Activation of immunocompetent cells	IFN affects NK and sensitized T lymphocytes and macrophages
Inhibition of multiplication of immunocompetent cells	IFN affects lymphocytes and macrophages

interferon (Svet-Moldavsky et al., 1974; Trinchieri and Santoli, 1978; Blalock, 1979), and (b) interferon can activate natural killer cells to destroy tumor cells. Trials of interferon in patients with cancer have been limited and as yet are uncontrolled (Galasso and Dunnick, 1977; Hill et al., 1979) but the results encourage further clinical trials. More effective application of interferon can be expected when recently discovered properties are exploited (e.g., potentiation, greater anti-tumor action of IFNγ, and removal of inhibition of interferon) and large scale synthesis in cells or bacteria is undertaken.

Hormonal Properties of Interferon

The interferon system bears a strong resemblance to glycoprotein hormone systems (Baron, 1966; Friedman et al., 1977). (a) Both interferon and hormones induce specific functions in cells other than that in the cells in which they are produced. (b) Cellular receptors for interferons and those for other glycoprotein hormones are related. (c) Hormones and interferon are glycoproteins in

Table 9.3. Anti-tumor Actions of Interferon.

Demonstrated:	
Direct inhibition of cell division	
Activation of:	sensitized T lymphocytes
	NK cells
	ADCC null cells
	macrophages
Possible:	
Regulation of immune sensitization	
Hormonal effects	
Direct cell killing	

the same size range. (d) Neither are consumed during their action on cells. (e) Both induce genetic derepression and synthesis of new protein(s) in cells. (f) Hormone and interferon-activated cells transfer cellular activity to surrounding cells. Recently it was shown that interferon may activate norepinephrine effects in cells, and norepinephrine may activate interferon-specified antiviral effects in treated cells (Blalock, 1980). Furthermore, the IFNα molecule may contain ACTH and MSH sequences (Blalock et al., 1980).

Summary

The genetically controlled interferon system is inducible in all somatic cells. When activated, the system can initiate several pathways which in turn can affect (a) viral replication, (b) the immune response, (c) cell growth, and (d) other cell functions. Three clearly distinct types of interferon have been identified. These are IFNα (leukocyte interferon), IFNβ (fibro-epithelial interferon), and IFNγ (immune [type II]) interferon. This chapter considers mechanisms for induction of these interferons and mechanisms by which they activate cells, along with the recent findings that the interferon-activated cell may transfer antiviral activity to adjacent, untreated cells without the continued presence of interferon. The interferon and immune systems interact in several important ways. A series of studies have shown that the specifically sensitized lymphocyte may be a unique cell type in its ability to produce the IFNγ, along with other lymphokines, in response to reaction with specific antigen. This immune interferon manifests major differences from other interferons. It is antigenically distinct. Its kinetics of cellular activation are dramatically slower. Metabolic inhibitor studies indicate that it activates cells through induction of intermediary proteins. Purification studies indicate that IFNγ is separable from many of the other lymphokines. Antibody to interferons has been used to classify the various interferons produced by cells of the immune system. Partially purified preparations of IFNγ can potentiate the antiviral activity of the other interferons. Recent evidence indicates that a regulator (inhibitor) of the action of interferon is produced during synthesis of lymphokines and IFN by spleen cells. Another interesting aspect of interferon is its strong resemblance to glycoprotein hormone systems. The mechanisms of interferon's anti-tumor action are complex, and are related to some of its other, better understood, effects.

References

Baron, S. (1963) Mechanism of recovery from viral infection. In *Advances in Virus Research*. Smith, D.M. and Lauffer, M.A. (eds.), New York: Academic Press, Inc., pp. 39–60.

Baron, S. (1966) The biological significance of the interferon system. In *Frontiers of Biology*, *Vol. 2.* Neuberger, A. and Tatum, E.L. (eds.), Amsterdam: North Holland Publishing Co., pp. 268–293.

Baron, S. and Dianzani, F. (1977) The interferon system: a current review to 1978. *Tex. Rep. Biol. Med.* 35:1–573.

Baron, S., Brunell, P.A., and Grossberg, S.E. (1979) Mechanisms of action and pharmacology: the immune and interferon systems. In *Antiviral Agents and Viral Diseases of Man*. Galasso, G.L. et al. (eds.), New York: Raven Press, pp. 151–208.

Blalock, J. E. and Baron, S. (1977) Interferon-induced transfer of viral resistance between animal cells. *Nature (London)* 269:422–425.

Blalock, J.E. and Baron, S. (1978) Mechanisms of interferon-induced transfer of viral resistance between animal cells. *J. Gen. Virol.* 42:363–372.

Blalock, J.E. and Smith, E.M. (1980) Human leukocyte interferon: structural and biological relatedness to adrenocorticotropic hormone and endorphins. *Proc. Natl. Acad. Sci.* 77:5972–5974.

Blalock, J.E. et al. (1979) Nonsensitized lymphocytes produce leukocyte interferon when cultured with foreign cells. *Cell Immunol.* 43:197–201.

Braun, W. and Levy, H.B. (1972) Interferon preparations as modifiers of immune responses. *Proc. Soc. Exp. Biol. Med.* 141:769–773.

Chany, C., Vignal, M., Couillin, P., Van-Cong, M., Boue, J., and Boue, A. (1975) Chromosomal localization of human genes governing the interferon-induced antiviral state. *Proc. Natl. Acad. Sci. U.S.A.* 72:3129–3133.

DeMaeyer, E. and DeMaeyer-Guignard, J. (1977) Effect of interferon on cell-mediated immunity. *Tex. Rep. on Biol. Med.* 35:370–374.

Dianzani, F., Salter, L., Fleischmann, W. R., Jr., and Zucca, M. (1978) Immune interferon activates cells more slowly than does virus-induced interferon. *Proc. Soc. Exp. Biol. Med.* 159:94–97.

Dianzani, F., Zucca, M., Scupham, A., and Georgiades, J. (1980) Immune virus-induced interferons may activate cells by different derepressional mechanisms. *Nature* 280:400–402.

Epstein, L.B. (1977) Mitogen and antigen induction of interferon *in vitro* and *in vivo*. *Tex. Rep. Biol. Med.* 35:42–56.

Finter, N.B. (ed.) (1973) *Interferons and Interferon Inducers*. New York: American Elsevier.

Fleischmann, W.R., Jr. (1979) Potentiation of interferon activity by mixed preparations of fibroblast and immune interferon. *Infect. and Immun.* 26:248–253.

Fleischmann, W.R., Jr., (1980) Potentiation of anti-tumor effect of virus-induced interferon by mouse immune interferon preparations. *JNCI* 65:963–966.

Fleischmann, W.R., Jr., Georgiades, J.A., Johnson, H.M., Dianzani, F., and Baron, S. (1978) An inhibitor of interferon action produced by mitogen-stimulated mouse spleen cells. *Bacteriol. Proc.* 247.

Friedman, R.M., Grollman, E.F., Chang, E.H., Kohn, L.D., Lee, G., and Jay, F.T. (1977) Interferon and glycoprotein hormones. *Tex. Rep. Biol. Med.* 35:326–329.

Galasso, G.J. and Dunnick, J.K. (1977) Interferon, an antiviral drug for use in man. *Tex. Rep. Biol. Med.* 35:478–482.

Georgiades, J.A., Osborne, L.C., Moulton, R.G., and Johnson, H.M. (1979) *Proc. Soc. Exp. Biol. Med.* 161:167–170.

Green, J.A., Cooperband, S.R., and Kibric, K.S. (1969) Immune specific induction of interferon production in cultures of human blood lymphocytes. *Science* 164:1415–1417.

Gresser, I. (1977) Anti-tumor effects of interferon. In *Cancer: A Comprehensive Treatise*, Vol. 5. Becker, F. (ed.), New York: Plenum Press.

Grossberg, S.E. (1972) The interferons and their inducers: molecular and therapeutic considerations. *N. Eng. J. Med.* 287:13–19; 287:79–85; 287:122–128.

Hill, N.O., Kahn, A., Loeb, E., Pardue, A., Aleman, C., Dorn, G., and Hill, J.M. (1979) Clinical trials of high dose human leukocyte interferon. In *Interferon, Properties, and Clinical Uses*. Kahn, A. and Dorn, G. (eds.), Dallas: Leland Fikes, pp. 667–677.

134

Joklik, W.K. (1977) Evidence for a translation-inhibitory ribosome-associated protein. *Tex. Rep. Biol. Med.* 35:264–269.

Johnson, H.M. (1977) Effect of interferon antibody formation. *Texas Rep. Biol. Med.* 35:357–369.

Johnson, H.M. and Baron, S. (1976) Interferon: effects on the immune response and the mechanism of activation of the cellular response. *CRC Crit. Rev. Biochem.* 4:203–227.

Jungwirth, C., Kroath, H., and Bodo, G. (1977) Effect of interferon on poxvirus replication. *Tex. Rep. Biol. Med.* 35:247–259.

Ohtsuki, K., Dianzani, F., and Baron, S. (1977) Decreased initiation factor activity in mouse L cells treated with interferon. *Nature* 269:536–538.

Ohtsuki, K., Masatuka, N., Tsuneaki, K., Nakao, I., and Baron, S. (1980) A ribosomal protein mediates eIF-2 phosphorylation by interferon-induced kinase. *Nature* 287:65–67.

Osborne, L.C., Georgiades, J.A., and Johnson, H.M. (1980) Classification of interferons with antibody to immune interferon. *Cell Immunol.* 53:65–70.

Paucker, K. (1977) Antigenic properties. *Tex. Rep. Biol. Med.* 35:23–28.

Revel, M. (1979) Molecular mechanisms involved in the antiviral effects of interferon. *Interferon* 1:101–163.

Riley, F.L. and Levy, H.B. (1977) Effect of interferon on cellular RNA synthesis and structure. *Tex. Rep. Biol. Med.* 35:239–246.

Salvin, S., Youngner, J.S., and Lederer, W.H. (1973) Migration inhibitory factor and interferon in the circulation of mice with delayed hypersensitivity. *Infect. and Immun.* 7:68–79.

Sonnenfeld, G., Mandel, A.D., and Merigan, T.C. (1977) The immunosuppressive effect of type II mouse interferon on antibody production. *Cell Immunol.* 34:193–206.

Stanton, G.J., Weigent, D.A., Langford, M.P., and Block, J.E. (1980) Human leukocyte transfer of viral resistance to heterologous cells. *Interferon: Properties and Clinical Uses.* Kahn, A., Hill, N.O., and Dorn, G.L. (eds.), Dallas: Leland Fikes, pp. 355–364.

Stewart, W.E., II. (1979) *The Interferon System.* New York: Springer-Verlag.

Svet-Moldavsky, G.J., Nemirovskaya, B.M., and Osipora, T.V. (1974) Interferonogenicity and antigen recognition. *Nature* 247:205–206.

Tan, Y.H., Tan, C., and Berthold, W. (1977) Genetic control of the interferon system. *Rep. Biol. Med.* 35:63–68.

Taylor, J. (1964) Inhibition of interferon action by actinomycin. *Biochem. Biophys. Res. Commun.* 14:447–451.

Trinchieri, G. and Santoli, D. (1978) Antiviral activity induced by culturing lymphocytes with tumor-derived or virus-transformed cells. Enhancement of human natural killer cell activity by interferon and antagonistic inhibition of susceptibility of target cells to lysis. *J. Exp. Med.* 147:1314–1333.

Vilcek, J. and Kohase, M. (1977) Regulation of interferon production: cell culture studies. *Tex. Rep. Biol. Med.* 35:57–62.

Youngner, J.S. (1977) Properties of interferon induced by specific antigens. *Tex. Rep. Biol. Med.* 35:17–22.

Published 1981 by Elsevier North Holland, Inc.
Saunders, Daniels, Serrou, Rosenfeld, and Denney, eds.
FUNDAMENTAL MECHANISMS IN HUMAN CANCER IMMUNOLOGY

CHAPTER 10

Activation and Cloning of T Lymphocytes[1]

Charles G. Orosz, Ph.D. and Fritz H. Bach, M.D.

Immunobiology Research Center, Departments of Laboratory Medicine/Pathology and Surgery, University of Minnesota, Minneapolis, Minnesota

The division of T lymphocytes into several functional subpopulations has complicated experimental questions regarding the activation of these cells, which in all probability involves non-T accessory cells as well as the different T lymphocyte subsets. Cloning of T lymphocytes in mouse (Baker et al., 1978; Fathman and Hengartner, 1978; Gillis and Smith, 1977; Nabholz et al., 1978) and man (Bach et al., 1979) has allowed isolation of both cytotoxic and helper (amplifier) T lymphocyte populations (Glasebrook and Fitch, 1979). This technological advance will no doubt greatly facilitate explorations of the area and bring to light critical information that has not been available in the past.

We shall deal with two separate topics in this paper: first, the signals that are required for the activation of T lymphocytes both in a primary and a secondary response, and second, some of the early results that have been obtained in our own laboratory and others on the cloning of T lymphocytes.

Signals Leading to Activation of Cytotoxic T Lymphocytes

The model which hypothesizes that precursor cytotoxic T lymphocytes (pT_c) require various signals for their activation (Bach et al., 1976) is based in large measure on experiments involving B lymphocytes. It has been hypothesized that for generation of a maximal cytotoxic response, T_c effector activation involves two signals, commonly referred to as signal 1 and signal 2. A minimal

[1] This work was supported by NIH Grants AI GM 17687, AI 15588, CA 27826, and March of Dimes Grant 6-214. This is paper number 261 from the Immunobiology Research Center, University of Minnesota.

model depicting the cells involved and the signals is shown in Figure 10.1. The pT_c recognizes the cytotoxic determinant (CD) that it is genetically pro-grammed to recognize (signal 1). This signal, in and of itself, is not sufficient to lead to the generation of a detectable cytotoxic response as ordinarily assayed. Rather, the pT_c must recognize the CD and also receive help, presumably from an activated T helper cell. The precursor helper T lymphocyte (pT_h) recognizes a lymphocyte defined (LD) foreign antigenic target determinant, which it is genetically programmed to recognize, and this recognition, possibly together with other signals to the T_h (Farrar et al., 1980; Shaw et al., 1980; Smith et al., 1980), leads to differentiation of the helper cell which in turn provides signal 2 to the T_c.

We previously hypothesized that recognition by the pT_c of the CD antigen to which it can respond does lead to some form of differentiation of that cell (Bach et al., 1976), albeit not the full differentiation which is possible if signal 2 is also present. The model proposed at that time (Bach et al., 1976) suggested that signal 1 leads to differentiation of the pT_c to a "poised" T_c which is "receptive to help." Although this model has not been fully substantiated, recent work supports the hypothesis (Larson and Coutinho, 1979).

Figure 10.1. Minimal model depicting the relationships between the functional lymphocyte subpopulations and the stimulating alloantigens involved in development of primary cytotoxic T cell activity *in vitro*. (CD: Allogeneic cytotoxic target determinant; LD: allogeneic lymphocyte-defined determinant; pT_c: cytotoxic T cell precursor; pT_h: helper T cell precursor; eT_c: effector cytotoxic T cell). For explanation, see text.

PRIMARY RESPONSE

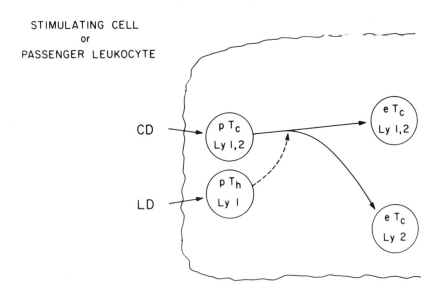

To explain more fully the experimental basis for the models just discussed, it will be helpful to review briefly the antigens encoded by genes of the Major Histocompatibility Complex (MHC). The general principles that appear to apply in mouse, the species most extensively used in these studies, also seem to apply in man. The mouse MHC, referred to as H-2, can be divided into a number of regions referred to as K, I, S, and D. A schematic representation of the H-2 complex is shown in Figure 10.2. Each region has a marker locus. Those loci of greatest concern to us are the H-2K and H-2D loci, related to the K and D regions respectively, as well as the Ia-1 locus, which serves as the marker for the I-A subregion of the I region. Antigenic determinants of the H-2K and H-2D phenotypic products serve as the primary target determinants for T_c.

By analogy with adoptive transfer experiments demonstrating T-B collaboration in antibody synthesis, we can utilize K and D encoded determinants as the structures which activate pT_c. The K/D encoded antigens can be presented in a variety of ways: for example, on x-irradiated or heat-treated thymocytes (Orosz et al., 1981; Scott et al., 1980). Such cells present the CD molecules so that they can be recognized by the pT_c, but they will not activate a detectable cytotoxic response, as measured by ^{51}Chromium assay on the fifth day of a primary mixed lymphocyte culture (MLC). Stimulation in the primary MLC with x-irradiated, I region disparate, stimulating cells carrying determinants particularly capable of stimulating pT_h will not yield effector T_c capable of lysing target cells that differ from the responding cells by only the K or D antigens. However, as illustrated in schematic fashion in Table 10.1, if the responding cells are simultaneously stimulated with thymocytes presenting allogeneic K region determinants, and with x-irradiated spleen cells bearing allogeneic I region encoded determinants, then a highly significant cytotoxic response is generated against the K region disparate target cells.

Figure 10.2. A schematic representation of the murine major histocompatibility (H-2) complex. For explanation, see text.

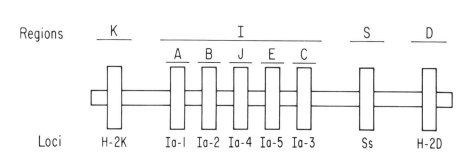

138

Table 10.1. Genetic Requirements for T_C Activation.

Responder cells	Irradiated stimulator cells	H-2 difference	Cytotoxicity on target cells differing from responders by K region
A	B spleen	K + I	++++
A	C spleen	K	+
A	C thym.	K	−
A	D spleen	I	−
A	C spleen + D spleen	K + I	++++
A	C thym. + D spleen	K + I	+++

Evidence of the cellular basis of this response, which relates to LD and CD determinants encoded by the MHC, supports the models depicted in Figure 10.1, and comes from studies in which anti-Ly sera are used to separate T_h from pT_c (Alter and Bach, 1979; Bach and Alter, 1978; Cantor and Boyse, 1975a; Roehm et al., 1981). In a series of studies, activation of T_h by LD determinants encoded by the I region was shown to markedly increase the magnitude of the cytotoxic response generated against antigenic determinants encoded by the K/D region. It would thus appear that the dichotomy of LD and CD antigen presentation is paralleled by a dichotomy in the cellular response to those antigens, in which pT_h respond to the LD determinants and provide the help (signal 2 of the T_c) which is needed for the generation of a maximal cytotoxic response by pT_c that recognize the K/D region encoded CD antigens.

A product of the Th, frequently referred to as "helper factor," "T cell growth factor" (TCGF), or "IL-2" may be sufficient to provide signal 2 to the developing T_c. Data supporting such a hypothesis, as shown in Table 10.2, demonstrates that the addition of a supernatant from a mixed leukocyte culture (MLC) which contains TCGF will substitute for the LD stimulus. That is, if responding cells are confronted with x-irradiated thymocytes differing by the K region, which by themselves do not generate a cytotoxic response as measured under routine conditions (see Table 10.1), generation of that cytotoxic response is allowed in the presence of the supernatant from the MLC.

Elicitation of a Secondary Cytotoxic Response

In contrast to the conditions necessary for a primary response to occur, where the generation of a maximal cytotoxic response is dependent on *both* the presence of the CD stimulus and help, a secondary cytotoxic response following *in vitro* "sensitization" is best elicited by restimulating the secondary population with an I region stimulus, presumably an LD stimulus (Alter et al., 1976; Grillot-Courvalin et al., 1977) as shown in Figure 10.3.

Table 10.2. Effects of TCGF on T_c Generation.

Responder cells	Irradiated stimulator cells	H-2 difference	Con A induced supernate	Cytotoxicity on target cells differing from responders by K region
A	B spleen	K + I	–	++++
A	C thymus	K	–	–
A	C thymus	K	+	+++
A	none	–	+	–

This finding is demonstrated in Table 10.3, in which cells from strain A are sensitized in the primary MLC to cells of strain B, which differs from A at both the K and I regions, and therefore provides both LD and CD stimuli. If these cells are allowed to remain in culture for 14 days, so that the cytotoxicity seen maximally on day 5 or 6 has decreased to almost background levels, then restimulation of the secondary cells with either strain B, the initial sensitizing cell, or strain C (which shares the I region with strain B but is identical with strain A for both the K and D regions) leads to the generation of an approximately equal amount of cytotoxicity. In fact, as Table 10.3 shows, stimulation with uv light treated stimulating cells of the sensitizing strain (which present their CD determinants in a manner analogous to those on thymocytes) does not elicit a very significant cytotoxic response. We have previously discussed a model (Bach, 1976) to explain these results, in which we hypothesize that stimulation of the secondary T_h led to the secretion of TCGF which could activate the secondary T_c.

In contrast with the results observed with *in vitro* sensitization, it has been demonstrated by several groups that following *in vivo* sensitization, an apparent CD stimulus, as presented on thymocytes or heat-treated cells, or in fact a sonicate of the sensitizing cells, will activate the secondary response system (Okada and Henney, 1980; Ryser et al., 1978). Further experiments will be required to determine whether this difference in responsiveness of *in vivo* and *in vitro* sensitized cells reflects the fact that, following *in vivo* sensitization, there is a true "memory T_c." This problem has been discussed recently (Bach et al., 1981), so we need not consider it here.

Cloning of T Lymphocytes

Cellular immunology advanced measurably when it was recognized that lymphocytes can be grown, in some cases for very prolonged periods of time, under appropriate conditions in the presence of the supernatant of a mitogen activated or allogeneically stimulated lymphocyte culture (Ruscetti et al., 1977). A variety of different methods have been described (Gillis et al., 1978; Inouye et al., 1980a; Ruscetti et al., 1977) to produce a supernatant containing T cell growth factor (TCGF), a substance to which some refer as IL-2.

SECONDARY RESPONSE

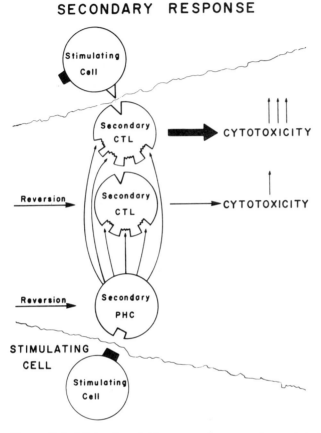

Figure 10.3. Minimal model for generating secondary cytotoxic responses from *in vivo* primed lymphocyte populations. (PHC: primed helper cell; CTL: cytotoxic T lymphocyte). For explanation, see text.

Cloning is usually accomplished in one of two ways. First, limiting numbers of responding cells are placed in wells of microtiter plates along with stimulator cells and/or "helper factor," and some days later the cells in a given well are tested for their ability to lyse the initial sensitizing cell. By obtaining a fit to the Poisson distribution, it is possible to state the probability with which the cytotoxic cells present in any given well may have originated from a single cell, i.e., represent a clone of T_c. The complex assumptions made in reaching such a conclusion cannot be discussed here. Alternatively, cells are activated in a bulk mixed lymphocyte culture for several days, after which (with or without isolation of the responding blast cells) the cells are placed at one or fewer cells per well under conditions permitting clonal expansion. Under either protocol, it is possible in the presence of TCGF and, in some cases, feeder cells of

Table 10.3. Restimulation of a Secondary Response.

Primary Response Responding cell	Initial sensitizing cell	H-2 difference	Cytotoxicity on K region disparate target
A	B	K + I	++
A	C	I	−

Secondary response	Restimulating cell		
	B	K + I	++++
	C	I	+++

various types, to obtain proliferation of the cloned cells and thus, as a first approximation, have a homogeneous population of cells fulfilling a given function.

We have concentrated much of our effort to clone human cells on obtaining cells that show primed lymphocyte typing (PLT) reactivity. The PLT test, first developed in our laboratories (Bach et al., 1977; Sheehy et al., 1975) as a cellular measure of HLA-D region encoded antigens, depends on the secondary proliferative response shown by a population of primed cells, when they are presented with the sensitizing antigen on test cells used as stimulators in PLT. A positive response of the "sensitized" cells to the test stimulating cells indicates that the test cells carry the antigen(s) recognized by the responding PLT cells.

Whereas the PLT test has provided valuable data in the past with regard to the analysis of HLA-D region encoded antigens, the ability to clone PLT reagents (Bach et al., 1979; Inouye et al., 1980b, 1981) has provided a much more powerful tool. Thus, for instance, in a situation where the initial responding and sensitizing cell donors were identical for the HLA-D antigens, as currently defined with the available homozygous typing cells, and were also identical for the serologically defined DR and MB antigens, it was possible to raise a PLT cell that still recognized an antigenic determinant(s) controlled by HLA-D and presumably present on the initial sensitizing cells and absent from the responding cells (Segall et al., 1980).

Table 10.4 shows the results of an experiment in which the PLT cell raised under such conditions was tested for its response to cells of a selected panel of individuals. As can be noted, the bulk PLT reagent generated in this manner reacted positively with cells of 14 unrelated individuals as well as the initial sensitizing cells and failed to react with a panel of cells of 14 other unrelated individuals (maximum response of 848 counts per minute). Several clones were derived from the sensitizing MLC which generated this bulk PLT reagent.

142

Table 10.4. Specificity of Restimulation of PLT Clones.

Stimulator	PLT	CL 1	CL 2	CL 3
C.S.[a]	3,342[b]	65,684	29,846	9,352
M.B.S.	2,222	212	100	15,694
F.S.	4,064	190	100	14,264
S.I.	5,980	67,678	42,948	22,902
M.H.	288	112	317	6,406
K.K.L.	2,938	161	123	12,392
E.M.	5,146	158	100	23,486
D.K.	4,312	486	192	20,514
N.J.	3,084	66,358	41,880	8,432
M.S.	2,884	320	262	13,070
W.M.	194	100	180	4,112
M.B.	4,408	176	111	16,652
K.H.	3,988	150	156	22,500
others	134-828	100-786	100-1,818	100-299

[a]Original stimulator in sensitizing culture.
[b]Median cpm of triplicate cultures.

Results using three of those clones are shown in the table. One clone showed a pattern of reactivity very similar to the bulk PLT reagent, although substantially higher counts per minute were incorporated by the cloned cells than by an equal number of cells in the bulk reagent. Very interestingly, however, two clones showed a very restricted pattern of reactivity in that they responded only to the initial sensitizing cells and cells from two of the unrelated individuals who tested positive with the bulk PLT reagent and with clone number 3. This very great discrimination by cloned PLT cells has been observed in many different situations and will no doubt allow a much finer structural analysis of determinants encoded by HLA-D than has been possible up to this time.

Similarly, the cloning of T_c has aided in antigen definition. Not only are determinants recognized that associate closely with the HLA-A and -B antigens, as defined serologically, but in some cases clones are derived which apparently recognize HLA encoded determinants that are not associated with the serologically defined determinants as currently recognized. Whether such clones will allow the definition of a CD polymorphism, i.e., the polymorphism recognized by T_c, as compared with that defined serologically, must be studied in future experiments.

Cloning of T lymphocytes has not only permitted a more exact definition of antigenic determinants, as might be expected, but has also allowed a reductionist approach to studying cellular interactions in the immune system. An elegant example of this, first described by Glasebrook and Fitch (1979), represents a clonal analysis of the phenomenon discussed earlier, where we were able to show several years ago that activation of cytotoxic T lymphocyte populations in secondary bulk cultures, i.e., after sensitization, was best accomplished by stimulating with LD antigens and thereby presumably activating the helper cells which in turn activated the T_c (Bach, 1976).

It has now been possible to show that T_c clones are not reactivated by antigens presented on the initial sensitizing cells. Rather, it is when one mixes the T_h (amplifier T cells) with the cloned T_c and then stimulates with the antigens to which the T_h are sensitized that one can obtain a marked increase in cytotoxic activity.

The findings from experiments with clones are totally in accord with the results of bulk culture experiments and closely fit the model devised to explain the earlier experiments. Nevertheless, the new results provide a much more elegant demonstration of the basic phenomenon, and demonstrate that it will be possible in the future to analyze the very complex interactions that take place at different times following the induction of immunity.

Summary

Antigenic and other requirements for the activation of cytotoxic T lymphocytes in both primary and secondary responses have been reviewed. In the primary response, activation of the precursor cytotoxic T lymphocyte requires both recognition of the antigenic determinant which it is genetically programmed to recognize on a clonal basis and help, presumably from an activated helper T lymphocyte. In the secondary response, depending on the method of sensitization (*in vitro* or *in vivo*), somewhat different stimuli and factors appear to play a role in generation of the cytotoxic response. The techniques for cloning of functionally disparate subpopulations of T lymphocytes are reviewed briefly, and some of the types of experiments made possible by cloning, including antigen definition and study of cellular interactions, are illustrated.

References

Alter, B.J. and Bach, F.H. (1979) Speculations on alternative pathways of T lymphocyte response. *Scand. J. Immunol.* 10:87–93.

Alter, B.J., Grillot-Courvalin, C., Bach, M.L., Zier, K.S., Sondel, P.M., and Bach, F.H. (1976) Secondary cell-mediated lympholysis: importance of H-2 LD and SD factors. *J. Exp. Med.* 143:1005–1014.

Bach, F.H. (1976) Differential function of MHC LD and SD determinants. In *Leukocyte Membrane Determinants Regulating Immune Reactivity*. Eijsvoogel, V.P., Roos, D., and Zeijlemaker, W.P. (eds.), New York: Academic Press, pp. 417–430.

Bach, F.H. and Alter, B.J. (1978) Alternative pathways of T lymphocyte activation. *J. Exp. Med.* 148:829–834.

Bach, F.H., Bach, M.L., and Sondel, P.M. (1976) Differential function of major histocompatibility complex antigens in T lymphocyte activation. *Nature* 259:273–281.

144

Bach, F.H., Jarrett-Toth, E.K., Benike, C.J., Shih, C.Y., Valentine, E.A., Sondel, P.M., and Bach, M.L. (1977) Primed LD typing: reagent preparation and definition of the HLA-D-region antigens. *Scand. J. Immunol.* 6:469–475.

Bach, F.H., Inouye, H., Hank, J.A., and Alter, B.J. (1979) Human T lymphocyte clones reactive in primed lymphocyte typing and cytotoxicity. *Nature* 281:307–309.

Bach, F.H., Alter, B.J., Dunlap, B., Koller, B., Orosz, C., Roehm, N., and Widmer, M. (1981) Allo-responsive T lymphocytes and their differentiation markers. *Federation Proceedings*, (in press).

Baker, P.E., Gillis, S., Ferm, M.M., and Smith, K.A. (1978) The effect of T cell growth factor on the generation of cytolytic T cells. *J. Immunol.* 121:2168–2173.

Cantor, H. and Boyse, E.A. (1975a) Functional subclasses of T lymphocytes bearing differing Ly antigens. I. The generation of functionally distinct T cell subclasses is a differentiative process independent of antigen. *J. Exp. Med.* 141:1376–1389.

Farrar, W., Mizel, J., and Farrar, J. (1980) Participation of lymphocytes activating factor (Interleukin 1) in the induction of cytotoxic T cell responses. *J. Immunol.* 124:1371–1377.

Fathman, C.G. and Hengartner, H. (1978) Clones of alloreactive T cells. *Nature* 272:617–618.

Gillis, S. and Smith, K.A. (1977) Long-term culture of tumor specific cytotoxic T cells. *Nature* 268:154–156.

Gillis, S., Ferm, M.M., Ou, W., and Smith, K.A. (1978) T cell growth factor: parameters of production and a quantitative microassay for activity. *J. Immunol.* 120:2027–2032.

Glasebrook, A.L. and Fitch, F.W. (1979) T cell lines which cooperate in generation of specific cytolytic activity. *Nature* 278:171–173.

Grillot-Courvalin, C., Alter, B.J., and Bach, F.H. (1977) Antigenic requirements for the generation of secondary cytotoxicity. *J. Immunol.* 119:1253–1259.

Inouye, H., Hank, J.A., Alter, B.J. and Bach, F.H. (1980a) TCGF production for cloning and growth of functional human T lymphocytes. *Scand. J. Immunol.* 12:149–154.

Inouye, H., Hank, J.A., Chardonnens, X., Segall, M., Alter, B.J., and Bach, F.H. (1980b) Cloned PLT reagents in the dissection of HLA-D. *J. Exp. Med.* 152:143s–155s.

Inouye, H., Hank, J., Chardonnens, X., Alter, B.J., Reinsmoen, N., Segall, M., and Bach, F.H. (1981) Cloned human T lymphocytes in PLT analysis of the HLA-D complex. *Trans. Proc.* (in press).

Larson, E.C. and Coutinho, A. (1979) The role of mitogenic lectins in T cell triggering. *Nature* 280:239–241.

Nabholz, M., Engers, H.D., Collavo, D., and North, M. (1978) Cloned T cell lines with specific cytolytic activity. *Curr. Top. Microbiol. Immunol.* 81:176–187.

Okada, M.Y. and Henney, C. (1980) The differentiation of cytotoxic T cells *in vitro*. III. The role of helper T cells from "memory" cell populations. *J. Immunol.* 125:850–857.

Orosz, C., Macphail, S., and Bach, F.H. (1981) H-2 I alloantigens and recall of memory cytotoxic responses. *J. Supramolec. Struct.* (in press).

Roehm, N., Alter, B.J., and Bach, F.H. (1981) Lyt phenotypes of alloreactive precursor and effector cytotoxic T lymphocytes. *J. Immunol.* 126:353–358.

Ruscetti, F.W., Morgan, D.A., and Gallo, R.C. (1977) Functional and morphologic characterization of human T cells continuously grown *in vitro*. *J. Immunol.* 119:131–138.

Ryser, J.-E., Ceroitini, J.-C., and Brunnek, K.T. (1978) Generation of cytotoxic T lymphocytes *in vitro*. IX. Induction of secondary CTL responses in primary long-term MLC by supernates from secondary MLC. *J. Immunol.* 120:370–377.

Scott, J., Ponzio, N., Orosz, C., and Finke, J. (1980) H-2K/H-2D and MLC and I region-associated antigens stimulated helper factor(s) involved in the generation of cytotoxic T lymphocytes. *J. Immunol.* 124:2378–2383.

Segall, M., Reinsmoen, N.L., Noreen, H.J., and Bach, F.H. (1980) Complexity of the HLA-D region studied by primed lymphocyte test. *J. Exp. Med.* 152:156s-163s.

Shaw, J., Caplan, B., Paetkau, V., Pilarski, L., Delovitch, T., and McKenzie, I. (1980) Cellular origins of co-stimulator (16-2) and its activity in cytotoxic T lymphocyte responses. *J. Immunol.* 124:2231–2239.

Sheehy, M.J., Sondel, P.M., Bach, M.L., Wank, R., and Bach, F.H. (1975) HL-A LD (lymphocyte defined) typing: a rapid assay with primed lymphocytes. *Science* 188:1308–1310.

Smith, K., Lachman, L., Oddenhein, J., and Fanata, M. (1980) The functional relationship of the interleukins. *J. Exp. Med.* 151:1551–1556.

Published 1981 by Elsevier North Holland, Inc.
Saunders, Daniels, Serrou, Rosenfeld, and Denney, eds.
FUNDAMENTAL MECHANISMS IN HUMAN CANCER IMMUNOLOGY

CHAPTER 11

Adoptive Chemoimmunotherapy of Murine Leukemia with Cells Secondarily Sensitized *In Vitro* and Cells Numerically Expanded by Culture with Interleukin 2[1]

Martin A. Cheever, Philip D. Greenberg,[2] and Alexander Fefer[3]

Division of Oncology, Department of Medicine, University of Washington School of Medicine and the Fred Hutchinson Cancer Research Center, Seattle, Washington

Adoptively transferred cells immune to tumor associated antigens have often been studied as a potential approach to experimental tumor therapy in animals. However, although immune lymphocytes are capable of using tumor cells *in vitro* and inhibiting the growth of transplanted tumors if administered either with, shortly before, or shortly after the inoculation of tumor, experimental therapy with adoptively transferred lymphocytes alone is with rare exceptions ineffective, once a tumor has become established (Rosenberg and Terry, 1977). Although transfer of immune cells provides the potential of unique anti-tumor specificity, it is limited by its inability to cope with a large tumor load. In contrast, chemotherapy can destroy a large tumor load but is limited by its relative non-specificity and toxicity.

We therefore have developed several murine models in which advanced disseminated leukemia can be eradicated by combining chemotherapy and adoptively transferred immune cells (adoptive chemoimmunotherapy) (Fefer et al., 1976). The leukemias employed have well defined antigenicity, have proven to be susceptible to immune manipulation, and are well suited for testing certain new approaches to specific immunotherapy. This report will describe some of these models and summarize our initial attempts to utilize secondary *in vitro* sensitization and long-term culture with Interleukin 2 (T cell

[1] This work was supported by Grant CA 10777 and Contract N01-CB-84247 from the National Cancer Institute of Health.
[2] Dr. Greenberg is an American Cancer Society Junior Faculty Fellow.
[3] Dr. Fefer is an American Cancer Society Professor of Clinical Oncology.

growth factor) to generate specifically immune T lymphocytes effective in adoptive tumor therapy.

FBL-3, a syngeneic Friend virus-induced leukemia of C57BL/6 origin was utilized for study. This tumor is antigenic and sensitive to specific immune attack (McCoy et al., 1967; Ting and Bonnard, 1976). If injected intraperitoneally (i.p.), as few as 100 FBL-3 cells grow progressively and kill 100% of adult mice. In the adoptive chemoimmunotherapy model, adult C57BL/6 mice are inoculated i.p. with 5×10^6 FBL-3 cells on day 0 and treated on day 5 with a combination of chemotherapy plus donor lymphocytes. At the time of therapy, mice have ascites, and disseminated tumor is detectable in both blood and spleen (Greenberg et al., 1980). The results of adoptive chemoimmunotherapy are exemplified by the cumulative results of 4 consecutive experiments presented in Figure 11.1 (Cheever et al., 1980). Mice receiving FBL-3 on day 0 and no treatment all died by day 13. Treatment with a single injection of cyclophosphamide (CY) i.p. at a dose of 180 mg/kg approximately doubles median survival time (MST), but all mice eventually died with tumor.

Immune spleen cells for therapy ($C57_{\alpha FBL}$) were derived from syngeneic C57BL/6 mice rendered immune by i.p. inoculation with irradiated FBL-3 6 to 8 weeks prior to therapy. Treatment on day 5 with $C57_{\alpha FBL}$ alone was totally

Figure 11.1. Adoptive chemoimmunotherapy of FBL-3. C57BL/6 mice inoculated i.p. on day 0 with 5×10^6 FBL-3 received either no therapy (NO TX) or treatment on day 5 with cyclophosphamide (CY ALONE) at 180 mg/kg, or 2×10^7 cells from mice immune to FBL-3 ($C57_{\alpha FBL}$ ALONE), or CY plus 5×10^6 or $2 \times 10^7 C57_{\alpha FBL}$ or CY plus 2×10^7 cells from normal non-immune mice or from mice immune to EL-4(G-), denoted as $C57_{normal}$ and $C57_{\alpha EL-4}$, respectively. The cumulative results of four experiments are presented with 32 mice per treatment group.

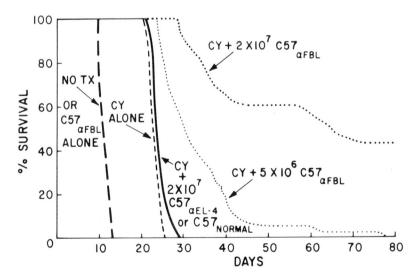

ineffective. However, as an adjunct to CY, such cells had significant dose-dependent effect. Thus, CY plus 5×10^6 C57$_{\alpha FBL}$ prolonged the MST to day 31 (p $<$ 0.01) and CY plus 2×10^7 C57$_{\alpha FBL}$ cells prolonged the MST to day 64 and cured 41% of mice (P $<$ 0.01). In contrast, normal non-immune C57BL/6 spleen cells (C57$_{normal}$) were ineffective as an adjunct to CY.

The specificity of adoptive chemoimmunotherapy with immune cells was confirmed by use of EL-4(G-) as a control (Cheever et al., 1980). EL-4(G-) is a subline of EL-4, a chemically-induced tumor of C57BL origin, and is negative for Gross cell surface antigens and mouse endogenous virus-associated surface antigen 1 and is antigenically distinct from FBL-3 and other tumors induced by Friend, Moloney, and Rauscher viruses (Herberman et al., 1974). Treatment of mice with advanced FBL-3 with CY plus cells from C57BL/6 mice immune to EL-4 (C57$_{\alpha EL-4}$) was no more effective than was treatment with CY alone (Figure 11.1). However, in concurrent reciprocal specificity experiments for the therapy of established EL-4(G-) (Figure 11.2), C57$_{\alpha EL-4}$ proved to be therapeutically effective in adoptive chemoimmunotherapy against established EL-4(G-), whereas C57$_{\alpha FBL}$ was no more effective than therapy with CY plus normal non-immune cells. Although normal non-immune cells had a modest

Figure 11.2. Adoptive chemoimmunotherapy of EL-4(G-). C57BL/6 mice inoculated i.p. on day 0 with 2×10^5 EL-4(G-) received either no therapy (NO TX) or treatment on day 5 with cyclophosphamide (CY ALONE) at 180 mg/kg, or CY plus 2×10^7 cells from normal non-immune mice (C57$_{normal}$) or mice immune to FBL-3 or EL-4, denoted as C57$_{\alpha FBL}$ and C57$_{\alpha EL-4}$, respectively. Fractions represent number of mice surviving 80 days/total.

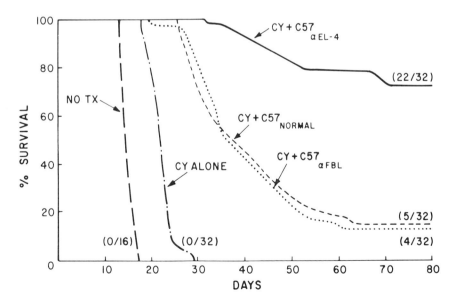

effect as an adjunct to CY, the enhancement of therapeutic efficacy resulting from *in vivo* exposure of donor to tumor was immunologically specific.

Several other characteristics of the effector cell in the FBL-3 model have been determined. To be therapeutically effective, $C57_{\alpha FBL}$ must contain T lymphocytes and must be capable of proliferation in the host (Fefer et al., 1976), as efficacy is abolished by incubation with anti-Thy plus C' and by x-irradiation to 2400 rads. Immune lymphocytes can be derived from peripheral blood or spleens of immune mice, and cells inoculated intravenously or intraperitoneally are equally effective. We have not yet identified the T lymphocyte subset(s) responsible for therapeutic efficacy and thus have not yet determined whether the anti-tumor effect of the infused immune T cells reflects direct cytotoxicity by the donor T cells themselves, or whether the donor cells help, amplify or recruit other cells, either donor or host, which may then in turn destroy the tumor.

The FBL-3 chemoimmunotherapy model was used to examine the therapeutic potential of immune cells secondarily sensitized *in vitro* (Cheever et al., 1977, 1978). Although adoptively transferred specifically immune cells are able to eradicate disseminated leukemia, animals bearing antigenic tumors often die from tumor progression despite the concurrent existence of documentable anti-tumor immunity (Hellström and Hellström, 1969). The progression of antigenic tumors may be the result of an inadequate quantity of effector cells. Theoretically, secondary sensitization *in vitro* of cells primed *in vivo* could be used to increase the number of anti-tumor effector cells and/or bypass mechanisms that would limit effective sensitization *in vivo*, such as tumor induced suppression (Friedman et al., 1976), blocking antibodies (Hellström and Hellström, 1974), or suppressor cells (Fujimoto et al., 1976).

To test the efficacy of secondary *in vitro* sensitization in generating cells effective in tumor therapy, spleen cells from mice immune to FBL-3 were cultured for 5 days with x-irradiated FBL-3. Secondary sensitization was confirmed by measuring direct anti-tumor cytotoxicity *in vitro* in a 4-hour chromium release assay, as depicted in Figure 11.3 (Cheever et al., 1978). Immune spleen cells tested directly without prior culture demonstrated no measurable cytotoxicity, whereas immune cells cultured with secondary tumor stimulation developed marked anti-tumor cytolytic reactivity and were significantly more cytotoxic than were cells cultured with control syngeneic spleen cells. The specificity of the cytolytic reactivity induced by culturing *in vivo* primed cells with tumor was confirmed by testing these cells against irrelevant tumor targets.

The *in vivo* efficacy of such secondarily sensitized cells was concurrently examined in the adoptive chemoimmunotherapy of FBL-3 (Figure 11.4; Cheever et al., 1978). Mice inoculated with FBL-3 and treated on day 5 with CY alone had an MST of 25 days. As an adjunct to CY, cells from mice immunized *in vivo* with FBL-3 ($C57_{\alpha FBL}$) prolonged the MST to day 35. Primed cells which were secondarily sensitized *in vitro* by culture with tumor

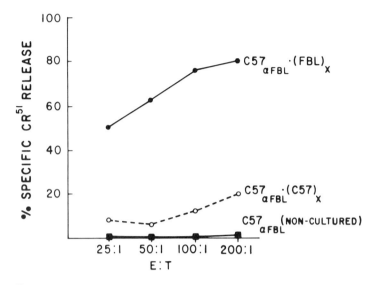

Figure 11.3. *In vitro* cytolytic reactivity of cells secondarily sensitized *in vitro*. Spleen cells from C57BL/6 mice immunized *in vivo* to FBL-3 [C57$_{\alpha FBL}$ (non-cultured)] were cultured for 5 days with x-irradiated FBL-3 [C57$_{\alpha FBL}$·(FBL)$_x$] or x-irradiated C57BL/6 spleen cells [C57$_{\alpha FBL}$·(C57)$_x$] and were tested for cytotoxicity to tumor in a 4-hour chromium release assay at variable effector to target (E:T) ratios.

were more effective and prolonged the median survival to day 52. In contrast, CY plus primed cells cultured without tumor were less effective and prolonged the MST to only day 27. Normal cells cultured with tumor (not depicted) were ineffective. Thus, *in vivo* primed cells that were effective in therapy were rendered significantly more effective by secondary sensitization *in vitro* (P < 0.01). In contrast, *in vivo* primed cells cultured without secondary sensitization were significantly less effective (P < 0.01).

Two problems which limit the efficacy of this culture system have been identified. First, culture-induced suppressor cells which are generated during the sensitization period co-exist with anti-tumor effector cells and are capable of inhibiting their *in vivo* therapeutic efficacy (Greenberg et al., 1979). Secondly, although cells secondarily sensitized *in vitro* for 5 days are therapeutically more effective on a cell for cell basis than are non-cultured primed cells, less than 30% of cells remain viable, and therefore the net change in therapeutic benefit is minimal (Cheever et al., 1981b).

Culture-induced suppressor cells have been described by others as radiosensitive T lymphocytes generated during *in vitro* culture of normal spleen cells which non-specifically suppress *in vitro* allogeneic responses (Hodes et al., 1977). We have shown that tumor immune cells cultured *in vitro* with or without tumor for 5 days contain similar non-specific suppressor cells (Greenberg et al., 1979).

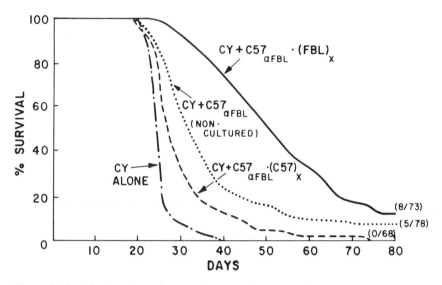

Figure 11.4. Adoptive chemoimmunotherapy of FBL-3 with cells secondarily sensitized *in vitro*. C57BL/6 mice inoculated i.p. with 5×10^6 FBL-3 on day 0 were treated on day 5 with cyclophosphamide (CY ALONE) at 180 mg/kg or with CY plus 5×10^6 non-cultured immune cells ($C57_{\alpha FBL}$) or CY plus 5×10^6 immune spleen cells cultured for 5 days with x-irradiated FBL-3 or x-irradiated C57BL/6 spleen cells denoted as $C57_{\alpha FBL} \cdot (FBL)_x$ and $C57_{\alpha FBL} \cdot (C57)_x$, respectively. Numbers represent number of mice surviving 80 days/total.

The effect on therapy of suppressor cells generated during secondary sensitization *in vitro* of tumor immune cells could not be directly tested in mixing experiments because of the co-existing anti-tumor effector cells. However, the effect of cultured normal cells on therapy was determined (Figure 11.5; Greenberg et al., 1979). Mice receiving no therapy all died by day 13 and therapy with CY alone or CY plus cultured normal cells prolonged the MST to day 25. Therapy with CY plus 5×10^6 cells secondarily sensitized *in vitro* further prolonged the MST to day 64. However their efficacy was significantly diminished ($P < 0.001$) by the concurrent inoculation at a separate i.p. site of an equal number of cultured normal cells. Thus, secondarily sensitized cells were made therapeutically less effective by the *in vivo* presence of culture-induced suppressor cells.

Thus, although secondary *in vitro* sensitization renders tumor primed spleen cells more effective in therapy, this culture system also generates culture-induced suppressor cells; and the *in vivo* therapeutic effect of the secondarily sensitized cells is diminished by concurrent inoculation of similar culture-induced suppressor cells. The *in vivo* suppression of effector cells from secondary *in vitro* sensitization cultures implies that secondarily sensitized cells must proliferate

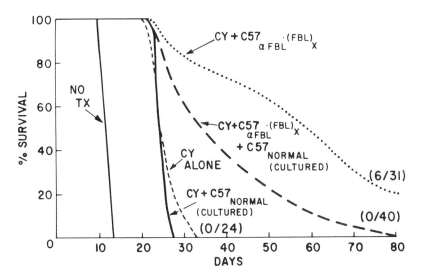

Figure 11.5. Effect of culture-induced suppressor cells on chemoimmunotherapy of FBL-3 with cells secondarily sensitized *in vitro*. C57BL/6 mice inoculated i.p. on day 0 with 5×10^6 FBL-3 received either no therapy (NO TX), treatment on day 5 with cyclophosphamide (CY ALONE) at 180 mg/kg, or treatment with CY plus 5×10^6 primed cells secondarily sensitized *in vitro* by culture for 5 days with x-irradiated FBL-3 [C57$_{\alpha FBL}$·(FBL)$_x$], 5×10^6 normal spleen cells cultured for 5 days [C57$_{normal}$ (cultured)] or both 5×10^6 secondarily sensitized cells and 5×10^6 cultured normal cells. Fractions represent number of mice surviving 80 days/total.

in vivo to be effective. This is consistent with our findings that x-irradiation of these cells inhibits their *in vivo* efficacy without affecting *in vitro* cytotoxicity (Greenberg et al., 1979).

To overcome the problem of inefficient expansion of effector cells during secondary *in vitro* sensitization, we have initiated studies to test the efficacy of cells numerically expanded *in vitro* by culture with T cell growth factor, now named Interleukin 2 (Mizel and Farrer, 1979). Culture with Interleukin 2 provides the potential of supplying large numbers of tumor-specific T lymphocytes.

Interleukin 2 (IL 2), a soluble protein produced by stimulated amplifier T lymphocytes (Wagner and Röllinghoff, 1978; Shaw et al., 1980), regulates T lymphocyte function, at least *in vitro*, through control of clonal expansion (Ruscetti et al., 1977; Gillis and Smith, 1977; Gillis et al., 1978). Activated T lymphocytes are induced to proliferate *in vitro* by IL 2 and can be maintained continuously even without the continued presence of activated antigen (Smith et al., 1979a; Bonnard et al., 1979). By continually supplementing cultures with IL 2, activated lymphocytes can be serially grown *in vitro* to large numbers

(Gillis and Smith, 1977; Rosenberg et al., 1978). Lymphocytes cytotoxic to alloantigens (Gillis and Smith, 1977; Nabholz et al., 1978), minor histocompatibility antigens (von Boehmer et al., 1979) or tumors (Gillis and Smith, 1977; Ryser et al., 1979; and Zarling and Bach, 1979), as well as noncytotoxic T lymphocytes expressing either helper function (Watson, 1979; Schreier and Tees, 1980) or an unknown function (Baker et al., 1979) have been maintained long-term in such cultures, some for greater than one year. These studies have suggested that culture with IL 2 may offer the means for generating large numbers of specific T lymphocytes of different functional subclasses.

Although long-term cultured T lymphocytes have been shown to be cytotoxic to tumor *in vitro* and have been shown to inhibit the growth of syngeneic tumors in a Winn assay, in which tumor and lymphocytes are mixed together *in vitro* and inoculated together *in vivo* (Smith et al., 1979b), it has not been shown that all the requisite subpopulations required for successful adoptive therapy survive long-term culture or that such cells are capable of mediating tumor therapy.

To test the efficacy and specificity of such long-term cultured T lymphocytes in adoptive therapy, spleen cells from mice immunized *in vivo* with FBL-3 or EL-4(G-) were activated by secondary sensitization *in vitro* by culture for 7 days with the sensitizing tumor. They were then numerically expanded *in vitro* through day 19 by repeated exposure to supernatants from Con A stimulated lymphocytes containing IL 2 (Cheever et al., 1981a).

Nineteen days of culture was chosen in initial experiments since at 3–4 weeks following initiation of culture, cells undergo a culture "crisis"—an unexplained culture phenomenon in which apparent growth rate falls off precipitiously and most cells die (Watson, 1979). After several weeks of net cell loss, some cultures recover with the resumption of a rapid growth rate. The cellular basis for this "crisis" has not been explained. However, since cells surviving this period may have markedly altered functional properies, we chose to first examine the therapeutic efficacy and specificity of cells tested prior to "crisis."

Activation of tumor specific cytotoxic T lymphocytes following 7 day culture of *in vivo* immunized spleen cells with the immunizing tumor was confirmed as described previously by measuring cytotoxicity *in vitro* (Table 11.1). Cells immune to FBL-3 and cultured for 7 days with irradiated FBL-3 became specifically cytotoxic to FBL-3 and not EL-4, and cells immune to EL-4 and cultured with irradiated EL-4 became specifically cytotoxic to EL-4 and not FBL-3.

Following culture for 7 days, cells were harvested, washed, recultured, and induced to proliferate through day 19 by repeated supplementation of media with supernatants from Con A stimulated lymphocytes containing IL 2. Following a lag period of several days, cells grew progressively and expanded in number by greater than 700%. Growth remained exquisitely dependent on

Table 11.1. Specific Cytolytic Reactivity Following *in Vitro* Activation and Long-Term Culture.

Responder	Stimulator	Day of culture	FBL-3 20:1	FBL-3 5:1	EL-4(G−) 20:1	EL-4(G−) 5:1
C57$_{normal}$	Non-cultured	0	−1	0	−1	0
C57$_{\alpha FBL}$	Non-cultured	0	−1	−1	−2	−1
C57$_{\alpha EL-4}$	Non-cultured	0	−1	0	1	0
C57$_{normal}$	(C57)$_x$	7	2	1	1	1
C57$_{normal}$	(FBL)$_x$	7	5	2	2	1
C57$_{normal}$	(EL-4)$_x$	7	7	3	5	2
C57$_{\alpha FBL}$	(C57)$_x$	7	1	1	1	1
C57$_{\alpha FBL}$	(FBL)$_x$	7	38	16	0	−3
C57$_{\alpha FBL}$	(EL-4)$_x$	7	4	1	4	2
C57$_{\alpha EL-4}$	(C57)$_x$	7	1	1	1	0
C57$_{\alpha EL-4}$	(FBL)$_x$	7	4	3	2	1
C57$_{\alpha EL-4}$	(EL-4)$_x$	7	3	−2	26	9
C57$_{\alpha FBL}$	(FBL)$_x$	19	61	40	13	7
C57$_{\alpha EL-4}$	(EL-4)$_x$	19	10	8	34	22

Note: Spleen cells from normal non-immune C57BL/6 mice (C57$_{normal}$), or from C57BL/6 mice which had been immunized *in vivo* with FBL-3 (C57$_{\alpha FBL}$) or with EL-4(G−) (C57$_{\alpha EL-4}$) were cultured for 7 days with irradiated (C57)$_x$, (FBL)$_x$, or (EL-4)$_x$. Then selected groups were further cultured to day 19 and induced to proliferate by supplementing media with Interleukin 2. Cytotoxicity against FBL-3 and EL-4(G−) was determined on days 7 and 19 in a 4-hr chromium release assay at effector to target ratios of 20:1 and 5:1. The data represent the means of 2 experiments.

repeated addition of IL 2, since cells similarly cultured without IL 2 supplementation progressively died and less than 1% remained viable on day 19. Following culture for 19 days, the expanded cell populations remained specifically cytotoxic to the immunizing tumor (Table 11.1).

These long-term cultured cells were concurrently tested *in vivo* in adoptive chemoimmunotherapy. As an adjunct to CY, therapy of FBL-3 with 2×10^7 non-cultured C57$_{\alpha FBL}$ cells prolonged the median survival to day 48, and an equal number of C57$_{\alpha FBL}$ which had been activated *in vitro* and numerically expanded by culture with IL 2 for 19 days prolonged the median survival to day 62 (Figure 11.6). Thus, following *in vitro* manipulation for 19 days, the resultant cells were expanded in number and were able to mediate *in vivo* therapy. To confirm specificity, cells immune to EL-4 were also tested. Non-cultured C57$_{\alpha EL-4}$ were totally ineffective and C57$_{\alpha EL-4}$ activated by culture with irradiated EL-4, then numerically expanded *in vitro*, demonstrated

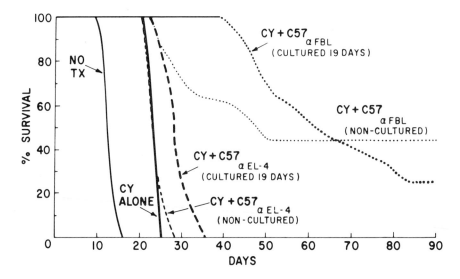

Figure 11.6. Adoptive chemoimmunotherapy of FBL-3 with long-term cultured cells. C57BL/6 mice inoculated i.p. on day 0 with 5×10^6 FBL-3 received either no therapy (NO TX), treatment on day 5 with cyclophosphamide (CY ALONE) at 180 mg/kg, or treatment with CY plus 2×10^7 cells from mice immunized *in vivo* to FBL-3 [C57$_{\alpha FBL}$ (non-cultured)] or EL-4(G-) [C57$_{\alpha EL-4}$ (non-cultured)] or CY plus 2×10^7 similar cells sequentially immunized *in vivo*, secondarily sensitized *in vitro*, and numerically expanded by culture through day 19 with Interleukin 2, denoted as [C57$_{\alpha FBL}$ (cultured 19 days)] and [C57$_{\alpha EL-4}$ (cultured 19 days)], respectively. The cumulative results of these experiments are represented with 16 mice per treatment group.

only a small effect. In concurrent experiments for the therapy of EL-4 (Figure 11.7) long-term cultured C57$_{\alpha EL-4}$ were effective, and long-term cultured C57$_{\alpha FBL}$ were ineffective. Thus, the *in vivo* therapeutic efficacy of long-term cultured lymphocytes was specific (Cheever et al., 1981a).

Previously, the therapeutic potential of *in vitro* sensitization has been markedly limited by problems apparently inherent to the technique, such as inefficient expansion of effector cells (Plata and Jongeneel, 1977), progressive loss of cells during culture (Cheever et al., 1981b), and the generation during culture of suppressor cells which inhibit tumor therapy (Greenberg et al., 1979). The current results underscore the therapeutic potential for IL 2 induced cell growth. With IL 2 induced cell growth in conjunction with recently developed techniques for T lymphocyte subset identification and selection and for cloning of continuously proliferating cells, it may ultimately be possible to modify conditions *in vitro*, so as to preferentially enhance the production of large numbers of the desired effector cells and to eliminate the generation of cells which exert a deleterious effect on therapy.

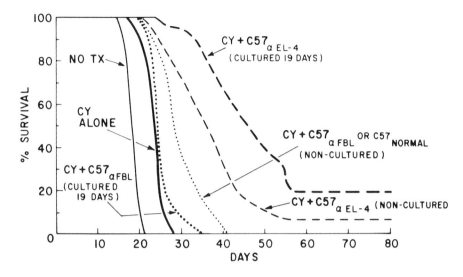

Figure 11.7. Adoptive chemoimmunotherapy of EL-4(G-) with long-term cultured cells. C57BL/6 inoculated i.p. on day 0 with 2×10^5 EL-4(G-) received either no therapy (NO TX), treatment on day 5 with cyclophosphamide (CY ALONE) at 180 mg/kg, or treatment with CY plus 2×10^7 cells from mice immunized *in vivo* to FBL-3 [C57$_{\alpha FBL}$ (non-cultured)] or EL-4(G-) [C57$_{\alpha EL-4}$ (non-cultured)] or CY plus 2×10^7 similar cells sequentially immunized *in vivo*, secondarily sensitized *in vitro*, and numerically expanded by culture through day 19 with Interleukin 2, denoted as [C57$_{\alpha FBL}$ (cultured 19 days)] and [C57$_{\alpha EL-4}$ (cultured 19 days)], respectively. The cumulative results of these experiments are represented with 16 mice per treatment group.

References

Baker, P.E., Gillis, S., and Smith, K.A. (1979) Monoclonal cytolytic T cell lines. *J. Exp. Med.* 149:273.

von Boehmer, H., Hengartner, H., Nabholz, M., Lernhardt, W., Schreier, M.H., and Haas, W. (1979) Fine specificity of a continuously growing killer cell clone specific for H-Y antigen. *Eur. J. Immunol.* 9:592.

Bonnard, G.D., Yasaka, K., and Jacobson, D. (1979) Ligand-activated T cell growth factor-induced proliferation: absorption of T cell growth factor by activated T cells. *J. Immunol.* 123:2704.

Cheever, M.A., Kempf, R.A., and Fefer, A. (1977) Tumor neutralization, immunotherapy, and chemoimmunotherapy of a Friend leukemia with cells secondarily sensitized *in vitro*. *J. Immunol.* 119:714.

Cheever, M.A., Greenberg, P.D., and Fefer, A. (1978) Tumor neutralization, immunotherapy, and chemoimmunotherapy of a Friend leukemia with cells secondarily sensitized *in vitro*. II. Comparison of cells cultured with and without tumor to non-cultured immune cells. *J. Immunol.* 121:2220.

Cheever, M.A., Greenberg, P.D., and Fefer, A. (1980) Specificity of adoptive chemoimmunotherapy of established syngeneic tumors. *J. Immunol.* 125:711.

158

Cheever, M.A., Greenberg, P.D., and Fefer, A. (1981a) Specific adoptive therapy of established leukemia with syngeneic lymphocytes sequentially immunized *in vivo* and *in vitro* and nonspecifically expanded by culture with Interleukin 2. *J. Immunol.*, in press.

Cheever, M.A., Greenberg, P.D., and Fefer, A. (1981b) Chemoimmunotherapy of a Friend leukemia with cells secondarily sensitized *in vitro*: effect of culture duration on therapeutic efficacy. *J. Natl. Cancer Inst.*, in press.

Fefer, A., Einstein, Jr., A.B., Cheever, M.A., and Berenson, J.R. (1976) Models for syngeneic adoptive chemoimmunotherapy of murine leukemias. *Ann. N.Y. Acad. Sci.* 276:573.

Friedman, H., Specter, S., Kamo, I., and Kately, J. (1976) Tumor-associated immunosuppressive factors. *Ann. N.Y. Acad. Sci.* 276:417.

Fujimoto, S., Greene, M.I., and Sehon, A.H. (1976) Regulation of the immune response to tumor antigens. I. Immunosuppressor cells in tumor-bearing hosts. *J. Immunol.* 116:800.

Gillis, S. and Smith, K.A. (1977) Long-term culture of tumor-specific cytotoxic T cells. *Nature* 268:154.

Gillis, S., Ferm, M.M., Ou, W., and Smith, K.A. (1978) T cell growth factor: parameters of production and a quantitative microassay for activity. *J. Immunol.* 120:2027.

Greenberg, P.D., Cheever, M.A., and Fefer, A. (1979) Suppression of the *in vitro* secondary response to syngeneic tumor and of *in vivo* tumor therapy with immune cells by culture-induced suppressor cells. *J. Immunol.* 123:515.

Greenberg, P.D., Cheever, M.A., and Fefer, A. (1980) Detection of early and delayed anti-tumor effects following curative adoptive chemoimmunotherapy of established leukemias. *Cancer Res.* 40:4428.

Hellström, K.E. and Hellström, I. (1969) Cellular immunity against tumor antigens. *Adv. Cancer Res.* 12:167.

Hellström, K.E. and Hellström, I. (1974) Lymphocyte-mediated cytotoxicity and blocking serum activity to tumor antigens. *Adv. Immunol.* 18:209.

Herberman, R.B., Aoki, T., Nunn, M., Lavrin, D.H., Soares, N., Gazdar, A., Holden, H., and Chang, K.S.S. (1974) Specificity of Cr release cytotoxicity of lymphocytes immune to murine sarcoma virus. *J. Natl. Cancer Inst.* 53:1103.

Hodes, R.J., Nadler, L.M., and Hathcock, K.S. (1977) Regulatory mechanisms in cell-mediated immune responses. III. Antigen-specific and non-specific suppressor activities generated during MLC. *J. Immunol.* 119:961.

McCoy, J.L., Fefer, A., and Glynn, J.P. (1967) Comparative studies on the induction of transplantation resistance in BALB/c and C57BL/6 mice in three murine leukemia systems. *Cancer Res.* 27:1743.

Mizel, S.B. and Farrar, J.J. (1979) Revised nomenclature for antigen-non-specific T cell proliferation and helper factors. *Cell Immunol.* 48:433.

Nabholz, M., Engers, H.D., Collavo, D., and North, M. (1978) Cloned T cell lines with specific cytolytic activity. *Current Topics in Microbiol. and Immunol.* 81:176.

Plata, F. and Jongeneel, C.V. (1977) Characterization of effector lymphocytes associated with immunity to murine sarcoma virus (MSV)-induced tumors. II. Repeated stimulation and proliferation *in vitro* of specific cytolytic T lymphocytes. *J. Immunol.* 119:623.

Rosenberg, S.A. and Terry, W.D. (1977) Passive immunotherapy of cancer in animals and man. *Adv. Cancer Res.* 25:323.

Rosenberg, S.A., Schwarz, S., and Spiess, P.J. (1978) *In vitro* growth of murine T cells. II. Growth of *in vitro* sensitized cells cytotoxic for alloantigen. *J. Immunol.* 121:1951.

Ruscetti, F.W., Morgan, D.A., and Gallo, R.C. (1977) Functional and morphologic characterization of human T cells continuously grown *in vitro*. *J. Immunol.* 119:131.

Ryser, J.-E., Cerottini, J.-C., and Brunner, K.T. (1979) Cell-mediated immunity to antigens associated with murine sarcoma virus-induced tumors: augmentation of cytolytic T lymphocyte activity by successive specific and non-specific stimulation *in vitro*. *Eur. J. Immunol.* 9:179.

Schreier, M.H. and Tees, R. (1980) Clonal induction of helper T cells: conversion of specific signals into non-specific signals. *Int. Archs. Allergy Appl. Immun.* 61:227.

Shaw, J., Caplan, B., Paetkau, V., Pilarski, L.M., Delovitch, T.L., and McKenzie, I.F.C. (1980) Cellular origins of co-stimulator (IL 2) and its activity in cytotoxic T lymphocyte responses. *J. Immunol.* 124:2231.

Smith, K.A., Gillis, S., Baker, P.E., McKenzie, D., and Ruscetti, F.W. (1979a) T cell growth factor mediated T cell proliferation. *Ann. N.Y. Acad. Sci.* 332:423.

Smith, K.A., Gillis, S., and Baker, P. (1979b) The inhibition of *in vivo* tumor growth by cytotoxic T cell lines. *Proc. of Am. Assoc. Ca. Res.* 20:93 (Abstract).

Ting, C.C. and Bonnard, G.D. (1976) Cell-mediated immunity to Friend virus-induced leukemia. IV. *In vitro* generation of primary and secondary cell-mediated cytotoxic responses. *J. Immunol.* 116:1419.

Wagner, H. and Röllinghoff, M. (1978) T-T cell interaction during *in vitro* cytotoxic allograft responses. I. Soluble products from activated Ly 1[+]T cells trigger autonomously antigen-primed Ly 23[+] T cells to cell proliferation and cytolytic activity. *J. Exp. Med.* 148:1523.

Watson, J. (1979) Continuous proliferation of murine antigen-specific helper T lymphocytes in culture. *J. Exp. Med.* 150:1510.

Zarling, J.M. and Bach, F.H. (1979) Continuous culture of T cells cytotoxic for autologous human leukemia cells. *Nature* 280:685.

Published 1981 by Elsevier North Holland, Inc.
Saunders, Daniels, Serrou, Rosenfeld, and Denney, eds.
FUNDAMENTAL MECHANISMS IN HUMAN CANCER IMMUNOLOGY

CHAPTER 12

Regulation of Natural Killer Cell Activity[1]

Hans Wigzell, Anders Örn, Magnus Gidlund, Inger Axberg, and Urban Ramstedt

Department of Immunology, Uppsala University Biomedical Center, Box 582, S-751 23, Uppsala, Sweden

Natural killer cells are "spontaneously" occurring cells endowed with a selective ability to lyse certain but not other target cells *in vitro* (Kiessling et al., 1975; Herberman et al., 1975). Several sets of experiments (summarized in Kiessling and Wigzell, 1981) appear to indicate that natural killer (NK) cells can also function *in vivo* in a presumably lytic manner. NK cells attracted attention at the time of their discovery because of their potential capacity to function *in vivo* as cells protecting against malignant disease. Evidence that NK cells contribute to oncogenic resistance is very scarce. Some suggestive preliminary data support the hypothesis (Loutit, 1980), but more experiments are required for confirmation. NK cells have been shown to be able to fulfill the necessary minimal requirements for a cell type which may function *in vivo* against spontaneous tumors. We will briefly discuss here some aspects of the *in vivo* and *in vitro* regulation of NK cells which bear upon their possible biological roles.

Distribution of NK Activity with Regard to Organ and Age of the Individual: Suppressing and Enhancing Humoral Factors

In particular in the mouse, to a lesser degree in the rat, and least conspicuously in humans, age influences the expression of NK activity (for summary, see Herberman, 1980). It has been found by several workers (see Kiessling and Wigzell, 1981, for summary) that in mice there is no or little NK activity before

[1] This work was supported by the Swedish Cancer Society and the NIH-Grant R01-CA-26752-01.

2–3 weeks of age, and that activity starts to decline after 3 months of age to reach quite low values in the aging animal. This drop in NK activity seems to occur in all lymphoid organs, whereas a select suppression, e.g., in the spleen, may occur subsequent to treatment with certain agents (Ojo et al., 1978). The sharpness of the "peak" of NK activity in relation to age is in part under genetic control. Whereas mouse strains such as AKR have quite a narrow peak (which makes the strain on the average a low level NK strain), other strains such as NZB display high activity even in the aging animals. One typical feature of NK cells is the characteristic profile of their distribution in various organs. Spleen and peripheral blood are rich in NK cells in every species analyzed, whereas lymph nodes and bone marrow have low NK activity, and thymus normally have undetectable activity. Possible explanations of this distribution profile will be presented later.

Variations in NK activity in relation to age have been shown to depend on the activity of stem cells in the bone marrow, as judged by chimera studies (Haller et al., 1977). Thus, stem cells from young donors transplanted into irradiated old individuals will lead to eventually high NK levels, whereas "old" marrow transplanted into irradiated young recipients will result in levels typical of old mice. One factor of major importance in the regulation of NK cells is interferon (Trinchieri et al., 1977, Gidlund et al., 1978), which appears to drastically enhance NK activity. Changes in endogenous levels of interferon, as regulated by external or internal stimuli for interferon production, may help to explain the age related profile of NK cells. Since levels of endogenous interferon are too low to be detectable by interferon assays, this possibility can not be directly addressed at present. One alternative approach is to search for NK suppressing factors, in particular in the newborn animal, where the absence of activity is close to absolute. We have found that one protein produced by certain tumors, namely alpha-fetoprotein, inhibited the ability of certain interferon inducers to initiate NK increases *in vitro* in adult spleen cells (Örn et al., 1980). Furthermore, the very same interferon inducer that failed (respectively functioned) to increase the NK levels of adult spleen cells in presence of AFP, also failed (functioned) in the absence of added AFP, when tested on newborn spleen cells. Table 12.1 presents these results in summary form. The data indicate that during the neonatal period, certain humoral substances may exist which could, at least in part, explain the low levels of NK activity during this time of ontogeny. It is intriguing that the interferon inducer, poly-I:C, which failed to initiate NK activity in the presence of AFP, is presumed to exert its activity largely via macrophages (Djeu et al., 1979). The activity of AFP, when acting as an immunosuppressive molecule for certain but not all T cell immune systems, may well also be mediated by adherent cells of an antigen-presenting nature (Peck et al., 1978).

It is thus clear that several humoral substances may enhance or suppress NK activities *in vitro* (and in several cases, also *in vivo*), and that local production of such factors may in part explain the organ distribution pattern of NK cells.

Table 12.1. Influence of Age of AFP on the Ability of Interferon or Interferon Inducers to Enhance NK Activity.

Target cells	AFP added	Inducer added	NK enhancement[a]
Newborn spleen	–	Interferon	++
_"_	–	NDV[b]	++
_"_	–	Poly-I:C	–
Adult spleen	–	Interferon	++++
_"_	–	NDV[b]	++++
_"_	–	Poly-I:C	++++
_"_	+	Interferon	++++
_"_	+	NDV[b]	++++
_"_	+	Poly-I:C	–

(Source: For conditions, see Örn et al., 1980.)

[a]Degree of enhancement in relation to lytic units induced.

[b]NDV = Newcastle Disease Virus

A summary of such factors can be studied in a recent book (Herberman, 1980).

In the following paragraphs, we will deal in more detail with the single most important enhancing molecule for NK cells so far found, namely interferon(s). It is now well established by many workers that interferon can function both *in vitro* and *in vivo* as an enhancing agent for NK activity. In our own studies, we have found that the action of interferon on NK cells is very rapid. It is caused by a direct reaction between the outer surface of NK cells (or pre-NK cells) and interferon (Senik et al., 1980). Thereafter, RNA and protein synthesis are required to allow the development of enhanced NK activity. Although this question is somewhat disputed, our data indicate that any interferon species can induce NK activity within the same species, but that immune interferon requires a longer time period to induce NK activity, compared to other types of interferon, just as it requires longer to induce interference with viral replication (Örn, unpublished experiments). Repeated administration of interferon *in vivo* can be shown to maintain high levels of NK activity in human beings over several months (Einhorn, 1980). *If* interferon treatment indeed can be shown to result in significant inhibition of tumor growth in man, it may be worthwhile to explore further the possibility of NK participation in such human systems.

Although the action of interferon can be shown to occur directly on NK cells (or pre-NK cells), debate is still raging as to the relative importance of its enhancement of the lytic ability of "mature" NK cells, as compared with its possible recruitment of pre-NK cells into lytic ability (for details, see Herberman, 1980). Our own interpretation of the available data would indicate that interferon can act upon both of these target groups, and the relative importance of each activity depends on the relative proportions of mature versus immature NK cells in the cell populations under study.

Table 12.2. Evidence that NK Cells are More Effective Against Cells of the Same Lineage but at an Earlier Stage of Differentiation.

Normal Cells

(a) *Thymocytes:* Immature cortical thymocytes are susceptible to NK lysis (Hansson et al., 1979). Fetal human and mouse thymocytes are more susceptible to NK cells than adult cells (Hansson et al., 1981).

(b) *Bone marrow cells:* Fetal bone marrow cells are more susceptible to NK lysis than adult marrow (Hansson et al., 1981). This fraction of marrow cells seems to contain the stem cells for colony formation (Hansson et al., to be published).

Malignant Cells

(a) *Teratocarcinomas:* Embryonic carcinoma cells are NK susceptible but endodermal lines derived from these cells are resistant (Stern et al., 1980). Controlled differentiation of embryonic carcinoma cells results in significant reduction in NK susceptibility (Stern et al., to be published).

(b) *Erythroid leukemia:* The human K562 line is highly susceptible to NK lysis. *In vitro* induced or spontaneous differentiation is always associated with a decrease in NK susceptibility (Gidlund et al., 1981). Likewise, Friend virus erythroid leukemia cells undergoing differentiation to lose their NK susceptibility (Gidlund et al., to be published).

(c) *Histiocytoma:* The human U937 line is highly NK susceptible but will lose this sensitivity upon differentiation *in vitro,* which will parallel appearance of Fc receptors and K cell activity (Gidlund et al., 1981).

The Specificity of NK Cells in Relation to the Activity and Distribution Pattern *in Vivo*

NK cells are well known to selectively lyse certain but not all kinds of target cells *in vitro* (for a discussion of their specificity, see Kiessling and Wigzell, 1981). Their fine specificity and its determination at the effector and the target cells is still a matter of argument. Protein as well as carbohydrate moieties have been suggested to play important roles in this respect (Roder, 1980; Durdik et al., 1980). During the last few years, we have been more and more impressed by the relative preference of NK cells to attack in a lytic manner "primitive" cells in relation to more differentiated cells. This preference, which may add to our understanding of the normal distribution pattern of NK cells *in vivo*, was first noted in some studies on the relative NK susceptibility of immature cortical thymocytes in mice (Hansson et al., 1979). The appearance of such NK normal targets was shown to be under genetic control. Low NK strains had high numbers of NK susceptible cortical thymocytes, while the opposite was true for high NK strains. Measures leading to an increase in *in vivo* NK activity were associated with a decrease in NK susceptible targets, indicating some common regulatory basis. Also, fetal bone marrow from human beings as well as fetal human thymocytes were also found to be more susceptible to NK attack than their corresponding cell populations obtained from adult human beings (Hansson et al., 1981). Similar results were obtained when studying tumor cells (Stern et al., 1980, Gidlund et al., 1981), where it could be shown that clones derived from a particular tumor line showing evidence of a more highly differentiated stage of function displayed a decrease in NK susceptibility. The tumor lines studied included human leukemias and histiocytomas as well as murine erythroid leukemias and embryonic carcinomas. Table 12.2 summarizes the evidence for the hypothesis that NK cells are prone to react even with certain autochthonous normal cells, provided they are of a "primitive" nature.

From the above, it is clear that the presence of normal cells able to function as targets for NK cells within the body may in itself have drastic consequences on the distribution patterns and detectability of NK cells for *in vitro* tests. Such natural "cold target" inhibition could thus well explain the absence of or very low levels of NK activity in the thymus, and low levels in bone marrow populations. In fact, suppressor cells that can be shown to exist by *in vitro* assays for NK cells (for summary, see Herberman, 1980) may well (among other activities) have the ability to function as competing targets for the NK effector cells. Be that as it may, the availability of controlled differentiation systems *in vitro* which allow the follow-up of cloned cells would provide a powerful tool for further analysis of NK cell specificity.

References

Djeu, J.Y., Heinbaugh, J.A., Holden, H.T., and Herberman, R.B. (1979) Role of macrophages in the augmentation of mouse natural killer cell activity by poly-I:C and interferon. *J. Immunol.* 122:182–188.

Durdik, J., Beck, B.N., and Henney, C.S. (1980) The use of lymphoma variants differing in their susceptibility to NK cell-mediated lysis to analyze NK cell-target cell interactions. In *Natural Cell-Mediated Immunity Against Tumors*. Herberman, R.B. (ed.), New York: Academic Press, pp. 805–818.

Einhorn, S. (1980) Enhancement of human NK activity by interferon (*in vivo* and *in vitro* studies). In *Natural Cell-Mediated Immunity Against Tumors*. Herberman, R.B. (ed.), New York: Academic Press, pp. 529–536.

Gidlund, M., Örn, A., Wigzell, H., Senik, A., and Gresser, I. (1978) Enhanced NK activity in mice injected with interferon and interferon inducers. *Nature* 273:759–760.

Gidlund, M., Örn, A., Pattengale, P., Wigzell, H., and Nilsson, K. (1981) Induction of differentiation in two human tumor cell lines is paralleled by a decrease in NK susceptibility. Submitted for publication.

Haller, O., Kiessling, R., Örn, A., and Wigzell, H. (1977) Generation of natural killer cells. An autonomous function of the bone marrow. *J. Exp. Med.* 145:1411–1416.

Hansson, M. and Kiessling, R. (1981) Human fetal thymus and bone marrow contain target cells for natural killer cells. Submitted for publication.

Hansson, M., Kärre, K., Kiessling, R., Roder, J.C., Andersson, B., and Häyry, P. (1979) Natural NK cell targets in the mouse thymus; characteristics of the sensitive cell population. *J. Immunol.* 123:765–773.

Herberman, R.B. (ed.) (1980) *Natural Cell-Mediated Immunity Against Tumors*. New York: Academic Press.

Herberman, R.B., Nunn, M.E., and Lavrin, D.H. (1975) Natural cytotoxic reactivity of mouse lymphoid cells against syngeneic and allogeneic tumors. I. Distribution of reactivity and specificity. *Int. J. Cancer* 16:216–229.

Kiessling, R. and Wigzell, H. (1981) Surveillance of primitive cells by natural killer cells. In *Current Topics in Microbiology and Immunology*. Haller, O. (ed.), in press.

Kiessling, R., Klein, E., and Wigzell, H. (1975) Natural killer cells in the mouse. I. Cytotoxic cells with specificity for mouse Moloney leukemia cells. Specificity and distribution according to genotype. *Eur. J. Immunol.* 5:112–117.

Loutit, J.F., Townsend, K.M., and Knowles, J.F. (1980) Tumor surveillance in beige mice. *Nature* 285:66.

Ojo, E., Haller, O., Kimura, A., and Wigzell, H. (1978) An analysis of the conditions allowing *Corynebacterium parvum* in mice to cause either augmentation of inhibition of natural cytotoxicity against tumor cells. *Int. J. Cancer* 21:444–452.

Örn, A., Gidlund, M., Ojo, E., Grönvik, K.-O., Andersson, J., Wigzell, H., Murgita, R.A., Senik, A., and Gresser, I. (1980) Factors controlling the augmentation of natural killer cells. In *Natural Cell-Mediated Immunity Against Tumors*. Herberman, R.B. (ed.), New York: Academic Press, pp. 581–592.

Peck, A.B., Murgita, R.A., and Wigzell, H. (1978) Cellular and genetic restrictions in the immunoregulatory activity of alpha-fetoprotein. II. Alpha-fetoprotein induced suppression of cytotoxic T lymphocyte development. *J. Exp. Med.* 148:360–372.

Roder, J.C. (1980) The specificity of NK cells at the level of target antigens and recognition receptors. In *Natural Cell-Mediated Immunity Against Tumors*. Herberman, R.B. (ed.), New York: Academic Press, pp. 939–948.

Senik, A., Kolb, J.P., Örn, A., and Gidlund, M. (1980) Study of the mechanism for *in vitro* activation of NK cells. *Scand. J. Immunol.* 12:51–60.

Stern, P., Gidlund, M., Örn, A., and Wigzell, H. (1980) Natural killer cells mediate efficient lysis of MHC-lacking embryonal carcinoma cells. *Nature* 285:341–2.

Trinchieri, G., Santoli, D., and Knowles, B. (1977) Tumor cell lines induce interferon in human lymphocytes. *Nature* 270:611–613.

Published 1981 by Elsevier North Holland, Inc.
Saunders, Daniels, Serrou, Rosenfeld, and Denney, eds.
FUNDAMENTAL MECHANISMS IN HUMAN CANCER IMMUNOLOGY

CHAPTER 13

Specific and Non-Specific Cellular Interactions Modulating Host Resistance to Tumors

R.W. Baldwin

Cancer Research Campaign Laboratories, University of Nottingham, University Park, Nottingham, NG7 2RD, England

Introduction

Studies of experimental animal tumors induced by chemical carcinogens or oncogenic viruses have suggested that malignant cells may be subject to control by the immunological network of the host. Immunological methods of cancer therapy have been developed, including treatment with so-called "immunomodulating agents" (Baldwin, 1980, Terry and Yamamura, 1979). But it is now recognized that the immune responses elicited against tumor cells are highly complex: they include the induction of specifically sensitized T lymphocytes following recognition of tumor associated antigens (Kitagawa et al., 1978), the generation and mobilization of natural killer cells (Herberman and Holden, 1978) and activated macrophages (Hibbs et al., 1978), and the stimulation of antibody formation. Tumor-host interactions also lead to the generation of suppressor lymphocytes and macrophages and the development of both specific and non-specific humoral factors which may interfere with cell-mediated immunity (Broder et al., 1978; Baldwin, 1980). This includes the release of tumor antigen and/or immune complexes into the circulation. Also tumor cells, either directly, or indirectly through interactions with host cells, may release immunosuppressive products (Baldwin et al., 1979a). It is most likely, therefore, that tumor rejection involves multiple host responses which offer several potential opportunities for manipulation of the tumor-host relationship in therapy.

Results

Tumor Antigen Expression on Carcinogen-Induced and Naturally Arising Tumors in WAB/Not Rats

In order for a tumor to generate immune rejection responses, it must express an appropriate cell surface antigen. This condition is fulfilled by many tumors induced by oncogenic viruses, where virus-related antigens, as well as virus-coded cell surface antigens, may be expressed (Moore, 1978; Kurth et al., 1979). Similarly, many, but by no means all, rodent tumors induced by chemical carcinogens express tumor rejection antigens (Embleton and Baldwin, 1980; Baldwin and Price, 1980). However, this type of neoantigen is not expressed by the great majority of naturally arising rodent tumors (Hewitt, 1979; Baldwin et al., 1979). The experiments summarized in Table 13.1 show that immunization of syngeneic WAB/Not rats with a range of naturally arising tumors did not in most cases produce any significant immunity to tumor cell challenge (Middle and Embleton, 1980). Immunization-challenge tests have been carried out with a wide range of naturally arising WAB/Not rat tumors and the results of these studies indicate that only 7 out of 44 tumors express neoantigens with the capacity to elicit a tumor rejection reaction (Baldwin et al., 1979b; Middle and Embleton, 1980).

Table 13.1. Induction of Immunity to Naturally Arising Tumors in WAB/Not Rats.

Tumor	Tissue type	Challenge: no. cells	Tumor growth after challenge	
			Excised rats	Controls
Sp1	Epithelioma	2×10^4	3/3	4/4
Sp4	Mammary carcinoma	10^5	0/6	4/6
Sp7	Fibrosarcoma	10^5	0/5	4/4
Sp24	Sarcoma	10^4	3/4	3/4
Sp41	Fibrosarcoma	10^5	0/4	4/4
Sp45	Nephroblastoma	10^6	3/3	5/5
Sp54	Leiomyosarcoma	10^4	3/4	4/4
SP59	Fibrosarcoma	Trocar Graft	4/4	4/4
Sp63	Nephroblastoma	5×10^4	5/5	3/4
Sp71	Chemodectoma	5×10^5	3/3	4/4
SP78B	Nephroblastoma	10^4	4/6	5/5

Note: Syngeneic subcutaneous grafts of tumors were surgically excised from experimental animals, and the treated rats and controls were challenged subcutaneously using doses of cells determined to be the minimum inoculum for consistent growth in controls. Figures indicate number of rats in which tumor growth was observed vs total number inoculated.

(Source: Middleton and Embleton, 1980).

These extensive studies with tumors in WAB/Not rats indicate that tumors induced with chemical carcinogens are more frequently immunogenic than naturally arising tumors. It has been proposed, however, that the neoantigens expressed upon carcinogen-induced tumors are not necessarily associated with malignant change, but may be altered cell products arising as a consequence of carcinogen-induced cell damage (Embleton and Baldwin, 1980). This hypothesis is supported by studies showing that immunization of WAB/Not rats with syngeneic 15-day-old embryo cells treated *in vitro* with 3-methylcholanthrene (MCA) elicit antibodies reacting with certain carcinogen-induced tumors (Embleton and Baldwin, 1979). Fifteen-day-old rat embryo cells treated with acetone used as solvent for MCA did not have detectable neoantigens (Embleton and Baldwin, 1979). Oncofetal antigens are expressed upon most of the carcinogen-induced and naturally arising tumors in WAB/Not rats (Rees et al., 1979; Baldwin and Price, 1980), but these differ from the neoantigens identified upon MCA treated rat embryo cells in that they are commonly expressed upon almost all tumors tested.

Generation of Tumor Specific Immunity

The nature of tumor antigen preparations used for immunization is critical for inducing a tumor rejection response, and this response can be augmented by incorporation of immunological adjuvants in the immunizing vaccine. Figure 13.1 compares the tumor rejection response elicited by vaccines containing viable or γ-radiation attenuated, MCA-induced sarcoma Mc7 cells, in combination with bacterial adjuvants. Subcutaneous injection of irradiated Mc7 cells did not produce sufficient immunological stimulation to prevent growth of a simultaneous contralateral challenge with viable tumor cells. The therapeutic response was enhanced following incorporation of Bacillus Calmette Guérin (BCG) or *Corynebacterium parvum* (the more effective agent of the two) in the immunizing vaccine. The most effective immune stimulation was obtained by a combination of viable sarcoma Mc7 cells admixed with BCG or *C.parvum*, used under conditions where the local immune response generated by the bacterial agents prevented tumor growth.

Of more importance to the design of future immunotherapeutic protocols is the finding that vaccines containing soluble (3MKCl) extracts of MCA-induced sarcomas or aminoazo dye (DAB)-induced hepatomas are completely ineffective in generating anti-tumor immunity (Price et al., 1978). This result may be attributed to inappropriate processing of tumor antigen preparations, since, as shown in Table 13.2, immunization with 3MKCl extracts of hepatoma D23 following pre-treatment of the rats with cyclophosphamide (40mg/kg body weight) leads to the development of tumor immunity. Cyclophosphamide is known to restrict the development of suppressor lymphocytes controlling the generation of delayed hypersensitivity to contact sensitizers (Asherson et al., 1979) and the induction of immunity to tumor cells (Glaser, 1979). This

170

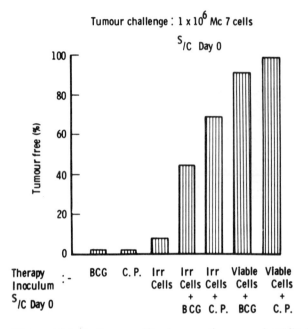

Figure 13.1. Active specific immunotherapy of MCA-induced sarcoma Mc7 in WAB/Not rats. Rats received a subcutaneous challenge with sarcoma Mc7 cells (1×10^6). Simultaneously and contralaterally, rats received tumor cell-containing vaccine to stimulate a tumor specific immune response. BCG: Glaxo percutaneous vaccine (0.5 mg moist weight). CP: *Corynebacterium parvum* (Wellcome CN6134 0.7 mg dry weight). Irradiated cells 2×10^6 — Sarcoma Mc7 cells inactivated by γ-irradiation (15,000R). These were administered alone or in combination with BCG or *C. Parvum*. Viable cells—Sarcoma Mc7 cells: 2×10^6 cells in admixture with BCG or *C. Parvum*. This inoculum did not produce a progressively growing tumor and the host responses generated prevented the growth of the contralateral tumor challenge.

conclusion is further substantiated by the experiments outlined in Table 13.3 which show that adoptive transfer of lysates of thymus derived cells from rats injected with 3MKCl extracts of hepatoma D23 abrogated the tumor rejection immunity which was elicited after immunization with irradiated D23 cells. This response was tumor specific, since thymus cells from rats treated with hepatoma D192A did not modify hepatoma D23-induced immunity (Price et al., 1980).

The induction of suppressor cells following immunization with soluble tumor antigen preparations further illustrates the important role of tumor-host interactions in the eventual influence of anti-tumor immune responses on tumor growth. There is an initial release of tumor antigen into the circulation following subcutaneous growth of hepatoma D23. The levels of free antigen are then rapidly reduced at the same time that tumor specific immune

Table 13.2. Induction of Immunity to Hepatoma D23 with Soluble 3MKCl Extracts of Tumor.

Group	Cyclophosphamide treatment (day 0)	Treatment[a] with 3MKCl extract of :	Tumor incidence after hepatoma D23 challenge[b]
1	40 mg/Kg, IV	Hepatoma D23	3/11
2	–	Hepatoma D23	10/10
3	40 mg/Kg, IV	–	5/5
4	40 mg/Kg, IV	Hepatoma D192A	6/6

[a]Rats were treated by intraperitoneal injection of doses of 1, 2, 3, and 4 mg soluble 3MKCl extract of tumor on days 3, 5, 7, and 9.

[b]Incidence measured after subcutaneous challenge on day 13 with 10^3 hepatoma D23 cells.

complexes appear (Figure 13.2). Comparably, as shown in Figure 13.3, thymus cells derived from hepatoma D23-bearing rats suppress the tumor immune response initiated by immunization with γ-irradiated hepatoma D23 cells.

Effector Cell Populations Mediating Tumor Rejection

The role of lymphocytes sensitized to tumor associated antigens in tumor rejection responses and their interaction with natural killer (NK) cells and activated macrophages has been evaluated in experiments with a series of aminoazo dye-induced hepatocellular carcinomas and MCA-induced sarcomas. These tumors express individually distinct tumor rejection antigens, and enhancement of the specific arm of the tumor immune response can lead to an effective tumor rejection reaction. Figure 13.4 summarizes experiments show-

Table 13.3. Abrogation of Immunity to Hepatoma D23 with Lysates of Thymus Cells from Rats Immunized with 3M KCL Extracts of Tumor.

Group	Immunization[a]	Thymus cell lysate[b] from rats immunized with 3M KCL extracts of :–	Tumor incidence in rats challenged with hepatoma D23 (5×10^2 cells)
I	D23 IR Cells	Hepatoma D23	4/4
II	D23 IR Cells	Hepatoma D192A	0/4
III	D23 IR Cells	Normal Thymus	1/5
IV	D23 IR Cells	–	0/5
V	–	–	3/4

[a]D23 cells (10^7) γ-irradiated (15000R) injected day −7 with respect to tumor challenge.

[b]Thymus cells from rats immunized with 3MKCL extracts of tumor. Cells lysed by freeze-thawing, centrifuged (100,000g, 60 min). Each recipient received lysate from one donor rat 24 hours before tumor challenge with hepatoma D23 (5×10^2 cells s/c).

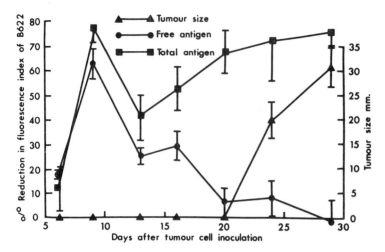

Figure 13.2. Serum levels of tumor antigen in rats developing subcutaneous growths following challenge with hepatoma D23 (5×10^2 cells). Circulating tumor specific antigen (free antigen) was determined by the capacity of tumor bearer serum to neutralize antibody in syngeneic tumor-immune serum, this being detected by membrane immunofluorescence reactions with hepatoma D23 cells. Total antigen was determined following dissociation of immune complexes at low pH and isolation of tumor antigen containing moieties by Sephadex G200 chromatography at low pH (Baldwin et al., 1979a). There was a rise in serum levels of free tumor antigen until 7 to 10 days after tumor cell challenge. Thereafter, free antigen levels decreased with a concomitant rise in immune complex levels. Both free tumor antigen and immune complexed products were detectable well before palpable tumors arose.

Figure 13.3. Suppression of immunity to hepatoma D23 by tumor-bearer thymocytes. WAB/Not rats were immunized by intraperitoneal injection of γ-irradiated hepatoma D23 cells. Seven days later, rats were challenged subcutaneously with hepatoma D23 (5×10^2 cells) and simultaneously received an intravenous injection of thymocytes (1×10^8) from normal or hepatoma D23-bearing donors.

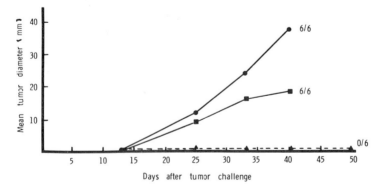

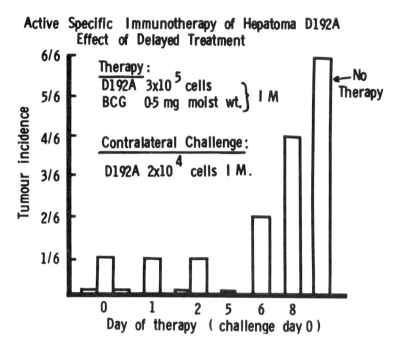

Active Specific Immunotherapy of Hepatoma D192A
Effect of Delayed Treatment

Figure 13.4. Active specific immunotherapy of rat hepatoma D192A. Hepatoma cells (2×10^4) were implanted intramuscularly and the rats received a tumor cell vaccine either simultaneously or up to 8 days after tumor challenge. The vaccine contained viable tumor cells (3×10^5) together with BCG (Glaxo percutaneous vaccine, 0.5 mg moist weight) and this mixed inoculum did not produce tumors. The immune response generated by this vaccine was highly effective in suppressing tumor growth when given up to 5 days after tumor challenge and was still partially effective even when given 8 days post tumor challenge.

ing that immunostimulation following intramuscular injection of vaccines containing viable hepatoma D192A cells mixed with BCG effectively suppresses tumor growth. In these three experiments, intramuscular growth of hepatoma D192A was effective, even when treatment was delayed until 6 days after tumor challenge. It is generally accepted that the responses produced by immunization with tumor cell-containing vaccines include the stimulation of specifically sensitized lymphocytes. The experiments summarized in Figure 13.5 show that lumbar lymph node cells draining an intramuscular implant of viable hepatoma D192A cells together with BCG suppress growth of hepatoma D192A when assayed by the Winn test. The D192A-stimulated lymph node cells were ineffective against another tumor, sarcoma Mc7. Conversely in the specificity control, lymph node cells sensitized to sarcoma Mc7 suppressed growth of this tumor, but not hepatoma D192A.

174

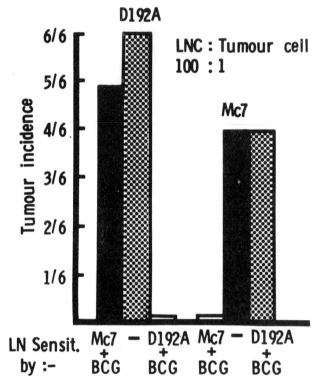

Figure 13.5. Adoptive transfer (Winn) test using rat hepatoma D192A sensitized lymph node cells. Growth of rat hepatoma D192A and sarcoma MC7 was inhibited by lumbar node cells obtained from rats immunized by intramuscular challenge with tumor cells admixed with BCG (Glaxco percutaneous vaccine). Lymph node cells from tumor immune donors mixed with tumor cells at a ratio of 100–1 were injected into normal rats and assayed for inhibitory activity (Winn test).

The immune response generated systemically following immunization with vaccines containing hepatoma D192A cells together with BCG is also directed specifically against hepatoma D192A; a contralateral challenge with hepatoma D192A is suppressed, while other tumors do not duplicate this effect (Jones et al., 1980). However, the cellular interactions leading to the destruction of tumor cells are less clearly understood. It has been found that immunization with tumor cell vaccines, especially in conjunction with bacterial agents, also generates NK cell activity and/or activated macrophages (Jones et al., 1980). Therefore, while Winn-type assays establish the requirement for specifically sensitized lymphocytes in the rejection of these carcinogen-induced hepatomas and sarcomas, there is no unequivocal evidence that these lymphocytes are the effector cells. A series of studies using both short- and long-term cytotoxicity tests with these tumors failed to demonstrate conclusively that immunization generated cytotoxic lymphocytes with individual specificity comparable to that detected by *in vivo* tumor rejection tests (Brooks et al., 1978; Robins et al., 1979b; Flannery et al., 1980). This uncertainty is illustrated by the data in Table 13.4, in which nylon column eluted normal spleen cells and sarcoma Mc7 derived tumor infiltrating lymphocytes (TIL) were tested in short- and long-term tests against NK-susceptible (Mc7) and relatively resistant (Mc57) target cells (Flannery et al., 1980). Spleen cells showed the same target cell specificity in both the 6-hr ^{51}Cr-release test and the 60-hr ^{75}Se-selenomethionine post-labeling test, although their reactivity as determined by slopes of regression lines for cytotoxicity (Brooks and Flannery, 1980) was increased in the long-term test. NK cell activity in sarcoma Mc7 TIL was revealed in the ^{51}Cr-release test, using Mc7 target cells. When tested in the long-term assay, however, TIL's were cytotoxic for both Mc7 and Mc57 target cells, with a reactivity far greater than that seen with spleen cells. In this context, analysis of host cells infiltrating subcutaneous growths of sarcoma Mc7 led to the identification of a highly reactive lymphocyte population which inhibited tumor growth in Winn assays using effector cell: tumor cell ratios as low as 1.5:1 (Robins et al., 1979a). Once again, however, lymphocyte populations did not display the characteristic specificities revealed by lymph node cells derived from tumor immune donors in Winn assays (Jones et al., 1980).

Non-Specific Anti-Tumor Responses

The finding that anti-tumor responses at the site of tumor deposits following

Table 13.4. Comparison of Cytotoxic Activity of Lymphocytes Infiltrating Rat Sarcoma Mc7 (TIL) in Short- (6 hr) and Long-Term (60 hr) Tests.

Duration of test	Effector cell[a]	Cytotoxic activity[b] against:					
		Sarcoma Mc7			Sarcoma Mc57		
6 hr	Spleen	3.79	4.00	5.23	0.88	0.67	1.35
	TIL	1.28	2.55	1.39	0.07	0.0	0.0
60 hr	Spleen	5.60	4.8	9.26	2.06	2.86	0.27
	TIL	16.0	16.0	18.4	12.0	13.3	10.1

[a]Lymphocytes infiltrating subcutaneous growths of sarcoma Mc7 were isolated by trypsin disaggregation of tumor and nylon column separation. Spleen lymphocytes were also isolated by nylon column elution and aliquots of these preparations used in the 6 hr or 60 hr cytotoxicity tests.
[b]Cytotoxicity determined in ^{51}Cr-release test (6 hr) or ^{75}Se-selenomethionine uptake test (60 hr). Figures represent slopes of regression lines ($\times 10^5$) in 3 separate experiments for each cell type. Each vertical column represents a complete experiment.

176

generation of specific immunity to tumor associated antigens on carcinogen-induced tumors may involve non-specific effector cells suggests that stimulation of natural immunity may have therapeutic potential. In most cases, however, systemic stimulation of NK cells and/or activated macrophages by treatment with bacterial agents such as BCG or *C. parvum* has not resulted in effective suppression of tumor growth (Baldwin and Byers, 1979; Baldwin, 1980). This result suggests that one of the functions of specifically-sensitized lymphocytes in tumor deposits is to induce infiltration and/or activation of NK cells and macrophages through the release of soluble factors (Baldwin, 1980; Hibbs et al., 1978). This hypothesis is consistent with the well-established finding that many agents, but particularly bacterial preparations used for tumor immunotherapy, are most effective when administered locally in tumor deposits. This technique is known as regional immunotherapy (Baldwin, 1980; Baldwin and Pimm, 1978; Milas and Scott, 1977). Many of the agents used for regional immunotherapy, such as BCG organisms and subcellular products including cell wall preparations, have multiple functions, including the capacity to elicit delayed hypersensitivity reactions (Baldwin and Byers, 1979; Kitagawa et al., 1978). The experiments summarized in Table 13.5 show that growth of naturally arising WAB/Not rat mammary carcinomas could be suppressed when tumor cells were injected in contact with BCG organisms, but only when the recipients were pre-sensitized to the organisms. These studies have been extended to show that growth of mammary carcinoma Sp15 is suppressed when tumor cells are contacted with tuberculin protein (PPD), but again only in BCG-sensitized recipients (Pimm and Baldwin, 1980).

Table 13.5. Adjuvant Contact Therapy of Mammary Carcinomas in WAB/Not Rats.

Mammary carcinoma	BCG sensitization[a]	Tumor cell challenge[b]	Tumor incidence in rats receiving:	
			Tumor cells	Tumor cells +BCG[c]
SP15	+	1×10^3	14/14	0/14
"	−	1×10^3	9/14	8/14
"	+	2×10^3	12/12	1/14
"	−	2×10^3	14/14	12/14
"	+	5×10^3	12/12	1/14
"	−	5×10^3	14/14	12/14
Sp22	+	2×10^3	11/13	0/14
"	−	2×10^3	12/13	10/13

[a]BCG Glaxo (0.5 μg moist weight), IP, day −14.
[b]Tumor challenge s/c, day 0.
[c]0.5 μg moist weight Glaxo BCG mixed with tumor cells.

The above findings have prompted a series of investigations to search for chemically defined agents with the capacity to elicit delayed hypersensitivity reactions within tumor deposits. One series of compounds selected for these studies are 3-n-alkylcatechols, which are analogues of the natural plant oil, urushiol, which causes poison oak/ivy dermatitis (Byers and Baldwin, 1980). These compounds are potent contact hypersensitizing agents (Friedlaender and Baer, 1972), and furthermore possess considerable lipophilicity, so that they incorporate into the lipid phase of cell membranes (Byers et al., 1979). The potential of this approach is illustrated by experiments showing that the intralesional injection of 3-n-pentadecylcatechol (PCD) in squalene into intradermal grafts of the guinea pig Line 10 hepatoma prevented growth of the local tumor and limited the development of regional lymph node metastases. (Pimm et al., 1980)

Discussion

One of the most effective means of manipulating the tumor-host relationship for therapy is to augment immunity to tumor associated antigens. This technique requires the generation of specifically sensitized T-lymphocytes, although the function of these effector cells is still unclear. Against some tumors, especially virus-induced lymphomas, these lymphocytes may be directly cytotoxic, but the mechanism for generating anti-tumor responses against solid tumors appears to be less simple. In tests with a range of rat tumors, *in vitro* cytotoxicity responses with sensitized lymphocytes could not be demonstrated (Flannery et al., 1980). So it may be that anti-tumor responses are mediated by other cell types which are triggered by factors which result from the interaction of sensitized lymphocytes and tumor cells. This hypothesis would reconcile the contradiction in findings which show that while cell-mediated responses to the individually distinct antigens on carcinogen-induced rat tumors are required for tumor rejection, the host cells derived from regressing tumors lack specificity (Robins et al., to be published).

Development of this therapeutic method depends upon the identification of tumor associated antigens on human tumors. While a large body of evidence for cell-mediated immunity has been derived from both *in vivo* and *in vitro* tests, much of this information is still equivocal (Baldwin, 1980). Preparation of monoclonal antibodies following fusion of antibody producing B lymphocytes from BALB/c mice immunized with tumor cells and murine myeloma cells offers an alternative approach to immunotherapy. This technique has led to the identification of tumor associated antigens on several tumor types, including malignant melanoma (Koprowski et al., 1978; Yeh et al., 1979) and osteogenic sarcoma (Embleton et al., 1980). At the present state of development of these studies, however, it appears that some of the antigens detected are not truly tumor specific, and so it remains to be established whether they will elicit immune responses in patients.

Another approach to immune manipulation involves stimulation of natural immunity, mediated by NK cells and/or activated macrophages. While this type of response can be induced by several immunomodulating agents, the therapeutic effect is generally small. In contrast, promotion of local responses by regional administration of immunomodulating agents frequently produces a strong anti-tumor effect, even with tumors lacking immunogenicity (Baldwin, 1980; Baldwin and Byers, 1979). For example, hypersensitizing agents can be used to stimulate local delayed type hypersensitivity responses. This type of response has been used to treat rat mammary carcinomas with PPD in tuberculin sensitized animals (Pimm and Baldwin, in preparation). However, chemically defined agents such as aklylcatechols, which are highly potent hypersensitizing agents, may be more effective.

ACKNOWLEDGMENTS

These investigations were carried out in collaboration with my colleagues and I wish to express my thanks for their permission to quote their studies. The work jointly carried out was supported by the Cancer Research Campaign.

I thank Dr. J.A. Jones for permission to reproduce her data on the treatment of rat hepatoma D192A.

References

Asherson, G.L., Perera, M.A.C.C., and Thomas, W.R. (1979) Contact sensitivity and the DNA response in mice to high and low doses of oxazolone; low dose unresponsiveness following painting and feeding and its prevention by pretreatment with cyclophosphamide. *Immunology* 36:449–459.

Azuma, I., Yamawaki, M., Ogura, T., Yoshimoto, T., Tokuzen, R., Hirao, F., and Yamamura, Y. (1978) Anti-tumor activity of BCG cell-wall skeleton and related materials. In *Cancer Immunotherapy and its Immunological Basis. Gann Monographs on Cancer Research*, 21. Yamamura, Y., Kitagawa, M., and Azuma, I. (eds.), Baltimore: University Park Press, pp. 73–86.

Baldwin, R.W. (1980) Immunotherapy of tumors. *Cancer Chemotherapy Annual*, 2. Pinedo, H.M. (ed.) Amsterdam: Exerpta Medica, pp. 150–175.

Baldwin, R.W. and Byers, V.S.(1979) Immunoregulation by bacterial organisms and their role in the immunotherapy of cancer. *Seminars in Immunopath.* 2:79–100.

Baldwin, R.W., Byers, V.S., and Robins, R.W. (1979a) Circulating immune complexes in cancer: characterization and potential as tumor markers. *Behring Inst. Mitt.* 64:63–77.

Baldwin, R.W., Embleton, M.J., and Pimm, M.V. (1979b) Host responses to spontaneous rat tumors. In *Antiviral Mechanisms in the Control of Neoplasia*. Chandra, P. (ed.), New York: Plenum Press, pp. 333–353.

Baldwin, R.W. and Pimm, M.V. (1978) BCG in tumor immunotherapy. *Adv. Cancer Res.* 28:91–147.

Baldwin, R.W. and Price, M.R. (1980) Neoantigen expression in chemical carcinogenesis. *Cancer Comprehensive Treatise*, Vol. 1. In press.

Broder, S., Muul, L, and Waldmann, T.A. (1978) Suppressor cells in neoplastic disease. *J. Nat. Cancer Inst.* 61:5–11.

Brooks, C.G., Flannery, G.R., Webb, P.J., and Baldwin, R.W. (1980) Quantitative studies of natural immunity to solid tumors in rats. Two types of cytotoxic cell detected in both short- and long-term assays. *Immunology*, submitted.

Brooks, C.G., Rees, R.C., and Robins, R.A. (1978) Studies on the microcytotoxicity test. II. The uptake of aminoacids (^{3}H-leucine or ^{75}Se-methionine) but not nucleosides (^{3}H-thymidine of ^{125}I-IUdR) or ^{51}CrO$_4$ provides a direct and quantitative measure of target cell survival in the presence of lymphoid cells. *J. Immunol. Meths.* 21:111-124.

Byers, V.S. and Baldwin, R.W. (1980) Modulation of tumor cell membranes with lipophilic haptens: and approach to modifying tumor immunogenicity. *J. Supramol. Struct.*, in press.

Byers, V.S., Epstein, W.L., Castagnoli, N., and Baer, H. (1979) *In vitro* studies of poison oak immunity. I. *In vitro* reaction of human lymphocytes to urushiol. *J. Clin. Invest.* 64:1437-1448.

Embleton, M.J. and Baldwin, R.W. (1979) Tumor-related antigen specificities associated with 3-methylcholanthrene-treated rat embryo cells. *Int. J. Cancer* 23:840-845.

Embleton, M.J. and Baldwin, R.W. (1980) Antigenic changes in chemical carcinogenesis. *Br. Med. Bull.* 36:83-88.

Embleton, M.J., Gunn, B., Byers, V.S., and Baldwin, R.W. (1980) Antigens on naturally occurring animal and human tumors detected by monoclonal antibodies. *Transplant. Proc.*, in press.

Flannery, G.R., Robins, R.A., and Baldwin, R.W. (1980) Quantitative studies of natural immunity to solid tumors in rats. Natural killer cells infiltrate transplanted chemically-induced sarcomas. *Cell Immunol.*, submitted.

Friedlaender, M.H. and Baer, H. (1972) The role of the regional lymph node in sensitization and tolerance to simple chemicals. *J. Immunol.* 109:1122-1130.

Glaser, M. (1979) Regulation of specific cell mediated cytotoxic response against SV40-induced tumor associated antigens by depletion of suppressor T cells with cyclophosphamide in mice. *J. Exp. Med.* 149:774-779.

Herberman, R.B. and Holden, H.T. (1978) Natural cell-mediated immunity. *Adv. Cancer Res.* 27:305-377.

Hewitt, H.B. (1979) The choice of animal tumors for experimental studies of cancer therapy. *Adv. Cancer Res.* 27:149-200.

Hibbs, J.B., Chapman, H.A., and Weinberg, J.B. (1978) The macrophage as an antineoplastic surveillance cell: biological perspectives. *J. Reticuloendothel Soc.* 24:549-570.

Jones, J.A., Brooks, C.G., Robinson, G., and Baldwin, R.W. (1980) In preparation.

Kitagawa, M., Fujiwara, H., Hamaoka, T., Yamamoto, H., and Teshima, K. (1978) T cell function in the induction of immune resistance against syngeneic murine tumor. In *Cancer Immunotherapy and its Immunological Basis, Gann Monograph on Cancer Research 21*. Yamamura, Y., Kitagawa, M., and Azuma, I. (eds.), Baltimore: University Park Press, pp. 37-47.

Koprowski, H., Steplewski, Z., Herlyn, D., and Herlyn, M. (1978) Study of antibodies against human melanoma produced by somatic cell hybrids. *Proc. Natl. Acad. Sci. U.S.A.* 75:3405-3409.

Kurth, R., Fenyö, E.M., Klein, E., and Essex, M. (1979) Cell surface antigens induced by RNA tumor viruses. *Nature* 279:197-201.

Middle, J.G. and Embleton, M.J. (1980) Naturally-arising tumors of the WAB/Not rat strain. II. Immunogenicity of transplanted tumors. *J. Natl. Cancer Inst.*, submitted.

Milas, L. and Scott, M.T. (1977) Anti-tumor activity of *Corynebacterium parvum*. *Adv. Cancer Res.* 26:257-306.

Moore, M. (1978) Antigens of experimentally-induced neoplasms: a conspectus. In *Immunological Aspects of Cancer*. Castro, J.E. (ed.), Lancaster, England: MTD Press, pp. 15-50.

Pimm, M.V., Baldwin, R.W., Basley, W.A., and Byers, V.S. (1980) Regional immunotherapy of guinea pig line-10 hepatoma with chemical hypersensitizers. *Br. J. Cancer* 42:175.

Price, M.R., Preston, V.E., Robins, R.A., Zöller, M., and Baldwin, R.W. (1978) Induction of immunity to chemically induced rat tumors by cellular and soluble antigens. *Cancer Immunol. Immunother.* 3:247-252.

Price, M.R., Hannant, D., Bowen, J.G., and Baldwin, R.W. (1980) Suppressor cells in rats immunized against solubilized hepatoma-specific antigen. *Br. J. Cancer* 42:176.

Rees, R.C., Price, M.R., and Baldwin, R.W. (1979) Oncodevelopmental antigen expression in chemical carcinogenesis. In *Methods In Cancer Research*, 18. Busch, H. (ed.) pp. 99–133.

Robins, R.A., Flannery, G.R., and Baldwin, R.W. (1979a) Tumor-derived lymphoid cells prevent tumor growth in Winn assays. *Br. J. Cancer* 40:946–949.

Robins, R.A., Rees, R.C., Brooks, C.G., and Baldwin, R.W. (1979b) Spontaneous development of cytotoxic activity in cultured lymph node cells from tumor bearing rats. *Br. J. Cancer* 39:659–666.

Terry, W.D. and Yamamura, Y. (eds.) (1979) *Immunobiology and Immunotherapy of Cancer*. Elsevier/New York: North Holland.

Yeh, M-Y., Hellstrom, I., Brown, J.P., Warner, G.A., Hansen, J.A., and Hellström, K.E. (1979) Cell surface antigens of human melanoma identified by monoclonal antibody. *Proc. Natl. Acad. Sci. U.S.A.* 76:2927–2931.

Published 1981 by Elsevier North Holland, Inc.
Saunders, Daniels, Serrou, Rosenfeld, and Denney, eds.
FUNDAMENTAL MECHANISMS IN HUMAN CANCER IMMUNOLOGY

CHAPTER 14

Modulation of Monocyte-Macrophage Cytotoxic Capacity[1]

Albert F. LoBuglio, David M. Garagiola, Maxine Solvay, and Thomas K. Huard

Simpson Memorial Research Institute, University of Michigan Medical Center, Ann Arbor, Michigan

Blood monocytes are the circulating precursors of most tissue macrophages and represent the cell population which responds to chemotactic stimuli to produce macrophage infiltration at sites of inflammation or tumor. Our laboratory has been examining the cytotoxic potential of these cells. In previously published studies, we have characterized their ability to lyse human tumor cell targets coated with either human (Shaw, 1978a) or rabbit antibody (Shaw, 1978b), and human red cells coated with human isoantibodies (Shaw, 1978c). We have compared their ability to carry out this antibody dependent cellular cytotoxicity (ADCC) with the other two Fc-receptor leukocyte populations, i.e., Fc-receptor lymphocytes and granulocytes (Shaw, 1978c; Levy, 1979).

These studies suggested that these three Fc-receptor cell populations shared many characteristics in carrying out ADCC. However, they also exhibited several notable differences in regard to expression of Fc-receptor activity toward antibody displayed on the target cell surface. For example, all three cell types could carry out ADCC to a human lymphoblastic cell line (CEM) coated with rabbit IgG, but granulocytes required 100 times more antibody/target cell in order to bind and lyse the target cell, as compared to lymphocytes and monocytes (Levy, 1979). We also noted that lymphocytes were unable to bind or lyse human red cell targets where the isoantibody was distributed randomly on the target cell, but lysed RBC's coated with the same number of IgG molecules distributed in a clustered arrangement. Monocytes lysed the red cell

[1] This work supported by National Cancer Institute Grant CA 25641-02.

targets regardless of the IgG distribution pattern (Shaw, 1978d, 1980). Thus, it would appear that these three cell types differ with respect to criteria for Fc-receptor interaction with antibody coated target cells.

Because of these findings, we have recently decided to examine whether cells at two different stages of differentiation in the same cell lineage might differ in their Fc-receptor activity toward antibody coated target cells. We used a rabbit model to examine the interaction of blood monocytes and tissue macrophages (alveolar macrophages) with both red cell and tumor cell targets coated with rabbit antibody. We have also examined the effect of mycobacteria or their active components on monocyte and alveolar macrophage ADCC to tumor cells. Concurrent with these animal model studies, we have been examining the ADCC and direct tumor cell cytotoxicity of blood monocytes from patients with cancer. The results of these human studies are briefly summarized in this report.

Methods

Cell Isolations

Monocytes were isolated from rabbit blood by methods previously described for the isolation of human monocytes (Shaw, 1978b). The procedure involved surface adherence of monocytes from mononuclear cell preparations obtained by Ficoll-Hypaque separation. The unbound lymphocytes were rigorously washed away and the adherent monocytes obtained by gentle scraping, after brief incubation with cold buffer containing EDTA and albumin. The monocyte preparations were >95% non-specific esterase positive and >95% viable by Trypan blue exclusion. Alveolar macrophages were harvested by the method of Myrvik (1961). Human monocytes were isolated as previously described (Shaw, 1978b).

Target Cells

For rabbit ADCC assays, ox RBC were ^{51}Cr labeled (Shaw, 1978c) and 50×10^6 cells sensitized with 50 ul of a $1:2$, $1:8$, $1:32$, or $1:128$ dilution of rabbit antisheep RBC antisera (Cordis Corporation, Miami, Florida) for 45 minutes at 37°C. Cells were washed and adjusted to 2×10^6 cells/ml. These dilutions of antisera resulted in a range of antibody density on the RBC surface from 60,000 IgG/cell ($1:2$ dilution) to 15,000 IgG/cell ($1:128$ dilution) as measured by an I^{125} Staphylococcus protein A (SPA) assay (Shaw, 1980). Tumor cell targets were CEM T lymphoblast cell lines coated with a rabbit anti-CEM antisera (Shaw, 1978b). The CEM targets were ^{51}Cr labeled and then 2.5×10^6 cells sensitized with 50 ul of undiluted, $1:8$, $1:32$, or $1:128$ dilutions of rabbit anti-CEM for 45 min at 37°C. The cells were then washed and resuspended to 2×10^5 cells/ml. These antisera dilutions produced a range of antibody density on the target cells from 400,000 IgG/cell (undiluted antisera) to 25,000 IgG/cell (1 : 128 dilution).

For human monocyte ADCC, human O+ RBC targets were sensitized with anti-D as previously described (Shaw, 1978c) and CEM targets were sensitized with rabbit anti-CEM antisera as previously described (Shaw, 1978b).

Antibody Dependent Cellular Cytotoxicity Assay

The assay used microtiter plates containing 200,000 RBC targets or 20,000 tumor cell targets incubated with varying numbers of effector cells as previously described (Shaw, 1978b). This was a 4-hr ^{51}Cr release assay system.

Direct Tumor Cell Cytotoxicity Assay

This assay has been briefly described previously (LoBuglio, 1979). Twenty thousand tritiated thymidine labeled HeLa cells are incubated alone or in the presence of varying numbers of monocytes in triplicate microwells containing RPMI 1640 and 5% FCS. The supernate is sampled at 48, 72, and 96 hours to determine the percent cytotoxicity at each of these time points. This cytotoxic assay requires viable, metabolically active monocytes, is not dependent on endotoxin, and produces lysis of a number of different human malignant target cells without lysing fibroblast target cells.

Mycobacteria Stimulation In Vivo

In vivo monocyte-macrophage activation was carried out in groups of 3 or 4 rabbits for each experimental observation. Animals were injected via ear vein with 0.1 cc of oil containing 100 μg dead M. bovis as previously described (Montarosso, 1979); 0.1 cc of oil containing 100 μg of Connaught living Bacillus Calmette Guerin (BCG) or 100 μg of muramyl dipeptide (Calbiochem Inc.); 0.1 cc normal saline containing 100 μg Connaught BCG or 100 μg muramyl dipeptide. Three weeks later, animals were bled for isolation of monocytes and sacrificed for alveolar macrophage isolation. The cells were then tested for cytotoxic capacity and the results expressed as mean ± 1 SD of at least 3 animals.

Monocyte and Macrophage Binding of Target Cells

We determined the ability of monocytes to bind antibody coated RBC (EA) or antibody coated tumor cells (TA) by methods previously described (Shaw, 1979). Optimally sensitized RBC's (1 : 2 dilution of antisera) and tumor cells (undiluted antisera) were mixed with effector cells at a 1 : 20 effector/target (E/T) ratio (to be sure target cell number was not limiting), centrifuged to initiate cell contact, incubated for 15 minutes at room temperature, resuspended, and examined microscopically to determine the percent of effector cells having >4, 1-4 or no bound target cells.

Results

Monocyte and Alveolar Macrophage ADCC to RBC and Tumor Cell Targets

As seen in Table 14.1, blood monocytes were effective at ADCC to the antibody coated RBC targets. The degree of target cell lysis was directly related to the number of effector cells present (E/T ratio) at all levels of target cell sensitization. Further, for any given E/T ratio, the amount of lysis was directly related to the amount of antibody used to sensitize the target cells. In contrast, the lysis of these same target cells by alveolar macrophages was unimpressive, with a maximum level of 7% at an E/T ratio of 20:1 with target cells sensitized with 60,000 IgG/rbc (1:2 dilution of antisera).

The same monocytes which were effective at ADCC to RBC targets were incapable of lysis of antibody coated CEM target cells (Table 14.2). In contrast, the macrophages carried out ADCC to these same targets. The amount of lysis was related to both the number of macrophage effector cells (E/T ratio) and the degree of antibody sensitization. The antisera dilutions used for the various target cell preparations produced a range of antibody sensitization from 400,000 IgG/cell (undiluted) to 25,000 IgG/cell (1:128 dilution), as determined by the ^{125}I-SPA assay.

We next determined if the different capacities of these two effector cell populations to carry out ADCC to the two different target cells was related to initial Fc-receptor recognition and binding of antibody coated target cells. As seen in Table 14.3, monocytes were very effective at binding antibody coated RBC. Forty percent of the monocytes formed large rosettes of at least 5

Table 14.1. Monocyte and Alveolar Macrophage ADCC to RBC Targets.

Effector/target ratio	Antiserum dilutions			
	1:2	1:8	1:32	1:128
Monocytes				
20:1	31 ± 1	29 ± 1	23 ± 5	9 ± 1
10:1	29 ± 6	17 ± 5	10 ± 2	7 ± 2
5:1	23 ± 2	18 ± 3	8 ± 3	7 ± 2
1:1	5 ± 4	3 ± 2	< 1	< 1
Alveolar macrophages				
20:1	7 ± 2	6 ± 1	5 ± 3	2 ± 1
10:1	4 ± 1	2 ± 1	3 ± 2	< 1
5:1	5 ± 3	3 ± 2	2 ± 2	< 1
1:1	2 ± 1	4 ± 3	< 1	< 1

Note: RBC targets were ox RBC sensitized with 50 ul/50 × 10⁶ RBC of varying dilutions of rabbit anti-sheep RBC antisera. Cytotoxicity is expressed as the mean ± SD of % ADCC of at least 3 animals.

Table 14.2. Monocyte and Alveolar Macrophage ADCC to CEM Targets.

Effector/target ratio	Antiserum dilutions			
	Neat	1:1	1:32	1:128
Monocytes				
20:1	2 ± 1	1 ± 1	3 ± 1	2 ± 1
10:1	< 1	< 1	< 1	< 1
5:1	< 1	< 1	< 1	< 1
1:1	< 1	< 1	< 1	< 1
Alveolar macrophages				
20:1	28 ± 4	15 ± 1	10 ± 1	5 ± 2
10:1	11 ± 4	7 ± 1	5 ± 2	3 ± 1
5:1	5 ± 3	6 ± 1	4 ± 3	2 ± 1
1:1	3 ± 2	4 ± 3	3 ± 1	2 ± 1

Note: Cytotoxicity is expressed as the mean ± SD % ADCC of at least 3 animals. CEM lymphoblast targets were sensitized with 50 ul/2.5 × 10^6 cells of varying dilutions of rabbit anti-CEM antisera.

attached RBC, while only 15% failed to bind the RBC targets. In contrast, 83% of the monocyte population failed to bind the tumor targets. The opposite pattern was seen with the alveolar macrophages. Seventy-four percent of the macrophages failed to bind the RBC targets while 71% of the macrophages bound 5 or more tumor targets.

These studies indicate that criteria for Fc-receptor interaction with antibody sensitized target cells can differ dramatically at different stages of differentia-

Table 14.3. Target Cell Binding by Rabbit Monocytes and Alveolar Macrophages.

Target cells[a]	Percent[b] of monocytes binding varying members of target cells		
	0	1-4	> 4
EA	15 ± 3	45 ± 5	40 ± 9
TA	83 ± 4	16 ± 4	1 ± 1
	Percent[b] of alveolar macrophages binding varying numbers of target cells:		
	0	1–4	> 4
EA	74 ± 5	22 ± 3	4 ± 3
TA	6 ± 2	23 ± 2	71 ± 5

[a]EA indicates RBC_{OX} sensitized with a 1:2 dilution of rabbit anti-sheep RBC antisera; TA indicates CEM tumor cells sensitized with undiluted rabbit anti-CEM antisera.
[b]Percent expressed as the mean ± SD of ⩾ 3 experiments.

tion in the monocyte-macrophage cell lineage. This may reflect different density, distribution, or affinity of Fc-receptors on the effector cells, or changes in Fc-receptor requirements for antibody density, distribution, subclass, or as yet undetermined factors which alter the Fc-receptor interaction with the Fc-portion of IgG displayed on cell surfaces.

Effect of Mycobacterial Stimulation In Vivo on Monocyte-Macrophage Fc-Receptor Activity

We next examined whether administration of mycobacteria might modulate monocyte-macrophage Fc-receptor interaction with antibody coated tumor cells. It has been previously reported that rabbit alveolar macrophages harvested 3 weeks after the intravenous injection of dead mycobacteria (100 μg) in oil had enhanced metabolic activity and Fc-receptor density (Montarosso, 1978, 1979). We chose this model to examine the effects of dead mycobacteria, an equivalent weight (100 μg) of live BCG suspended in oil or in saline, as well as 100 μg of muramyl dipeptide (MDP) in either oil or saline. Blood monocytes and alveolar macrophages were harvested three weeks after injection. The animals appeared to have no alteration in health during the three weeks of observation. Table 14.4 lists the effects of these agents on monocyte ADCC to CEM target cells. Dead mycobacteria in oil caused a modest but significant increase in monocyte ADCC. The monocytes harvested from animals receiving live BCG or MDP in oil had cytotoxicity comparable to or greater than that seen with normal alveolar macrophages (see Table 14.2). MDP in saline produced no alterations in monocyte or macrophage ADCC.

We examined the effects of these agents further by varying the effector: target ratios and by using target cells sensitized with varying dilutions of antisera. As seen in Tables 14.5 and 14.6, alveolar macrophages harvested from animals receiving BCG in saline or MDP in oil had a striking activation of ADCC ability. This activation affected several aspects of the cytotoxic event. First, at a 20:1 E/T ratio and optimally sensitized targets, the amount of cytotoxicity was almost doubled. More impressive is the fact that activated

Table 14.4. Effect of Mycobacteria on Monocyte-Macrophage ADCC to CEM Tumor Cells.

Activator	Monocytes	Alveolar macrophages
None	2 ± 1	28 ± 4
CFA (100 μg)	13 ± 3	47 ± 10
BCG/oil (100 μg)	28 ± 3	52 ± 5
BCG/NS (100 μg)	25 ± 10	48 ± 4
MDP/oil (100 μg)	43 ± 4	51 ± 7

Note: Cells were harvested 3 weeks after a single intravenous injection of mycobacteria. Cytotoxicity is expressed as mean ± 1 SD % ADCC of cells harvested from at least 3 animals.

Table 14.5. Effect of BCG on Monocyte and Alveolar Macrophage ADCC to CEM Targets.

Effector/target ratio	Antiserum dilutions			
	Neat	1:8	1:32	1:128
Monocytes				
20:1	25 ± 10	11 ± 5	4 ± 2	1 ± 1
10:1	12 ± 5	4 ± 4	2 ± 1	1 ± 1
5:1	6 ± 3	2 ± 2	1 ± 1	< 1
1:1	1 ± 1	1 ± 1	1 ± 1	< 1
Alveolar macrophages				
20:1	48 ± 4	44 ± 5	34 ± 8	25 ± 1
10:1	44 ± 3	42 ± 6	32 ± 8	25 ± 2
5:1	36 ± 2	35 ± 4	26 ± 5	20 ± 1
1:1	25 ± 2	21 ± 4	20 ± 5	13 ± 2

Note: 100 µg of Connaught BCG in normal saline was injected i.v. and effector cells harvested 3 weeks later. Cytotoxicity is expressed as the mean ± 1 SD % ADCC of at least 3 animals. CEM targets are identical to those in Table 14.2.

macrophages at a 1:1 E/T ratio (20,000 macrophages) were able to lyse as many target cells as normal macrophages at a 20:1 E/T (400,000 macrophages). In addition, target cells coated with only 25,000 IgG/target cells were lysed by activated macrophages to a degree requiring 400,000 IgG/target cell by normal macrophages.

We were surprised at the degree of monocyte activation. These cells have a half-life in the circulation of 4–7 days (possibly shorter with inflammation)

Table 14.6. Effect of Muramyl Dipeptide on Monocyte and Alveolar Macrophage ADCC to CEM Targets.

Effector/target ratio	Antiserum dilutions			
	Neat	1:8	1:32	1:128
Monocytes				
20:1	43 ± 4	32 ± 6	19 ± 2	8 ± 1
10:1	34 ± 4	25 ± 6	16 ± 1	4 ± 1
5:1	25 ± 3	19 ± 4	13 ± 2	3 ± 1
1:1	8 ± 3	7 ± 3	5 ± 2	2 ± 1
Alveolar macrophages				
20:1	51 ± 7	45 ± 11	37 ± 14	23 ± 1
10:1	45 ± 6	40 ± 13	35 ± 18	25 ± 5
5:1	39 ± 7	33 ± 13	25 ± 11	17 ± 2
1:1	24 ± 13	22 ± 14	16 ± 12	11 ± 5

Note: 100 µg muramyl dipeptide in oil was injected i.v. and effector cells harvested 3 wk later. Cytotoxicity is expressed as the mean ± 1 SD % ADCC of at least 3 animals. CEM targets same as in Table 14.2.

Table 14.7. Monocyte Binding of Antibody Coated CEM Targets.

	Percent[a] of monocytes binding varying numbers of tumor cells:		
Activator	0	1-4	> 4
None	83 ± 4	16 ± 4	1 ± 1
CFA	44 ± 6	52 ± 3	4 ± 2
BCG/oil	22 ± 4	55 ± 3	23 ± 4
BCG/NS	34 ± 8	35 ± 7	31 ± 10
MDP/oil	12 ± 3	60 ± 3	28 ± 4

[a]Expressed as the mean ± 1 SD % of cells harvested from at least 3 animals.

and yet three weeks after injection were still being modulated to an activated state. The mycobacteria activation transformed the monocyte population from a noncytotoxic state (Table 14.2) to a population which exceeded the cytotoxic activity of normal alveolar macrophages (comparison of Tables 14.2 and 14.6). Once again the activation was reflected in greater cytotoxicity with fewer

Figure 14.1. Human monocyte ADCC to RBC targets. 200,000 anti-D coated O+ RBC were incubated with varying numbers of monocytes from normal donors or patients with lymphoma or solid tumors. Results are expressed as mean ±1 SD ADCC for each group at each effector/target (E/T) ratio.

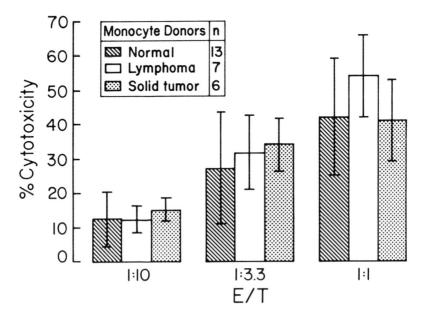

effector cells (low E/T ratios) and increased recognition and lysis of lightly sensitized target cells.

Finally, we examined the ability of these activated monocytes to bind antibody coated tumor cells. As seen in Table 14.7, the enhanced cytotoxic potential correlated with an increase in monocyte Fc-receptor binding of antibody coated tumor cells.

Thus, it is clear that mycobacteria or their products are capable of activating both blood monocytes and alveolar macrophages, enhancing their cytotoxic capacity (increased lytic units) as well as their capacity to recognize and lyse target cells with lower antibody density on their surface.

Effect of Cancer on Human Monocyte Cytotoxic Capacity

Concurrent with these animal model studies, we examined the cytotoxic potential of monocytes from patients with untreated malignant lymphoma and metastatic solid tumors. Monocytes from patients with cancer had cytotoxic activity to antibody coated red cell targets (Figure 14.1) and antibody coated tumor cells (Figure 14.2) comparable to that of normal individuals. Furthermore, their direct monocyte cytotoxicity to HeLa tumor cells was similar to that seen in normal donors (Figure 14.3). Thus, malignancy did not seem to

Figure 14.2. Human monocyte ADCC to tumor cell targets. 20,000 CEM lymphoblasts coated with rabbit anti-CEM antibody were incubated with varying numbers of monocytes from normal donors or patients with lymphoma or solid tumors. Results are expressed as mean ±1 SD ADCC for each group at each effector/target (E/T) ratio.

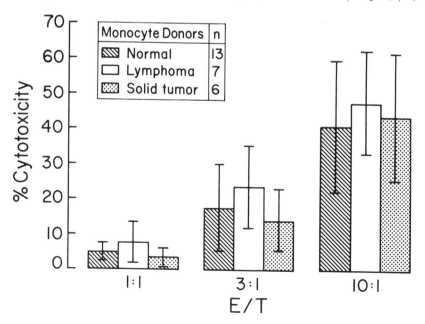

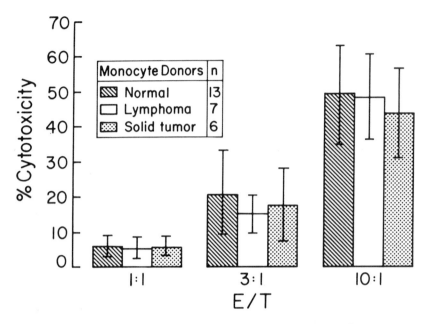

Figure 14.3. Human monocyte direct tumor cell cytotoxicity to human tumor cells. 20,000 tritiated thymidine labeled HeLa cells were incubated with varying numbers of monocytes from normal donors or patients with lymphoma or solid tumors. Results are expressed as mean ±1 SD cytotoxicity at 96 hours for each group of patients at each effector/target (E/T) ratio.

impair the cytotoxic potential of blood monocytes in either ADCC or direct cytotoxicity assay systems.

ACKNOWLEDGMENTS
The authors wish to thank Ms. Helen Ilc for her assistance in the preparation of this manuscript.

References

Levy, P.C., Shaw, G.M., and LoBuglio, A.F. (1979) Human monocyte, lymphocyte, and granulocyte antibody-dependent cell-mediated cytotoxicity toward tumor cells. I. General Characteristics of cytolysis. *J. Immunol.* 123:594–599.

LoBuglio, A.F., Solvay, M.D., and Weiss, S.J. (1979) Characterization of human monocyte direct tumor cell cytotoxicity. *Blood* 54:103a.

Montarosso, A.M. and Myrvik, Q.N. (1978) Effect of BCG vaccination on the IgG and complement receptors on rabbit alveolar macrophages. *J. Reticuloendothel. Soc.* 24:93–98.

Montarosso, A.M. and Myrvik, Q.N. (1979) Oxidative metabolism of BCG-activated alveolar macrophages. *J. Reticuloendothel. Soc.* 25:559–574.

Myrvik, Q.N., Leake, E.S., and Fariss, B. (1961) Studies on pulmonary alveolar macrophages from the normal rabbit. *J. Immunol.* 86:128–135.

Shaw, G.M., Levy, P.C., and LoBuglio, A.F. (1978a) Human monocyte cytotoxicity to tumor cells. I. Antibody dependent cytotoxicity. *J. Immunol.* 121:573–578.

Shaw, G.M., Levy, P.C., and LoBuglio, A.F. (1978b) Human monocyte antibody-dependent cell-mediated cytotoxicity to tumor cells. *J. Clin. Invest.* 62:1172–1180.

Shaw, G.M., Levy, P.C., and LoBuglio, A.F. (1978c) Human lymphocyte, monocyte, and neutrophil antibody-dependent cell-mediated cytotoxicity toward human erythrocytes. *Cell Immunol.* 41:122–133.

Shaw, G.M., Levy, P.C., and LoBuglio, A.F. (1978d) Human lymphocyte antibody-dependent cell-mediated cytotoxicity toward human red blood cells. *Blood* 52:696–705.

Shaw, G.M., Levy, P.C., and LoBuglio, A.F. (1979) Reexamination of the EA rosette assay ("Ripley") for Fc-receptor leukocytes. *Clin. Exp. Immunol.* 36:496.

Shaw, G.M., Aminoff, D., Balcerzak, S.P., and LoBuglio, A.F. (1980) Clustered IgG on human red blood cell membranes promotes human lymphocyte antibody-dependent cell-mediated cytotoxicity. *J. Immunol.* 125:501–507.

Published 1981 by Elsevier North Holland, Inc.
Saunders, Daniels, Serrou, Rosenfeld, and Denney, eds.
FUNDAMENTAL MECHANISMS IN HUMAN CANCER IMMUNOLOGY

CHAPTER 15

Interrelationships Between Immunoregulatory Cells, Neoplastic Diseases and Immunodeficiency States

Samuel Broder, M.D. and Mary Megson, M.S.

Metabolism Branch, National Cancer Institute, National Institutes of Health, Bethesda, Maryland

Introduction

Experimental murine systems have generated most of our information about the characterization and functional manipulation of T cell regulatory subsets. In mice, it has been shown that there exists an Ly-system of surface membrane alloantigens which has bearing upon both suppressor and helper T cell function (Cantor and Gershon, 1979). In the T cell Ly-system, three subsets have been identified. One subset bears all three relevant Ly determinants (Ly-123$^+$). Another subset bears only Ly-determinants (Ly-1$^+$), and a third subset bears predominantly LY-23 determinants (Ly-23$^+$). (Even cells which previously had been classified as Ly-23$^+$ express *some* Ly-1 antigens when sensitive detection methods are used [Ledbetter et al., 1980].) Data from three different laboratories indicate that Ly-123$^+$ auxiliary T cells (with adherent properties) promote the maturation of Ly-23$^+$ suppressor cell precursor T cells into fully functional suppressor effector cells (Feldman et al.., 1977; Tada et al., 1977; Basten et al., 1978). Recent data indicate an even higher level of complexity in the Ly-system. A subset of immune (antigen-specific) Ly-1$^+$ helper cells, which bear the major histocompatibility-linked marker Qa-1, may act upon a non-immune Qa-1$^+$ subset of Ly-123$^+$ T cells to induce *feedback suppressor* Ly-23$^+$ cells (Cantor and Gershon, 1979; McDougal et al., 1979; Eardley et al., 1979). More complexity in this system will emerge in the very near future. We will touch upon these issues again in discussing immunoregulatory neoplasms.

As discussed elsewhere (Reinherz et al., 1979a,b; Reinherz et al., 1980) a panel of monoclonal antibodies reactive with human T cell subset antigens has been developed using somatic cell hybridization and cloning technology. One such monoclonal antibody, termed OKT4, appears to detect a human T cell subset with helper activity (Reinherz et al., 1979a, b). Other monoclonal antibodies termed OKT5 and OKT8, and a panel of conventional heteroantiserums, termed TH_2, may detect a human T cell subset with suppressor activity (Reinherz et al., 1980). It is not established whether these antigens have a direct immunoregulatory function and whether some types of regulatory T cells have unusual antigenic profiles. We shall return to additional potential antigenic markers for human regulatory cells later in the article.

I-Subregion Systems

In mammals, the major histocompatibility complex is a chromosomal segment containing genes that control the strongest allotransplantation antigens (Bach and Van Rood, 1976). Genes within this region also profoundly influence several functions of the immune system, including the capacity to generate immune responses to certain well-defined antigens (Schrefler and David, 1975; Benacerraf and Dorf, 1976; Benacerraf and Germain, 1978). The major histocompatibility complex in mice is called H-2 and is located on chromosome 17. At present, five major H-2 regions are recognized: *K*, *I*, *S*, *G*, and *D*. The genetic information for a number of distinct immune functions in mice can be assigned to one (or more) subregions of the *I*-region. Cell surface antigens encoded by genes which map within the *I*-region are called Ia (immune response associated) antigens (McDevitt et al., 1976; Sachs, 1976). Unlike determinants encoded within the *K* and *D* regions, Ia antigens appear predominantly on B cells and monocytes. However, T cells may express Ia antigens under a variety of activating conditions. There are unequivocal data that T cell helper and suppressor regulatory activities are associated with the *I*-region.

By using strains of mice with recombinant events within this region, five *I*-subregions have previously been described. These are designated *I-A*, *I-B*, *I-J*, *I-E*, and *I-C*. There has been a suggestion that *I-A* should be divided into two subregions by assigning a new subregion, *I-N*, between *K* and *I-A* (Hayes et al., 1980). This is still an evolving field of research.

Different *I*-subregions may govern different T regulatory functions. There is evidence that at least some of the structural information for soluble helper T cell factors may be encoded in the *I-A* subregion (Tada et al., 1977; Taussig and Munro, 1976; Mozes, 1976). On the other hand, antibodies to *I-A* antigens may favor the activation of suppressor T cells (see Discussion in Perry et al., 1980). Other *I*-subregions participate in suppressor-cell function. For example, Rich and Rich (1976) have found suppressor T cells and their factors capable of inhibiting mixed lymphocyte reactions of responder cells with the same *I-C* subregion genotype. Perhaps the most important genes known to be associated with suppressor function reside within the *I-J* subregion. The *I-J* subregion contains the genetic information for surface-membrane markers found on suppressor T cells (and a special subset of helper T cells) and also for a portion of the antigen-specific suppressor factors secreted by certain T cells (Benacerraf and Germain, 1978; Tada et al., 1976; Thèze et al., 1977; Greene et al., 1977c; Tada et al., 1978). These *I-J*-encoded factors may profoundly depress both humoral and cellular immune reactions. Recent data indicate that certain *I-J*-related suppressor substances are composed of two distinct molecules, which are independently synthesized in the cytoplasm and then secreted in an associated form (Taniguchi et al., 1980). One of these associated molecules is involved in specific antigenic binding and presumably contains immunoglobulin V_H structural determinants. The other associated molecule contains *I-J*-encoded structural determinants that could conceivably serve as restricting elements in suppressor cell interactions.

I-J-encoded suppressor factors were initially considered to be antigen-specific (and histocompatibility-restricted) mediators of suppressor T cell activity. However, as with a great many immune reactions, there is a significant non-specific component in the *I-J* suppressor system. The *I-J* suppressor system seems to depend on interaction with a T cell that produces the relevant soluble factor and another T cell that accepts the factor (Taniguchi and Tokuhisa, 1980). The accepting T cell (in the presence of antigen) probably responds as an intermediary in achieving the final suppressor activity, perhaps by generating a new set of suppressor T cells that actually implements the inhibitory effect. In certain strains of mice, it has been possible to show the existence of discrete H-2-linked genetic deficits in either the actual generation of T cell suppressor factor, or the capacity to respond to T cell suppressor factor (Germain et al., 1980). At least in some systems, the apparent antigen specificity and *I-J* histocompatibility requirement occurs at the level of soluble factor/acceptor T cell interaction. However, the suppressor effector T cells induced following this interaction are no longer antigen-specific, and they can suppress both syngeneic and allogeneic immune responses. These observations underscore the importance of non-specific elements in the physiological regulation of immunity.

Pierres and his co-workers have proved that the intravenous injection of alloantiserums directed against *I-J* determinants can potentiate certain immune responses by diminishing suppressor-cell function (Pierres et al., 1978). They reported that the administration of alloantiserums to appropriate *I-J*-related antigens could actually reverse a form of genetic non-responsiveness to certain synthetic polymers, which is mediated by suppressor cells. Thus, genetically non-responsive mice could acquire immune reactivity to the relevant synthetic polymers, presumably as a direct consequence of the serologic disruption of their suppressor system. We shall return later in the article to the *I-J* subregion and some of the immunologic perturbations caused by antibodies directed against Ia or Ia-like antigens.

Concepts evolving out of studies of the murine *I*-region are already and will continue to be applicable to human systems. In man, the major histocompatibility genes map within the *HLA*-complex on chromosome 6, and genes closely linked to the *HLA-D* subregion control the expression of antigens that appear to be homologous (and analogous) to murine Ia antigens (Van Rood et al., 1976; Lunney et al., 1979). By analogy to murine systems, human Ia-like antigens are most readily evident on normal (or neoplastic) B cells and monocytes. Activated human T cells also express Ia-like antigens (Evans et al., 1978; Metzgar et al., 1979; Ko et al., 1979; Greaves et al., 1979). *HLA-D*-associated products may serve as structures permitting certain types of suppressor T cells to recognize appropriate target cells for the exertion of inhibitory activity (Engleman and McDevitt, 1978). Antibodies to Ia-like antibodies can sterically block certain crucial cellular interactions needed for immune reactivity. Moreover, certain antibodies to human Ia-like framework molecules can activate suppressor cells (Broder et al., 1980) via a mechanism which probably requires an initial interaction between antibodies and target molecules on the surface membrane of monocytes. This effect is critically dependent on the concentration of the relevant antibodies to Ia-like antigens.

Regulatory Cell Abnormalities in Cancer

Suppressor Cells As Mediators of Immunologic Enhancement

Host/tumor relationships represent some of the most complex systems in biology. One aspect of this complexity is the growing experimental evidence that different kinds of suppressor cells and their secreted factors may undermine effective anti-tumor immune responses and enhance tumor growth. The activation of suppressor cells provides one (but definitely not the only) explanation for the paradoxical reduction of host resistance to tumor growth and dissemination in certain animals, given treatments which superficially resemble active immunization. One carefully studied tumor model illustrating this point involves the use of 3-methylcholanthrene-induced sarcomas transplanted into A/J mice. A critical factor favoring tumor growth in this syngeneic system is the development of suppressor T cells (Fujimoto et al., 1975, 1976a,b; Green et al., 1977b). In this system, Fujimoto, Green, and Sehon found that tumor cells implanted into normal mice caused death within 40 days, whereas tumor cells implanted into mice previously rendered immune to this tumor were rejected in approximately 14 days. Mice were rendered highly immune to the tumor by complete surgical excision of the tumor mass seven days after subcutaneous injection of 1×10^6 neoplastic cells, followed by several additional immunizations with such cells. When thymocytes or spleen cells from tumor-bearing animals were injected intravenously into immune mice at the same time that they received live tumor cells, tumor growth was enhanced. Therefore, the thymus glands and spleens of host animals with growing tumors contained suppressor cells. Moreover, such suppressor cells could actually counteract host immune defenses when injected into immune mice during the time of ongoing rejection, thereby suggesting that suppression at the efferent limb of tumor immunity is possible. The suppressor cells active in the recipient mice were detectable and remained effective for as long as net tumor growth occurred. However, suppressor cell activity disappeared rapidly after surgical removal of the tumor.

The suppressor activity of these tumor-bearing hosts was totally abolished *in vitro* by treatment with antisera against T cells. These studies were extended by testing the effect of *in vivo* antithymocyte serum treatment on the growth of primary transplantable syngeneic tumors. Repeated injections of antithymocyte serum at appropriate intervals after tumor cell challenge markedly reduced primary tumor growth. This reduction of tumor growth probably occurred because suppressor T cells had been interfering with the capacity of most effector cells to halt tumor growth. Therefore, the elimination of such suppressor cells promoted tumor regression. It should be noted that the suppressor T cells involved in the enhancement of tumor growth in this system were specific in that they did not affect the growth of unrelated tumors.

Fujimoto and his co-workers have recently shown that splenic T cells from animals carrying methylcholanthrene-induced sarcomas or a spontaneous lymphoma specifically inhibited the effector phase of tumor cell lysis by preformed cytotoxic T cells *in vitro* (Fujimoto et al., 1978). These workers discovered that the suppressor activity was strictly specific for the individual tumor involved during the *in vivo* generation of suppressor cells. However, in some cases, cytotoxic T cells generated *in vitro* against two closely related sarcomas exhibited a certain degree of cross-reactivity. These observations underscore the principle that suppressor T cells and cytotoxic T cells need not necessarily recognize and respond to the same antigenic determinants. Furthermore, these studies should dispel the widely held misconception that suppressor cells act only to prevent the generation of certain kinds of effector lymphocytes. Clearly, suppressor cells can act at the final effector phase of immunity in certain experimental models.

There are recent data from other murine studies (Berendt and North, 1980) which support the hypothesis that protective immunity to tumors may progressively decay because of the generation of suppressor cells. This hypothesis is supported by two main findings. First, complete regression of large established fibrosarcomas could be achieved by intravenously infusing sensitized effector spleen cells from immune donors, if the tumors were growing in thymectomized, T cell-depleted recipients. (Sensitized effector spleen cells were obtained from mice whose 6-day-old intradermal tumors had undergone complete regression following intravenous endotoxin treatment.) There was about a one-week delay in the onset of regression induced by such sensitized spleen cells, but once initiated, the regression was rapid and complete. However, these workers could not cause regression of established tumors in T cell intact hosts under comparable conditions.

The second major finding by Berendt and North was that when spleen cells from T cell intact mice bearing tumors in a late stage of growth were administered to T cell-depleted, tumor-bearing recipients a few hours before the administration of the sensitized effector spleen cells, tumor regression did *not* take place. Taken together, these observations provide proof that the tumor-bearing hosts acquired a tumor-induced population of suppressor cells, which could nullify the protective activity of immune effector cells. These suppressor cells expressed Thy 1.2 antigens and could, therefore, be characterized as T cells. The potency of the suppressor T cell effect increased as tumor growth progressed.

One of the implications of the observations discussed above is that late in the course of tumor growth, attempts to cause regression of neoplasms simply by transferring immune T cells will likely fail, because an activated suppressor T cell population is functionally dominant. Indeed, Berendt and North have made a convincing case that their observations account for the rarity of published reports documenting regression of established tumors by the passive transfer of sensitized T cells. Therefore, clinical trials involving the administration of activated autologous cytotoxic T cells may fail if host suppressor cells are ignored.

Greene, Fujimoto, and Sehon were able to extract a soluble factor from the lymphoid cells of tumor-bearing mice that had essentially the same tumor growth-promoting effect as intact suppressor T cells. This soluble suppressor T cell factor bore strikingly similar immunochemical and biologic features to the *I-J*-encoded suppressor factors, which were discussed earlier in this article as potent inhibitors of humoral and cellular immune function.

We have already discussed studies (Pierres et al., 1978) proving that the *in vivo* administration of antibodies directed against certain Ia antigens (i.e., the products of genes within the *I-J* subregion) can increase immune responses by reducing suppressor-cell activity. Other research (Green et al., 1977a) extended this concept by demonstrating that the *in vivo* administration of anti-*I-J* antibodies would reduce the function of suppressor T cells in tumor-bearing mice. The predictable net effect of such a maneuver would be to inhibit tumor growth. Indeed, Green and his co-workers found a major retardation of tumor growth in mice treated daily with anti-*I-J* antisera in microliter quantities. Spleens from tumor-bearing mice given anti-*I-J* antiserum no longer contained specific suppressor cells. These experiments provide an important model for the serologic inactivation of suppressor T cells in neoplastic states, and provide a firm experimental precedent for inducing the host to mount a more effective immune response against lethal tumors by a process of selective T cell depletion.

Probably within the next 5 to 10 years, the true clinical relevance of these observations will be understood. It may be valuable to emphasize two points. First, the T cell system as a whole plays a critical role in host defenses against microorganisms and neoplastic cells in a number of settings. Therefore, interventions that nonselectively impair overall T cell function will probably not contribute to the survival of tumor-bearing patients. Secondly, the success of serologic (or pharmacologic) therapeutic manipulations designed to disrupt the suppressor T-cell network will probably require attention to very subtle experimental details. For example, while we have just discussed murine experiments indicating that certain anti-Ia antibodies (those directed against *I-J*-encoded products) may protect tumor-bearing hosts, certainly not all antibodies reactive with Ia or Ia-like determinants can be expected to achieve the same result. There are data indicating that the *in vivo* administration of anti-Ia antibodies directed against *I-A*-encoded antigens can interfere with tumor rejection in immune mice (Perry et al., 1979). Furthermore, lymphoid cells from hyperimmune mice pretreated *in vivo* with antibodies reactive with *I-A* determinants are no longer capable of adoptively transferring tumor immunity to non-immune recipients. (The observation that certain kinds of antibodies to Ia-like antigens can activate, rather than inhibit, suppressor cells could be relevant here.)

The data discussed thus far (taken together) strongly imply that a subset of host T cells may contribute to tumor growth and, accordingly, might be an appropriate target for certain experimental therapeutic maneuvers. The literature describes a great number of additional systems in which suppressor cells might contribute to tumor growth (e.g., see Reinisch et al., 1977; Treves et al., 1974; Levy et al., 1976; Fisher and Kripke, 1977; Spellman and Daynes, 1977; Hodes and Hathcock, 1976; Yu et al., 1977). Moreover, suppressor cells of non-T cell origin are commonly seen in tumor-bearing animals and can non-specifically suppress a wide spectrum of immunologic functions.

Recent data (Ting and Rodrigues, 1980) indicate that tumor cells can suppress the generation of cytotoxic T cells through the collaboration of splenic *and* peritoneal populations of macrophages. Ting and Rodrigues showed that a specific sequence of interaction was required for the suppressor effect. Splenic macrophages had to be pre-exposed to tumor cells prior to the addition of peritoneal macrophages in order to bring about suppressor effects.

It is known that many human tumors lead to impaired cellular immune function (Herberman, 1976). Certain neoplastic states, such as the syndrome of thymoma combined with hypogammaglobulinemia and multiple myeloma, are especially associated with abnormalities of humoral immunity that may predispose patients to infection with highly pathogenic organisms even before the underlying tumor is documented (Jeunet and Good, 1968; Waldmann et al., 1975; Broder and Waldmann, 1979).

There are data to suggest that suppressor cells play a role in the pathogenesis or perpetuation of impaired antibody formation in a subgroup of patients with congenital or acquired immunodeficiency disease. Suppressor cells have also been implicated in the impaired immunity associated with widespread fungal and mycobacterial infections (Stobo et al., 1976; Ellner, 1978). Moreover, there are recent data to suggest that suppressor cells have an impact upon host/parasite interactions (Ottesen, 1979; Piessens et al., 1980). These demonstrations of suppressor cells in nonneoplastic diseases reinforce the need to reevaluate the forces responsible for immune impairment in some cancer patients. Indeed, a wide range of experimental evidence suggests that non-specific suppressor cells of both T cell and macrophage origin do participate in the immunodeficiency state associated with certain human neoplasms (Broder and Waldmann, 1978; Engleman et al., 1978; Goodwin et al., 1977; Hillinger and Herzig, 1978; Schecter and Soehnlen, 1978; Twomey et al., 1975; Zembala et al., 1977). Excessive suppressor T cell function has been demonstrated in patients with the syndrome of thymoma combined with hypogammaglobulinemia and in patients with certain solid tumors. Excessive macrophage-like suppressor-cell function that inhibits immunoglobulin synthesis has been demonstrated in patients with multiple myeloma. Moreover, macrophage-like cells that inhibit T cell proliferative function have been demonstrated in the circulation of patients with certain solid tumors and also in anergic patients with Hodgkin's disease. In some forms of cancer, suppressor cells of *both* T cell and macrophage origin have been observed. Even if such suppressor-cell abnormalities do not contribute directly to neoplastic growth, an understanding of how such cells are activated and how they function could prove useful, since diminished resistance against microbal pathogens becomes a serious clinical problem in the management of many cancer patients.

Neoplasms Comprised of Cells that Retain Immunoregulatory Activity

A number of useful insights into the nature of the humoral immune response in humans were made possible by studying neoplasms of the B cell/plasma cell series. The recognition that paraproteins derived from patients with multiple myeloma represent extremely homogeneous immunoglobulins was a truly indispensible step in illuminating the structural, functional, metabolic, and genetic aspects of humoral immunity. Malignancies of T cell origin are of exceptional interest because in some cases the neoplastic T cells retain immunoregulatory properties. For this reason, the study of malignant T cells (and their products) could eventually be as rewarding in resolving questions regarding cellular immunity, and in particular the cellular control of immunoglobulin production, as myelomas and their paraprotein products have proved to be in resolving questions concerning humoral immunity. In the remaining portion of this chapter, we shall describe the use of neoplastic T cells from a variety of patients as a resource for studying human helper and suppressor T cell activity.

Neoplasms in Which Helper Activity May Be Evident

The Sézary Syndrome

Mycosis fungoides and the Sézary syndrome may be viewed as part of a spectrum of lymphoproliferative disorders for which the term cutaneous T cell lymphoma has recently been proposed (Lutzner et al., 1975; Bunn and Lamberg, 1979). Such cutaneous lymphomas have been systematically characterized for nearly 175 years, in large measure through the efforts of French clinical investigators (Alibert, 1835; Vidal and Brocq, 1885; Sézary and Bouvrain, 1938; Brouet et al., 1973). The Sézary syndrome is a serious disorder characterized by exfoliative erythroderma, generalized lymphadenopathy, and circulating malignant lymphocytes with a propensity to infiltrate epidermis. The bone marrow is relatively spared. These circulating neoplastic lymphocytes (referred to as Sézary cells) have a deeply folded or cerebriform nucleus as their key morphologic feature. In the epidermis, the neoplastic cells may form distinctive nests known as Pautrier's microabscesses. Skin biopsies from patients with the Sézary syndrome are essentially indistinguishable from those of patients with mycosis fungoides. The Sézary cells from most patients studied have a T cell origin, as demonstrated by their capacity to form spontaneous sheep erythrocyte rosettes and susceptibility to lysis in the presence of complement and specific heterologous antisera raised against thymic lymphocyte antigens.

Most investigators would now agree that the Sëzary syndrome is not truly a separate entity but rather is a clinical variant of mycosis fungoides. Overt transitions between these two clinical subsets are common. For a variety of purposes, it is extremely useful to view these diseases as subtypes of a unified cutaneous T cell lymphoma syndrome (Broder and Bunn, 1980).

In 1966, Blaylock et al. provided what might have been one of the first clues that some patients with cutaneous T cell lymphomas have a neoplasm that represents an expansion of cells with an immunoregulatory capacity. These investigators observed that many patients with what would now be considered a cutaneous T cell lymphoma syndrome had exceedingly high serum levels of IgA. IgA is an important immunoglobulin which is found in both serum and external secretions. There is a large body of data to suggest that those B cells which ultimately mature into IgA-secreting plasma cells depend heavily on T cell helper influence before final maturation can occur (Clough et al., 1971). In our own laboratory, we have observed that lymphocytes from patients with low leukemic forms of the Sëzary syndrome spontaneously secrete large amounts of IgA *in vitro*, without activation by polyclonal lectins, such as pokeweed mitogen (Broder et al., 1977). Thus, the striking overproduction of a highly thymic-dependent isotype might have been the first indication that the neoplastic lymphocytes found in certain patients with cutaneous T cell lymphoma had retained an important immunoregulatory function. We have observed elevations of serum immunoglobulin classes other than IgA (e.g., striking elevations of IgE may be seen in lymphocytes from some patients). Moreover, there have been reports of patients with the Sëzary syndrome who developed monoclonal serum immunoglobulin abnormalities (Puissant et al., 1976; Kövary et al., 1977; Dupré et al., 1977; Joyner et al., 1979). Monoclonal IgM, IgG, and IgA serum abnormalities have been documented. We have observed one patient with a circulating low-molecular weight form of IgA. It is conceivable that such examples of excessive B cell activity could represent the *in vivo* expression of overactive helper T cell function. There is a real possibility that certain subsets of neoplastic T cells can express helper activity for a specific B cell clone (so-called idiotype-specific helper function), while other neoplastic T cell subsets can express polyclonal B cell helper activity.

Results in our laboratory over the past four years have led us to conclude that some (but *not* all) patients with the Sézary syndrome variant of cutaneous T cell lymphoma have a disease that represents a homogeneous expansion of polyclonal active helper T cells (Broder et al., 1976). Highly purified normal B cells do not undergo a transition into immunoglobulin-secreting cells *in vitro* after stimulation with certain lectins, such as pokeweed mitogen, unless a source of helper T cells is provided. The neoplastic T cells from certain patients with the Sézary syndrome provide such a helper effect by promoting the maturation of normal indicator B cells (rigorously depleted of T cells) into immunoglobulin-secreting cells following stimulation with pokeweed mitogen *in vitro* (Figure 15.1). Furthermore, recent experiments by Berger et al. (1979) have suggested that cytogenetically monoclonal neoplastic lymphocytes from involved nodes in certain patients with aleukemic cutaneous T cell lymphomas (mycosis fungoides) can exhibit an exceptional degree of polyclonal helper-like activity.

In collaboration with Drs. Uchiyama and Waldmann, we have examined the surface membrane phenotype of Sézary cells using the monoclonal reagents OKT4 and OKT8 discussed earlier. Sézary T cells from all six patients studied expressed the OKT4 antigen (thought to be present on normal helper T cells), but did not express the OKT 8 antigen thought to be present on normal suppressor T cells. We consider these membrane-marker studies as supplements to *functional* studies. At this time, we do not believe that membrane-marker studies alone can be used to ascribe immunoregulatory characteristics to neoplastic cells.

We are continuing our research efforts to learn whether neoplastic T cells with idiotype-specific helper activity exist, and also whether normal T cells augment or modify some neoplastic helper effects.

We recently studied a patient with the Sézary syndrome in whom the neoplasm evolved and could be histopathologically classified as a T cell immunoblastic sarcoma. Although the lymphomatous cells formed spontaneous sheep red cell rosettes (and could thus be classified as having a T cell origin), they did not have the cerebriform nuclei characteristically associated with Sézary cells, but rather, had round to oval nuclear contours. Nonetheless, these lymphomatous cells could mediate a helper T cell function (Lawrence et al., 1978). These observations suggest that neoplastic T cells from neoplasms with histopathologic features entirely different from the Sézary syndrome may eventually be found to mediate helper-cell immunoregulatory activity. Roder et al. (1978) have preliminary data that the permanently transformed T cells of a murine leukemia line maintain a carrier-specific type of helper activity under conditions of antigen activation. Finn et al. (1979) have carefully described a

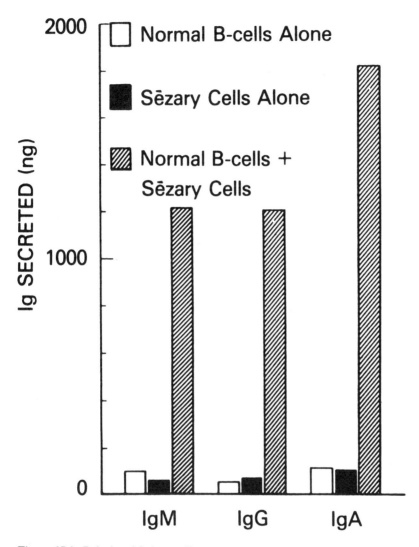

Figure 15.1. Polyclonal helper cell activity mediated by the neoplastic T cells from a patient with a cutaneous T cell lymphoma (Sézary syndrome). Pokeweed mitogen is the polyclonal activator used. Normal B cell populations, after rigorous T cell depletion, do not produce immunoglobulins *in vitro*. The addition of Sézary T cells restores immunoglobulin-producing capacity. (For details, see Broder et al., 1976.)

method involving the infection of immune T cells with radiation leukemia virus to produce murine lymphoma cell lines that can provide antigen-specific help to appropriately primed B cells in secondary antibody production. Later in this article, we shall discuss other systems in mice that could yield additional information about neoplasms of immunoregulatory T cells.

Suppressor Cell Neoplasms

Subacute T Cell Leukemia in Japan

Recently, the clinical and hematologic features of an apparently new kind of adult T cell leukemia were described (Uchiyama et al., 1977). This disease has several interesting features, and although it has certain similarities to the cutaneous T cell lymphoma syndrome discussed earlier, this entity should be considered a distinct disease category. It occurs in adults. There is generally a subacute leukemic course with a rapidly progressive terminal phase. The disease appears resistant to conventional chemotherapy. As with the neoplastic cells found in the cutaneous T cell lymphoma syndrome discussed earlier, the leukemic cells in this disorder form spontaneous sheep red cell rosettes and can be killed by heterologous antisera against human T cell membrane antigens. Moreover, the leukemic cells in this syndrome frequently have lobulated nuclei. Under electron microscopic examination, however, the nuclei are generally not as convoluted as those of typical Sézary cells. There is frequent leukemic involvement of the dermis and subcutaneous layers, but true *epidermal* infiltration and the formation of Pautrier's microabscesses are unusual. Lymphadenopathy and hepatosplenomegaly are common. These patients do not have mediastinal masses, but about 25% have significant parenchymal infiltration of the lungs.

Perhaps the most striking finding described by Uchiyama and co-workers is the geographic clustering of the patients' birth in the south of Japan. Thirteen of 16 patients reported were born on Kyushu, an island on which the city of Nagasaki is located. The role of atomic radiation and other environmental or genetic factors in the epidemiology of this disease has not been resolved.

The leukemic T cells from three of six patients with this disease inhibited immunoglobulin production by equal numbers of co-cultured normal (unfractionated) lymphocytes under conditions of polyclonal activation (Uchiyama et al., 1978). Furthermore, supernatant fluids obtained from a short-termed culture of leukemic cells from one of these three patients showed a marked suppressive effect on the capacity of normal lymphocytes to produce immunoglobulins. This supernatant fluid did not appear to mediate the suppressor effect through a mechanism of direct cytotoxicity. The suppressor effect was lost when the supernatant was heated at 56°C for 30 minutes. In collaboration with Dr. Uchiyama and Dr. Waldmann, we have developed a hybridoma antibody which detects activated regulatory T cell effectors. The antigen detected by this reagent (termed *Tac*) was expressed *in vivo* by these subacute Japanese T cells in preliminary experiments. Thus, by contrast to the immunoregulatory capacity found in certain patients with the Sézary syndrome, patients with the Japanese form of subacute adult T cell leukemia may have a neoplasm that originates from suppressor cells.

It may prove important to screen carefully cases of acute or subacute adult T cell leukemia in other nations to learn whether this type of leukemia is available for clinical investigation outside Japan. There is a report of one American patient with apparent Sëzary syndrome (and a monoclonal gammopathy) whose circulating cells induced a suppressor effect when cultured with normal B cell/T cell combinations, but only when a very great excess of the patient's cells were provided (Kansu and Hauptman, 1979). Hopper and Haren (1980) have reported another American patient with Sëzary syndrome whose neoplastic cells induced a potent suppressive effect in co-culture with normal peripheral blood lymphocytes, even at relatively low neoplastic:normal cell ratios. These investigators did not formally test helper activity using purified normal indicator B cells. Thus, a feedback form of suppressor cell induction (similar to the effect brought about by Ly-1$^+$ Qa-1$^+$ T cells) cannot be excluded.

It is crucial to bear in mind the complexity of murine regulatory circuits when evaluating human regulatory cell neoplasms. Normal and neoplastic human immunoregulatory circuits are likely to reveal at least as much complexity.

Neoplastic Pro-Suppressor Cells from a Child with Acute Lymphoblastic Leukemia and Hypogammaglobulinemia

We recently investigated an infant boy with acute lymphoblastic leukemia who had hypogammaglobulinemia at initial presentation (Broder et al., 1978). The neoplastic cells were of T cell origin. One of the most striking features of this child's unusual disease was a profound depression of serum IgM and IgG concentrations. The child received successful multimodal inductive therapy for acute lymphoblastic leukemia, after which the serum immunoglobulin levels temporarily rose. During the preterminal relapse of the leukemia, there was once again a depression of serum IgM and IgG levels.

Our studies of this patient indicated that the leukemic cells had a potent suppressor effect under suitable conditions of pokeweed mitogen activation. However, the leukemic cells could not bring about a suppressor effect without the cooperation of a radiosensitive subset of normal T cells. In more recent experiments, we found that these leukemic T cells appear to function as a population of *pro-suppressor* T cells which can mature into suppressor effector T cells following interaction with a population of normal suppressor activator or inducer T cells (Broder et al., 1979). This maturation did not occur when another polyclonal activator (Nocardia water-soluble mitogen) was used unless pokeweed mitogen was also provided. In some settings, the neoplastic pro-suppressor T cells could mature into fully functional suppressor effector T cells under the influence of a soluble factor secreted by pokeweed mitogen-triggered cooperating normal T cells. We believe this particular form of regulatory-cell leukemia is rare, but probably not unique.

In more recent studies, we found that these pro-suppressor leukemic suppressor cells could be used to raise antibodies that react with a new group of high-molecular weight glycoproteins found on the surface of certain cultured normal T cells exhibiting an *in vitro* suppressor activity for immunoglobulin production (Figure 15.2).

Based on our studies with these neoplastic pro-suppressor T cells, we have constructed a general hypothesis for the induction of human suppressor

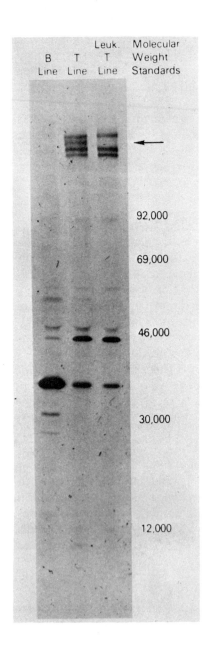

effector cells. According to this hypothesis, human suppressor T cells have an interim existence as pro-suppressor cells. At this stage of maturation, such cells do not have significant immunoregulatory capacity. Under the proper circumstances, pro-suppressor T cells may interact with a different set of activating T cells, or soluble factors derived from these cells. It is likely that the pro-suppressor T cells must be capable of synthesizing DNA *de novo* in order to mediate suppression fully. Once the pro-suppressor T cell subset has differentiated into a suppressor effector T cell subset, further DNA synthesis is probably no longer necessary for suppressor function. To allow further tests of this hypothesis, it would be important to identify other children and adults with T cell lymphoproliferative disorders whose neoplastic cells retain regulatory activity. Several laboratories are doing research in this area.

The hypothesis developed from the use of the leukemic cells with pro-suppressor T cell properties generates at least two predictions which can be tested by future clinical investigation. The first is that neoplastic diseases characterized by proliferations at different steps in suppressor-cell differentiation will eventually be discovered. Exactly where the Japanese form of subacute T cell leukemia with suppressor properties fits into the construct cannot be fully resolved at this time. The second prediction is that those patients with a neoplasm composed largely of suppressor effector cells will very likely have a degree of immune impairment directly related to their total tumor cell burden,

---

Figure 15.2. A newly defined, high-molecular weight group of related glycoproteins appears on the surface membrane of cultured suppressor-like T cells from normal individuals and can be revealed using *unabsorbed* heteroantibodies from early bleeds of rabbits inoculated with human pro-suppressor leukemic T cells (see text). These studies were done in collaboration with Drs. Warren Judd, Jack Strominger, Takashi Uchiyama, and Dean Mann. The figure shows the autoradiographic profile of membrane antigens derived from cultures of a growth factor-dependent normal T cell line with suppressor activity (T-line); for comparison, the simultaneous profile of membrane antigens from cultures of leukemic T cells (Leuk. T-line) that had lost the capacity to mediate suppression (sometime during the establishment of the culture) is shown. An autologous normal B-line is shown as a control.

Cells were pulsed with ^{35}S-methionine. Endogenously radiolabeled proteins were sequentially precipitated using the rabbit antibodies to pro-suppressor T cell leukemia antigens and protein A from *Staphylococcus aureus*. Immunoprecipitated membrane proteins were then subjected to sodium dodecyl sulfate polyacrylamide gel analysis using 7–15% gradients under reducing conditions.

The T line with suppressor cell activity reveals a new complex of four antigenic bands (top of figure) with a molecular weight in the range of 1.5×10^5 to 2.0×10^5 daltons. None of these four bands is detected using syngeneic Epstein-Barr virus transformed B cells. The antigenic bands represent glycoproteins since, for the most part, they can be removed by a mannose- or galactose-binding lectin precipitation step. The nonfunctional leukemic T cell line appears to be deficient in one of these high-molecular weight glycoproteins (see arrow). However, more research is necessary to define the biologic or clinical implications of these results.

while those patients with a neoplasm of pro-suppressor cells or suppressor activator cells will very likely have immune impairment related to the residual number or efficiency of nonneoplastic cooperating T cells, as well as their leukemic cells. In such patients, it should not be surprising to learn that the serum immunoglobulin levels may not bear a simple relationship to the patient's neoplastic disease status and, indeed, may sometimes appear normal in spite of strong *in vitro* evidence for suppressor activity. As an added complexity for future clinical investigation, the neoplastic cells from a patient with ataxia telangiectasia and a T-leukemia have recently been reported to mediate both helper and suppressor activity (Saxon et al., 1979). How neoplasms which appear to have mixed immunoregulatory properties will affect host-immune status cannot be predicted at this time. In addition, neoplastic T cells which retain certain cytotoxic effector functions have been reported (Bom-Van Noorloos et al., 1980). While such cells do not have an immunoregulatory activity per se, it is conceivable that such neoplastic cells can disturb normal immune regulatory circuits in certain patients.

Neoplastic thymic-derived suppressor cells have also been demonstrated in mice. The AKR strain of mice is noted for a very high incidence of spontaneous thymic lymphomas. There are recent data indicating that the neoplastic cells derived from mice bearing such lymphomas suppress the *in vitro* generation of humoral immune responses (Roman and Golub, 1976, 1978; Mulder et al., 1978; Russell and Golub, 1978). Suppression in this system appears to require cell contact. In about 80% of the spontaneous lymphomas studied, a suppressor effect can be observed only when syngeneic or semi-allogeneic target responder cells are used. In the remaining 20%, suppression is effective against both allogeneic and syngeneic target responder cells. A subset of the AKR suppressor lymphoma cell population appears to synthesize a form of surface-membrane-associated DNA, and this cell-surface DNA may be essential for the actual suppressor effect mediated by these neoplastic cells. The precise analogies between human and murine immunoregulatory T cell neoplasms are critical topics for continued research.

Possible Significance of Immunoregulatory Neoplasms to Clinical and Basic Research

The recognition that some T cell leukemias or lymphomas may produce a homogeneous proliferation of T cells which are committed to either helper or suppressor function is important for a number of reasons. For example, certain forms of humoral immunodeficiency may be due to a helper cell defect and not to either intrinsically defective B cells alone or exclusively activated suppressor cells. It is possible that an analysis of neoplastic T cell membrane-associated products or soluble helper factors released by neoplastic T cells will prove useful in the treatment of selected immunodeficiency states related to thymic impairment. By the same token, if such helper-cell factors could be identified and synthesized, they might be useful in those situations in which it is desirable to amplify a physiologic immune response, for example, following immunizations in overwhelming infections or, theoretically, even in certain forms of cancer.

The use of human neoplastic T cells as starting immunogens for raising conventional heteroantibodies or monoclonal (hybridoma) antibodies against T cell subsets may expedite the establishment of a serologic marker system, analogous to the murine Ly or *I-J* systems, for human helper and suppressor T cell subsets. Certain patients quite conceivably could present with neoplasms which arise from as yet unrecognized kinds of regulatory cells that would not be found among accessible normal lymphoid populations. Indeed, the availability of large numbers of homogeneous human T cells with known immunoregulatory capacity might eventually help define significant lymphoid antigenic markers for which there are as yet no *fully defined* murine equivalents (see Figure 15.2). Neoplastic T cells with known functional properties might also be extremely useful as reference targets for antisera from multiparous women or individuals with multiple transfusions in the search for alloantisera that can affect immunoregulatory cell function. There is a very real possibility that immunoregulatory T cell neoplasms may make it practical to serologically manipulate human immune responses.

Even when patients with immunoregulatory neoplasms are rare or relatively inaccessible, several new approaches may still make them important resources for clinical and basic investigation. It is worth reemphasizing that it is technically practical to establish functioning culture lines from both normal and neoplastic T cells using T cell growth factors (Maca et al., 1979; Gazdar et al., 1980), and in theory, clonally expanded immunoregulatory cell lines could be made available on a wide scale. Also, the technology for making T cell hybrid clones (hybridomas) *in vitro* is available, and hybrid cell lines which produce *I-J*-encoded factors with both specific and non-specific immunoregulatory activity have been developed in murine systems (Taniguchi and Miller, 1978; Taniguchi et al., 1980). The use of neoplastic T cells with established immunoregulatory functions may provide an important resource for making available large numbers of monoclonal T cell hybrid lines that bring about defined kinds of immunoregulatory activity. Somatic cell hybridization between regulatory neoplastic cells and appropriate functionally inert, T cell lines is feasible with currently available technology for the selection of hybridomas.

Taking a somewhat different perspective, recombinant DNA technology has made it feasible to isolate and clonally expand several mammalian genes through an insertion in the genomes of bacteria, which may then be used as *in vitro* biologic factories for the large-scale production of mammalian gene-products (Fiddes et al., 1979). Indeed, very recent applications of recombinant DNA technology have made it possible to insert selected genes into murine bone marrow cells, which can then be introduced *in vivo*, thereby altering the genetic repertoire of the intact murine host (Cline et al., 1980). Neoplastic T

210

cells with known immunoregulatory function could conceivably provide an important starting resource for isolating specific human genes involved in regulating normal immunity or in rectifying the regulatory-cell imbalances that cause or perpetuate certain immunodeficiency states.

References

Alibert, J.L.M. (1835) *Monographie de Dermatoses.* Bailiere, G. (ed.), Paris: France.

Bach, F.H. and van Rood, J.J. (1976) The major histocompatibility complex—genetics and biology. *N. Eng. J. Med.* 295:806–813, 872–878, 927–936.

Basten, A., Miller, J.F.A.P., Loblay, R., Johnson, P., Gamble, J., Chia, E., Pritchard-Briscoe, H., Callard, R., and McKenzie, I.F.C. (1978) T cell-dependent suppression of antibody production. I. Characteristic of suppressor T cells following tolerance induction. *Eur. J. Immunol.* 8:360–370.

Benacerraf, B. and Dorf, M. (1976) The nature and function of specific H-linked response genes and immune suppression genes. In *The Role of Products of Products of the Histocompatibility Gene Complex in Immune Responses.* Katz, D.H. and Benacerraf, B. (eds.), New York: Academic Press, pp. 225–248.

Benacerraf, B. and Germain, R.N. (1978) The immune response genes of the major histocompatibility complex. *Immunol. Rev.* 38:70–119.

Berendt, M.J. and North, R.J. (1980) T cell-mediated suppression of anti-tumor immunity: an explanation for progressive growth of an immunogenic tumor. *J. Exp. Med.* 151:69–80.

Berger, C.L., Warburton, D., Raafat, J., LoGerfo, P., and Edelsen, R.L. (1979) Cutaneous T cell lymphoma: neoplasm of T cells with helper activity. *Blood* 53:642–651.

Blaylock, W.K., Clendenning, W.E., Carbone, P.P., and Van Scott, E.J. (1966) Normal immunologic reactivity in patients with the lymphoma mycosis fungoides. *Cancer* 19:233–236.

Bom-van Noorloos, A.A., Pegels, H.G., van Oers, R.H.J., Silberbusch, J., Feltkamp-Vroom, T.M., Goudsmit, R., Zeijlemaker, W.P., von dem Borne, A.E.G., and Melief, C.J.M. (1980) Proliferation of T cells with killer-cell activity in two patients with neutropenia and recurrent infections. *N. Eng. J. Med.* 302:933–937.

Broder, S. and Bunn, P.A. (1980) Cutaneous T cell lymphomas. *Seminars in Oncology* 7:310-331.

Broder, S. and Waldmann, T.A. (1978) The suppressor-cell network in cancer (two parts). *N. Eng. J. Med.* 299:1281–1284, 1335–1341.

Broder, S. and Waldmann, T.A. (1979) Immunologic defects in patients with plasma cell neoplasms. In *Clinical Immunology Update.* Franklin, E. (ed.), New York: Elsevier Publishing Co., pp. 1–22.

Broder, S., Edelson, R.L., Lutzner, M.A., Nelson, D.L., MacDermott, R.P., Durm, M.E., Goldman, C.K., Meade, B.D., and Waldmann, T.A. (1976) The Sézary syndrome: a malignant proliferation of helper T cells. *J. Clin. Invest.* 58: 1297–1306.

Broder, S., Dobbins, W.O., and Waldmann, T.A. (1977) Excessive IgA production by lymphocytes with the Sézary syndrome and low numbers of circulating neoplastic T cells. *Fed. Proc.* 36:1210.

Broder, S., Poplack, D., Whang-Peng, J., Durm., Goldman, C., Muul, L., and Waldmann, T.A. (1978) Characterization of a suppressor cell leukemia: evidence for the requirement of an interaction of two T cells in the development of human suppressor effector cells. *New Engl. J. Med.* 298:66–72.

Broder, S., Muul, L., Durm, M., Goldman, C., Mann, D., and Waldmann, T.A. (1979) T-T interactions in the generation of human suppressor effector cells *in vitro.* In *In Vitro Induction and Measurement of Antibody Synthesis in Man.* Fauci, A. and Ballieux, R. (eds.), New York: Academic Press, pp. 69–84.

Broder, S., Mann, D.L., and Waldmann, T.A. (1980) Participation of suppressor T cells in the immunosuppressive activity of a heteroantiserum to human Ia-like antigens (*p. 23, 30*). *J. Exp. Med.* 151:257–262.

Brouet, J-C., Flandrin, G., and Seligmann, M. (1973) Indications of the thymus-derived nature of the proliferating cells in six patients with Sézary's syndrome. *New Engl. J. Med.* 289:341–344.

Bunn, P.A. and Lamberg, S.I. (1979) Report of the committee on cutaneous T cell lymphoma: staging classification. *Cancer Treat. Rep.* 63:725–728.

Cantor, H. and Gershon, R.K. (1979) Immunological circuits: cellular composition. *Fed. Proc.* 38:2058–2064.

Cline, M.J., Stang, H., Mercola, K., Morse, L., Ruprecht, R., Browne, J., and Salser, W. (1980) Gene transfer in intact animals. *Nature* 284:422–425.

Clough, J.D., Mims, L.H., and Strober, W. (1971) Deficient IgA antibody responses to arsanilic acid bovine serum albumin (BSA) in neonatally thymectomized rabbits. *J. Immunol.* 106:1624–1629.

Dosch, H., Percy, M.E., and Gelfand, E.W. (1977) Functional differentiation of B lymphocytes in congenital agammaglobulinemia. I. Generation of hemolytic plaque-forming cells. *J. Immunol.* 119:1959–1964.

Dupré, A., Bonafé, J.L., Lassère, J., Courret, B., Pieraggi, M.T., and Fédou, R. (1977) Syndrome de Sézary et dysglobulinemie monoclonale. *Rev. Med. Toulouse* 13:803–808.

Eardley, D.D., Shen, F.W., Cantor, H., and Gershon, R.K. (1979) Genetic control of immunoregulatory circuits: genes linked to the Ig locus govern communication between regulatory T cell sets. *J. Exp. Med.* 150:44–50.

Ellner, J.J. (1978) Suppressor adherent cells in human tuberculosis. *J. Immunol.* 121:2573–2579.

Engleman, E.G. and McDevitt, H.O. (1978) A suppressor T cell of the mixed lymphocyte reaction specific for the *HLA-D* region in man. *J. Clin. Invest.* 61:828–838.

Engleman, E.G., Hoppe, R., Kaplan, H., Comminskey, J., and McDevitt, H.D. (1978) Suppressor cells of the mixed lymphocyte reaction in healthy subjects and patients with Hodgkin's disease and sarcoidosis. *Clin. Res.* 26:513A.

Evans, R.L., Faldetta, T.J., Humphreys, R.E., Pratt, D.M., Yunis, E.J., and Schlossman, S.F. (1978) Peripheral human T cells sensitized in mixed leukocyte culture synthesize and express Ia-like antigens. *J. Exp. Med.* 148:1440–1445.

Feldmann, M., Beverley, P.C.L., Woody, J., and MacKenzie, I.F.C. (1977) T-T interactions in the introduction of suppressor and helper T cells: analysis of membrane phenotype of precursor and amplifier cells. *J. Exp. Med.* 145:793–801.

Fiddes, J.C., Seeburg, P.H., DeNoto, F.M., Hallewell, R.A., Baxter, J.D., and Goodman, H.M. (1979). Structure of genes for human growth hormone and chorionic somatomammotropin. *Proc. Natl. Acad. Sci. U.S.A.* 76:4294–4298.

Finn, O.J., Boniver, J., and Kaplan, H.S. (1979) Induction, establishment *in vitro*, and characterization of functional, antigen-specific, carrier-primed murine T cell lymphomas. *Proc. Natl. Acad. Sci. U.S.A.* 76:4033–4037.

Fisher, M.S., and Kripke, M.L. (1977) Systemic alteration induced in mice by ultraviolet light irradiation and its relationship to ultraviolet carcinogenesis. *Proc. Natl. Acad. Sci.* 74:1688–1692.

Fujimoto, S., Greene, M., and Sehon, A.H. (1975) Immunosuppressor T cells and their factors in tumor-bearing hosts. In *Suppressor Cells in Immunity*. Singhal, S.K. and Sinclair, N.R. (eds.), London, Ontario: University of Western Ontario Press, pp. 136–148.

Fujimoto, S., Greene, M., and Sehon, A.H. (1976a) Regulation of the immune response to tumor antigens. I. Immunosuppressor cells in tumor-bearing hosts. *J. Immunol.* 116:791–799.

Fujimoto, S., Greene, M., and Sehon, A.H. (1976b) Regulation of the immune response to tumor antigens. II. The nature of immunosuppressor cells in tumor-bearing hosts. *J. Immunol.* 116:800–806.

Fujimoto, S., Matsuzawa, T., Nakagawa, K., and Tada, T. (1978) Cellular interaction between cytotoxic and suppressor T cells against syngeneic tumors in the mouse. *Cell. Immunol.* 38:378–387.

Gazdar, A.F., Carney, D.N., Bunn, P.A., Russell, E.K., and Jaffe, E.S. (1980) Mitogen-requirement for the *in vitro* propagation of cutaneous T cell lymphoma. *Blood* 55:409–417.

Gelfand, E.W. and Dosch, H. (1979) *In vitro* functional heterogeneity of humoral and cellular immune deficiency states. In *In Vitro Induction and Measurement of Antibody Synthesis in Man.* Fauci, A. and Ballieux, R. (eds.), New York: Academic Press, pp. 309–324.

Germain, R., Waltenbaugh, C., and Benacerraf, B. (1980) Antigen-specific T cell-mediated suppression. V. H-2-linked genetic control of distinct antigen-specific defects in the production and activity of L-glutamic^{50}-L-tyrosine^{50} suppressor factor. *J. Exp. Med.* 151:1245–1259.

Goodwin, J.S., Messner, R.P., Bankhurst, A.D., Peake, G.T., Saiki, J.H., and Williams, R.C., Jr. (1977). Prostaglandin-producing suppressor cells in Hodgkin's disease. *New. Engl. J. Med.* 297:963–968.

Greaves, M.F., Verbi, W., Festenstein, C., Papasteriadis, C., Jaraquemada, D., and Hayward, A. (1979) "Ia-like" antigens on human T cells. *Eur. J. Immunol.* 9:356–362.

Greene, M.I., Dorf, M.E., Pierres, M., and Benacerraf, B. (1977a) Reduction of syngeneic tumor growth by an anti-*I-J* alloantiserum. *Proc. Natl. Acad. Sci. U.S.A.* 74:5118–5121.

Greene, M.I., Fujimoto, S., and Sehon, A.H. (1977b) Regulation of the immune response to tumor antigens. III. Characterization of thymic suppressor factor(s) produced by tumor-bearing hosts. *J. Immunol.* 119:757–764.

Greene, M.I., Pierres, A., Dorf, M.E., and Benacerraf B. (1977c) The *I-J* subregion codes for determinants on suppressor factor(s) which limit the contact sensitivity response to picryl chloride. *J. Exp. Med.* 146:293–296.

Hayes, C.E. and Bach, F.H. (1980) *I-N*: a newly described H-2 *I*-subregion between *K* and *I-A*. *J. Exp. Med.* 151:481–485.

Herberman, R.B. (1976) Immunologic approaches to the diagnosis of cancer. *Cancer* 37:549–561.

Hillinger, S.M. and Herzig, G.P. (1978) Impaired cell-mediated immunity in Hodgkin's disease mediated by suppressor lymphocytes and monocytes. *J. Clin. Invest.* 61:1620–1627.

Hodes, R.J. and Hathcock, K.S. (1976) *In vitro* generation of suppressor cell activity: suppression of *in vitro* induction of cell-mediated cytotoxicity. *J. Immunol.* 116:167–177.

Hopper, J.E. and Haren, J.M. (1980) Studies on a Sézary lymphocyte population with T-suppressor activity: suppression of Ig synthesis of normal peripheral blood lymphocytes. *Clin. Immunol. Immunopath.* 17:43–54.

Jeunet, F.S. and Good, R.A. (1968) Thymoma: immunologic deficiencies and hematological abnormalities. *Birth Defects* 4:192–206.

Joyner, M.V., Cassuto, J.P., Dujardin, P., Barety, M., Duplay, H., and Audoly, P. (1979). Cutaneous T cell lymphoma in association with a monoconal gammapathy. *Arch. Dermatol.* 115:326–328.

Kansu, E. and Hauptman, S.P. (1979) Suppressor cell population in Sézary syndrome. *Clin. Immunol. Immunopath.* 12:341–350.

Ko, H.S., Fu, S.M., Winchester, R.J., Yu, D.T.Y., and Kunkel, H.G. (1979) Ia determinants on stimulated human T lymphocytes: occurrence on mitogen and antigen-activated T cells. *J. Exp. Med.* 150:246–255.

Kövary, P.M., Niedorf, H., Breu, H., Kamanabroo, P., Büchner, T., and Mader, E. (1977) Paraproteinemia in Sézary syndrome. *Dermatologica* 154:138–146.

Lawrence, E.C., Broder, S., Jaffe, E.S., Braylan, R.C., Dobbins, W.O., Young, R.C., and Waldmann, T.A. (1978) Evolution of a lymphoma with helper T cell characteristics in Sézary syndrome. *Blood* 52:481–492.

Ledbetter, J.A., Rouse, R.V., Micklem, H.S., and Herzenberg, L.A. (1980) T cell subsets defined by expression of Lyt-1, 2, 3 and Thy-1 antigens. Two-parameter immunofluorescence and cytotoxicity analysis with monoclonal antibodies modifies current views. *J. Exp. Med.* 152:280–295.

Levy, R.B., Waksal, S.D., and Shearer, G.M. (1976) Correlation of suppressor cell development in parental and F₁ hybrid mouse strains with the growth of a parental tumor *in vivo. J. Exp. Med.* 144:1363–1368.

Lunney, J.K., Mann, D.L., and Sachs, D.H. (1979). Sharing of Ia antigens between species. III. Ia specificities shared between mice and human beings. *Scand. J. Immunol.* 10:403–413.

Lutzner, M., Edelson, R., Schein, P., Green, I., Kirkpatrick C., and Ahmed, A. (1975) Cutaneous T cell lymphomas: The Sézary syndrome, mycosis fungoides, and related disorders. *Ann. Intern. Med.* 83:534–552.

Maca, R.D., Bonnard, G.D., and Herberman, R.B. (1979) The suppression of mitogen and alloantigen-stimulated peripheral blood lymphocytes by cultured human T lymphocytes. *J. Immunol.* 123:246–251.

McDevitt, H.O., Delovitch, T.L., Press, J.L., and Murphy, D.B. (1976) Genetic and functional analysis of the Ia antigens: their possible role in regulating the immune response. *Transplant. Rev.* 30:197–235.

McDougal, J.S., Shen, F.W., and Elster, P. (1979) Generation of T helper cells *in vitro*. V. Antigen-specific Lyl⁺ T cells mediate the helper effect and induce feedback suppression. *J. Immunol.* 122:437–442.

Metzgar, R.S., Bertoglio, J., Anderson, J.K., Bonnard, G.D., and Ruscetti, F.W. (1979) Detection of HLA-Drw (Ia-like) antigens on human T lymphocytes grown in tissue culture. *J. Immunol.* 122:949–958.

Mozes, E. (1976) The nature of antigen-specific T cell factors involved in the genetic regulation of immune responses. In *The Role of Products of the Histocompatibility Gene Complex in Immune Responses.* Katz, D.H. and Benacerraf, B. (eds.), New York: Academic Press, pp. 485–505.

Mulder, A.M., Durdik, J.M., Toth, P., and Golub, E.S. (1978) Leukemia in AKR mice. III. Size distribution of suppressor T cells in AKR leukemia and neonatal mice. *Cell. Immunol.* 40:326–335.

Ottesen, E.A. (1979) Modulation of the host response in human schistosomiasis. I. Adherent suppressor cells that inhibit lymphocyte proliferative responses to parasite antigens. *J. Immunol.* 123:1639–1644.

Perry, L.L., Dorf, M.E., Benacerraf, B., and Greene, M.I. (1979) Regulation of immune responses to tumor antigen: interference with syngeneic tumor immunity by anti-*I-A* alloantisera. *Proc. Natl. Acad. Sci. U.S.A.* 76:920–924.

Perry, L.L., Dorf, M.E., Bach, B.A., Benacerraf, B., and Greene, M.I. (1980) Mechanisms of regulation of cell-mediated immunity: anti-*I-A* alloantisera interfere with induction and expression of T cell-mediated immunity to cell-bound antigen *in vivo. Clin. Immunol. Immunopath.* 15:279–292.

Pierres, M., Germain, R.N., Dorf, M.E., and Benacerraf, B. (1978) *In vivo* effects of anti-Ia alloantisera. I. Elimination of specific suppression by *in vivo* administration of antisera specific for *I-J* controlled determinants. *J. Exp. Med.* 147:656–666.

Piessens, W.F., Ratiwayanto, S., Tuti, S., Palmieri, J.H., Piessens, P.W., Kaiman, I., and Dennis, D.T. (1980) Antigen-specific suppressor cells and suppressor factors in human filariasis with *Brugia Malayi. New Engl. J. Med.* 302:833–837.

Puissant, A., Saurat, J.H., Lassarovici, M.C., and Delanoe, J. (1976) Eritrodermia con piccole cellule di Sézary-Baccaredda e immunoglobulina M monoclonale. *Giornale Italiano di Dermatoligia* 111:398–400.

Reinherz, E.L., Kung, P.C., Goldstein, G., and Schlossman, S.F. (1979a) Further characterization of the human inducer T cell subset defined by monoclonal antibody. *J. Immunol.* 123:2894–2896.

214

Reinherz, E.L., Kung, P.C., Goldstein, G., and Schlossman, S.F. (1979b) Separation of functional subsets of human T cells by a monoclonal antibody. *Proc. Natl. Acad. Sci. U.S.A.* 76:4061–4065.

Reinherz, E.L., Kung, P.C., Goldstein, G., and Schlossman, S.F. (1980) A monoclonal antibody reactive with the human cytotoxic/suppressor T cell subset previously defined by a heteroanti-serum termed TH_2. *J. Immunol.* 124:1301–1307.

Reinisch, C.L., Andrew, S.L., and Schlossman, S.F. (1977) Suppressor cell regulation of immune response to tumors: abrogation by adult thymectomy. *Proc. Natl. Acad. Sci. U.S.A.* 74:2989–2992.

Rich, S.S., and Rich, R.R. (1976) Regulatory mechanisms in cell-mediated immune responses. III. *I*-region control of suppressor cell interaction with responder cells in mixed lymphocyte reactions. *J. Exp. Med.* 143:672–677.

Roder, J.C., Tyler, L., Singhal, S., and Ball, J.K. (1978) Are T cell lymphomas immunocompetent? *Nature* 273:540–541.

Roman, J.M. and Golub, E.S. (1976) Leukemia in AKR mice. I. Effects of leukemic cells of antibody-forming potential of syngeneic and allogeneic normal cells. *J. Exp. Med.* 143:482–496.

Roman, J.M. and Golub, E.S. (1978) Leukemia in AKR mice. II. Two modes of suppression of *in vitro* antibody formation by leukemic cells. *Cell Immunol.* 40:316–325.

Russell, J.L. and Golub, E.S. (1978) Leukemia in AKR mice: a defined suppressor cell population expressing membrane-associated DNA. *Proc. Natl. Acad. Sci. U.S.A.* 75:6211–6214.

Sachs, D.H. (1976) The Ia antigens. *Contemp. Top. Molec. Immunol.* 5:1–34.

Saxon, A., Stevens, R.H., and Golde, D.W. (1979) Helper and suppressor T lymphocyte leukemia in ataxia telangiectasia. *New Engl. J. Med.* 300:700–704.

Schechter, G.P. and Soehnlen, F. (1978) Monocyte-mediated inhibition of lymphocyte blastogenesis in Hodgkin's disease. *Blood* 52:261–271.

Schreffler, D.C. and David, C.S. (1975) The H-2 major histocompatibility complex and the *I* immune response region: genetic variation, function, and organization. *Adv. Immunol.* 20:125–195.

Sézary, A. and Bouvrain, Y. (1938) Erythrodermie avec presence de cellules monstrueses dans le derme et dans le sang circulant. *Bull. Soc. Fr. Dermatol. Syph.* 45:254–260.

Siegal, F.P., Siegal, M., and Good, R.A. (1976) Suppression of B cell differentiation by leukocytes from hypogammaglobulinemic patients. *J. Clin. Invest.* 58:109–122.

Soothill, J.F., Hill, L.E., and Rowe, D.S. (1968) A quantitative study of the immunoglobulins in the antibody deficiency syndrome. In *Immunologic Deficiency Diseases in Man*. Bergsma, D. and Good, R.A. (eds.), New York: National Foundation Press, pp. 71–79.

Spellman, C.W. and Daynes, R.A. (1977) Modification of immunological potential by ultraviolet radiation. II. Generation of suppressor cells in short-term UV-irradiated mice. *Transplantation* 24:120–126.

Stobo, J.D., Paul, S., Van Scoy, R.E., and Hermans, P.E. (1976) Suppressor thymus-derived lymphocytes in fungal infection. *J. Clin. Invest.* 57:319–328.

Tada, T., Taniguchi, M., and David, C.S. (1976) Properties of the antigen-specific suppressive T cell factor in the regulation of the antibody response of the mouse. IV. Special subregion assignment of the gene(s) that codes for the suppressive T cell factor in the H-2 histocompatibility complex. *J. Exp. Med.* 144:713–725.

Tada, T., Taniguchi, M., and Okumura, K. (1977) Regulation of antibody response by antigen-specific factors bearing *I*-region determinants. *Prog. Immunol.* 3:369–377.

Tada, T., Takemori, T., Okumura, K., Nonaka, M., and Tokuhisa, T. (1978). Two distinct types of helper T cells involved in the secondary antibody response: independent and synergistic effects of Ia^- and Ia^+ helper T cells. *J. Exp. Med.* 147:446–458.

215

Taniguchi, M. and Miller, J. (1978) Specific suppressive factors produced by hybridomas derived from the fusion of enriched suppressor T cells and a T lymphoma line. *J. Exp. Med.* 148:373–382.

Taniguchi, M. and Tokuhisa, T. (1980) Cellular consequences in the suppression of antibody by the antigen-specific T cell factor. *J. Exp. Med.* 151:517–527.

Taniguchi, M., Takei, I., and Tada, T. (1980) Functional and molecular organization of an antigen-specific suppressor factor from a T cell hybridoma. *Nature* 283:227–228.

Taussig, M.J. and Munro, A.J. (1976) Antigen-specific T cell factor in cell cooperation and genetic control of the immune response. *Fed. Proc.* 35:2061–2066.

Thèze J., Waltenbaugh, C., Dorf, M., and Benacerraf, B. (1977) Immunosuppressive factor(s) specific for L-glutamic acid^{50}-L-tyrosine^{50} (GT). II. Presence of *I-J* determinants on the GT-suppressive factor. *J. Exp. Med.* 146:287–292.

Ting, C.C. and Rodrigues, D. (1980) Switching on the macrophage-mediated suppressor mechanism by tumor cells to evade host immune surveillance. *Proc. Natl. Acad. Sci. U.S.A.* 77:4265–4269.

Treves, A.J., Carnaud, C., Trainin, N., Feldman, M., and Cohen, I.R. (1974) Enhancing T lymphocytes from tumor-bearing mice suppress host resistance to a syngeneic tumor. *Eur. J. Immunol.* 4:722–727.

Twomey, J.J., Laughter, A.H., Farrow, S., and Douglass, C.C. (1975) Hodgkin's disease: an immunodepleting and immunosuppressive disorder. *J. Clin. Invest.* 56:467–475.

Uchiyama, T., Yodoi, J., Sagawa, K., Takatsuki, K., and Uchino, H. (1977) Adult T cell leukemia: clinical and hematologic features in 16 cases. *Blood* 50:481–492.

Uchiyama, T., Sagawa, K., Takatsuki, K., and Uchino, H. (1978) Effect of adult T cell leukemia cells on pokeweed mitogen-induced normal B cell differentiation. *Clin. Immunol. Immunopath.* 10:24–34.

Van Rood, J.J., Van Leeuwen, A., Termijtelen, A., and Keuning, J.J. (1976) B cell antibodies, Ia-like determinants, and their relation to MLC determinants in man. *Transplant. Rev.* 30:122–139.

Vidal, E. and Brocq, L. (1885) Etude sur le mycosis fungoide. *France Medical* 2:946–1085.

Vogler, L.B., Pearl, E.R., Gathings, W.E., Lawton, A.R., and Cooper, M.D. (1976) B lymphocyte precursors in bone marrow in immunoglobulin deficiency states. *Lancet* 2:376.

Waldmann, T.A., Broder, S., Durm, M., Blackman, M., Krakauer, R., and Meade, B. (1975) Suppressor T cells in the pathogenesis of hypogammaglobulinemia associated with thymoma. *Trans. Assoc. Am. Physicians* 88:120–134.

Yu, A., Watts, H., Jaffee, N., and Parkman, R. (1977) Concomitant presence of tumor-specific cytotoxic and inhibitor lymphocytes in patients with osteogenic sarcoma. *N. Engl. J. Med.* 297:121–127.

Zembala, M., Mytar, B., Popiela, T., and Asherson, G.L. (1977) Depressed *in vitro* peripheral blood lymphocyte response to mitogens in cancer patients: the role of suppressor cells. *Int. J. Cancer* 19:605–613.

Published 1981 by Elsevier North Holland, Inc.
Saunders, Daniels, Serrou, Rosenfeld, and Denney, eds.
FUNDAMENTAL MECHANISMS IN HUMAN CANCER IMMUNOLOGY

CHAPTER 16

Modulation of the Immune Reactions in Patients Bearing Solid Tumors[1]

B. Serrou, D. Cupissol, A. Rey, F. Favier, C. Thierry, C. Esteve, and C. Rosenfeld[+]

Department of Immuno-Chemotherapy and Laboratoire d'Immunopharmacologie des Tumeurs, INSERM U-236-ERA-CNRS n°844, Centre Paul Lamarque, Hôpital Saint-Eloi, BP. 5054, 34033 Montpellier Cedex, France and +Department of Human Cell Cultures and Production, I.C.I.G.-Hôpital Paul Brousse, 14-16 Av. Paul Vaillant Couturier, 94800 Villejuif, France

The therapeutics of solid tumors remains difficult despite recent progress linked to adjuvant therapy (Mathe et al., 1980). Certain recent studies (Cuttner et al., 1980; Jones et al., 1980; Klefstrom et al., 1980; Pavlovsky et al., 1980; Pouillart et al., 1978; Verhegen et al., 1980) suggest that response to chemotherapy may depend on the patient's immunological status. The more immunodepressed a patient, the worse will be his response to this type of treatment.

Evaluation of the immune response in the cancer patient, particularly in the solid tumor patient, has proved difficult for two reasons (Table 16.1). First, the antigens which characterize these tumors are either poorly- or un-defined. The existence of specific antigens to solid tumors remains an investigative dilemna. If such antigens do exist, they are probably weak, or are modifications of normally occurring autologous antigens altered by chemical or viral carcinogenic agents. It is nevertheless probable that virus-exposed (but not chemically altered) antigens permit an adequate immune response (Herberman et al., 1974; Zoller et al., 1975; Doherty et al., 1976). Secondly, lymphocyte subpopulations are poorly defined (Chess et al., 1977). Recent monoclonal antibody studies (Kung et al., 1979) have provided an improved functional definition of these subpopulations as well as a more revealing characterization of suppressor, amplifier, and cytotoxic subpopulations. Subpopulation markers should lead to more accurate evaluation of immune imbalance in solid tumor patients

[1]This work was supported by Grants from INSERM 71-78-103, CNRS, DGRST 79-7-0670, and 79-7-0674, Association pour la Recherche sur le Cancer de Villejuif (ARCV) and the Coordinating Council for Cancer Research (CCCR).

218

Table 16.1. Immune Status of the Cancer Patient
Related to Treatment.

Impairment of the immune status
Need for evaluation of new markers and new functions:
   Leukocytes
   Monocytes and macrophages
   Lymphocytes (monoclonal antibodies)
Tumor associated antigens and autologous immune responses
Impairment of the immune status and response to chemotherapy

(Serrou et al., 1980a; Cobleigh et al., 1980; Serrou et al., 1980g). Furthermore, functional subpopulation definitions, such as exist for NK activity, could prove useful if, for example, NK cells have *in vivo* biological significance (Riccardi et al., 1980).

Up until the last two years, few substances were capable of modifying the immune response, and these usually corresponded to particularly complex agents, such as Bacille Calmette Guerrin (BCG) and *Corynebacterium parvum*. More and more such agents are becoming available which are better or completely defined biochemically. Some of these have been subsequently synthesized, and their site of action on lymphocyte subpopulations, macrophages or leukocytes is now open to investigation (Serrou et al., 1980i,j).

Today the concept of immunomodulation is gradually replacing that of immunotherapy in the treatment of the tumor patient, due to better understanding of a certain autologous-like anti-tumor response (at least for chemically-induced tumors or those linked to the environment), combined with the availability of lymphocyte subpopulation functional markers and well characterized drugs which modulate this response. During the last two years, an increased number of phase I and phase II trials of new drugs providing a more precise chemoimmunomodulation have produced encouraging results (Terry et al., 1980).

Immunomodulating Agents

Numerous recently developed drugs have been proposed as modulators of the immune response. Among them, our work has mostly centered around thymus extracts (thymosin), human fibroblast interferon, bestatin, a retinoic acid derivative, isoprinosine, and cyclomunine.

Thymosin

Thymosin is a thymus extract first prepared by A.L. Goldstein et al. (1972). Fraction V Thymosin is a combination of several subfractions, including thymosin alpha-1 (Thurman et al., 1979). Based on preliminary results, it is probable that each subfraction may act on different lymphocyte functions (Thurman et al., 1979).

We evaluated the possible benefits of fractions V and alpha-1 thymosin in animal models applicable to man and in *in vitro* human lymphocyte protocols (Serrou et al., 1979a, b, 1980h). Our results based on an animal tumor (Lewis tumor) model are the following (Serrou et al., 1980n). Splenocytes from tumor-bearing animals were capable of facilitating tumor growth when obtained 10 days after tumor implantation, then injected intravenously into syngeneic animals implanted with the same tumor. If one treats these splenocytes beforehand with serum anti-Thy 1-2, the facilitating effect disappears and tumor growth advances at the same rate as is observed in animals receiving physiological saline. In contrast, if the cells are instead treated with fraction V thymosin, not only does facilitation cease, but regional tumor mass is diminished and the number of pulmonary metastases (common with Lewis tumor) decreases. These results suggest that thymosin modulates the immune response and is capable of controlling tumor growth as well as other thymic factors (Cupissol et al., 1981a).

In subsequent studies, we employed a model which more closely approximated the human situation and is directly applicable to the treatment of solid tumors in man. It has been demonstrated that thymic factors permit T lymphocyte differentiation from immature bone marrow cells (Scheid et al., 1975). We have developed a technique for autologous bone marrow grafts for malignant melanoma or metastasized breast cancer patients. The bone marrow of the patient to be treated is removed prior to intensive chemotherapy and placed in liquid nitrogen, assuming it has not been infiltrated by tumor cells. This marrow is then reinjected intravenously 2 or 3 days after chemotherapy. We noted that these patients were severely immunodepressed for approximately 3 weeks, due to the continued presence of immature cells which were probably null cells. We have previously shown that null cells can exert a suppressor effect (Serrou et al., 1980m). This finding led us to the hypothesis that prior *in vitro* induced differentiation of immature lymphocytes with agents such as thymosin could reduce the risk and duration of the observed immunosuppression.

We developed an animal model to test this hypothesis (Cupissol et al., 1981a). The tumor employed was chemically induced by methylcholanthrene and injected intravenously, either on the day of tumor implantation or 10 days post-implantation, accompanied by 30×10^6 marrow cells, either preincubated or not with thymosin. The results showed that the animals treated with thymosin preincubated cells demonstrated decreased regional tumor growth with a significant increase in survival time. On the other hand, the cells responsible for the observed effect were T cells, while NK cells played no role whatsoever (Tables 16.2 and 16.3). Analysis of these results indicates that thymosin permits marrow cell differentiation to T lymphocytes, and this effect is therapeutically advantageous. The next point of investigation will be to determine if marrow cells preincubated with thymosin subsequent to intensive chemotherapy can improve upon the results obtained by intensive chemotherapy alone.

Table 16.2. T-Dependence of Bone Marrow Cell Thymosin Effect on Syngeneic Mouse Tumor Growth.

Groups	Days after tumor implantation Tumor volume (cm³ ± SD)			
	7	14	21	28
1. Control medium	1.20 ± 0.1	3.9 ± 0.1	8.7 ± 0.5	11 ± 0.2
2. BMC[a] alone	1 ± 0.2	4.0 ± 0.1	9.1 ± 0.1	10 ± 0.3
3. BMC pretreated with thymosin fraction 5	0.7 ± 0.1(S)[b]	3 ± 0.6(S)	6.5 ± 0.1(S)	8 ± 0.1(S)
4. BMC pretreated with an anti Thy 1.2 antiserum	1.4 ± 0.2(S)	4.8 ± 0.4(S)	9.8 ± 0.7(S)	12.3 ± 0.4(S)
5. BMC pretreated with an anti Thy 1.2 antiserum, then preincubated with thymosin fraction 5	1.45 ± 0.12(S)	5.0 ± 0.15(S)	9.9 ± 0.15(S)	13.07 ± 0.7(S)

[a] BMC: Bone marrow cells. BMC were preincubated with thymosin (1 hour at 37°C), then i.v. reinjected into syngeneic tumor bearing mice. 6 mice per group.

[b] S: Significant – Day 7: 3 and 5 vs 1 and 2: $p < 0.05$. Day 14: 3 and 5 vs 1 and 2: $p < 0.01$. Days 21 and 28: 3 and 5 vs 1 and 2: $p < 0.001$.

Table 16.3. NK Independence of Bone Marrow Cell Thymosin Effect on Syngeneic Mouse Tumor Growth.

Groups	Days after tumor implantation			
	7	14	21	28
		Tumor weight (gm ± SD)		
1. Control medium	1.09 ± 0.27	4.27 ± 0.18	9.64 ± 0.29	11.26 ± 0.12
2. BMC[a] alone	0.89 ± 0.21	4.38 ± 0.25	9.2 ± 0.3	10.9 ± 0.20
3. BMC pretreated with thymosin fraction 5	0.65 ± 0.18(S)[b]	3.12 ± 0.18(S)	6.7 ± 0.22(S)	8.1 ± 0.16(S)
4. Strontium treated tumor bearing mice	1.1 ± 0.21	4 ± 0.38	9.8 ± 0.2	11.3 ± 0.15
5. Strontium treated mice injected with thymosin preincubated BMC	0.69 ± 0.16(S)	3 ± 0.1(S)	7.1 ± 0.15(S)	8 ± 0.2(S)

[a]BMC: Bone marrow cells. BMC were preincubated with thymosin (1 hour at 37°C), then i.v. reinjected into syngeneic tumor bearing mice. 6 mice per group.

[b]S: Significant – day 7: 3 and 5 vs 1 and 2: $p < 0.05$. Day 14: 3 and 5 vs 1 and 2: $p < 0.01$. Days 21 and 28: 3 and 5 vs 1 and 2: $p < 0.001$.

We also studied *in vitro* treatment of human lymphocytes with thymosin (Serrou et al., 1979a; Touraine et al., 1980a) and showed that thymosin fraction V and especially alpha 1 thymosin could modulate the number of human peripheral blood auto-rosette forming cells (ARFC), particularly if the number were subnormal (Serrou et al., 1980k). Solid tumor patients with ARFC levels under 15% showed the most remarkable *in vitro* rebound, using this type of drug (Serrou et al., 1980h). In a parallel experiment, we showed an *in vitro* T cell suppressor population from solid tumor patients, purified on an anti-Fab'2 immunoabsorbent column, was less suppressive following thymosin incubation (Serrou et al., 1980h).

Taken as a whole, these *in vitro* results reinforce those obtained *in vivo* in animals and point to thymosin as a drug capable of modulating and restoring the immune response, thereby acting on tumor growth *in vivo*. These findings and published results from *in vitro* (Hersh et al., 1978; Patt et al., 1979; Wolf et al., 1980) and *in vivo* human studies (Chretien et al., 1980) of this agent, have prompted the human phase I and II trials presently under way (Chretien et al., 1979).

Interferon

Numerous recent investigations have supported the idea that the antiviral substance, interferon, acts not only on cell multiplication but on differentiation as well. This information helps to illuminate its effect on diverse tumor systems and its potential action on tumor cell multiplication and lymphocyte differentiation (Krim, 1980; Bloom, 1980).

Our attention has centered on human fibroblast interferon, which we used to treat metastatic breast cancer patients (Serrou et al., 1980b, d, e). In one patient treated for 5 weeks (3.3×10^6 I.U. injected intravenously 3 times a week), we obtained complete remission of pelvis and shoulder bony metastases. This result persisted throughout 7 treatment-free months. Subsequently, the patient suffered a relapse of bony metastases which is presently being treated by chemotherapy. During interferon therapy, the patient demonstrated improved delayed hypersensitivity skin tests, as evaluated by the Merieux system (Table 16.4). This test is based on response to seven antigens, and it allows one to classify a subject as anergic, hypoergic or hyperergic (Cupissol et al., 1979). We also observed a strong increase in NK activity and peripheral blood ARFC levels and noted an increase in immune complexes, particularly IgG and IgM. These complexes did not contain anti-interferon antibodies.

In vitro studies were performed to determine the effect of human fibroblast interferon on human lymphocytes (Serrou et al., 1980e). The results showed that this drug was able to increase NK activity and reestablish normal ARFC levels (or at least cause a significant ARFC increase). Above all, it influenced suppressor function, as evaluated on Concanavalin A (Con A) induced suppressor cells. It was established that suppressor cell induction could be facilitated or inhibited by varying the *in vitro* concentration of interferon

Table 16.4. Evaluation of Human Fibroblastic Interferon in One
Metastatic Breast Cancer Patient.

	Skin tests score mm	ARFC %	NK activity % cytotoxicity[a]
Before treatment	3	10	30
After treatment	18	15	90

Note: This patient has been in complete remission for 7 months after 5 weeks
interferon treatment.

[a]Lytic units per 10^7 cells (25:1).

(Table 16.5). These results suggest that interferon may be capable of modulating the immune response. In the present case, its effects were dose-dependent.

These results converge toward those reported in the literature (Blomgren et al., 1980a; Krim, 1980; Fridman et al., 1980; Herberman, 1980; Peter et al., 1980). Nevertheless, the impact of this drug on different lymphocyte subpopulation still remains undefined, and clinical applications have yet to be ascertained.

Bestatin

Bestatin is an immunomodulatory substance purified by Umezawa et al. (1976) from *Streptomyces olivoreticuli*. In animals, this drug acts on tumor growth but can also modulate different immunological activities such as NK activity. Bestatin studies have shown that it can significantly repress the onset of spontaneous tumors in older mice (Bruley-Rosset et al., 1979). This drug has been studied in man by various Japanese research teams (Umezawa, personal communication) and Blomgren et al. (1980b), who report low toxicity for the doses employed as well as complete patient tolerance. *In vivo*, the drug restored normal levels of circulating T cells and amplified certain types of immune response, particularly NK activity. At present, several clinical trials are in progress. We conducted our phase I trials as part of the EORTC Immunology and Immunotherapy Group (GI2C) (Serrou et al., 1980c,g). We have found that 40 mg/m2 bestatin given to immunodepressed patients, 3 times per week for 2 weeks, significantly ameliorated immune function in these advanced solid tumor patients as evaluated by the Merieux 7-antigen skin test system. Results showed a very significant improvement in the score value, increased numbers of circulating ARFC's and higher NK activity. No side-effects were noted, but no change in tumor volume was observed. The tumors remained quite large in these advanced patients. These results are based on a 30-patient study and appear sufficiently remarkable, even more so since they entirely corroborate the Japanese findings (Umezawa 1980, personal communication) as well as those of Blomgren et al. (1980b). These promising results

Table 16.5. *In Vitro* Suppressor Effect of Human Fibroblast Interferon.

HFI doses	Spon. inc.	PHA dpm ± SD	PWM dpm ± SD	Con A dpm ± SD
No interferon	908 ± 134	115,850 ± 5912	110,957 ± 2805	96,095 ± 2280
Interferon 5 U/ml	12,720 ± 1314	72,895 ± 1028	65,420 ± 2179	66,850 ± 831
% inhibition		38	41	32
Interferon 50 U/ml	14,828 ± 490	32,423 ± 2677	36,423 ± 1281	24,495 ± 592
% inhibition		72	57	75
Interferon 500 U/ml	8,786 ± 280	50,505 ± 1237	45,302 ± 475	53,548 ± 2286
% inhibition		57	60	45

amply justify initiation of randomized trials in immunodepressed patients either in evolution or on therapy. A randomized trial has been approved using bestatin as a post-radiotherapeutic adjuvant in head and neck cancers. Randomized trials are currently underway in Sweden for both bladder and prostate cancers (Blomgren, 1980, personal communication).

The results reported thus far suggest that bestatin may prove of considerable interest as a non-toxic, well tolerated immunomodulator. This drug seems to act primarily on T lymphocytes and cells presenting NK activity. However, the effect on NK cells does not seem to depend on the production of interferon (Blomgren et al., 1980a). Several lines of research are presently in progress to evaluate better the clinical impact of this drug, especially as a pre-treatment to chemotherapy for the immunodepressed patient, and also to determine its effects on lymphocyte subpopulations, which can now be functionally defined by means of monoclonal antibodies.

Retinoic Acid Derivatives

Vitamin A plays an important role in maintaining the cellular differentiation process (Bollay, 1979). Recent findings suggest that vitamin A acts as a neuraminidase-like substance by decapping the cell surface to allow more effective expression of hidden antigens (Hogan-Ryan and Fennely, 1978). However, one must keep in mind that the toxicity of long-term or strong dose vitamin A therapy gives rise to poorly tolerated side-effects. Under such conditions, the drug loses its effectiveness. Several derivatives have been synthetized. Among them is RO 10-9359, which we evaluated in advanced solid tumor patients who were judged by the Merieux system to be immunodepressed.

This well characterized, synthetic substance was administered at 5 mg per kg per day for 21 days. As with bestatin, we evaluated the *in vivo* immunorestorative capability of this drug in the immunodepressed patient. We focused on immunorestoration prior to chemotherapy, since evidence suggests that the immunodepressed patient is less responsive to chemotherapy.

Results show that the drug is well tolerated at the test dose employed, and no major side-effects were encountered (Table 16.6). There was no effect on tumor volume, but it should be kept in mind that treatment was only short-term and the patients had very advanced tumors. Immunologically, there was a very significant change in delayed hypersensitivity, which reached normal levels, and a strong increase in the number of circulating ARFC's. A lesser effect was noted for NK activity which in this small sample of 25 patients was not significant. It is possible that retinoic acid derivatives may exert only a minimal effect on NK activity, as compared to bestatin or interferon.

The results suggest that certain retinoic acid derivatives may act on lymphocyte differentiation. Presently, little is known about the mechanism of action at this level (Dennert and Lotan, 1978; Mickshe et al., 1977; Patek et al.,

Table 16.6. Side-Effects of RO 109359.

Skin rash	2 patients
Nausea and vomiting	no effect
Renal toxicity	no effect
Hematologic toxicity	no effect
Liver toxicity	no effect
Cardiac toxicity	no effect
Neurologic toxicity	no effect

1979), but the availability of functional markers should lead to a better understanding of the drug's site of action. Toxicity after long-term use remains a problem, particularly at the 5 mg/kg dose employed in the present short-term study. The concentration used in long-term treatment is approximately 1 mg/kg (Lutzner and Blanchet-Bardin, 1980; Peck and Yoder, 1976; Peck et al., 1979).

These results appear encouraging enough to justify new phase I and II trials for new retinoic derivatives as they become available, since they appear to possess immunomodulatory properties.

Isoprinosine

Isoprinosine is a new antiviral drug with immunostimulatory properties (Simon and Glasky, 1978). It is made up of 1:3 molar ratio of P acetaminobenzoic acid to dimethyl amino-isopropanol. In animals, this drug facilitates monocyte, T lymphocyte, and probably neutrophil functions (Ginsberg and Glasky, 1977; Hadden et al., 1976, 1977; Morin et al., 1980; Renoux et al., 1979; Wybran et al., 1978, 1980).

We evaluated the *in vitro* isoprinosine effects on ARFC and suppressor activity (Serrou et al., 1980). In an overall sense, isoprinosine does not alter the number of ARFC's. However, if these results are studied with respect to the initial ARFC level, one notes that isoprinosine can increase subnormal ARFC values, although very high or very low values remain relatively unaffected (Table 16.7). It therefore appears that isoprinosine acts to increase normal ARFC values.

In contrast, it was shown that isoprinosine can modulate the activity of Con A induced suppressor T cells. When isoprinosine is added to the induction phase, it significantly reduces and can even totally block suppressor cell induction. This phenomenon was completely independent of cytotoxicity and was most evident at 200 µg/ml (Table 16.8).

Overall, these results confirm those of other investigators, who found that isoprinosine can modulate suppressor or non-suppressor T lymphocyte functions (Renoux et al., 1979; Wybran et al., 1980). However, some workers have shown that isoprinosine can induce a suppressor cell-dependent activity (Touraine et al., 1980b). This result does not contradict our findings, since it is

Table 16.7. Effect of Isoprinosine on Autorosette Forming Cells (ARFC).

ARFC %	0-15		15-25		25-50		Total	
	NI	I	NI	I	NI	I	NI	I
Mean	11	10.8	20.17	20.8	27.25	32.5	21.83	24.63
SD	2.39	3.49	3.06	3.9	4.7	3.5	9.71	9.87
p value	0.99		0.80		0.05		0.53	

Note: NI: No isoprinosine; I: isoprinosine in the test. Lymphocytes were incubated 1 hour at 37°C with 100 μg/ml isoprinosine.

becoming more and more apparent that substances which modulate immune activity can enhance or inhibit a given function, depending on both the moment at which the substance comes in contact with the lymphocytes and the dose administered. This phenomenon, has already been demonstrated for thymosin (Horowitz et al., 1977; Serrou et al., 1979).

Therefore, isoprinosine is a modulator of the immunological equilibrium and in this respect is of clinical interest for the treatment of viral diseases, as preliminary results have shown. New derivatives (NPT 15392) are now available which may be of ever greater interest in the treatment of tumors, and these are presently under study in both animals and man (phases I and II). These trials should indicate if a drug of this chemical definition possesses *in vitro* immunorestorative capability.

Cyclomunine

Cyclomunine (Simon-Lavoine, 1980) is a new immunomodulating agent. It is a hexacyclodepsipeptide extracted from *Fusarium equiseti*. It is insoluble in water and has a molecular weight of approximately 500 daltons. In low doses (10^{-6}

Table 16.8. Effect of Isoprinosine on Con A Induced Suppressor Cell Activity.

Populations		dpm ± 2SE	% inhibition	p value[a]
A. ST Lys. + fresh Lys.	PHA	133263 ± 1094		
	Con A	178534 ± 4220		
B. S$_2$ Lys. + fresh Lys.	PHA	101136 ± 11098	23	< 0.001
	Con A	73316 ± 5963	59	< 0.001
C. Isoprinosine	PHA	185939 ± 8650	–	< 0.001
S$_2$ + fresh Lys.	Con A	123171 ± 4860	32	< 0.001

Note: Lys.: Lymphocytes; ST: 72-hr culture lymphocytes without mitogen; S$_2$: Con A induced suppressor lymphocytes (200 μg/ml/2 × 10^6 Lys.) Isoprinosine: 200 μg/ml/2 × 10^6 Lymphocytes added at the induction phase.

[a]p value: B vs A and B vs C.

228

to 10^{-3} µg/ml *in vitro*; 1.25 and 500 µg/kg *in vivo*), cyclomunine stimulates immunological metabolic activity of macrophages, increases primary response to sheep red blood cells, facilitates Con A suppressor T cell induction in mixed culture, and potentiates interferon mediated protection against FMC virus. At higher doses (5 to 10 µg/ml *in vitro* and 12.5 mg/kg *in vivo*) it suppresses mitogen and antigen induced lymphocyte transformation, prolongs kidney and skin allografts, reduces graft versus host reactions, and decreases PFC response to sheep red blood cells (Simon-Lavoine, 1980). It therefore appears to be an immunomodulator. Moreover, cyclomunine very significantly increases the level of circulating Facteur Thymique Serique (FTS; Dardenne et al., 1980) in both young and old mice as well as NZB mice or those with thymus grafts. FTS (Bach et al., 1979) was measured by indirect immunofluorescence, based on purified anti-FTS antibody against synthetic FTS. The results suggest that cyclomunine can modulate overall immune system activity, but since it stimulates thymic function, this effect may merely be a reflection of thymic stimulation.

We have shown (Serrou et al., in preparation) that cyclomunine did not significantly alter ARFC levels in normal subjects (where the level exceeds 20%). However, cyclomunine caused a significant increase in ARFC'S for patients whose level was under 20% (Table 16.9)

We have already begun human phase I trials and have shown that there is no toxicity associated with cyclomunine administration per os and that cyclomunine augments the number of circulating ARFC's as well as NK activity (Table 16.10). We have also observed a smaller change in delayed hypersensitivity in the small number of patients studied thus far. Taken as a whole, these results underline the potential interest of cyclomunine, whose thymic effect will have to be further investigated. These studies may eventually lead to development of the first drug capable of *in vivo* induction of thymic factors, one whose therapeutic benefit could be significant.

Modulation of Markers and Functions

We have discussed several biochemically characterized drugs now available which are capable of modulating the immune response (Mathe and Serrou,

Table 16.9. *In Vitro* Effects of Cyclomunine on the Level of Autorosette Forming Cells (ARFC).

Drug	Before treatment	After treatment	p value
Healthy donors	24 ± 0.95	38.44 ± 1.93	< 0.001
Cancer patients bearing solid tumors	8 ± 0.7	10	NS

Table 16.10. Phase I Evaluation of Cyclomunine.

	Skin tests score mm	p Value	ARFC %	p value	NK activity lytic units per 10^7 cells (30:1)	p value
Patient number	5		5		5	
Before treatment	5.0 ± 0.5	–	6.6 ± 1.3	–	10.2 ± 3.7	–
After treatment	6.1 ± 0.7	0.05	17 ± 3.1	< 0.001	41.5 ± 2.1	< 0.001

Note: Side-effects: Diarrhea in 2 patients.

1979). A fuller appreciation of lymphocyte subpopulations and their functions
have led to the hope of finding drugs capable of affecting a specific subpopulation function, thereby modulating the immune response to respond specifically
to a given pathological situation. In order to achieve this goal, we have focused
on three types of markers which follow functional activity: T lymphocyte
ARFC's, NK activity, and Con A induced suppressor T cell activity *in vitro*.

Autorosette Forming Cells (ARFC)

Identification of this cell subset involves contact between lymphocytes, autologous red cells, and serum. The technique has already been described in detail
(Caraux et al., 1978, 1979a). Under test conditions, we have determined the
normal level of the ARFC T cell subset is 26%.

These cells are characterized (Serrou et al., 1980l) as T cells which lack the
Fc receptor for IgG, do not react with antibodies from Juvenile Rheumatoid
Arthritis (JRA), and have no suppressor activity. In fact, they include two
subpopulations. One group includes immature T lymphocytes expressing no
IgG or IgM-Fc receptors on their surface. These are associated with thymus,
since 70% of thymocytes are ARFC's. The other subpopulation consists of
mature T lymphocytes with IgM-Fc receptors. Recently, we were able to purify
this subpopulation (95% ARFC's), which allowed us to study its function
(Rucheton et al., 1981). These cells respond well to phytohemagglutinin (PHA),
but only weakly to pokeweed mitogen (PWM) or Concanavalin A (Con A)
(Table 16.11). They possess no NK or antibody dependent cell mediated
cytotoxicity (ADCC) activities but demonstrate autologous (Figure 16.1) and
allogenic mixed lymphocyte culture (MLC) response (Rey et al., 1981a,b). We
have not as yet determined the precise function(s) of ARFC subpopulations.

Table 16.11. Mitogen Responsiveness of Enriched Autologous Rosette Forming Cell
(ARFC) Fractions.

		Peripheral blood lymphocytes dpm ± 2 SE	ARFC depleted fraction dpm ± 2 SE	ARFC enriched fraction dpm ± 2 SE
PHA	10 μg/ml	45129 ± 3914	118155 ± 2665	88113 ± 5773
	100 μg/ml	34157 ± 2065	113158 ± 2743	44350 ± 2857
	1000 μg/ml	2758 ± 364	22354 ± 1077	4757 ± 167
PWM	10 μg/ml	12004 ± 496	60958 ± 3821	11987 ± 250
	100 μg/ml	11404 ± 1200	65995 ± 5514	10442 ± 40
	1000 μg/ml	830 ± 50	32553 ± 845	506 ± 174
Con A	10 μg/ml	11429 ± 1798	93083 ± 9617	4252 ± 1018
	100 μg/ml	8961 ± 4302	100473 ± 4248	6934 ± 374
	1000 μg/ml	208 ± 32	32001 ± 3548	178 ± 17

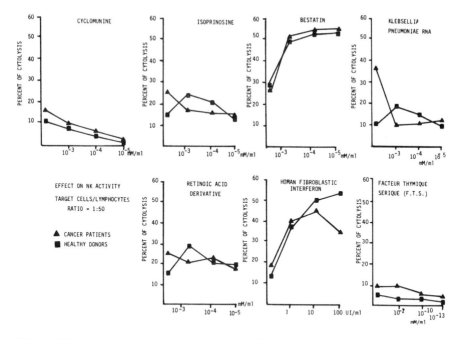

Figure 16.1. Autologous mixed lymphocyte culture response of autorosette forming cells. This figure suggests that the autologous mixed lymphocyte stimulation depends, for a large part, on autologous rosette forming cells.

Cytological examination shows that autorosettes are a homogenous population, slightly activated or in the early stages of activation. They present a distinct Golgi apparatus and endoplasmic reticulum. They are lysosome poor and show weak lysosomal activity for enzymes such as acid phosphatase and beta-glucuronidase (Serrou et al., 1980l).

Measurement of ARFC levels are of significant utility in clinical follow-up of the solid tumor patient (Caraux et al., 1979b). We have found that the relapsed patient produced a significantly lower level of ARFC's than the patient in remission. Furthermore, ARFC levels drop several weeks prior to clinical relapse. In the weeks preceding solid tumor patient relapse, one observes a very significant increase in one hour autorosettes, but a marked decrease in overnight rosettes (Table 16.12).

These cells not only appear sensitive to a changing pathological context, but also to different pharmacological agents (Rey et al., 1981b; Serrou et al., 1980k). Both thymosin and FTS can reestablish normal ARFC levels *in vitro*. The same was found to be true of cortisol, diethyl thiocarbamate (DTC) and a derivative of retinoic acid. In contrast, these cells appear unaffected by irradiation. Certain agents such as cyclomunine were only capable of increas-

Table 16.12. Early and Late Autorosette Forming Cells (ARFC) in Healthy Donors and Cancer Patients.

ARFC (%)	Healthy donors	Patients in remission	Patients 8-12 weeks before relapse	Patients in relapse
Early (1 hour)	5.43 ± 1.55	6.93 ± 2.09	14.62 ± 3.06	2.67 ± 1.07
Late (overnight)	23.86 ± 2.18	24.36 ± 2.47	9.08 ± 2.83	7.42 ± 1.53
Difference (late-early)	+ 18.43	+ 17.43	− 5.54	+ 4.75
p value	—	NS	p < 0.001	p < 0.001

ing ARFC levels in subjects with initially normal levels. This characteristic differs from the properties of drugs such as thymosin or FTS, interferon, cis-platinum (Serrou et al., 1981) and cimetidine (Serrou et al., 1980q), which are active in the cancer patient with low ARFC levels.

The ARFC cell assay may prove to be a valuable *in vitro* screening test for new immunorestorative drugs which could eventually lead to a simplified two group classification: those drugs acting on low ARFC levels, and those acting in normal levels. We have not as yet been able to ascertain the impact of these drugs on early and delayed ARFC's, a finding which would certainly help to define their potential impact on T lymphocyte subpopulations. In addition, we are presently evaluating the relationship between changes in ARFC levels *in vitro* and autologous mixed culture responses. However, as we previously pointed out, the observed *in vitro* effects correlate well with *in vivo* results in human phase I and II trials (Serrou et al., 1980a, c, d).

NK Activity

The NK test was used as a potential evaluation of both *in vivo* and *in vitro* immunorestoration. Most of the drugs tested *in vitro* for their effect on ARFC levels were also evaluated for NK activity. We were able to show *in vivo* that certain drugs (Figure 16.2), such as interferon, bestatin, and to a lesser extent, retinoic acid derivative, modulated and increased NK activity, whereas substances such as purified RNA from *Klebsiella pneumoniae* (Serrou et al., 1980p) decreased this activity. Thymosin and FTS, cimetidine (Serrou et al., 1980q), muramyl dipeptide (Mdp) (Chedid, 1980), and theophylline (Limatibul et al., 1978) have little or no effect on this activity. Cortisol may provoke a marked NK activity in normal subjects, but exerts no effect in the cancer patient who demonstrates an initial weak response. Cis-platinum could significantly alter NK activity. Cyclomunine causes a slight depression of NK activity.

These results suggest that relatively few drugs are available which increase NK activity as effectively as interferon. Among such drugs, bestatin, which shows minimal toxicity, appears to be particularly promising, as indicated by *in vivo* human trials. This drug has been shown to modulate NK activity, both *in vivo* and *in vitro*.

Concanavalin A (Con A) Induced Suppressor T Cell Activity

Several investigators studying the cancer patient have reported an immune imbalance and alteration of the helper cell/suppressor cell ratio (Serrou et al., 1980a; Cobleigh et al., 1980). A better definition of this imbalance may arise from experiments using monoclonal antibodies (Kung et al., 1979). Some investigators, including ourselves (Serrou et al., 1980a), have shown that advanced solid tumor patients exhibit a marked increase in suppressor activity. Since this activity is observed in patients with evolving tumor growth it would seem, *a priori*, worthwhile to be able to modulate this type of activity (Hersh et al., 1978; Patt et al., 1979; Chretien et al., 1979).

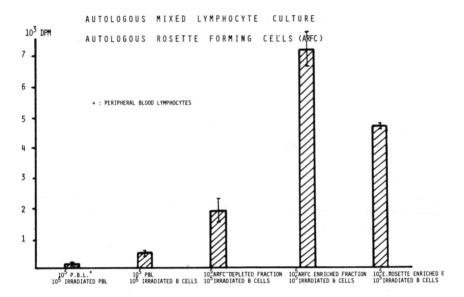

AUTOLOGOUS MIXED LYMPHOCYTE CULTURE

AUTOLOGOUS ROSETTE FORMING CELLS (ARFC)

Figure 16.2. *In vitro* effects of different drugs on NK activity. One should note the marked increase of NK activity due to bestatin and fibroblastic interferon. A slight effect was observed for lymphocytes from healthy donors in response to retinoic acid derivative and isoprinosine. *Klebsiella pneumoniae* RNA preparation dramatically decreases NK activity of lymphocytes from cancer patients. Other drugs tested showed no significant effect.

We have evaluated a small number of drugs to determine their effect on suppressor activity in the Con A induced T cell suppressor system. In addition, in a small sample of solid tumor patients, we were able to demonstrate this same activity on T cells purified on an anti-(Fab')2 immunoabsorbent column. We studied the modulation of this activity *in vitro* (Serrou et al., 1980a) and showed that thymosin fraction V and fraction alpha-1 significantly decrease this type of activity (Figure 16.3). The most remarkable effects were observed in the suppressor cell effector phase, whereas thymosin had little effect on the induction phase. If thymosin is added to both phases, there is a potentiation of the decrease in suppressor activity which had previously been very markedly decreased. The same effect was noted when levamisole was added during the induction phase and thymosin during the effector phase. Although levamisole has little effect on the effector phase, it significantly blocks suppressor activity in the induction phase of Con A suppressor cell induction (Figure 16.3). The exactly opposite effect was noted for thymosin. These effects were not due to a cytotoxic effect and were noted for all of the following effector systems: PHA, PWM, Con A, or allogenic mixed culture. Suppressor activity was also significantly reduced by isoprinosine added to the induction phase (Table 16.8). This effect was likewise not due to cytotoxicity.

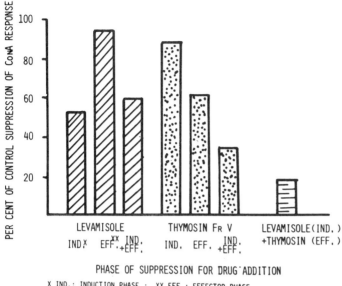

Figure 16.3. Effect of thymosin and levamisole on suppressor activity of Con A induced suppressor cells. Thymosin significantly decreases the suppressor activity of Con A induced suppressor cells when added during the effector phase but has no effect on the induction phase. The inverse is observed for levamisole. There is an additive effect when levamisole is introduced during the induction period and thymosin during the effector period.

These results are corroborated by the fact that thymosin fraction V and alpha-1 were also capable of significantly inhibiting at least 25% of T cell suppressor activity in advanced solid tumor patients (Serrou et al., 1980a).

The overall importance of these results lies not only in the potential modulation of *in vitro* suppressor activity in tumor patients (by drugs such as thymosin, levamisole, and isoprinosine) and *in vitro* artificially induced suppressor activity, but also the *in vivo* control by thymosin of T cell suppressor activity in solid tumor patients. It should be recalled that interferon can either induce or inhibit suppressor activity depending on the dose (Table 16.5), as previously demonstrated for thymosin and isoprinosine.

Conclusions

The points presented above bear witness to a new era in immunotherapy. Immunostimulation, as we know it today, using extremely complex substances such as BCG and *Corynebacterium parvum*, will probably eventually disappear to make way for immunomodulation which includes immunorestoration.

A fuller understanding of immunomodulatory drugs and a better regulatory control of the immune system should ensue from: (1) precise definition of human autologous responses, at least those against weak tumor-associated differentiation antigens in humans; (2) availability of functional markers for human lymphocyte subpopulations; and (3) biochemically defined or at least better characterized immunomodulatory drugs. Achievement of these goals should lead to *in vitro* dissection of the intimate mechanism(s) of action of these drugs at the lymphocyte subpopulation level, eventually making possible phase I and II trials in man.

It appears that most of these drugs are short-acting, demonstrate minimal toxicity (except for the retinoic acid derivative), and may soon assume their place in human therapy, either for treatment of cancer or for general use in treating bacterial or viral infections. For the latter, only a few effective drugs presently exist. However, these trials will have to be undertaken carefully by cooperating research teams, guided by ethics similar to those defined for chemotherapy. This approach should yield the most interpretable results and avoid the hasty conclusions which marred early studies of interferon, which not only detracted from the treatment in question but slowed progress of the entire field.

In adapting the chemotherapy guidelines for human phase I and II trials in man, new definitions will have to be formulated to accommodate immunomodulatory drugs. In Europe, this re-definition for such trials has been undertaken by two EORTC groups: the Cancer Immunology and Immunotherapy Group (CI2G) and the Tumor Immunology Project Group (TIPG). Potentially useful drugs in man are being reviewed by these groups for evaluation in experimental animal and *in vitro* human lymphocyte systems. If, after this initial stage, a drug produces sufficiently encouraging results, randomized phase I and II trials are designed for therapeutic use, either alone or as a preparation for chemotherapy in the immunodepressed patient.

The results of early tests of immunomodulatory drugs have been sufficiently encouraging that serious consideration of immunomodulation as an associative treatment for cancer seems warranted. Before this can occur, however, it will be necessary to functionally define the different subpopulations of lymphocytes, design appropriate screening tests, and stimulate the synthesis of an increasing number of biochemically characterized drugs directed at specific activities within the immune system.

References

Bach, J.F., Bach, M.A., Charreire, J., Dardenne, M., and Pleau, J.M. (1979) The mode of action of thymic hormones. *Ann. N.Y. Acad. Sci.* 332:23–32.

Blomgren, H., Einhorn, S., and Strander, H. (1980a) Modulation of the immune response by interferon *in vivo* and *in vitro*. In *New Trends in Human Immunology and Cancer Immunotherapy. Vol. 1 Biological Response Modifiers.* Serrou, B. and Rosenfeld, C. (eds.), Paris, London: Doin-Saunders, pp. 875–886.

Blomgren, H., Strander, L., and Edsmyr, F. (1980b) The influence of bestatin on the lymphoid system in the human. In *Small Molecular Immunomodulators*. Umezawa, H. (ed.), in press.

Bloom, B.R. (1980) Interferon and the immune system. *Nature* 284:593–595.

Bollag, W. (1979) Retinoids and cancer. *Cancer Chemoth. Pharmacol.* 3:207–215.

Bruley-Rosset, M., Forentin, I., Kiger, N., Schulz, G., and Mathe, G. (1979) Restoration of impaired immune functions of aged animals by chronic bestatin treatment. *Immunology* 38:75–83.

Caraux, J. and Serrou, B. (1978) The binding of autologous erythrocytes by human lymphocytes. *Biomedicine* 29:315.

Caraux, J., Thierry, C., Esteve, C., Flores, G., Lodise, R., and Serrou, B. (1979a) Human autologous rosettes. I. Mechanism of binding of autologous erythrocytes by T. cells. *Cell Immunol.* 45:36–48.

Caraux, J., Thierry, C., and Serrou, B. (1979b) Human autologous rosettes. II. Prognostic significance of variations in autologous rosette-forming cells in the peripheral blood of cancer patients. *J. Nat. Cancer Inst.* 63:593–597.

Chedid, L. (1980) Use of Mdp derivatives in experimental tumor immunotherapy. In *New Trends in Human Immunology and Cancer Immunotherapy. Vol. 1. Biological Response Modifiers*. Serrou, B. and Rosenfeld, C. (eds.), Paris, London: Doin-Saunders, pp. 995–1009.

Chess, L. and Schlossman, S.F. (1977) Human lymphocyte subpopulations. *Adv. Immunol.* 25:213–231.

Chretien, P.B., Lipson, S.D., Makuch, R., Kenady, D.E., and Cohen, M.H. (1979) Effects of thymosin *in vitro* in cancer patients and correlation with clinical course after thymosin immunotherapy. *Ann. N.Y. Acad. Sci.* 332:135–147.

Cobleigh, M., Braun, D., and Harris, J. (1980) Quantification of lymphocytes and T cell subsets in patients with disseminated cancer. *J. Natl. Cancer Inst.* 1041–1045.

Cupissol, D., Dabouis, G., Decroix, G., Fière, A., Hayat, M., Israel, L., Khouri, S., Kuss, R., Lang, J.M., Le Mevel, B., Lesourd, B., Martin, A., Moulias, R., Schneider, M., Serrou, B., and Thivolet, J. (1979) Delayed cutaneous hypersensitivity (DCH) reactions in cancer patients by multitest. In *Medical Oncology*. Berlin, Heidelberg, New York: Springer Intern. Abstract 118.

Cupissol, D., Rey, A., Goldstein, A., and Serrou, B. (1981a) Thymosin treated bone marrow cells suppress tumor growth in mice. Submitted.

Cupissol, D., Touraine, J.L., and Serrou, B. (1981b) Ability of lymphocytes treated with thymic factor to decrease lung metastasis in tumor bearing mice. *Thymus*, in press.

Cuttner, J., Glidewell, O., and Holland, J. (1980) A controlled trial of chemoimmunotherapy in acute myelocytic leukemia (AML). In *Immunotherapy of Cancer: Present Status of Trials in Man*. Terry, W.D. (ed.), Amsterdam: Elsevier/North-Holland, in press.

Dardenne, M., Niaudet, P., Simon-Lavoine, N., and Bach, J.F. (1980) Stimulation of thymic humoral function by cyclomunine, a cyclic peptide, in mice. *Intern. J. Immunopharmacol.* 2:154–157.

Dennert, G. and Lotan, R. (1978) Effects of retinoic acid on the immune system: stimulation of T killer cell induction. *Eur. J. Immunol.* 8:23–29.

Doherty, P.C., Blanden, R.V., and Zinkernagel, R. (1976) Specificity of virus-immune effector T cells for H-2k and H-2D compatible interactions: implications for H antigen diversity. *Transplant. Rev.* 29:89–124.

Fridman, H., Gresser, I., Auguet, M., and Neauport-Sautes, C. (1980) Interferon induced effects on lymphocyte membrane. In *New Trends in Human Immunology and Cancer Immunotherapy. Vol. 1. Biological Response Modifiers*. Serrou, B. and Rosenfeld, C. (eds.), Paris, London: Doin-Saunders, pp. 856–864.

Ginsberg, T. and Glasky, A.J. (1977) Inosiplex: an immunomodulation model for the treatment of viral disease. *Ann. N.Y. Acad. Sci.* 284:128–138.

Goldstein, A.L., Guha, A., Zatz, M.M., Hardy, M.A., and White, A. (1972) Purification and biological activity of thymosin, a hormone of the thymus gland. *Proc. Natl. Acad. Sci. U.S.A.* 69:1800–1806.

Hadden, J.W., Hadden, E.M., and Goffey, R.G. (1976) Isoprinosine augmentation of phytohemagglutinin induced lymphocyte proliferation. *Infect. Imm.* 13:382–385.

Hadden, J.W., Lopez, C., O'Reilly, R.J., and Hadden, E.M. (1977) Levamisole and inosiplex: antiviral agents with immunopotentiating action. *Ann. N.Y. Acad. Sci.* 284:139–150.

Herberman, R.B. (1974) Cell-mediated immunity to tumor cells. *Adv. Cancer Res.* 19:207–263.

Herberman, R. (1980) Human Lymphocyte Differentiation, in press.

Hersh, E.M., Patt, Y.Z., Mavligit, G.M., Murphy, S.G., Gutterman, J.U., Dicke, K., and Spitzer, G. (1978) Studies of cell-mediated immunity in man and the effects of immunotherapy. In *Human Lymphocyte Differentiation. Its Application to Cancer*. Serrou, B. and Rosenfeld, C. (eds.), Amsterdam, New York: North-Holland Publ. Co., 8:375–382.

Hogan-Ryan, A. and Fennely, J.J. (1978) Neuraminidase-like effect of vitamin A on cell surface. *Europ. J. Cancer* 14:113–116.

Horowitz, S., Borcherding, W., Moorthy, A.V., Chesney, R., Schulme-Wasserman, H., Hong, R., and Goldstein, A. (1977) Induction of suppressor T cells in systemic lupus erythematosus by thymosin and cultured thymic epithelium. *Science* 197:999–1002.

Jones, S., Salmon, S., and Haskins, C. (1980) Chemoimmunotherapy of non-Hodgkin's lymphoma. In *Immunotherapy of Cancer: Present Status of Trials in Man*. Terry, W.D. (ed.), Elsevier, North-Holland, in press.

Klefstrom, P., Holsti, P., Grohn, P., and Heinonen, E. (1980) Combination of levamisole immunotherapy with conventional treatments in breast cancer. In *Immunotherapy of Cancer: Present Status of Trials in Man*. Terry, W.D. (ed.), Elsevier, North-Holland, in press.

Krim, M. (1980) Towards therapy with interferons. In *New Trends in Human Immunology and Cancer Immunotherapy. Vol. 1 Biological Response Modifiers*. Serrou, B. and Rosenfeld, C. (eds.), Paris, London: Doin-Saunders, pp. 831–843.

Kung, P. Goldstein, G., Reinherz, E., and Schlossman, S. (1979) Monoclonal antibodies defining distinctive human T cell surface antigens. *Science* 206:347–349.

Limatibul, S., Shore, A., Dosh, H.M., and Gelfand, E.W. (1978) Theophylline modulation of E-Rosette formation: an indicator of T cell maturation. *Clin. Exp. Immunol.* 33:503–513.

Lutzner, M.A. and Blanchet-Bardon, C. (1980) Oral retinoid treatment of human papillomavirus type 5-induced epidermodysplasia verruciformis. *N. Engl. J. Med.* 19:1091.

Mathe, G. and Serrou, B. (1979) Immunomodulateurs à visée cancérolytique et/ou cancérostatique. In *Pharmacologie Clinique. Bases de le Thérapeutique 2*. Giroud, J.P., Mathe, G., and Meyniel, G. (eds.), Paris: Expansion Scientifique, 2:1797–1830.

Mathe, G., Bonadonna, G., and Salmon, S. (1980) *Adjuvant Therapies of Cancer*. Berlin, Heidelberg, New York: Springer-Verlag, in press.

Micksche, M., Cerni, C., Kokron, O., Titscher, R., and Wrba, H. (1977) Stimulation of immune response in lung cancer patients by vitamin A therapy. *Oncology* 34:234–238.

Morin, A., Griscelli, C., and Daguillard, F. (1979) Effets de l'isoprinosine sur l'activation des lymphocytes humains *in vitro*. *Ann. Immunol.* (Inst. Pasteur) 130C:541–551.

Morin, A., Touraine, J.L., Touraine, F., and Hadden, J. (1980) Isoprinosine as an immunomodulating agent. In *New Trends in Human Immunology and Cancer Immunotherapy. Vol. 1 Biological Response Modifiers*. Serrou, B. and Rosenfeld, C. (eds.), Paris, London: Doin-Saunders, pp. 1021–1031.

Patek, P.Q., Collins, J.L., Yogeeswaran, G., and Dennert, G. (1979) Anti-tumor potential of retinoic acid: stimulation of immune mediated effectors. *Int. J. Cancer* 24:624–628.

Patt, Y.Z., Hersh, E., Adebile, M., Goldman, R., and Mavligit, G. (1979) New approaches to the evaluation of immunomodulation by thymic hormones. *Ann. N.Y. Acad. Sci.* 332:160–171.

Pavlovsky, S., Garay, G., Sackmann, F.M., Svarch, E., et al. (1980) Levamisole therapy during maintenance of remission in patients with acute lymphoblastic leukemia. In *Immunotherapy of Cancer: Present Status of Trials in Man*. Terry, W.D. (ed.), Elsevier, North-Holland, in press.

Peck, G.L. and Yoder, F.W. (1976) Treatment of lamellar ichthyosis and other keratinizing dermatoses with an oral synthetic retinoid. *Lancet* 2:1172–1174.

Peck, G.L., Olsen, F.G., and Yoder, F.W. (1979) Prolonged remissions of cyctic and conglobate acne with 13-cis-retinoic acid. *N. Engl. J. Med*. 300:329–333.

Peter, H., Dallugge, H., Zawatzki, R., Euler, S., Kirchner, H., and Leibold, W. (1980) Human peripheral null lymphocytes are producers of type 1 interferon upon stimulation with herpes virus, *Corynebacterium parvum*, and tumor cell lines. In *New Trends in Human Immunology and Cancer Immunotherapy. Vol. 1 Biological Response Modifiers*. Serrou, B. and Rosenfeld, C. (eds.), Paris, London: Doin-Saunders, pp. 844–855.

Pouillart, P., Palangic, P., Huguenin, P., Morin, P., Gauthier, H., Baron, A., Mathe, G., Lededente, A., and Botto, G. (1978) Cancers épidermoides bronchiques inopérables. Etude de la signification pronostique de l'état immunitaire et résultats d'un essai d'immunorestauration par BCG. *Nouv. Presse Med*. 7:265–269.

Renoux, G., Renoux, M., and Guillaumain, J.M. (1979) Isoprinosine as an immunopotentiator. *J. Immunopharmac*. 1:337–356.

Rey, A., Rucheton, M., Caraux, J., Esteve, C., Thierry, C., and Serrou, B. (1981a) Autorosette forming cells: functional evaluation. Submitted.

Rey, A., Duclos, B., Ilnicky, C., Esteve, C., and Serrou, B. (1981b) Human autologous rosettes. III. Pharmacology of autologous rosette-forming cells. Submitted.

Riccardi, C., Santoni, A., Barlozzari, T., Puccetti, P., and Herberman, R. (1980) *In vivo* natural reactivity of mice against tumor cells. *Int. J. Cancer* 25:475–486.

Rucheton, M., Rey, A., Esteve, C., Mazauric, J.P., Thierry, C., and Serrou, B. (1981) Human autologous rosettes. IV. Purification of autologous rosette forming cells. Submitted.

Scheid, M.P., Goldstein, G., and Boyse, E.A. (1975) Differentiation of T cells in nude mice. *Science* 190:1211–1244.

Serrou, B., Goldstein, A., Thierry, C., and Caraux, J. (1979a) Regulation of human suppressor cell function by thymosin. *Biomedicine* 31:89.

Serrou, B., Rosenfeld, C., Caraux, J., Thierry, C., Cupissol, D., and Goldstein, A. (1979b) Thymosin modulation of suppressor function in mice and man. *Ann. N.Y. Acad. Sci*. 332:95–100.

Serrou, B., Gauci, L., Caraux, J., Thierry, C., Cupissol, D., and Rosenfeld, C. (1980a) Immune imbalance in cancer patients. In *Cancer Chemo and Immunopharmacology. Recent Results in Cancer Research*. Mathe, G. and Muggia, F. (eds.), Heidelberg, New York: Springer-Verlag, in press.

Serrou, B., Cupissol, D., Gauci, L., Thierry, C., Caraux, J., Rosenfeld, C., and Horoszewicz, J. (1980b) *In vivo* and *in vitro* modulation of the immune response by human fibroblast interferon (HFI). *Intern. J. Immunopharmacol*. 2:159 (abstract).

Serrou, B., Cupissol, D., Flad, H., Goutner, A., Lang, J.M., Spirzglas, H., Plagne, R., Beltzer, M., Chollet, P., Nameur, M., and Mathe, G. (1980c) Phase 1 evaluation of bestatin in patients bearing advanced solid tumors. In *Immunotherapy of Cancer: Present Status of Trials in Man*. Terry, W.D. (ed.), Elsevier, North-Holland, in press.

Serrou, B., Cupissol, D., Gauci, L., Thierry, C., Caraux, J., Rosenfeld, C., and Horoszewicz, J. (1980d) *In vitro* and *in vivo* modulation of the immune response by human fibroblast Interferon. In *New Trends in Human Immunology and Cancer Immunotherapy. Vol. 1 Biological Response Modifiers*. Serrou, B. and Rosenfeld, C. (eds.), Paris, London: Doin-Saunders, pp. 921–928.

Serrou, B., Cupissol, D., Thierry, C., Caraux, J., Gerber, M., Pioch, Y., Estève, C., and Lodise, R. (1980e) *In vivo* and *in vitro* modulation of helper, suppressor, and NK activities by human Interferon. *Interferon: Prop. Clin. Uses (Proc. Int. Symp.)* S.621-31.

Serrou, B., Cupissol, D., Flad, H., Goutner, A., Lang, J.M., Spirzglas, H., Plagne, R., Beltzer, M., Chollet, P., and Mathe, G. (1980f) Phase I evaluation of bestatin in patients bearing advanced solid tumors. *Intern. J. Immunopharmacol.* 2:168 (abstract).

Serrou, B., Cupissol, D., and Rosenfeld, C. (1980g) Immune imbalance and immune modulation of solid tumor patient. New Insights. *In Adjuvant Therapies of Cancer.* Mathe, G., Bonadonna, G. and Salomon, J.C. (eds.), Heidelberg, Berlin, New York: Springer-Verlag. In press.

Serrou, B., Cupissol, D., Caraux, J., Thierry, C., Rosenfeld, C., and Goldstein, A.L. (1980h) Ability of thymosin to decrease *in vivo* and *in vitro* suppressor cell activity in tumor bearing mice and cancer patients. In *Cancer Chemo and Immunopharmacology. Recent Results in Cancer Research.* Mathe, G. and Muggia, F. (eds.), Heidelberg, New York: Springer-Verlag, 75:110–114.

Serrou, B., Cupissol, D., Touraine, J.L., Rosenfeld, C., and Goldstein, A.L. (1980i) Thymosin modulates suppressor cell activity. In *Thymus, Thymic Hormones, and T Lymphocytes.* Aiuti, F. (ed.), New York, San Francisco, London: Academic Press, pp. 257–262.

Serrou, B., Cupissol, D., Caraux, J., Thierry, C., and Rosenfeld, C. (1980j) New immunomodulating agents with immunorestorative potential in cancer patients. In *Prospects of Manipulation of Host-Tumor Relationship.* Salomon, J.C. and Israel, L. (eds.), Paris: Inserm Publ. In press.

Serrou, B., Rucheton, M., Rey, A., Caraux, J., Estève, C., and Thierry, C. (1980k) Autorosette forming cells: further characterization and immunopharmacology. *Clinical Immunology News Letter.* In press.

Serrou, B., Cupissol, D., Thierry, C., and Estève, C. (1980l) Isoprinosine as modulator of non-suppressor and suppressor T cells. *Intern. J. Immunopharmacol.*, in press.

Serrou, B., Rosenfeld, C., Thierry, C., and Rucheton, M. (1980m) Suppressor activity of Reh human ALL non-B/non-T cell line. In *New Trends in Human Immunology and Cancer Immunotherapy. Vol. 1 Biological Modifiers.* Paris, London: Doin-Saunders, pp. 656–660.

Serrou, B., Cupissol, D., Goldstein, A., and Rosenfeld, C. (1980n) T lymphocytes from Lewis tumor-bearing mice lose their *in vivo* enhancing effect and inhibit syngeneic tumor growth following *in vitro* preincubation in thymosin. Submitted.

Serrou, B. and Rosenfeld, C. (1980o) *New Trends in Human Immunology and Cancer Immunotherapy. Vol. 1 Biological Response Modifiers.* Serrou, B. and Rosenfeld, C. (eds.), Paris-London: Doin-Saunders, p. 920.

Serrou, B., Rey, A., Cupissol, D., Estève, C., Dussourd-d'Hinterland, L., Normier, G., Pinèle, A.M., and Rosenfeld, C. (1980p) Efficacy of *Klebsiella pneumoniae* RNA on tumor growth in mice. In *Human Cancer Immunology. Vol. 4. New Immunomodulating Agents.* Serrou, B. and Rosenfeld, C. (eds.) Guest editors: Wybran, J. and Meyer, G. Amsterdam, New York: North-Holland. In press.

Serrou, B., Rey, A. Cupissol, D., Thierry, C., Estève, C., and Rosenfeld, C. (1980q) Modulation of the immune response by cimetidine. In *Human Cancer Immunology. Vol. 4. New Immunomodulating Agents.* Serrou, B. and Rosenfeld, C. (eds.) Guest Editors: Wybran, J. and Meyer, G. Amsterdam, New York: North-Holland. In press.

Serrou, B., Rey, A., Cupissol, D., Thierry, C., and Estève, C. (1981) *In vitro* effects of cis-platinum on the immune response. Submitted.

Simon-Lavoine, N. (1980) Cyclomunine. An overview. In *Human Cancer Immunology. Vol. 4. New Immunomodulating Agents.* Serrou, B. and Rosenfeld, C. (eds.) Guest Editors: Wybran, J., and Meyer, G. Amsterdam, New York: North-Holland. In press.

Simon, L.N. and Glasky. A.J. (1978) Isoprinosine an overview. *Cancer Treat. Rep.* 62:1963–1969.

Terry, W.D. (1980) *Immunotherapy of Cancer: Present Status of Trials in Man.* Amsterdam, New York: North-Holland. In press.

Touraine, J.L., Serrou, B., Thierry, C., Caraux, J., De Bouteiller, O., and Touraine, F. (1980a) Human suppressor T lymphocytes active on T cell proliferative responses. *In vitro* effects of some immunopharmacological agents. In *Human Cancer Immunology. Vol. 2 Human Suppressor Cells in Cancer Patients*. Serrou, B. and Rosenfeld, C. (eds.), Amsterdam, New York: North-Holland Publ. In press.

Touraine, J.L., Serrou, B., Hadden, J.W., Morin, A., and Touraine, F. (1980b) Modulation of suppressor T cell activity by isoprinosine. In *New Trends in Human Immunology and Cancer Immunotherapy. Vol. 1 Biological Response Modifiers*. Serrou, B. and Rosenfeld, C. (eds.), Paris, London: Doin-Saunders, pp. 1032–1037.

Thurman, G.B., Chincarini, C., Mc Clure, J.E., Marshall, G.D., Hu, S.H., and Goldstein, A. (1979) Current status of thymosin research: evidence for the existence of a family of thymic factors that control T cell maturation. *Ann. N.Y. Acad. Sci.* 332:33–48.

Umezawa, H., Hoyagi, T., Suda, H., Hamada, M., and Takeuchi, T. (1976) Bestatin a new aminopeptidase B inhibitor produced by actinomycites. *J. Antibiot.* 29:97–99.

Verhaegen, H., De Cree, J., De Cock, W., and Verhaegen-Declercq, M.L. (1980) Levamisole therapy in patients with colorectal cancer. In *Immunotherapy of Cancer: Present Status of Trials in Man*. Terry, W.D. (ed.), Elsevier, North-Holland. In press.

Wolf, G. and Chretien, P.B. (1980) Immunological reconstitution *in vitro* with thymosin fraction V and alpha 1. In *New Trends in Human Immunology and Cancer Immunotherapy. Vol. 1 Biological Response Modifiers*. Serrou, B. and Rosenfeld, C. (eds.), Paris, London: Doin-Saunders, pp. 773–788.

Wybran, J., Govaerts, A., and Appelboom, T. (1978) Inosiplex, a stimulating agent for normal human T cells and human leucocytes. *J. Immunol.* 121:1184–1187.

Wybran, J. (1980) Recent observation regarding the immunostimulating properties of isoprinosine and lynestrenol in man. In *New Trends in Human Immunology and Cancer Immunotherapy. Vol. 1 Biological Response Modifiers*. Serrou, B. and Rosenfeld, C. (eds.), Paris, London: Doin-Saunders, pp. 1010–1020.

Zoller, M., Price, M., and Baldwin, R. (1975) Cell-mediated cytotoxicity to chemically-induced rat tumors. *Int. J. Cancer* 16:593–606.

Published 1981 by Elsevier North Holland, Inc.
Saunders, Daniels, Serrou, Rosenfeld, and Denney, eds.
FUNDAMENTAL MECHANISMS IN HUMAN CANCER IMMUNOLOGY

CHAPTER 17

The Interrelationship of Immune Complexes and Suppressor T Cells in the Suppression of Macrophages[1]

Macolm S. Mitchell, M.D. and V. Srinivasa Rao, Ph.D.

Departments of Medicine and Microbiology, University of Southern California School of Medicine and the U.S.C. Cancer Center, 2025 Zonal Avenue, Los Angeles, California

Introduction

Tumors and successful allografts may avoid destruction by the host through an exaggeration of normal immunoregulatory controls rather than through completely unique mechanisms. In this presentation, we will focus on how the interaction of T lymphocytes and antigen-antibody complexes, which are akin to serum blocking factors, ultimately produce suppression of macrophages. We will emphasize the importance of receptors for the Fc portion of antibody, presumably on a subpopulation of T cells, and the induction by the immune complexes of an activated subpopulation of Lyt 1 T cells, which then interact with other T cells to generate suppressor T cells.

In the course of investigating the effects of alloantibody to leukemia L1210 ($H-2^d$) on that tumor and on the syngeneic or allogeneic ($H-2^b$ or $H-2^k$) host bearing the tumor, we found that both spleen cell-mediated cytotoxicity to $H-2^d$ antigens and macrophage-mediated reactivity to L1210 were impaired (Mitchell, 1972; Mitchell and Mokyr, 1972). Further investigations revealed that both specific antibody and specific (L1210) antigens were required to impair both types of cell-mediated immunity, and that the receptors for cytophilic antibody to L1210 on macrophages were somehow inhibited in an apparently specific manner. Thus, the attachment of other cytophilic antibodies to the macrophages inhibited by anti-L1210 and L1210, such as leukemia $EL4(H-2^b)$ cells, was unimpaired (Mitchell et al., 1975). Soluble immune

[1]Supported by Research Grant IM 50, American Cancer Society.

complexes formed *in vitro* of anti-L1210 and 3M KCl-extracted antigen from L1210 cells could entirely reproduce the effects of antibody and L1210 cells, administered separately. Neither antibody nor antigen alone was sufficient to produce the inhibition (Rao et al., 1979). It is our hypothesis that immune complexes formed *in vivo* cause the inhibition of macrophages (i.e., make them unable to attach cytophilic antibody to L1210).

The suppressed macrophages not only do not attach cytophilic antibody, indicating a blocked, absent or perhaps defective receptor on their membrane, but have other abnormal functions too. Phagocytosis and cytocidal activity are also probably impaired, as judged by our preliminary observations. The suppressed macrophages in fact appear small, poorly vacuolated, and stain poorly for acid phosphatase granules (Mitchell, 1972). We have used their inability to attach cytophilic antibody as a convenient indicator of their suppressed state.

Our reasons for studying this phenomenon are several. First, the important role of macrophages in rejection of allografts and tumors has been increasingly appreciated, and it is likely that cytophilic antibodies from B lymphocytes, or perhaps a qualitatively similar substance from T cells, permit the macrophage to identify foreign cells in the initial phase of the rejection process. Secondly, the similarity of "blocking factors" obtained from the serum of patients with syngeneic tumors (Sjogren et al., 1971) to the immune complexes we have prepared *in vitro* suggests that such factors may act to inhibit cell-mediated immunity by similar mechanisms. Finally, it seems likely to us that the normal regulation of the immune response to a variety of antigens may involve mechanisms like those that we can elucidate in our model system.

In support of these statements, it may be useful first to mention a few observations in the literature that appear to bear upon the inhibitory phenomenon we have reported. Birbeck and Carter (1972) and Chantler (1967) found that hamsters or mice containing "enhancing" antibody had apparently inactivated monocytic cells at the site of the tumor, (hamster: metastasizing lymphoma; mouse: BP8 sarcoma). Dullens et al. (1975), in attempting to treat murine leukemia with macrophages "armed" with antibody, found instead that the adherent antibody led to inhibition of macrophage cytotoxicity *in vivo*. More recently, Hellstrom et al. (1978, 1979) have described the effects of passively transferred serum "blocking factors" on the rejection of a methylcholanthrene-induced, syngeneic tumor, concluding that those factors initiated cellular interactions like those we will be discussing. Finally, in studies of regulation of antibody synthesis by antibody, Sinclair (1979) and Gershon and his colleagues (Eardley et al., 1978) have amply demonstrated the intermediary involvement of lymphoid cells and membrane receptors. These results closely parallel our studies of the macrophage. We have studied the inhibition of macrophage receptors, therefore, not only for its immediate application to tumor immunology and transplantation, but because it may provide a paradigm for basic study of immunoregulation by antibodies.

Results and Discussion

Eight to 10 days after an intraperitioneal injection of soluble immune complexes of anti-L1210 and soluble 3M KCl-extracted antigens from L1210 cells (SA-L1210) prepared in a zone of slight antigen excess, macrophages from the peritoneal cavity were found to lack the ability to attach cytophilic antibody to L1210, and thus to form rosettes when L1210 cells were added (Figure 17.1). This inhibition lasted until approximately day 30 after injection of the complexes, at which time macrophages formed rosettes normally. That is, in the presence of cytophilic antibody to L1210, approximately 50% of the macrophages formed rosettes of at least 2–6 macrophages per tumor cell, or vice versa, depending upon the relative sizes of macrophages and tumor cells (Figure 17.2). At the other end of the spectrum, "activated" macrophages from immunized mice given L1210 cells were greatly enlarged and more than 80% of them formed rosettes, often with 6 or more tumor cells on their surface (Figure 17.3).

Figure 17.1. "Suppressed" peritoneal macrophages from a mouse given anti-L1210 and L1210 cells, sequentially, 10 days earlier. Cytophilic anti-L1210 and additional L1210 cells were injected to test for their ability to form rosettes. The small size of the macrophages, the absence of refractile granules, and the failure of the macrophages to attach to nearby tumor cells are shown. (Phase-contrast)

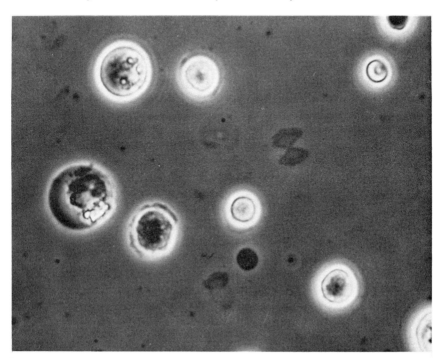

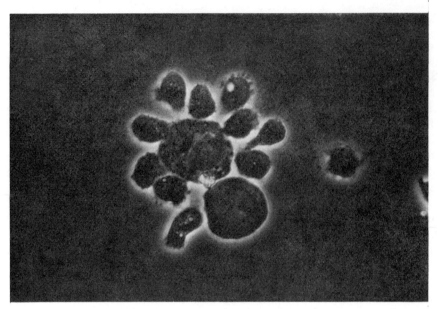

Figure 17.2. Normal peritoneal macrophages attached to a central tumor cell, after arming by cytophilic anti-L1210. (Phase-contrast)

Figure 17.3. "Activated" peritoneal macrophages from a mouse immunized 10 days earlier with (allogeneic) L1210 cells alone, with several rosettes of leukemic cells and some ingested, partially digested tumor cells. (Phase-contrast)

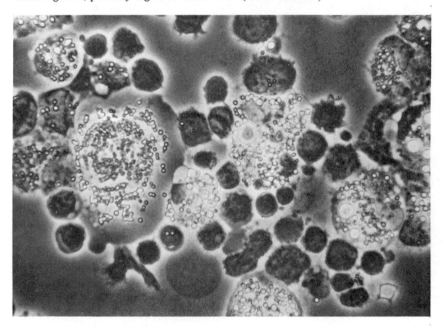

The Fc portion of antibody was required for the immune complexes to inhibit macrophages. (Table 17.1). Immune complexes prepared with $F(ab')_2$ fragments derived from anti-L1210 IgG were ineffective, as was the Fc portion by itself. The $F(ab'_2)$ fragments were of course unable to lyse L1210 cells in the presence of complement, but were not denatured, since ^{125}I-labeled fragments specifically and avidly attached to L1210 cells. We injected $F(ab')_2$ or Fc fragments sequentially with L1210 cells or SA-L1210 (Tables 17.1 and 17.2) and gave large amounts (4- to 6-fold excess over complexes with intact

Table 17.1. Effect of $F(ab')_2$ Immune Complexes of IgG Antibody on Cytophilic Antibody Receptors of Macrophages *In Vivo*.

A. Treatment with immune complexes

Group	Immune complexes[a] Antibody class	Dose (ml)		Rosettes on day 10 %	Score
1	IgG	0.3		8.7 ± 0.9[b]	0
2	$F(ab')_2$	1.2		40.0 ± 3.9	2+
3	$F(ab')_2$	1.8		39.7 ± 4.2	2+

B. Treatment with antibody and SA-L1210 sequentially

Group	Antibody[c] Class	Dose (ml)	SA-L1210[d] dose (mg)	Rosettes on day 10 %	Score
4	IgG	0.1	12	9.1[a] ± 1.0[b]	0
5	$F(ab')_2$	0.4	48	38.5 ± 5.7	2+
6	$F(ab')_2$	0.6	72	37.2 ± 4.1	2+
7	$F(ab')_2$	0.6	5×10^6 cells[e]	85.2 ± 2.0	4+
8	Nil	Nil	5×10^6 cells	90.5 ± 2.2	4+

Note: There was no difference in the effects on macrophages caused by several injections of $F(ab')_2$ fragments compared to those of a single injection.

[a]Immune complexes prepared with IgG of $F(ab')_2$ and SA-L1210 were injected i.p. into different groups of mice as indicated. Each group received 4 injections of immune complexes (days − 3 to 0); 0.3 ml of immune complex injected into Group 1 mice contained 0.1 ml of IgG and 0.2 ml of SA-L1210 (32 mg). The other doses of immune complexes given to Groups 2 and 3 mice contained proportionally more $F(ab')_2$ and SA-L1210.

[b]Mean ± SE.

[c]IgG or $F(ab')_2$ antibody of different concentrations were given to other groups (Groups 4 to 7) in 4 i.p. injections starting on day -4.

[d]On day 0, different concentrations of SA-L1210 were injected i.p. as shown in the table: 1 ml of SA-L1210 contained 160 mg of protein.

[e]Five $\times 10^6$ L1210 cells in 0.2 ml were given i.p. to C3H mice.

Table 17.2. Effect of Fc Fragments on Cytophilic Antibody Receptors of Macrophages *in Vivo*.

	Antibody[a]			Rosettes on day 10	
Group	Class	Dose (ml)	L1210[b] dose (× 10^6)	%[c]	Score
1	IgG	0.1	Nil	41.3 ± 4.6	2+
2	IgG	0.1	5	9.2 ± 1.1	0
3	Fc	0.4	5	90.2 ± 2.3	4+
4	Fc	0.6	5	84.9 ± 4.6	4+
5	Fc	0.6	Nil	38.6 ± 4.2	2+
6	Nil	Nil	5	90.5 ± 2.0	4+

[a]Groups 1 and 2 mice received 4 injections of IgG i.p. starting on day -4 to -1. Groups 3, 4, and 5 received 4 daily injections of Fc fragments of various concentrations as indicated starting on day -4. The Fc fragments used were reconstituted to the original volume of IgG antibody.
[b]On day 0, Groups 2, 3, 4, and 6 were given a single injection of 5 × 10^6 L1210 cells i.p.
[c]Mean ± SE.

antibody) in an attempt to compensate for the more rapid excretion of fragments, but in no instance was suppression observed (Rao et al., 1979a).

Several years ago we had ruled out a direct blockade of the macrophage's receptors for cytophilic antibodies, presumably involving receptors for the Fc portion, by experiments showing that an intact thymus was necessary for inhibition to occur (Gershon et al., 1974; Mitchell, 1976). Normal thymocytes upon transfer to suppressed mice could perpetuate suppression and antagonize the restorative effects of normal bone marrow cells, probably by being recruited into the suppressor mode (Mitchell et al., 1975). Thymocytes from mice given a non-specific antigenic stimulation intraperitoneally not only failed to perpetuate suppression, but in fact led to reversal of suppression (Rao et al., 1977). We therefore concluded that the requirement for an intact Fc portion in immune complexes indicated that a Fc receptor-bearing T cell might be involved in initiating the events leading to suppression of macrophages.

As shown in Table 17.3, we have have been able to adoptively transfer suppression of macrophages *in vivo* with 4×10^7 thymocytes obtained from mice treated with immune complexes. When tested 4 days after intravenous injection of suppressor-containing thymocytes, macrophages from the peritoneal cavity were unable to affix cytophilic antibody to L1210, in contrast to normal macrophages. Thymocytes treated with anti-Thy 1 and complement lost their ability to transfer suppression. The same transfer of suppression was achieved with nylon wool-non-adherent splenic T lymphocytes, also proved to be T cells by treatment with anti-Thy 1 and complement. Nylon wool-adherent spleen cells were consistently unable to transfer suppression (Rao et al., 1979b).

249

Table 17.3. Suppression of Cytophilic Antibody Receptors on Macrophages by Adoptive Transfer of Thymocytes from Suppressed to Normal Mice.

Group	Type	Thymocytes injected Number (× 10⁷)	Rosettes on day 4 after transfer[a] Mean ± SE	Score
1	Suppressed[b]	1	36.2 ± 1.8	2+
2	Suppressed	2	40.1 ± 2.1	2+
3	Suppressed	4	8.6 ± 0.8	0
4	Suppressed	5	8.0 ± 0.9	0
5	Suppressed[c] (anti-Thy 1 + C)	5	42.3 ± 2.8	2+
6	Normal	5	35.4 ± 3.0	2+

[a]Four days after transfer of suppressor thymocytes into normal C3H mice, the peritoneal monocytes of these mice were tested for rosetting *in vivo* in the presence of L1210 via the cytophilic antibody to L1210. Similar results were observed with suppressor thymocytes obtained from mice suppressed with anti-L1210 (0.4 ml) and 4 × 10⁶ L1210 cells.

[b]C3H mice were injected with immune complexes i.p. on 4 consecutive days. Ten days later, the thymocytes from the suppressed mice were processed and injected i.v. into normal C3H mice.

[c]Suppressor thymocytes were treated with Anti-Thy 1 and complement. Anti-Thy 1 (1 ml, 1:30 dil) was used per 1 × 10⁷ thymocytes.

An interesting result was obtained when we attempted to transfer suppression to T cell deprived mice which had been thymectomized, lethally irradiated, and then reconstituted with bone marrow cells from syngeneic donors (Rao et al., 1979b). As shown in Table 17.4, when these T cell depleted ("B") mice were given 6×10^7 thymocytes from donor treated with immune complexes, their macrophages were not suppressed, whereas even 4×10^7 thymocytes were sufficient to cause maximal suppression in normal recipients. The interaction of normal thymocytes or T cells with the suppressor-inducing thymocytes or T cells was conclusively demonstrated in experiments (Table 17.5) in which various numbers of normal T cells were admixed before injection into the B mice. Ten to 20 million ($1-2 \times 10^7$) normal T cells or thymocytes were required to restore the suppressive effect of transferred T cells; five million (5×10^6) normal T cells or fewer were ineffective. This result indicated that an interaction of suppressor-inducing T cells generated by immune complexes with a normal population of T cells was required to produce the suppressor T cells that ultimately suppressed macrophages.

At this point, we surmised that either the transferred T cells recruited additional suppressors from the immunologically naive cooperator T cells with which they were mixed, or that the transferred cells were somehow rendered functionally active after interaction with the normal T cells. The remainder of

Table 17.4. Lack of Macrophage Suppression by Suppressor Thymocytes in "B" Mice (T Cell Deficient).

	Cells injected[a]			Rosettes on day 4 after transfer	
Group	Type	Dose (× 10^7)	Recipient (C3H mice)	Mean + SE	Score
1	Supp Thy	2	B mice[b]	43.0 ± 2.9	2+
2	Supp Thy	4	B mice	32.5 ± 2.1	2+
3	Supp Thy	6	B mice	30.1 ± 2.5	2+
4	Supp Spl T cell	4	B mice	42.5 ± 3.1	2+
5	Supp Spl T cell	6	B mice	31.5 ± 2.4	2+
6	Supp Thy	4	Normal	9.2 ± 0.7	0
7	Supp Spl T cell	4	Normal	11.3 ± 1.1	0

[a]C3H mice were suppressed with anti-L1210 and L1210 cells as detailed in the text. Ten days later, the thymocytes from the suppressed mice were used as suppressor thymocytes (Supp Thy). Spleen cells from the suppressed mice were fractionated on nylon column. The nylon non-adherent cells were used as suppressor spleen T cells (Supp Spl T cell).

[b]Thymectomized, lethally irradiated, and bone marrow reconstituted C3H mice ("B" mice) or T cell depleted mice.

Table 17.5. Cooperation of Suppressor and Normal T Cells in Macrophage Suppression in "B" Mice.

	Suppressor cells injected (4 × 10^7)[a]	Normal cells injected			Rosettes on day 4 after transfer	
Group		Type	Number (× 10^7)	Recipient	Mean + SE	Score
1	Thy	Nor Thy	2.5	B mice[b]	35.4 ± 2.4	2+
2	Thy	Nor Thy	5	B mice	37.2 ± 2.4	2+
3	Thy	Nor Thy	10	B mice	13.1 ± 1.2	0
4	Thy	Nor Thy	20	B mice	9.8 ± 0.8	0
5	Thy	Nor Spl T cell[c]	5	B mice	42.8 ± 2.8	2+
6	Thy	Nor Spl T cell	10	B mice	12.1 ± 1.0	0
7	Thy	Nor Spl T cell	20	B mice	13.8 ± 1.1	0
8	Thy	Supp Spl T cell	20	B mice	34.2 ± 2.5	2
9	Thy	Nil	Nil	B mice	39.2 ± 2.6	2+
10	Thy	Nil	Nil	Normal	10.4 ± 0.9	0

[a]C3H mice were suppressed with immune complexes and/or anti-L1210 and SA-L1210 as detailed in the text. Ten days later, the thymocytes from the suppressed mice were used as suppressor thymocytes (Supp Thy).

[b]Thymectomized, lethally irradiated, and bone marrow reconstituted mice.

[c]Spleen cells from normal C3H mice were fractionated on nylon wool column and the nylon non-adherent splenocytes were used as normal splenic T cells (Nor Spl T cell).

the experiments we will describe concerns the phenotypes of the cells participating in this T-T interaction. These studies have given us both a conception of the sequence of interactions that occur and a sense of their mechanism, although much remains to be learned about that.

We studied the Lyt phenotypes of the participating cells by treating either the inducer thymocytes or splenic T cells with anti-Lyt 1.2 or anti-Lyt 2.2, and complement, or by treating the cooperating (acceptor) thymocytes or peripheral T cells similarly before adoptive transfer into appropriate animals. Although our recovery of Lyt 1-resistant or Lyt 2-resistant cells from the thymus was very low, (10% of total thymocytes or less) after treatment with anti-Lyt sera and complement, we adjusted the final concentration to $1-2 \times 10^8/\text{ml}$ in all instances. Splenic T cells were treated similarly and adjusted to the same concentration.

Four $\times 10^7$ viable inducer cells and 2×10^7 cooperator cells were injected in all experiments. Table 17.6 shows that only Lyt 1 thymocytes were capable of transferring suppression to normal mice; Lyt 2 + cells were ineffective. Similar results were found for Lyt 1 splenic T cells. The cooperating normal T cells bore both Lyt 1 and Lyt 2 markers, that is, they were Lyt 123 cells, since treatment with either antiserum abrogated cooperation (Table 17.7). In this experiment, both types of T cell, inducer and cooperator, were injected into T cell deprived mice to analyze the contribution of each, as in our previous experiments. It was of interest that treatment with cyclophosphamide, a compound known to inhibit suppressor T cells, failed to inhibit the activity of Lyt 1 suppressor inducer cells when given 5 or 9 days *after* immune complexes had already generated such inducers. In contrast, treatment with cyclophosphamide 1 day *before* administration of complexes prevented the formation of the inducer cells. These results indicated that precursors or amplifiers of

Table 17.6. Characterization of Suppressor Inducers (T Cells) Induced by Soluble Immune Complexes in Macrophage Suppression.

Cells transferred[a]	Rosettes on day 4 after transfer (mean % ± SE)
Unselected thymic	10.7 ± 0.8[b]
Lyt 1 thymic	12.4 ± 1.2[b]
Lyt 2 thymic	43.8 ± 1.8
Unselected splenic	13.8 ± 0.9[b]
Lyt 1 splenic	15.6 ± 2.1[b]
Lyt 2 splenic	48.2 ± 2.1
None	42.6 ± 1.7

[a] Mice were treated with immune complexes 10 days previously. 4×10^7 cells were transferred per mouse i.v.

[b] Significantly different from mice not receiving cells at $P < 0.05$.

Table 17.7. Characterization of the Normal T Cells that Interact with Suppressor Inducers (T cells) to Induce Macrophage Suppression in "B" Mice.[a]

Cell transferred		Rosettes on day 4 after transfer
Inducers[b]	Normal[c]	(Mean % ± SE)
Thymic	None	39.6 ± 1.5
Thymic	Splenic Lyt 1 + Lyt 2	32.9 ± 1.7
Thymic	Thymic Lyt 1 + Lyt 2	33.8 ± 1.8
Thymic	Unselected Thymus	12.3 ± 0.8[d]
Splenic	None	42.5 ± 1.9
Splenic	Splenic Lyt 1 + Lyt 2	37.8 ± 2.2
Splenic	Thymic Lyt 1 + Lyt 2	38.2 ± 2.1
Splenic	Unselected Spl T cells	14.8 ± 0.9[d]
None	None	39.2 ± 1.8

[a]Thymectomized, lethally irradiated (750R) and bone marrow reconstituted mice.

[b]Mice were given immune complexes 10 days previously. 4×10^7 cells were transferred per mouse i.v.

[c]2×10^7 normal T cells were transferred (ratio of 1:1 Lyt 1 and Lyt 2 viable cells). Injection of either Lyt 1 or Lyt 2 splenic or thymic cells alone with suppressor inducer cells did not elicit suppression of macrophages.

[d]Significantly different from "B" mice not receiving cells, at $P < 0.05$.

the activity of the Lyt 1 suppressor inducers were cyclophosphamide sensitive, but not the inducers themselves (Table 17.8). In similar experiments, it was shown that the Lyt 123 cooperator cells were also cyclophosphamide sensitive. Whether the ultimate suppressor cells, presumably Lyt 23 or 123, were sensitive to cyclophosphamide could not be determined from these experiments.

One of several conclusions stemming from these experiments was that not only peripheral T cells but also thymocytes could transfer suppressor function to normal hosts and could induce suppressor activity from normal thymocytes or splenic T cells. Also, the failure of Lyt 2^+ cells to transfer suppression probably indicated that they are poor inducers of additional suppressor cells, or that the expression of their activity requires the presence of an additional inducer cell. Most important, the experiments demonstrated that immune complexes did not induce suppressor T cells directly, but principally elicited Lyt 1 inducers of suppressor cells. The precise role of antibody in this process, which may be to directly induce suppressor cells or in addition inhibit helper pathways, is a matter for further scrutiny. Finally, the sensitivity of cooperating T cells and of the precursors of Lyt 1 cells to cyclophosphamide but not of the Lyt 1 suppressor inducers themselves, pinpoints the sites of action of this immunomodulator in at least one system.

Our most recent work has dealt with the role of I-region determinants in the T-T interaction. We treated suppressor inducer thymocytes or splenic T cells

Table 17.8. Cyclophosphamide (Cy) Sensitivity of the Inducer T Cells
that Adoptively Transfer Macrophage Suppression.

Cells transferred[a]	Day of Cy treatment[b]	Rosettes on day 4 after transfer (mean % ± SE)
Thymic	None	13.2 ± 0.6[c]
Thymic	−1	38.4 ± 2.1
Thymic	5	10.2 ± 0.7[c]
Thymic	9	9.8 ± 0.6[c]
Splenic	None	14.1 ± 0.7[c]
Splenic	−1	35.8 ± 1.8
Splenic	5	12.8 ± 0.9[c]
Splenic	9	13.4 ± 0.6[c]
None	−	37.6 ± 0.9

[a]Mice were given with immune complexes on day "0" and 10 days later 4×10^7 cells were transferred to normal mice.

[b]20 mg/kg cyclophosphamide administered.

[c]Significantly different from mice not receiving cells at P < 0.05.

with anti-Ia serum and complement and transferred 4×10^7 viable cells to normal recipients, testing them for suppressed macrophages 4 days later. This treatment abolished the ability of the T cells to transfer suppression, demonstrating the presence of Ia antigens on their surface (Table 17.9). Similarly, treatment of the normal T cells from thymus or spleen with anti-Ia and complement made them unable to cooperate. Furthermore, anti-Ia serum given *in vivo* before antigen-antibody complexes were administered blocked the

Table 17.9. Characterization of Inducer T Cells Generated by Soluble Immune Complexes.

Inducers transferred[a]	Rosettes on day 4 after transfer (mean % ± SE)
Untreated thymic	16.7 ± 1.0
Untreated splenic	14.4 ± 0.6
Anti-Ia + C treated splenic	41.2 ± 2.9[b]
Anti-Ia + C treated thymic	40.4 ± 3.2[b]
None	39.8 ± 2.8

[a]Mice were treated with immune complexes on day 0. Ten days later 4×10^7 thymocytes or spleen T cells from these mice were injected into normal mice, i.v.

[b]Significantly different from mice receiving untreated inducer cells, at p < 0.05

generation of suppressor inducer cells. In contrast, however, when anti-Ia serum was injected 5 or 9 days after immune complexes, it was ineffective in blocking inducer activity, as demonstrated by adoptive transfer (Table 17.10). Finally, anti-Ia serum given to normal mice failed to block their T cells from cooperating with suppressor inducer cells to produce suppression of macrophages (Table 17.11). These results indicate that the Lyt 1^+ inducer cells in this system bear Ia antigens and come from Ia^+ precursors. Cooperating normal Lyt 123 cells are also Ia^+. However, the Ia antigens do not seem to be involved in the process of cooperation that leads to the ultimate suppressor T cells and beyond that to suppression of the macrophages, since blocking of Ia antigens with anti-Ia *in vivo* was ineffectual.

It has become increasingly apparent to us that what at first might have appeared a simple "blockade" of receptors for cytophilic antibodies by immune complexes is instead yet another example of immunological regulation involving T cells, set in motion by a humoral influence. Although we have persistently studied the allogeneic system with which we began several years ago, we must point out that the Hellstroms have recently begun to corroborate many of the findings we have presented here with a syngeneic tumor. With a methylcholanthrene-induced tumor, Hellstrom et al. (1979) found, in the spleen and thymus of mice that had rejected the tumor T cells that enhance the growth of the tumor in syngeneic recipients. These T cell "inducers" require the additional presence of normal T cells in the recipient mice. Broder, Waldmann, and colleagues showed that the generation of suppressor cells from

Table 17.10. Effects of Anti-Ia Serum on *In Vivo* Inducer T Cells that Adoptively Transfer Macrophage Suppression.

Inducers transferred[a]	Day anti-Ia serum injected[b]	Rosettes on day 4 after transfer (mean % ± SE)
Thymic	(−1)	43.2 + 2.9[c]
Thymic	5	16.8 + 1.2
Thymic	9	11.3 ± 0.9
Thymic	None	12.1 ± 0.7
Splenic	(−1)	34.6 ± 2.7[c]
Splenic	5	14.4 ± 0.9
Splenic	9	12.7 ± 0.8
Splenic	None	15.8 ± 0.8
None	None	41.5 ± 2.1

[a]Mice were injected with immune complexes on day 0 and 10 days later 4×10^7 cells were transferred to normal mice, i.v.

[b]100 μl of anti-Ia serum was administered i.p.

[c]Significantly different from mice receiving inducer cells obtained from donors treated with immune complexes alone, at $p < 0.05$.

Table 17.11. *In vivo* Effect of Anti-Ia Serum on Cooperating
Normal T Cells.

Inducers injected[a]	Recipient mice[b]	Rosettes on day 4 after transfer (mean % ± SE)
Thymic	Anti-Ia treated	14.8 ± 0.8
Splenic T cells	Anti-Ia treated	15.1 ± 0.6
Thymic	Normal	10.4 ± 0.7
Splenic T cells	Normal	12.9 ± 0.7
None	Normal	34.8 ± 2.9

[a]Mice were treated with immune complexes on day 0. Ten days later thymocytes or splenic T cells from the suppressed mice were injected into recipient mice.

[b]Recipient mice were treated with anti-Ia serum (100 μl) one day before they received inducer cells.

peripheral blood in man also required T-T cooperation, and that immune complexes interacting with T cells bearing Fc receptors for IgG were the initiators (Broder et al., 1978; Pichler et al., 1978).

The chain of induction of functional cytotoxic and suppressor T cells by Lyt 1 cells has been demonstrated by Cantor and Boyse (1975), Cantor et al. (1978), and by Stout et al. (1976). Thus Lyt 1 cells are not simply helpers for antibody formation, but are general inducers of fully functional B and T effectors, including those T cells that terminate (suppress) ongoing immune responses. Since the inducer cells we have studied are Lyt 1^+, but not Lyt 123, it is very unlikely that they acquired functional capacity as suppressors from their subsequent interactions with normal Lyt 123 cells, because Lyt $1+2$-suppressor cells have not been identified in any system yet studied. Whether the final suppressor cells are Lyt 23 or 123 has yet to be determined; examples of each have been found in other systems.

Summary

We have described a series of experiments on the *in vivo* effects of immune complexes formed of antigens from L1210 tumor cells and antibodies to them. These complexes can inhibit the activity of peritoneal macrophages after administration *in vivo*, as measured by defective attachment of cytophilic antibodies. The inhibition lasts approximately 30 days, which suggests a mechanism more profound than simple blockade of the receptors of the macrophages. Inhibition of macrophages has been shown to involve the induction of suppressor T cells in a chain of events (Figure 17.4) comprising: (1) activation of cyclophosphamide-resistant, Lyt 1, Ia$^+$ T cells (thymocytes and splenic T cells) from Fc receptor positive, Ia+, cyclophosphamide-sensitive Lyt 123 precursors, (2) interaction of the Lyt 1 cells with Lyt 123, Ia$^+$,

IMMUNE COMPLEX–T CELL–MACROPHAGE INTERACTIONS

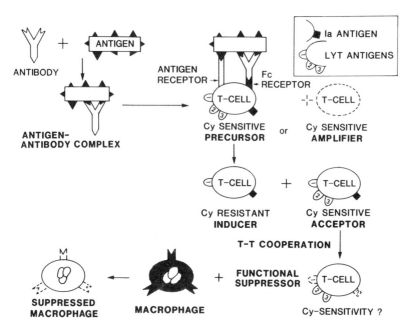

Figure 17.4. Schema of the interrelationship of immune complexes and subsets of T cells in thymus and spleen in the production of suppressed peritoneal macrophages. Known characteristics of the interacting cells are indicated. The amplifier cell shown in dotted lines has not yet been conclusively identified, nor is it known whether cytophilic antibody receptors similarly drawn are absent or inhibited.

cyclophosphamide-sensitive normal T cells (thymocytes and splenic T cells) to generate suppressor effector cells, and (3) subsequent interaction of the ultimate suppressor T cell (of unknown phenotype and cyclophosphamide sensitivity) with the macrophage. Whether one or more lymphocyte-derived soluble "factors" are involved in these processes is uncertain. What is now becoming clear is that such things as antibodies, soluble tumor antigens, and serum "blocking factors" probably exert their considerable *in vivo* influence on the host's immunity to the tumor through exaggeration of normal T cell immunoregulatory mechanisms, rather than by any sort of peripheral blockade, regardless of the methods used for demonstrating their presence *in vitro*.

ACKNOWLEDGMENTS

We gratefully acknowledge the collaboration at various times during these investigations of the following individuals (listed chronologically): Margalit B. Mokyr, Danielle J. Goldwater, Robert L. Grodzicki, James A. Bennett, F.W. Shen, Richard K. Gershon, Margaret Eyler, and Jeffrey A. Frelinger.

References

Birbeck, M.S.C. and Carter, R.L. (1972) Observations on the ultrastructure of two hamster lymphomas, with particular reference to infiltrating macrophages. *Int. J. Cancer* 9:249–257.

Broder, S., Poplack, D., Whang-Peng, J., Durm, M., Goldman, C., Muul, L., and Waldmann, T.A. (1978) Characterization of a suppressor cell leukemia. Evidence for the requirements of an interaction of two T cells in the development of human suppressor effector cells. *New Engl. J. Med.* 298:66–72.

Cantor, H. and Boyse, (1975) Functional subclasses of T lymphocytes bearing different Ly antigen. II. Cooperation between subclasses of Ly+cells in the generation of killer activity. *J. Exp. Med.* 141:1390–1399.

Cantor, H., McKay-Boudreau, L., Hugenberger, J., Naidorf, K., Shen, F.W., and Gershon, R.K. (1978) Immunoregulatory circuits among T cell sets. II. Physiologic role of feedback inhibition *in vivo*: absence in N2B mice. *J. Exp. Med.* 147:1116–1125.

Chantler, S.M. (1967) Characteristics of the cellular response in pretreated recipients exhibiting enhanced tumor growth. *Transplantation* 5:1400–1408.

Dullens, H.F.J., DeWeger, R.A., Woutersen, R.A., and Den Otter, W. (1975) Therapy with antibody-coated immune and hyperimmune peritoneal cells in a murine lymphoma system. *J. Natl. Cancer Inst.* 54:77–82.

Eardley, D.D., Hugenberger, J., McVay-Boudreau, L., Shen, F.W., Gershon, R.K., and Cantor, H. (1978) Immunoregulatory circuits among T cell sets. I. T helper cells induce other T cell sets to exert feedback inhibition. *J. Exp. Med.* 147:1106–1115.

Gershon, R.K., Mokyr, M.B., and Mitchell, M.S. (1974) Activation of suppressor T cells by tumor cells and specific antibody. *Nature (New Biol.)* 250:594–596.

Hellstrom, K.E., and Hellstrom, I. (1978) Evidence that tumor antigens enhance tumor growth *in vivo* by interacting with a radiosensitive (suppressor?) cell population. *Proc. Natl. Acad. Sci. U.S.A.* 75:436–40.

Hellstrom, I., Hellstrom, K.E., and Bernstein, I.D. (1979) Tumor-enhancing suppressor activator T cells in spleens and thymuses of tumor immune mice. *Proc. Natl. Acad. Sci. U.S.A.* 76:5294–5298.

Mitchell, M.S., Mokyr, M.B., and Goldwater, D.J. (1975) Analysis and reversal of the suppression of cytophilic antibody receptors produced by antibody. *Cancer Res.* 35:1121–1127.

Mitchell, M.S. (1972) Central inhibition of cellular immunity to leukemia L1210 by isoantibody. *Cancer Res.* 32:825–831.

Mitchell, M.S. (1976) Role of "suppressor" T-lymphocytes in antibody-induced inhibition of cytophilic antibody receptors. *Ann. N.Y. Acad. Sci.* 276:229–241.

Mitchell, M.S. and Mokyr, M.B. (1972) Specific inhibition of receptors for cytophilic antibody on macrophages by isoantibody. *Cancer Res.* 32:832–838.

Pichler, W.J., Lum, L., and Broder, S. (1978) Fc receptors on human T lymphocytes. I. Transition of T_G to T_M cells. *J. Immunol.* 121:1540–1548.

Rao, V.S., Grodzicki, R.L., and Mitchell, M.S. (1979a) Specific *in vivo* inhibition of macrophage receptors for cytophilic antibody by soluble immune complexes. *Cancer Res.* 39:174–182.

Rao, V.S., Bennett, J.A., Grodzicki, R.L., and Mitchell, M.S. (1979b) Suppressor T cells induced by immune complexes can adoptively transfer inhibition of cytophilic antibody receptors on macrophages. *Cell Immunol.* 46:227–238.

Rao, V.S., Mokyr, M.B., Gershon, R.K., and Mitchell, M.S. (1977) Specific T cell dependent, antigen-antibody induced suppression of macrophages: abrogation by non-specifically stimulated T cells. *J. Immunol.* 118:2117.

Sinclair, N.R. St.C. (1979) Modulation of immunity by antibody, antigen-antibody complexes, and antigen. *Pharmac. Ther.* 4:355–432.

Sjogren, H.O., Hellstrom, I., Bansal, S.C., and Hellstrom, K.E. (1971) Suggestive evidence that the "blocking antibodies" of tumor-bearing individuals may be antigen-antibody complexes. *Proc. Nat. Acad. Sci.* 68:1372–1375.

Stout, R.D., Waksal, S.D., and Herzenberg, L.A. (1976) The Fc receptor on thymus-derived lymphocytes. III. Mixed lymphocyte reactivity and cell-mediated lympholytic activity of Fc⁻ and Fc⁺ lymphocytes. *J. Exp. Med.* 144:54–68.

CHAPTER 18

"The Motor of Phagocytic Leukocytes" [1]

Thomas P. Stossel, M.D., John H. Hartwig, and Helen L. Yin, Ph.D.

Hematology-Oncology Unit, Department of Medicine, Massachusetts General Hospital and Harvard Medical School, Boston, Massachusetts

The motor of phagocytic leukocytes is of potential importance in cancer biology for several reasons. First, if phagocytes destroy or contain tumors, as is often speculated, the motor is an important part of the mechanism whereby phagocytes find, attach to, and possibly engulf tumor cells. Second, the components governing tumor cell and phagocyte movements are probably qualitatively similar or identical. Furthermore, the machinery controlling cell movement certainly functions in other cell activities such as endocytosis, exocytosis, and cell division. Therefore, development of novel strategies that act on these components to impair tumor spread and influence the very integrity and growth of tumors might be possible. Third, alterations in cell shape, movement, and ultrastructure accompany malignant transformations (Nicolson, 1976) and transformed epithelial cells and fibroblasts come more or less to resemble mobile phagocytic leukocytes in morphology and movement (Armstrong and Lackie, 1975). Therefore, knowledge of the motor of phagocytes relates to the tumor cell phenotype.

This review summarizes information concerning the biochemical components of the motor of mammalian phagocytes and how they can interact to generate directional movement. The phagocytic leukocyte is only one prototype of a motile cell, and many of the concepts summarized here are applicable to other cells. However, a comparison of the state of knowledge of this macrophage motor with that of other cells is beyond the scope of this review, and for such a comparison the reader is referred to other articles (Goldman et al., 1979; Korn, 1978).

[1]Supported by Grants from the USPHS (HL19429 and CA 09032), from the Council for Tobacco Research, as U.S.A., from the Edwin S. Webster Foundation, and gifts from Edwin W. Hiam and Charles L. and Jane D. Kaufman.

and for such a comparison the reader is referred to other articles (Goldman et al., 1979; Korn, 1978).

The "motor" region of phagocytic leukocytes appears to reside in the peripheral cytoplasm beneath the plasma membrane. The cortical region ordinarily excludes lysosomes and other organelles and although evident around the entire cell circumference, it is particularly prominent in veils, pleats, and pseudopodia extended by the cell (Lewis, 1939).

Transmission electron micrographs of thin sections of fixed phagocytic leukocytes reveal that this cortical cytoplasm consists primarily of filamentous material and that the filaments have the dimensions of actin polymers (Reaven and Axline, 1973). The existence of actin in the cell periphery has been confirmed by means of histochemical procedures (Allison et al., 1971; Berlin and Oliver, 1978). The actin filaments in the cortical cytoplasm of phagocytes seem to form a meshwork in which the filaments intersect or overlap at random intervals. Electron micrographs of these cortical meshworks, after critical point drying, show remarkable perpendicularity of the intersection angles of the cortical filaments (Boyles and Bainton, 1979). Phagocytic leukocytes only rarely have cortical actin filaments aligned in parallel aggregates (Reaven and Axline, 1973), in contrast to less motile fibroblast and epithelial cells in tissue culture which contain long actin filaments, many of which become organized in bundles called "stress fibers" (Buckley and Porter, 1967). These stress fibers tend to disappear after malignant transformation or during mitosis in cultured cells (Nicolson, 1976). The lack of bundles therefore seems to correlate with increased cell movement.

Actin constitutes about 10% of the total protein of phagocytic leukocytes, and the phagocyte actin molecules are not distinguishable from muscle actin in any functions. This finding is typical for nonmuscle cell actins and probably is a consequence of the high degree of conservation in the primary structure of actins throughout phylogeny (Vanderkerckhove and Weber, 1978). Actin molecules exist in a dynamic equilibrium between free monomers and linear double helical filaments, the distribution of molecules between monomer and filament states being determined by the ambient ionic conditions, temperature, and various exogenous proteins and other factors. Recently, considerable interest has focused on the idea that the two ends of an actin polymer have different rates of loss and addition of monomers (Wegner, 1976). Actin polymers are easily fragmented by mechanical forces, but the fragments anneal rapidly when the force is removed (Oosawa and Kasai, 1977). There is evidence that a relatively high proportion of actin may be unpolymerizable in extracts of nonmuscle cells (Blikstad et al., 1978) in conditions under which purified actin is easily polymerized. However, the aggregation state of actin in the intact cell is not precisely known. In any case, the transmission electron micrographs of thin sections of phagocyte cortices engaged in phagocytosis and locomotion do show that many filaments are present.

Myosin molecules comprise about 1% of the total protein of phagocytic leukocytes. The myosin molecules are asymmetrical hexamers composed of a pair of heavy chains (of 200,000 daltons) and two pairs of light chains of about 20,000 and 15,000 daltons (Hartwig and Stossel, 1975; Boxer and Stossel, 1976). Myosin molecules are diffusely localized throughout the cytoplasm of phagocytic leukocytes as determined by immunofluorescence microscopy. However, these molecules are apparently concentrated in the cell periphery and are present in ruffles, blebs and pseudopods, regions of active movement (Davies et al., 1977; Hartwig et al., 1977; Stendahl et al., 1980; Valerius et al., 1981).

In striated muscle, myosin molecules exist as bipolar aggregates and generate force by their interactions with actin filaments. The myosin heavy chains have globular domains, or "heads," on flexible stems that can bend away from long helical domains, or "tails," that aggregate colinearly to form the shaft of the myosin filament. The light chains are located near the heads. The heads make repetitive contacts with the actin monomers in filaments and drive them toward the center of the myosin filament. This sliding filament or crossbridge mechanism of force generation derives its energy from the hydrolysis of ATP (Huxley, 1969; Tregear and Marston, 1979).

In vertebrate striated muscle, the interaction between myosin crossbridges and actin filaments is regulated by calcium and a complex of proteins, tropomyosin, and the troponins, which are associated with the actin filaments. At low calcium concentrations ($>\mu$M), these regulatory proteins inhibit crossbridge formation; when the calcium concentration is in the μM range, the inhibition is removed, and cyclic crossbridge formation generates tension. A subunit of troponin, troponin C, is the calcium binding moiety in this control system. Variations of the mechanism exist in invertebrates in which the myosin light chains together with tropomyosin bound to the actin filaments regulate contraction. These muscles lack troponins, and one of the myosin light chains binds calcium and confers control on crossbridge formation (Lehman, 1976). The mechanism of regulation of crossbridge activity in nonmuscle and smooth muscle cells is somewhat controversial. Considerable circumstantial evidence suggests that phosphorylation and dephosphorylation of the 15,000 dalton myosin light chains by protein kinase and phosphate enzymes, respectively, turn crossbridge activity on (phosphorylation) and off (dephosphorylation). The myosin light chain kinases are activated by μM calcium concentrations in the presence of the heat-stable cytoplasmic calcium-binding protein, calmodulin (Adelstein and Eisenberg, 1980). However, some believe that the phosphorylation mechanism is either insufficient for or irrelevant to control of crossbridge activity, and that other regulatory proteins govern this interaction (Hirata et al., 1980).

The myosin molecules of phagocytic leukocytes can form bipolar filaments at physiologic pH and ionic strength, and these myosin filaments bind to actin filaments. However, relatively little is known about the regulation of the crossbridge cycle in these cells. Solutions containing macrophage actin and myosin have high rates of ATP hydrolysis and undergo a "contraction" (also called superprecipitation) in the presence of a crude protein fraction isolated from macrophage extracts (Stossel and Hartwig, 1975, 1976). Trotter and Adelstein, (1979) have offered evidence to support the idea that this factor could be a protein kinase that phosphorylates the 20,000-dalton myosin light chain. The activities of both the phosphorylation and myosin-activating reactions are equivalent in the presence or absence of calcium ions.

Another uncertainty concerns the state of aggregation of myosin filaments in phagocytic leukocytes. Recent evidence suggests that the degree of phosphorylation of smooth muscle and nonmuscle cell myosins might affect the extent to which they aggregate (Suzuki et al., 1978). Although phagocyte myosin forms bipolar filaments, these filaments have not been observed with certainty in the cell cortex. It has been argued that the relatively low myosin concentration in such cells is the basis of this failure (Niederman and Pollard, 1976).

Even if the factors regulating the assembly and function of myosin in phagocytic leukocytes were fully known, this information would not explain how the crossbridge cycle could generate tension with directionality in the actin lattice in the cortex of phagocytic leukocytes. Nevertheless, it may be feasible now to explain how the filament organization of cortical cytoplasm, so unlike the architecture of actin filaments in the muscle sarcomere, could be responsible for directional movement in cortical cytoplasm. The explanation incorporates components associated with actin in the phagocyte. It is argued that: (1) the macrophage cortex is an isotropic lattice of actin filaments cross-linked by a protein called actin-binding protein. (2) Myosin filaments, dispersed together with magnesium and ATP throughout the lattice, exert tension on it by means of the crossbridge mechanism. (3) Depending on the calcium concentration, gelsolin, a recently discovered macrophage protein, regulates the structure of the lattice. Gelsolin weakens the lattice in the presence of submicromolar calcium concentrations. At very low (less than 2×10^{-8}) calcium concentrations, the lattice restructures itself, as gelsolin is reversibly inactivated. (4) The lattice moves from regions of lesser to domains of greater network structure, that is from high to low calcium concentrations. This formulation is called the "tug of war" hypothesis.

Actin filament solutions of physiologic ionic strength and pH form a weak network structure, probably because of entanglements between the long filaments and weak bonds between monomers of overlapping filaments (Kasai et al., 1960). This network is easily destroyed by low shear forces which cause the filaments to align in parallel (Kasai et al., 1960). In fact, the filaments tend to orient in parallel spontaneously (Kasai et al., 1960), a property of very long filaments of limited flexibility (Flory, 1956).

Actin-binding protein binds to actin filaments with high affinity ($Ka = 2 \times 10^6 M^{-1}$) (Hartwig and Stossel, 1981). It forms a rigid isotropic network when added to actin polymers or when copolymerized with monomeric actin. Actin-binding protein composes about 1% of the phagocyte protein (Hartwig and Stossel, 1975). Its distribution as determined by immunofluorescence microscopy is similar to that of myosin, in that it resides in the cell periphery (Boxer et al., 1976; Stendahl et al., 1980; Valerius et al., 1981). Actin-binding protein has a molecular weight of 540,000, is composed of two 270,000 dalton subunits and is an asymmetrical molecule in 0.1 M KCl solution (frictional coefficient, $f/f_0 - 2.56$) (Hartwig and Stossel, 1975, 1981; Stossel and Hartwig, 1976).

The radius of gyration of 17 nm estimated for actin-binding protein dimers from hydrodynamic studies agrees with the corresponding radius determined from the configurations of actin-binding protein dimers in electron micrographs. Electron micrographs of actin-binding protein reveal that its dimeric subunits are long and flexible and are joined at their ends, arbitrarily designated "heads." The opposite ends, defined as "tails," bind to actin filaments during cross-linking (Hartwig and Stossel, 1981).

Classical network theory (Flory, 1946) predicts that the rigidity of polymer solutions rises abruptly at a critical cross-linker concentration, ν_c/N_0 where ν_c is the critical number of cross-linking molecules, and N_0 is the number of actin monomers in the polymer being cross-linked. The critical cross-linker concentration is very sensitive to the length distribution of polymers and is inversely proportional to the weight average degree of polymerization ($\overline{X}_w$).

$$\frac{\nu_c}{N_0} = \frac{1}{\overline{X}_w} \text{ or } M_c = \frac{c}{\overline{M}_w} \tag{18.1}$$

where M_c is the critical cross-linker concentration in moles/L, c is the concentration of actin in polymers in G/L and $\overline{M}_w$ is the weight-average molecular weight of actin polymers. The formation of actin networks by actin-binding protein conforms with the theory. The rigidity of actin polymers rises suddenly at a critical actin-binding protein concentration close to that predicted by theory (Brotschi et al., 1978; Hartwig and Stossel, 1979, 1981; Yin et al., 1980). The abruptness of this transition renders the sol to gel transformation an excellent mechanism for controlling cytoplasmic structure. The close agreement between experiment and theory indicate that actin-binding protein dimers are very efficient gelation factors. This efficiency arises from their high affinity for actin filaments, their large subunits, and the flexibility of the subunits. The size and flexibility of the subunits permit actin-binding protein molecules to bind to specific sites in the actin filament helices without distorting the filament orientation. The maintenance of filament isotropy minimizes parallel alignment of the actin polymers and the resulting propensity of redundant or incestuous cross-linking between such filaments.

Low concentrations of actin-binding protein sufficient to solidify dilute actin filament solutions do not perceptibly alter the relatively random orientation of the long actin filaments (Hartwig and Stossel, 1981). However, when actin is copolymerized with actin-binding protein, short filaments branch with striking perpendicularity, reminiscent of the morphology of the phagocyte cortex (Hartwig et al., 1981). In the latter case, actin-binding protein subunits act as nucleation sites for the growth of actin filaments, and the nucleation function of actin-binding protein results in shortening of average filament lengths (Hartwig et al., 1981). The bipolarity of actin-binding protein acts to create branching. The perpendicular branching also would be expected to maintain the isotropy of the networks and thereby minimize alignment of filaments and intramolecular cross-linking.

In principle, cross-linking of preexisting polymers by addition of cross-linking molecules and a branching condensation polymerization, where cross-linking and polymerization occur simultaneously, can generate the same network structure (Flory, 1946). The effect of actin-binding protein in nucleating actin assembly shortens the polymer length distribution, resulting in the rapid formation of a highly branched structure with short segments. Networks formed by the addition of actin-binding protein to long actin filaments do not have this appearance initially (Hartwig et al., 1981), although redistribution of actin monomers could eventually lead to the same structure as is observed in the case of copolymerization.

Theoretically, addition or removal of actin-binding protein cross-links from actin filaments or the reversible separation of the dimeric subunits of actin-binding protein could regulate actin network structure. However, experiments performed at physiological ionic strength provide no evidence of such changes. The logic behind regulating actin lattice structure by a mechanism other than removing actin-binding protein may be that the inherent isotropy of the actin filaments is preserved even during deformation. This isotropy limits the tendency toward parallel alignment of the filaments and the formation of bundles.

Rearrangement of Equation 1 yields Equation 2:

$$\nu_c = \frac{N_0}{\overline{X}_w}, \tag{18.2}$$

which shows that the critical cross-linking density for incipient gelation can be changed by altering the filament length distribution, provided that the number of monomers and polymers remains unchanged. These events are efficiently accomplished by breaking and annealing of actin filaments. Gelsolin, a 91,000 dalton, heat-labile, globular calcium-binding protein of rabbit lung macrophages, regulates the lattice structure in this fashion (Yin and Stossel, 1979, 1980; Yin et al., 1980).

Gelsolin binds 2 moles of calcium per mole of subunit with a K_a of 0.92 μM^{-1} (Yin and Stossel, 1980). In the presence of calcium ($>2 \times 10^{-8} M$), gelsolin binds to actin filaments and shortens them, as evidenced by a decrease in the flow birefringence and viscosity of actin solutions and by shortening of actin filament contour lengths viewed in the electron microscope. The calcium-gelsolin complex increased in a concentration-dependent manner the ν_c, the critical concentration of actin-binding protein for gelation of actin filaments, by a magnitude consistent with that predicted from shorting of $\overline{X}_w$, the degree of polymerization. This result indicates that gelsolin shortens actin filaments without extensive depolymerization (no change in N_0), and this conclusion is verifiable by sedimentation analysis and measurement of the turbidity of actin filament solutions. The effect of gelsolin is reversed rapidly by lowering of the calcium concentration (Yin and Stossel, 1979; Yin et al., 1980).

Actin and myosin filaments purified from skeletal muscle and mixed together in a solution containing magnesium and ATP will contract or "superprecipitate" away from the walls of the container into a compact aggregate (Szent-Györgyi, 1949). The contraction is driven by the crossbridge mechanism reviewed above and indicates that actin and myosin can perform mechanical work in the absence of sarcomeric structures. Entanglements between actin filaments are important for the net centripetal contraction of protein, because without them, actin filaments would simply slide past one another (Hayashi and Maruyama, 1975). Cross-linking of the actin filaments would be expected to be more effective than this entanglement in promoting tension development and contraction. α-actinin, a muscle protein which has the capacity to cross-link actin filaments, accelerates the rate of superprecipitation of solutions of actin and myosin (Ebashi et al., 1964), and actin-binding protein reduces the ratio of myosin to actin required to initiate such a contraction (Stendahl and Stossel, 1970). Therefore, cross-linking of actin filaments amplifies the contraction. The calcium-gelsolin complex reverses the amplifying effect (Stendahl and Stossel, 1970). This phenomenon indicates that the degree of cross-linking of actin influences the power of contraction by myosin, a concept that can be called gelation-contraction coupling (for a different interpretation of the relationship between actin gelation and contraction, see Hellewell and Taylor, 1979).

The importance of gelation contraction coupling for the cortical motor is that it can explain directional movement of cortical actin. If the degree of cross-linking varies from one domain of the cortex to another, movement will precede from regions of less to regions of greater cross-linking, that is, from high to low calcium concentrations (Figure 18.1). It has been shown experimentally that the directional movement of an actin lattice cross-linked by actin-binding protein and containing myosin and gelsolin does indeed orient from high to low calcium concentration (Stendahl and Stossel, 1970). In the cell, one can hypothesize that structures tethered to actin filaments would move with the actin in response to the actin gradient, although the molecules that anchor actin filaments to membranes in phagocytes remain to be identified.

The actin of the fungal metabolite, cytochalasin B, provides evidence tying actin lattice structure to phagocyte motor activity. This and related compounds alter the morphology of cortical cytoplasm, inhibit phagocytosis, and enhance the exocytosis of lysosomal enzymes by cells exposed to various stimuli (Allison et al., 1971; Allison, 1973; Axline and Reaven, 1974). Cytochalasin B

A. Superprecipitation

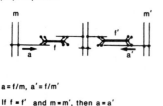

$a = f/m, a' = f/m'$

If $f = f'$ and $m = m'$, then $a = a'$

B. Directional Movement

1.

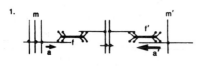

If $f = f'$ and $m > m'$, then $a < a'$

2.

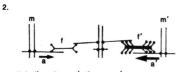

If $f < f'$ and $m = m'$, then $a < a'$

3.

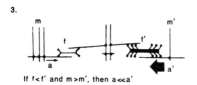

If $f < f'$ and $m > m'$, then $a \ll a'$

Figure 18.1. Schemes compare the superprecipitation of actomyosin (A) to directional movement of an actin lattice (B). In the equation, $a = f/m$, f is the contractile force per myosin crossbridge, m is the mass of a cross-linked actin filament lattice, and a is the rate of movement of the lattice. Arrow size designates the relative rate and direction of lattice movement. If, as shown in A, the lattice is considered to be divided into identical repeat units of equal mass, m and m′, and if adjacent units are subject to comparable contractile forces, f and f′, the lattice units will move toward each other equal rates, where $a = a'$. Superprecipitation of actomyosin solutions occurs by this mechanism. Myosin dispersed in the actin filament solution exerts contractile tension via cyclic crossbridging of the actin filaments, causing a centrifugal contraction of the actin filaments as a unit which moves the actin filament mass equally from all directions. Directional movement of the lattice requires localized changes in the mass and/or contractile force within the lattice. As shown in B1, when the mass of one lattice unit is diminished in one region $(m > m')$, or in B2 where the contractile force is increased in a region $(f < f')$, directional movement of the lattice will result $(a < a')$. Since the structure of the lattice directly reflects the level of cytoplasmic calcium (through gelsolin), movement is always toward the lowest concentration of free cytoplasmic calcium. B3 shows that, if increasing the free calcium were to activate both gelsolin and myosin cross-bridge activity, the same directionality takes place as in B2, but with amplified acceleration.

does not interact substantially with monomeric actin (Flanagan and Lin, 1980), but in a solution of actin filaments, cytochalasin B binds to each filament with high affinity ($K_a = 10^7 M^{-1}$) (Brown and Spudich, 1979; Hartwig and Stossel, 1979). Under conditions which are not optimal for actin assembly, cytochalasin B slows the rate of polymerization (Brenner and Korn, 1979; Brown and Spudich, 1979). However, in 0.1 M KCl solutions, cytochalasin B enhances the initial rate of actin assembly (Löw and Dancker, 1974), and, at equilibrium, the filaments are shorter than filaments polymerized in the absence of cytochalasin B without a large increase in the actin monomer concentration. Addition of cytochalasin B to actin filaments also shortens filaments without increasing the monomer concentration (Hartwig and Stossel, 1979; Maruyama et al., 1977). As predicted by Equation 18.2 the shortening of $\overline{X}_w$ without a change in N_0 should raise ν_c, the density of actin-binding protein required for incipient gelation of the actin filaments. Such an increase has been verified experimentally (Hartwig and Stossel, 1979).

The effects of cytochalasin B are quite complex but are consistent with a mechanism wherein the drug "caps" one of the ends of actin filaments and competitively inhibits the binding of monomers or annealing of polymers to the capped end. At physiologic ionic strength, the effects of cytochalasin are quantitatively reduced because of the high affinity of actin-actin interactions that lead to assembly and annealing. Therefore, relatively high concentrations of cytochalasin B ($\sim 10^{-4}$ M) are required for substantial shortening of the polymers (Spudich, 1972). However, the subtle effects of lower ($\sim 10^{-6} - 10^{-5}$ M) cytochalasin B concentrations on actin fragmentation can have important effects on living cells.

The effect of μM cytochalasin B concentrations in disrupting actin networks cross-linked by actin-binding protein (Hartwig and Stossel, 1976, 1979) can explain the inhibition of phagocyte motility, alteration of morphology, and enhancement of stimulated secretion. Cytochalasin B, by disrupting the actin lattice, disorganizes the cortical contractile activity ordinarily regulated by cytoplasmic calcium gradients. Addition of cytochalasin B is effectively similar to irreversible activation of gelsolin. Cytochalasin B will cross the plasmalemma and effectively sever peripheral filaments. The membrane barrier therefore causes the drug to act nonrandomly on cortical filaments. Aggregation of actin filaments in the presence of myosin will be inhibited in domains where cytochalasin B has disrupted the network structure, but not in regions where the network remains intact. The result of this unregulated actin-myosin interaction is focal aggregation of actin. Filament aggregates are seen in transmission electron micrographs of cytochalasin B treated cells (Axline and Reaven, 1974). Disorganization of cortical contraction can account for the inhibition of locomotion and phagocytosis, because the pseudopodia involved in these movements cannot be established. The depletion of cortex from focal regions can also account for the approach of secretory granules to the plasma membrane and the enhancement of exocytosis by cytochalasin B in suitably stimulated cells.

In conclusion, information currently available permits a biochemical explanation for directional movement of the motor of the macrophage cortex. However, important questions need to be answered to clarify our understanding of the cortical motor.

First, is there control over the force-generating mechanism involving actin and myosin, and, if there is, how does it affect directional movement? As shown in Figure 18.1, alteration of the crossbridge activity alone could affect directional movement of the lattice, but in the presence of changes in lattice structure, the predicted directionalities obtain, whether or not crossbridge activities vary from one domain to another. However, regulation of crossbridge activity could modulate or amplify movements and limit ATP consumption to regions of active contraction.

Second, do changes in the distribution of actin between its monomeric and polymeric forms have an important function? There is strong evidence for the rapid polymerization of actin as the basis for the extension of the acrosomal process in starfish sperm (Tilney et al., 1973). The branching structure that occurs when actin polymerizes in the presence of actin-binding protein is a possible mechanism for the expansions of cortical cytoplasm that form pseudo-podia. Actin monomers or oligmers could assemble on demand upon the actin-binding sites on the tails of actin-binding protein dimers. The branching polymer would enlarge in all directions, and structures in the cell center such as organelles, intermediated filaments, or microtubules would provide a fulcrum against which the expanding polymer could push to extrude plasma membrane in the opposite direction.

Several proteins have been isolated from cells that increase the fraction of subunits that are monomeric or oligomeric rather than organized in long polymers (Kuroda and Maruyama, 1976; Maruyama, 1978; Carlsson et al., 1977; Southwick and Stossel, 1981). However, it is not currently known what physiologic signals could be involved in regulating how these proteins control the equilibrium between monomeric and polymeric actin in cytoplasm of phagocytic leukocytes.

Third, what is the structure of the actin filament-plasmalemma attachments?

Finally, what controls calcium concentrations in the cortex of phagocytes? Substances that stimulate directional movement and alter the cortical morphology of phagocytic leukocytes stimulate the efflux of cell-associated calcium ions (Naccache et al., 1979). Phagocytic vesicles (inverted plasma membrane sacs) purified from rabbit lung macrophages have a magnesium- and ATP-dependent high-affinity calcium pump that transports calcium against an electrochemical gradient from the cytoplasmic to the external face of the plasma membrane. Calmodulin stimulates the activity of this pump (Lew and Stossel, 1980). These findings indicate that a membrane calcium pump could control the level of cytoplasmic calcium in the cell periphery. However, it remains to be shown how the activity of these pumps or of the peripheral calcium concentrations influenced by the pumps are coupled to environmental signals acting on cell surfaces.

As stated previously, a feature of cells subjected to malignant transformation *in vitro* is that they acquire certain characteristics of phagocytic leukocytes. One of these features is an absence of dense actin bundles (stress fibers) customarily present in the corresponding untransformed cells (Ash et al., 1976; Rifkin et al., 1979; Tucker et al., 1978; Wang and Goldberg, 1976; Pollack et al., 1975). It has even been reported that cultured cells from individuals with a genetic propensity to develop neoplasms have fewer actin-containing stress fibers than cells from normal persons (Kopelovich et al., 1979). Results correlating with the lack of an ordered filamentous conformation of actin in transformed cells show that more actin in extracts of transformed cells appears to be in a monomeric or oligomeric form than in normal cells (Wickus et al., 1975; Markey and Soriano, 1980).

The conformation of actin in tumor cells *in vivo* is understandably more difficult to ascertain than the state of actin in cultured cells. However, some electron microscopy and immunofluorescence studies of tumor cells have also indicated that the malignant cells contained isotropic networks of actin-like filaments but few filament bundles (Malech and Lentz, 1974; Gabbiani et al., 1976). It is difficult to explain the finding that tumor cells treated with antibodies to actin or myosin stain more heavily than normal cells (Gabbiani et al., 1976). The proteins being stained could be present in increased quantities or be altered so as to react more readily with the antibodies, or some other factors may be involved.

From what has been learned concerning actin and related proteins of phagocytic leukocytes and other cells, certain inferences can be made about the basis of the relatively disaggregated state of actin filaments in tumor cells. Actin disaggregation could arise from changes in the molecular structure of actin molecules that effect the equilibrium between their monomeric and polymeric forms. Some, but not all, transformed cells have different isoelectric variants of actin compared with the corresponding untransformed cell (Weber et al., 1977; Leavitt and Kakunaga, 1980; Leavitt et al., 1980). However, there is no evidence that these isoactins have different properties with respect to assembly. An increase in the concentrations or activities of actin-associated proteins in tumor cells that alter the supramolecular state of actin, such as gelsolin, could also explain the form of actin in these cells. Finally, differences between normal and transformed cells in the distribution of ionized calcium could affect actin architecture in the presence of normal quantities of gelsolin-like proteins. Presently, there is no information bearing on these possibilities.

The network state of actin exerts significant control over cytoplasmic structure and movement in phagocytic leukocytes. If this control is also important in motile tumor cells, then drugs, such as cytochalasin B or the chaetoglobosins (Löw et al., 1979), which alter this network structure, might be examined further for their capacity to interfere with tumor cell movement and function.

References

Adelstein, R.S. and Eisenberg, E. (1980) Regulation and kinetics of the actin-myosin-ATP interaction. *Ann. Rev. biochem.* 49:921–956.

Allison, A.C. (1973) The role of microfilaments and microtubules in cell movement, endocytosis, and exocytosis. In *Locomotion of Tissue Cells*. Abercrombie, M. (ed.), Amsterdam: Elsevier North Holland, pp. 109–148.

Allison, A.C., Davies P., and De Petris, S. (1971) Role of contractile microfilaments in macrophage movement and endocytosis. *Nature New Biol.* 232:153–155.

Armstrong, P.B. and Lackie, J.M. (1975) Studies on intercellular invasion *in vitro* using rabbit peritoneal neutrophil granulocytes (PMNS). *J. Cell. Biol.* 65:439–462.

Ash, J.F., Vogt, P.K., and Singer, S.J. (1976) Reversion from transformed to normal phenotype by inhibition of protein synthesis in rat kidney cells infected with a temperature-sensitive mutant of Rous sarcoma virus. *Proc. Natl. Acad. Sci. U.S.A.* 73:3603–3607.

Axline, S.G. and Reaven, E.P. (1974) Inhibition of phagocytosis and plasma membrane mobility of the cultivated macrophage by cytochalasin B. Role of subplasmalemmal microfilament. *J. Cell. Biol.* 62:647–659.

Berlin, R.D. and Oliver, J.M. (1978) Analogous ultrastructure and surface properties during capping and phagocytosis in leukocytes. *J. Cell. Biol.* 77:789–804.

Blikstad, I., Markey, F., Carlsson, L., Persson, T., and Lindberg, U. (1978) Selective assay of monomeric and filamentous actin in cell extracts, using inhibition of deoxyribonuclease I. *Cell* 15:935–943.

Boxer, L.A., Floyd, A., and Richardson, S. (1976) Association of actin-binding protein with membrane in polymorphonuclear leukocytes. *Nature* 263:259–261.

Boxer, L.A. and Stossel, T.P. (1976) Interactions of actin, myosin, and an actin-binding protein of chronic myelogenous leukemia leukocytes. *J. Clin. Invest.* 57:964–976.

Boyles, J. and Bainton, D.F. (1979) The changing patterns of plasma membrane associated filaments during the initial phases of polymorphonuclear leukocyte adherence. *J. Cell. Biol.* 82:347–368.

Brenner, S.L. and Korn, E.D. (1979) Substoichiometric concentrations of cytochalasin D inhibit actin polymerization. Additional evidence for an F-actin treadmill. *J. Biol. Chem.* 254:9982–9985.

Brotschi, E.A., Hartwig, J.H., and Stossel, T.P. (1978) The gelation of actin by actin-binding protein. *J. Biol. Chem.* 255:8988–8993.

Brown, S.S. and Spudich, J.A. (1979) Cytochalasin inhibits the rate of elongation of actin filament fragments. *J. Cell. Biol.* 83:657–662.

Buckley, I.K. and Porter, K.R. (1967) Cytoplasmic fibrils in living cultured cells. *Protoplasma* 64:349–362.

Carlsson, L., Nyström, L-E, Sundkvist, I., Markey, F., and Lindberg, U. (1977) Actin polymerizability if influenced by profilin, a low-molecular weight protein in nonmuscle cells. *J. Mol. Biol.* 115:465–463.

Davies, W.A. and Stossel, T.P. (1977) Peripheral hyaline blebs (podosomes) of macrophages. *J. Cell. Biol.* 75:941–955.

Ebashi, S., Ebashi, F., and Maruyama, K. (1964) A new protein factor promoting contraction of actomyosin. *Nature* 203:645–646.

Flanagan, M.D. and Lin, S. (1980) Cytochalasins block actin filament elongation by binding to high affinity sites associated with F-actin. *J. Biol. Chem.* 255:835–838.

Flory, P.J. (1946) Fundamental principles of condensation polymerization. *Chem. Rev.* 39:137–197.

Flory, P.J. (1956) Statistical thermodynamics of semi-flexible chain molecules. *Proc. Roy. Soc. (London) Ser. A* 234:60–72.

Gabbiani, G., Csank-Brassert, J., Schneeberger, J-C, Kapanci, Y., Trenchev, P., and Holborow, E.J. (1976) Contractile proteins in human cancer cells. Immunofluorescent and electron microscopic study. *Am. J. Path.* 83:457–465.

Goldman, R.D., Milsted, A., Schloss, J.A., Starger, J., and Yerna, M-J (1979) Cytoplasmic fibers in mammalian cells: cytoskeletal and contractile elements. *Ann. Rev. Physiol.* 41:703–722.

Hartwig, J.H. and Stossel, T.P. (1975) Isolation and properties of actin, myosin, and a new actin-binding protein in rabbit alveolar macrophages. *J. Biol. Chem* 250:5696–5705.

Hartwig, J.H. and Stossel, T.P. (1976) Interactions of actin, myosin, and an actin-binding protein of rabbit pulmonary macrophages. III. Effects of cytochalasin. *J. Cell. Biol.* 71:295–303.

Hartwig, J.H. and Stossel, T.P. (1979) Cytochalasin B and the structure of actin gels. *J. Mol. Biol.* 134:539–554.

Hartwig, J.H. and Stossel, T.P. (1981) Structure of actin-binding protein molecules in solution and interacting with actin filaments. *J. Mol. Biol.* 145:163–181.

Hartwig, J.H., Davies, W.A., and Stossel, T.P. (1977) Evidence for contractile protein translocation in macrophage spreading, phagocytosis, and phagolysosome formation. *J. Cell. Biol.* 75:956–967.

Hartwig, J.H., Tyler, J., and Stossel, T.P. (1981) Actin-binding protein promotes the bipolar and branching polymerization of actin. *J. Cell. Biol.* In press.

Hayashi, T. and Maruyama, K. (1975) Myosin aggregates as a requirement for contraction and a proposal to the mechanism of contration of actomyosin systems. *J. Biochem.* 78:1031–1038.

Hellewell, S.B. and Taylor, D.L. (1979) The contractile basis of ameboid movement. VI. The solation-contraction coupling hypothesis. *J. Cell. Biol.* 83:633–648.

Hirata, M., Mikawa, T., Nonomura, Y., and Ebashi, S. (1980) Ca^{2+} regulation in vascular smooth muscle. II. Ca^{2+} binding of aorta leiotonin. *J. Biochem.* 87:369–378.

Huxley, H.E. (1969) The mechanism of muscular contraction. *Science* 164:1356–1366.

Kasai, M., Kawashima, H., and Oowawa, G. (1960) Structure of F-actin solutions *J. Polymer. Sci.* 44:51–69.

Kopelovich, L., Conlon, S., and Pollack, R. (1977) Defective organization of actin in cultured skin fibroblasts from patients with inherited adenocarcinoma . *Proc. Natl. Acad. Sci.* 74:3019–3022.

Korn, E.D. (1978) Biochemistry of actomyosin-dependent cell motility, a review. *Proc. Natl. Acad. Sci. U.S.A.* 75:588–599.

Kuroda, M. and Maruyama, K. (1976) α-actinin, a new regulatory protein from rabbit skeletal muscle. II. Action on actin. *J. Biochem.* 80:323–332.

Leavitt, J. and Kakunaga, T. (1980) Expression of a variant form of actin and additional polypeptide changes following chemical-induced *in vitro* neoplastic transformation of human fibroblasts. *J. Biol. Chem.* 255:1650–1661.

Leavitt, J., Leavitt, A, and Attallah, A.M. (1980) Dissimilar modes of expression of β- and α-actin in normal and leukemic human T lymphocytes. *J. Biol. Chem.* 255:4984–4987.

Lehman, W. (1976) Phylogenetic diversity of the proteins regulating muscular contradiction. *Int. Rev. Cytol.* 44:55–92.

Lew, P.D. and Stossel, T.P. (1980) Calcium transport by macrophage plasma membranes. *J. Biol. Chem.* 255:5841–5846.

Lewis, W.H. (1939) Some cultural and cytological characteristics of normal and malignant cells *in vitro. Arch. Exp. Zellforsch.* 23:8–26.

Löw, I., Jahn, W., Wieland, T., Sekita, S., Yoshira, K., and Natori, S. (1979) Interactions between rabbit muscle actin and several chaetoglobosins or cytochalsins. *Anal. Biochem.* 95:14–18.

McClain, D.A., Maness, P.F., and Edelman, G.M. (1978) Assay for early cytoplasmic effects of the src gene product of Rous sarcoma virus. *Proc. Natl. Acad. Sci. U.S.A.* 75:2750–2754.

Malech, N.L. and Lentz, T.L. (1974) Microfilaments in epidermal cancer cells. *J. Cell. Biol.* 60:473–482.

Markey, F. and Soriano, L. (1980) Actin pools in extracts of teratocarcinoma cells, assayed by inhibition of DNAse I. *FEBS Lett.* 110:05–307.

Maruyama, K., Kimura, S., Ishii, T., Kuroda, M., Ohashi, K., and Muramatsu, S. (1977) β-actinin, a regulatory protein of muscle. Purification, characterization, and function. *J. Biochem.* 81:215–232.

Naccache, P.H., Showell, H.J., and Becker, E.L. (1979) Involvement of membrane calcium in the response of rabbit neutrophils to chemotactic factors as evidenced by the fluorescence of chlorotetracycline. *J. Cell. Biol.* 83:179–186.

Nicolson, G.L. (1976) Trans-membrane control of the receptors on normal and tumor cells. II. Surface changes associated with transformation and malignancy. *Biochim. Biophys. Acta* 458:1–72.

Oosawa, F. and Kasai, M. In *Subunits in Biological Systems*, Part A. Timasheff, S.N. and Fasman G.D. (eds.), New York: Marcel Dekker, Inc., pp. 261–322.

Pollack, R., Osborn, M., and Weber K. (1975) Patterns of organization of actin and myosin in normal and transformed cultured cells. *Proc. Natl. Acad. Sci. U.S.A.* 72:994–998.

Reaven, E.P. and Axline, S.G. (1973) Subplasmalemmal microfilaments and microtubules in resting and phagocytizing cultivated macrophages. *J. Cell. Biol.* 59:12–27.

Rifkin, D.B., Crowe, R.M., and Pollack, R. (1979) Tumor promotors induce changes in the chick embryo fibroblast cytoskeleton *Cell* 18:361–368.

Scholey, J.M., Taylor, K.A., and Kendrick-Jones, J. (1980) Regulation of nonmuscle myosin assembly by calmodulin-dependent light chain kinase. *Nature* 287:233–234.

Southwick, F.S. and Stossel, T.P. (1981) Isolation of an inhibitor of actin polymerization from human polymorphonuclear leukocytes. *J. Biol. Chem.* In press.

Spudich, J.A. (1972) Effects of cytochalasin B on actin filaments. *Cold Spring Harbor Symp. Quant. Biol.* 37:585–593.

Stendahl, O.I. and Stossel, T.P. (1970) Actin-binding protein amplifies actomyosin contraction and gelsolin confers calcium control on the direction of contraction. *Biochem. Biophys. Res. Commun.* 92:675–681.

Stendahl, O.I., Hartwig, J.H., Brotschi, E.A., and Stossel, T.P. (1980) Distribution of actin-binding protein and myosin in macrophages during spreading and phagocytosis. *J. Cell. Biol.* 84:215–224.

Stossel, T.P. and Hartwig, J.H. (1975) Interactions of actins, myosin, and an actin-binding protein of rabbit alveolar macrophages. macrophage myosin Mg^{++}-adenosine triphosphatase requires a cofactor for activation by actin. *J. Biol. Chem.* 250:5706–5712.

Stossel, T.P. and Hartwig, J.H. (1976) Interactions of actin, myosin, and a new actin-binding protein of rabbit pulmonary macrophages. II. Role in cytoplasmic movement and phagocytosis. *J. Cell. Biol.* 68:602–619.

Suzuki, H., Onishi, H., Takahashi, K., and Watanabe, S. (1978) Assembly of myosin filaments *J. Biochem.* 84:1529–1542.

Szent-Györgyi, A. (1949) *Chemistry of Muscular Contraction*. New York: Academic Press.

Tilney, L.D., Hatano, S., Ishikawa, H., and Mooseker, M.S. (1973) The polymerization of actin: its role in the generation of the acrosomal process of certain echinoderm sperm. *J. Cell. Biol.* 59:109–126.

Tregear, R.T. and Marston, S.B. (1979) the crossbridge theory. *Ann. Rev. Physiol.* 41:723–736.

Tucker, R.W., Sanford, K.K., and Frankel, F.R. (1978) Tubulin and actin in paired nonneoplastic and spontaneously transformed neoplastic cell lines *in vitro*: fluorescent antibody studies. *Cell* 13:629–642.

Valerius, N.H., Stendahl, O.I., Hartwig, J.H., and Stossel, T.P. (1981) Distribution of actin-binding protein and myosin in polymorphonuclear leukocytes during locomotion and phagocytosis. *Cell*, in press.

Vanderkerckhove, J. and Weber K. (1978) At least six different actins are expressed in a higher mammal: an analysis based on the amino acid sequence of the amino-terminal tryptic peptide. *J. Mol. Biol.* 126:783–802.

Wang, E. and Goldberg, A.R. (1976) Changes in microfilament organization and surface topography upon transformation of chick embryo fibroblasts with Rous sarcoma virus. *Proc. Natl. Acad. Sci. U.S.A.* 73:4065–4069.

Weber, K., Koch, R., Herzog, W., and Vandekerckhove, J. (1977) The isolation of tubulin and actin from mouse 3T3 cells transformed by simian virus 40 (SV3T3 cells), an established cell line growing in culture. *Eur. J. Biochem.* 78:27–32.

Wegner, A. (1976) Head to tail polymerization of actin. *J. Mol. Biol.* 108:139–150.

Weihing, R.R. (1976) Cytochalasin B inhibits axtin-related gelation of HeLa cell extracts. *J. Cell. Biol.* 71:303–307.

Wickus, G, Gruenstein, E., Robbins, P.W., and Rich A. (1975) Decrease in membrane-associated actin of fibroblasts after transformation by Rous sarcoma virus. *Proc. Natl. Acad. Sci. U.S.A.* 72:746–749.

Yin, H. and Stossel, T.P. (1979) Control of cytoplasmic actin gel-sol transformation by gelsolin, a calcium-dependent regulatory protein. *Nature* 281:538–586.

Yin, H. and Stossel, T.P. (1980) Purification and structural properties of gelsolin, a Ca^{2+}-activated regulatory protein of macrophages. *J. Biol. Chem.* 255:9490–9493.

Yin, H., Zaner, K.S., and Stossel, T.P. (1980) Ca^{2+} control of actin gelation. Interaction of gelsolin with actin filaments and regulation of actin gelation. *J. Biol. Chem.* 255:9494–9500.

CHAPTER 19

Effects of Immunotherapy and Chemotherapy on Various Host Defense Parameters: Development of a Multiparameter Analysis Approach to the Study of Biological Response Modifiers[1]

Evan M. Hersh, M.D., Marvin L. Powell, M.D.,
Jordan U. Gutterman, M.D., and
Raymond Alexanian, M.D.

Department of Developmental Therapeutics, M.D. Anderson Hospital and Tumor Institute, Houston, Texas

Immunotherapy of human cancer is now considered to be entering its second generation. The first phase involved mainly crude materials such as intact microbial adjuvants (Hersh et al., 1977). The second phase involves purified subcomponents of these microbial adjuvants and, in addition, synthetic substances which mimic some of the actions of the crude preparations. One of the major problems encountered in the first decade of clinical immunotherapy trials was the lack of suitable assays to monitor the dose, schedule, and timing of the immunotherapy. In consequence, the dose and schedule were often arbitrary and were not based on host defense modification.

Currently, a number of newly developed assays are available to characterize patients receiving augmenting agents as well as other modalities of immunotherapy (Hersh et al., 1980). These include assays of cell-mediated cytotoxicity such as natural killer (NK) cell activity and antibody dependent cell-mediated cytotoxicity (ADCC), assays of serum lysozyme, which are useful as a rough measure of the mass and activity of the monocyte-macrophage-reticuloendothelial (RES) system, and assays of monocyte adherence which are

[1]Supported by Grants CA14528 and CA05831 from the National Cancer Institute, National Institutes of Health, Bethesda, Maryland.

useful in counting the numbers of adherent monocytes in the peripheral blood. Furthermore, there are a number of assays useful in identifying and characterizing suppressor cell activity which are relevant to the study of augmenting agents, since a number of these are known to activate suppressor cell mechanisms (Rosenthal, 1980).

We initially applied the multiparameter approach to the phase I study of the methanol extraction residue (MER) of Bacillus Calmette Guerin (BCG) (Hersh et al., 1980). We were able to demonstrate that MER boosted NK cell activity, ADCC to chicken erythrocytes and human erythrocytes, levels of serum lysozyme, and monocyte adherence, without activating suppressor cells. The maximal tolerated dose, as measured by clinical symptoms and side-effects, was found to be an immune stimulating dose. To follow up this study, we have started phase II studies of MER.

We have now applied components of this multiparameter assay to the study of patients receiving interferon, poly-ICLC, a complex of polyriboinosinic-polyribocytodylic acid with poly-L-lysine and carboxymethyl cellulose, and MVE-2 biological response modifier therapy as well as FAC (5-FU, adriamycin, and cytoxan) combination chemotherapy. These assays have detected differences between effects on the host's defenses of these various agents and treatments, and the data suggest that the assay system will be useful in the phase I-II development of newer augmenting agents. It will need to be demonstrated, however, that the optimal immune augmenting dose is in each case also the optimal anti-tumor dose.

Methods

Monocyte Adherence

The monocyte adherence assay is carried out by the method of Currie and Headley (1977). Washed peripheral blood mononuclear cells from a Ficoll-Hypaque gradient are prepared at a concentration of 1×10^6/ml and are set up at 1×10^5 mononuclear cells per well in media and 50% autologous serum with 5 replicate points in microtest plates. Plates are incubated for 7 days, washed 6 times, and the adherent cells are released with citric acid and enumerated microscopically or with a coulter counter. Results are expressed as the number of adherent macrophages per ml of blood.

ADCC Assays

The ADCC assays are conducted according to the method of Poplack and co-workers (1976). Human red blood cell (HRBC) and chicken red blood cell (CRBC) targets are utilized. Effector cells are mononuclear leukocytes collected by Hypaque-Ficoll density solution centrifugation. Chromium[51]-labeled target cells, antisera, and effector cells are incubated in microwells for four hours with effector cells at 1×10^6 per well, and target:effector ratios of 1:1, 3:1, and 10:1. Chromium release is measured by conventional methods with the final results being recorded as percent specific target cell lysis. More recently, we have also used a heteroantibody coated nucleated human leukemia cell target (CEM) at a target:effector ratio of 1:25.

Natural Killer Cell Assay

Spontaneous cell-mediated cytotoxicity is determined using the K562 cell line as well as the CEM cell line as targets. Target cells are labeled with chromium[51] in the standard fashion, with target cell concentration of 1×10^4 cells per well which represents approximately 2000 counts per minute. The length of the assay is 3 hours. Effector:target cell ratios are 10:1 and 25:1 for the K562 cell line, giving approximately 25–35% target cell lysis. The activity against CEM is approximately 15% with an effector:target ratio of 25:1.

Serum Lysozyme

Serum lysozyme determinations are performed using the Worthington Diagnostic Lysozyme reagent kit. The test measures the rate at which a cell suspension of *Micrococcus lysodictatus* is lysed. The kit contains a vial of lyophilized substrate and a vial of lysozyme standard which are reconstituted with distilled water. The standard is used to prepare a standard curve for the substrate, and all subsequent determinations using the substrate are based on the curve generated. The absorbance of an aliquot of 300 µl of substrate is read at 400 nanometers after a 0.5 minute interval, and again after 3 minutes. The difference in optical densities is computed and the amount of lysozyme present is determined from the standard curve.

Suppressor Cell Assays

Suppressor cells are evaluated in several ways. One is a co-culture system for lymphocyte blastogenesis involving mixtures of equal numbers of normal or indicator and patient lymphocytes (Hersh et al., 1980). The latter are either used untreated, are irradiated, or treated with thymic hormones. Suppression of the normal subjects' lymphocyte proliferative responses to concanavalin A (Con A), phytohemagglutinin (PHA) and pokeweed mitogen (PWM) by the patients' cells are measured by the usual lymphocyte blastogenesis technique. Appropriate controls are utilized. Depression of lymphocyte proliferative responses which can be abrogated by irradiation or thymic hormone treatment of patient cells is taken as evidence of suppressor cell activity. Lymphocyte proliferative responses are also evaluated in the presence or absence of indothemacin (Goodwin, 1981) and cimetidine (Avella et al., 1978), both of which have been documented to abrogate suppressor cell activity. These tests are also utilized to detect this activity in peripheral blood leukocyte cultures.

Results

Five patients with advanced, chemotherapy refractory malignancy received 3×10^6 units of partially human leukocyte interferon (Cantell) daily. This schedule of study and data are shown in Table 19.1. Two out of three monocyte-associated parameters, namely, monocyte adherence and ADCC to HRBC, were progressively depressed by interferon. As anticipated from the earlier work of others, there was a striking increase in NK cell activity which was noted mainly during the first seven days of interferon therapy. After this time, NK cell activity tended to return towards the baseline.

Eight patients with advanced chemotherapy refractory multiple myeloma were evaluated during treatment with 15 doses of weekly poly ICLC. The two monocyte associated parameters which were depressed by interferon were also depressed within 24 hours after the dose of poly ICLC, with a trend towards recovery by 48 to 72 hours. However, in contrast to results of the interferon study, NK cell activity was significantly depressed at 24 hours after poly ICLC, with a subsequent return towards the baseline (Table 19.2). The dose of poly ICLC was active in that it induced a mean peak serum interferon titer of 569 IU. However, the depression of monocyte adherence (or other parameters) did not correlate with the peak serum interferon titer in these patients treated with poly ICLC (Table 19.3).

We have recently initiated studies of a new biological response modifier, namely MVE-2, the 15,500 molecular weight fraction of pyran copolymer. This is a polymer of maleic-anhydride and divinyl ether (Breslow, 1976). Approximately thirty patients have been entered on a study with dose levels ranging from 25 to 650 mg/m^2 of body surface area. The drug has been administered

Table 19.1. Effect of Interferon Therapy on Host Defense Parameters in Patients with Various Advanced Malignancies.

Parameter	Pre-therapy	Day of therapy				
		2	4	7	14	21
Monocyte adherence	22.50	9.35[a]	11.96[a]	2.82[a]	4.09[a]	2.53[a]
Serum lysozyme	17.2	14.3	13.6	15.9	13.3	12.8
ADCC-CRBC	25.2	27.4	30.4	24.5	22.2	30.2
ADCC-HRBC	15.0	15.7	10.9[a]	5.5[a]	5.4[a]	4.2[a]
ADCC-CEM	45.7	51.4	55.4	52.9	49.8	53.4
NK-K562	17.7	40.4[a]	28.4[a]	27.0[a]	22.9	19.9

Note: Monocyte adherence: adherent cells/ml blood $\times$ 10^4; serum lysozyme: μg/ml; ADCC and NK: % target cell lysis. ADCC: antibody dependent cell-mediated cytotoxicity; CRBC: chicken red blood cells; HRBC: human red blood cells; CEM: heteroantibody coated nucleated human leukemia cell target.
[a]Significant difference compared to pre-therapy.

Table 19.2. Changes in Host Defense Parameters Associated with Poly ICLC
Therapy in Patients with Advanced Refractory Multiple Myeloma.

Parameter	Pre-therapy	24 hr post-therapy	48 hr post-therapy	3-7 d post-therapy
		Timing of Study		
Monocyte adherence	3.52	0.36^a	0.42^a	3.52
Serum lysozyme	14.10	14.05	11.00	15.75
ADCC-CRBC	10.7	12.5	12.6	10.2
ADCC-HRBC	5.3	2.6^a	4.8	7.9
ADCC-CEM	22.6	15.6	18.3	23.4
NK-K562	11.8	4.9^a	8.3	8.9

Note: Units of parameters and abbreviations same as in Table 19.1.
[a] Significant depression compared to pre-therapy.

weekly intravenously to patients with advanced refractory solid tumors. Thus far, no significant side effects have been observed and no depression of immunological parameters has been observed, but we have noted significant or near significant increases in ADCC to CRBC, ADCC to CEM, and NK cell activity (Table 19.4). These results should be considered tentative, as these studies are at an early stage of development.

Contrasting results have been obtained from studies conducted in patients with breast cancer receiving 5 fluoruracil, adriamycin, and cytoxan (FAC) combination chemotherapy (Table 19.5). A major selective depression of monocyte-associated parameters has been noted. Thus, monocyte adherence, serum lysozyme, and ADCC to HRBC were markedly depressed, while ADCC to CRBC and to the CEM cell line were not depressed. Furthermore, while the PHA response was not affected or was actually slightly augmented, the PWM and Con A responses were significantly but transiently depressed. The latter two, but not the former are strongly dependent on monocytes for their activity (Hersh et al., 1980).

Table 19.3. Correlations Between Suppression of Monocyte Adherence,
Lymphocyte Count and Peak Serum Interferon Titer During Poly ICLC Therapy.

	Adherent monocytes per ml blood × 10^4	Absolute lymphocytes per mm^3	Peak interferon (INF) Titer (units/ml)
Pre-therapy	4.55 ± 1.01	1180.1 ± 288.6	−
Post-therapy	1.11 ± 0.46	586.6 ± 143.5	569.7 ± 158.5
Correlation coefficient with INF level	−.136	+.023	
P value	> .30	> .50	−

Table 19.4. Effect of Therapy with MVE-2 on Host Defense Parameters in Patients with Advanced Malignancy.

Parameter	Pre-therapy	Host defense on inducted day of therapy normalized to the pre-therapy value				
		D2	D4	D7	D14	D21
Monocyte adherence	0	.6	.9	2.6	3.2	1.3
Serum lysozyme	0	.1	−.4	−.2	.2	−2.2
ADCC-CRBC	0	3.9	9.4	0.3	5.9	4.6[a]
ADCC-HRBC	0	.9	.9	3.0	.1	.9
ADCC-CEM	0	1.1	4.7	7.9	4.5	8.3[a]
NK-K562	0	2.3	3.4	5.6	2.6	6.5[a]

Note: Units of parameters and abbreviations same as in Table 19.1.
[a] Significant difference (by ANOVA and linearity test).

These findings, plus our earlier work with MER, are summarized in Table 19.6, which indicates the various host defense parameters studied in each therapy group and compares the changes in each during therapy. The unique patterns of change for each therapeutic agent, indicate their different mechanisms of action, and also demonstrate the ability of this multiparameter host defense assay to characterize the therapeutic agent.

Table 19.5. Changes in Host Defense Parameters Associated with FAC Combination Chemotherapy in Patients with Advanced Breast Cancer.

Parameter	Timing of study			
	Pre-therapy	D7	D14	D21
Monocyte adherence	13.15	0.93[a]	2.06[a]	8.30
Serum lysozyme	8.24	3.70[a]	3.70[a]	4.99
ADCC-CRBC	12.94	10.90	8.71	18.16
ADCC-HRBC	8.23	3.30[a]	3.93[a]	6.28
ADCC-CEM	51.76	45.69	44.89	49.20
NK-K562	35.98	36.45	31.39	26.35
PHA response	52.93	64.62	91.51	57.68
PWM response	25.23	5.82[a]	16.24	24.98
Con A response	31.68	16.03[a]	20.85	22.30

Note: Units of parameters and abbreviations same as Table 19.1 plus the following: FAC: 5FU, adriamycin and cytoxan chemotherapy; PHA: phytohemagglutinin; PWM: pokeweed mitogen. PHA, PWM and Con A responses in counts per minute of H^3 thymidine incorporation per culture $\times\ 10^3$.
[a] Significant depression.

Table 19.6. Summary of Effects of Selected Biological Response Modifiers and Chemotherapy Regimens on Selected Host Defense Parameters.

Host defense	Therapy				
	MER	MVE-2	IFN	Poly ICLC	FAC
Serum lysozyme	I	NC	NC	NC	D
Monocyte adherence	I	NC	D	D	D
ADCC-HRBC	I	NC	D	D	D
ADCC-CRBC	I	I	NC	NC	NC
ADCC-CEM	ND	I	NC	NC	NC
NK-K562	I	I	I	D	D

Note: Abbreviations same as Table 19.1 plus the following: IFN: interferon; FAC: 5FU, adriamycin and cytoxan chemotherapy; I: increase; NC: no change; D: decrease; ND: not done.

Discussion

During the last few years, a number of assay systems have been developed which facilitate assessment of immunotherapy and related approaches to biological therapy by augmenting agents. Augmenting agents can be defined as drugs or products which stimulate intrinsic, non-specific host defense mechanisms against cancer, e.g., BCG, *C. parvum*, interferon inducers, and macrophage activators. The assays outlined in this paper are important as they are relevant to the major mechanisms of action of augmenting agents: namely, macrophage activation, NK cell activation, and interferon induction. These assays are also relatively simple, reproducible, and relatively easily controlled with appropriate standards, and the data from most of them can be available within 24 hours.

Using these assay systems, we have detected unique patterns of change induced by individual therapeutic agents. For example, while interferon itself induced an increase in NK cell activity, the interferon inducer poly ICLC resulted in a decrease in this parameter. Furthermore, the tests have been demonstrated to detect the effects of different doses of agents and to discriminate between different doses.

The need for such an evaluation is obvious. Not only can it quantitate induced changes in host defense parameters, but it can also determine the maximum immune stimulating dose and differentiate it from the maximally tolerated dose. Furthermore, serial studies will allow the appropriate timing of agent administration to be determined. The anticipated outcome of this approach will be more a effective development of biological therapy agents for the clinic. This approach will also help to avoid the problems which arose during the early years of immunotherapy research, when the dose and schedule of therapy were arbitrary and little meaningful data on host defense modification was accumulated. The doses used in these early studies may have been either too high or too low for host defense augmentation or have been in the range where suppressor cells activity would have been induced.

References

Avella, J., Binder, H.J., Madsen, J.E., and Askenase, P.W. (1978) Effect of histamine H_2-receptor antagonists on delayed hypersensitivity. *Lancet* 1:624–625.

Breslow, D.S. (1976) Biologically active synthetic polymers. *Pure and Applied Chem.* 46:103–113.

Currie, E.A. and Headley, G.W. (1977) Monocytes and macrophages in malignant melanoma. I. Peripheral blood macrophage precursors. *Brit. J. Cancer* 36:1–6.

Goodwin, J.S. (1981) Prostaglandin E and cancer growth: potential for immunotherapy with prostaglandin synthetase inhibitors. In *Augmenting Agents in Cancer Therapy* Hersh, E.M. (ed.), Raven Press, in press.

Hersh, E.M., Gutterman, J.U., Alexanian, R., Lotzova, E., and Murphy, S.G. (1980) A seven parameter host defense assay system for evaluating biological response modifiers (BRM) therapy of human cancer. (Abstract) *Proc. Amer. Assoc. Cancer Res.*, in press.

Hersh, E.M., Gutterman, J.U., and Mavligit, G.M. (1977) Immunotherapy of human cancer. *Adv. Int. Med.* 22:145–185.

Hersh, E.M., Murphy, S., Quesada, J., Gutterman, J.U., Mavligit, G.M., Gschwind, C.R., and Morgan, J. (1980) The effect of immunotherapy with *C. parvum* and MER administered intravenously on host defense function in cancer patients. Submitted to *J. Natl. Cancer Inst.*, in press.

Hersh, E.M., Murphy, S., Zander, A., Dicke, K., Stewart, D., Toki, H., and Latreille, J. (1980) Host defense deficiency in hairy cell leukemia and its correction by leukocyte transfusion. *Blood* 56(3):526–533.

Hersh, E.M., Patt, Y.Z., Murphy, S.G., Dicke, K., Zander, A., Washington, M., and Goldman, R. (1980) A radiosensitive thymic hormone sensitive suppressor cell in the peripheral blood of cancer patients. *Cancer Res.* 40:3134–3140.

Poplack, D.O., Bonnard, G.D., Holiman, B.J., and Balese, R.M. (1976) Monocyte-mediated antibody-dependent cellular cytotoxicity: a clinical test of monocyte function. *Blood* 48:809–816.

Rosenthal, A.S. (1980) Regulation of the immune response—role of the macrophage. *New Engl. J. Med.* 303:1153–1156.

Copyright 1981 by Elsevier North Holland, Inc.
Saunders, Daniels, Serrou, Rosenfeld, and Denney, eds.
FUNDAMENTAL MECHANISMS IN HUMAN CANCER IMMUNOLOGY

CHAPTER 20

Genetic Studies in Experimental Tumor Resistance

R. Michael Williams, M.D., Ph.D.

Professor of Medicine, Chief, Medical Oncology, Department of Medicine and the Cancer Center, Northwestern University, Evanston, Illinois

In 1967, Amiel's reports of his studies of Hodgkin's Disease established the first solid link between HLA and disease, but indications of the significance of the major histocompatibility complex (MHC) to fundamental mechanisms in cancer immunology emerged much earlier. Two major prognostic events were the discovery of linkage between specific immune responses and the MHC of animals (reviewed in Benacerraf and McDevitt, 1972) and the description of the H-2 linked resistance to Gross virus leukemogenesis by Lilly and collaborators (Lilly et al., 1964).

A third, somewhat under-recognized discovery was reported by Snell in 1958, well before publication of any of these reports. Snell's observation had most significance to the present topic, the genetics of the resistance to tumors. He reported that F_1 hybrids had greater than expected resistance to transplanted, apparently histocompatible tumors. He called this the hybrid effect. The phenomenon was shown to involve the H-2 complex, but extensive studies by the Möllers (Möller and Möller, 1965) and then by their colleagues the Hellströms (Hellström and Hellström, 1967) led to the impression that immunity was not involved in the hybrid effect. They called it syngeneic preference or allogeneic inhibition. Barbara Sanford (1967) and Daniel Oth (Oth et al., 1969) studied the same phenomenon and concluded that the resistance of the F_1 hybrid was due to a hybrid vigor of the immune response. In the early 1970's, when the focus of tumor immunology shifted to the exciting studies of cytotoxic T lymphocyte function, specificity, and regulation, immunologists reflected on the immunological consequences of interactions between *non*-histocompatible lymphoid cells (the allogeneic effect, Katz, 1972) and occasionally confused this with allogeneic inhibition.

At about this time, Cudkowicz and Bennett (1971) began to explore the immunobiology of bone marrow grafts. This hybrid or hematopoietic histocompatibility (Hh) phenomenon, which seemed possibly related to the hybrid effect for tumor resistance, had already been shown to be related to H-2 (Cudkowicz and Stimpfling, 1964). At that time, however, very few immunologists or immunogeneticists appreciated the significance of their observation. Even today, there is no good explanation for why two identical alleles must be expressed at the same locus to produce a functional antigen. However, the potential importance of natural killer (NK) cells in tumor resistance, and the experiments with the *beige* mutant (Kaminsky and Cudkowicz, 1980), which provide solid evidence to corroborate the many associations between the Hh resistance mechanism and NK cells, underscore the importance of this phenomenon.

Katz and Benacerraf (1976) and Kindred and Shreffler (1972) correctly seized on the allogeneic effect data as the key to an understanding of the original observation by Claman's group (Claman et al., 1966) that thymocytes and bone marrow cells could somehow collaborate to produce immunity. The revelations which followed from the observation of MHC restriction by Zinkernagel and Doherty (1975) served to focus even more importance on the MHC. Much attention was also directed toward a "new" gene product, Ia (Frelinger et al., 1974), and Amos and Yunis, VanRood, Svejgaard, Bach, Dausset and others related this fundamental work on H-2 in mice to studies of the human counterpart, HLA.

During this period, as a student of genetics and disease from a thymologist's laboratory, this author was trying to learn about tumor immunology and immunogenetics, particularly *Ir*-genes. The hybrid effect system of Snell was, and still is, the focus of our work. Tumors were studied because anti-tumor immunity was clearly T-cell dependent, and many immunologists were trying to find the *Ir* gene product on a T cell.

The summary data presented here are based on studies of the tumor P815-X2, which has provided one of several hybrid effect systems. This tumor was chosen for in depth study because it is used by many investigators to analyze the mechanism of cytotoxic T lymphocyte killing and because it appears to be free of the numerous known viruses expressed by most experimental mouse tumors. The only absolutely unequivocal *in vivo* parameter of tumor resistance is survival. Therefore, genetic differences in histocompatible tumor resistance are determined by an animal's survival time after a standard inoculum of tumor cells is administered.

Since P815-X2 arose in a DBA/2 mouse, the basic hybrid system is to compare DBA/2 with an F_1 hybrid which has DBA/2 as one parent (i.e., a D2 hybrid). Among the readily available D2 hybrids which were simultaneously inoculated with P815-X2, C3H×DBA/2 (C3D2F1) mice appeared to die at the same time as DBA/2, while C57BL/6×DBA/2 (B6D2F1) consistently survived the longest.

To focus on the H-2 complex, hybrids were constructed utilizing H-2 congenics on a C57BL/10 (B10) background (Williams et al., 1975). To eliminate a direct role for non-H-2 genes, all hybrids were compared with (D2×B10.D2)F$_1$, the hybrid which was homozygous at the major histocompatibility complex. Like the H-2^k/H-2^d C3D2F1 hybrid, the D2×B10.BR which is also heterozygous for the same H-2 alleles was no more resistant than the H-2^d/H-2^d homozygous controls. Contrary to our initial expectations, further dissection of the H-2 complex utilizing intra-H-2 recombinants failed to localize the effect to a single I-region gene. In fact, the data suggested that there may be a role for more than one H-2 gene. Also, since P815-X2 injected (D2×B10.BR)F$_1$ mice lived longer than similarly treated C3D2F1 mice, we also had early evidence for participation by non-H-2 genes (Williams, 1977).

Faced with such obvious genetic complexity in the basic phenomenon, namely two or more H-2 genes and at least one non-H-2 gene, we were forced to develop new approaches. Either we had to create simpler *in vivo* genetic models by selective breeding, or (ideally) find mutants, rather than congenics, which showed similar effects.

Fortunately, mutants at H-2K^b were readily available, and several comparisons of D2×B6 versus D2×B6^m (m=H-2 mutant) showed highly significant survival differences (Williams et al., 1981). Also, D2×B6.C-H-2^{bm12} mice died sooner than D2×B6 hybrids. The bm12 mutation has been shown to involve the I-A^b subregion of H-2^b (McKenzie et al., 1979; Hansen et al., 1980). Thus, there is now evidence, based on mutation studies, for participation by the H-2K and I-A genes in hybrid resistance to P815. Combined with the earlier evidence suggesting a role for the H-2D end and for non-H-2 genes, this means that this single hybrid effect system could depend on at least four separate genes, acting alone or in combination.

While early genetic analysis of this system was in progress, we sought to test the hypothesis that the relatively resistant hybrids produced more cytotoxic T lymphocyte-mediated P815-X2 killing. B6D2F1 and C3D2F1 mice were chosen as examples of high and low resistance respectively, and *in vivo* P815-X2 specific cytotoxicity was evaluated throughout the lifetime of tumor bearing mice.

The system used was shown previously to detect *in vivo* generated P815-X2 specific cytotoxic T cells in the node draining the site of tumor inoculation (Germain et al., 1976). The *most* resistant B6D2F1 hybrid appeared to have the *lowest* level of P815-X2 specific cytotoxic activity.

This was true even when corrections were made for cell number and tumor burden. Thus, we still have no evidence to link cytotoxic T cells (CTL) to genetically controlled resistance to P815-X2. Indeed, the data could be interpreted to suggest that the most resistant hybrids have the least P815-X2 specific CTL activity.

In the P815-X2 model system, the presence of cytolytic T cells that can be detected using P815-X2 as the test antigen, *in vitro*, is not formal proof that the physiological role of these cells *in vivo* is to eliminate the tumor. If this were the case, one might expect more easily demonstrable cytolytic T lymphocytes at earlier times in the course of tumor growth. Similarly, the decline in cytotoxic T lymphocytes against P815 occurs many days before the general health of the animal is detectably compromised by the presence of growing tumor. We have also observed viable tumor cells in the draining lymph node as early as 5–7 days after inoculation, so it is also likely that cytotoxic T lymphocytes can exist in a draining lymph node that itself contains viable P815-X2 cells. That these P815-X2 cells may be inhibiting cytolysis in the assay system is a strong possibility, yet we must also ask why such cells are not destroyed *in vivo*.

We have proposed (Singer and Williams, 1978, 1980) an alternative hypothesis for the physiological role of cytolytic T lymphocytes, which is more consistent with the regulation of the immune response to meet an expanding antigen load, but does not contain any teleological implications that the cytotoxic cells are "there in order to destroy the tumor." The fact that the tumor cell mass is expanding, despite continuing destruction, strongly suggests that the animal is being bombarded with an increasing tumor antigen load. If this antigen is treated like any other antigen, one may presume that the immune response to it is regulated through a network of positive and negative signals, each with a precise specificity. If the host response to P815-X2 increases with time, then we would expect to find large numbers of cells bearing a receptor specific for the P815-X2 antigen. These may include cells with cytotoxic and cytostatic activity when tested on P815-X2, but physiologically they serve to regulate other lymphoid cells bearing P815 antigen.

If the response to an antigen is to be regulated, then the immune system must have a network of positive and negative controls which would be expected to turn off the response to P815-X2 antigen in a specific manner. We have postulated that such regulation of the immune response occurs through the action of T lymphocytes, which are therefore suppressor cells with respect to an antigen, even though they may also be cytotoxic cells for that same antigen when presented in another context (for example, when presented on P815-X2 tumor cells). Thus, we propose that in the P815-X2 model, the cytolytic T cells are in fact physiologically present to turn off the response to the P815-X2 antigen that itself is being mediated by other lymphoid cells of host origin. The cytotoxic cells detected using ^{51}Cr-labeled P815-X2 are then considered cross-reactive cells. Their physiological specificity is against anti-P815-X2 antigen. Thus, the cytotoxic cell activity might well be expected to depend on host histocompatibility antigen and/or immunoglobulin determinants, depending on the precise nature of the antigen specific idiotype. In preliminary experiments, it has been possible to detect significant activity against host lymphoid cells which have been cultured with nonviable P815-X2 cells. These effector cells also have significant cytolytic activity against ^{51}Cr-labeled P815-X2 cells (Figure 20.1).

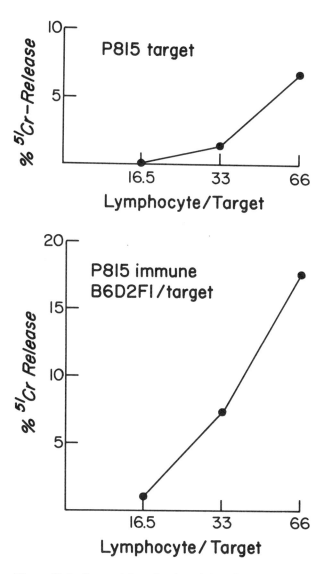

Figure 20.1. Cytotoxicity of cultured lymphocytes from P815 bearing B6D2F1 mice tested against ^{51}Cr-labeled P815 cells (upper panel) and against B6D2F1 cells which are themselves responding to P815 (lower panel). Values represent percent ^{51}Cr-release in 4 hours at the lymphocyte/target ratios depicted.

Also, using the DBA/2 and B6D2F1 system and the bone marrow/thymus epithelium chimera approach to study genetic restriction, we have demonstrated that P815-X2 resistance depends on the genotype of each element: bone marrow, thymus epithelium, and the host (Williams et al., 1980). Further studies of the genetics and the immunobiology of this system must consider each level of complexity in turn. Fortunately, the genetic tolls are improving, albeit less rapidly than immunological theory has demanded.

Concerning our original attempt to use the hybrid effect to find H-2 linked *Ir*-genes for tumor specific antigens, the accumulated experimental data combined with the regulatory circuit concept force the conclusion that *Ir*-gene phenomena can be seen with many products of the MHC. Our first experiments with an A strain leukemia pointed to the K-end of H-2 and to non-H-2 genes as the possible site for the genes controlling resistance (Williams, 1973). The data generated with a methylcholanthrene induced fibrosarcoma implicated H-2 controlled suppression of host resistance to tumor growth because some hybrids died *sooner* than the parent, and the P815-X2 data implicated at least two H-2 genes for one response (Williams et al., 1975).

All these findings seemed paradoxical until they were also observed using the same H-2 recombinant haplotypes and the random polymer systems GLΦ (Dorf et al., 1975) and GT (Debre et al., 1975). Now biochemical studies of Ia molecules (Uhr et al., 1979) have even provided support for the α and β gene complementation model of Dorf and collaborators. The immune suppression (*Is*) gene, like the immune response (*Ir*) gene, is a concept which must ultimately be elucidated with biochemical analysis of the proteins and the DNA. At present, the data support the conclusion that Ia molecules themselves can function as *Is* and *Ir* gene products. The I-J region now seems more relevant to suppression, but it is the fact of antigen specific regulation of immunity, not necessarily the direction of regulation, which should form the basis for further investigation.

The mechanisms of regulation probably involve the interaction of a single antigen with an MHC molecule, with or without a V-region gene product. What is defined as idiotype in this context depends on the system being analyzed. However, it is clear that antigen specificity is the cornerstone.

Despite our claim that two H-2 genes may interact to regulate resistance to a single tumor and the elegant biochemical support for the α and β gene concept, there is no proof that only a single antigenic determinant is involved in any of these systems.

There are no strong data to implicate any molecule as the relevant tumor associated antigen in a hybrid effect system. Except for virus-induced or infected tumors and the virus determined antigens, this statement might be made for all experimental tumor systems. Differentiation or oncofetal antigens may be relevant to tumor resistance, but we have no strong data to implicate differentiation antigens as targets in the hybrid effect model. It is possible to immunize F_1 hybrids against leukemia by injecting normal parental bone marrow cells (Haynor et al., 1979). This model is analogous in part to the Hh system, where the effector appears to be a natural killer cell (Cudkowicz and Hochman, 1979). Unfortunately, there is no biochemical evidence for an Hh antigen. Nevertheless, the theoretical complexity of such antigens is unlikely to exceed that of random terpolymers.

For the same reasons that our optimal biochemical understanding of H-2 linked *Ir* gene function cannot rely on complex antigens, we may no longer base all our important conclusions on H-2 recombinants. H-2 mutants are being analyzed widely, and there are *Ir* gene phenomenon differences among many (Kohn et al., 1978).

There may be a number of differences between the qualitative immunoregulatory functions of K/D and I or Class I and Class II H-2 products (Klein, 1979). It is likely, however, that each immune response gene function will involve antigen presentation or recognition. Thus, there may be no way precisely to identify a specific *Ir* or *Is* gene for a single antigen, except by using that specific antigen or an analogous anti-idiotype reagent. This also means that single MHC gene products will be the *Ir* gene product for responses to numerous different antigens.

Available data favor the generalization that cytotoxic and, at least for lymphocyte targets, "off" signals are generated preferentially when antigen is presented in association with or in the context of a Class I histocompatibility antigen. This phenomenon plus other data about suppressor factors and network theory led us to postulate that the predominant *in vivo* physiologic function of CTL's was to act as suppressor cells which could kill normal immune cells bearing the relevant antigen. The fact that a CTL can also kill antigen expressing tumor cells does not mean that the physiologic function of such cells is to eliminate antigen. In fact, the kinetics of CTL production in histocompatible tumor bearing animals is consistent with that of suppressor cell development in response to very long or frequent challenges with antigen.

Helper T cells are stimulated preferentially by antigen in association with class II histocompatibility antigens (Ia). This same Ia dependent MHC restriction holds for *in vivo* delayed type hypersensitivity phenomena (Miller and Vadas, 1976). *In vivo* delayed type hypersensitivity is initiated by T cells (Williams and Waksman, 1969), but most cells in these reactions are not antigen specific, and need not be T cells (McClusky et al., 1963; Najarian and Feldman, 1963). Specific tumor immunity is T cell dependent but not necessarily CTL dependent. Evidence for the importance of lymphokines, natural killer cells, macrophages, and other cells in tumor rejection is continually increasing, while evidence for a unique anti-tumor role for CTL's remains unimpressive. As the details of humoral and cellular immunity against tumors continue to be identified and interrelated, the well characterized examples of the genetic control of tumor resistance will continue to provide a touchstone to relate *in vivo* resistance and survival to the myriad of measurable parameters, immunological and otherwise.

References

Amiel, J.F. (1967) Study of the leukocyte phenotypes in Hodgkin's disease. In *Histocompatibility Testing*. Curtoni, E.S., Nattioz, P.L., and Tosi, R.M. (eds.), Copenhagen: Munksgaard, pp. 79–81.

290

Benacerraf, B. and McDevitt, H.O. (1972) The histocompatibility linked immune response genes. *Science* 175:273–278.

Claman, H.N., Chaperon, E.A., and Triplett, R.F. (1966) Thymus-marrow cell combinations. Synergism in antibody production. *Proc. Soc. Exp. Biol. Med.* 122:1167–1171.

Cudkowicz, G. and Bennett, M. (1971) Peculiar immunobiology of bone marrow allografts. I. Graft rejection by irradiated "responder" mice. *J. Exp. Med.* 134:83–97.

Cudkowicz, G. and Hochman, P.S. (1979) Do natural killer cells engage in regulated reactions against self to ensure homeostasis? *Immunol. Rev.* 44:13–41.

Cudkowicz, G. and Stimpfling, J.H. (1964) Deficient growth of C57BL marrow cells transplanted in F_1 hybrid mice. Association with the histocompatibility -2 locus. *Immunology* 7:291–306.

Debre, P., Kapp, J.A., Dorf, M.E., and Benacerraf, B. (1975) Genetic control of specific immune suppression. II. H-2-linked dominant genetic control of immune suppression by the random copolymer L-glutamic acid ^{50}-L-tyrosine ^{50}(GT). *J. Exp. Med.* 142:1447–1454.

Dorf, M.E., Stimpfling, J.H., and Benacerraf, B. (1975) Requirement for two H-2 complex *Ir* genes for the immune response to the L-Glu, L-Lys, L-Phe terpolymer. *J. Exp. Med.* 141:1459–1463.

Frelinger, J.A., Niederhuber, J.E., David, C.S., and Shreffler, D.C. (1974) Evidence for the expression of Ia (H-2 associated) antigens on thymus derived lymphocytes. *J. Exp. Med.* 140:1273–1284.

Germain, R.N., Williams, R.M., and Benacerraf, B. (1976) Specific and non-specific anti-tumor immunity. III. Specific T lymphocyte-mediated cytolysis of P815 mastocytoma and SL2 lymphoma by draining lymph node cells from syngeneic tumor bearing DBA/2J mice. *Amer. J. Pathol.* 85:661–673.

Hansen, T.H., Melvold, R.W., Arn, J.S., and Sachs, D.H. (1980) Evidence for mutation of an I-A locus. *Nature* 285:340–341.

Haynor, D.R., Singer, D.E., and Williams, R.M. (1979) Resistance to BN myelogenous leukemia in LBNF1 rats preinjected with BN bone marrow. *Fed. Proc.* 38:1069.

Hellström, K.E. and Hellström, I. (1967) Allogeneic inhibition of transplanted tumor cells. *Progr. Exptl. Tumor Res.* 9:40–76.

Kaminksy, S. and Cudkowicz, G. (1980) Natural killing and resistance to marrow grafts: correlations in four beige mutant mouse lines. *Fed. Proc.* 39:359.

Katz, D.H. (1972) The allogeneic effect on immune responses: model for the regulatory influences of T lymphocytes on the immune system. *Transplant. Rev.* 12:141–179.

Katz, D.H. and Benacerraf, B. (1976) Genetic control of lymphocyte interactions and differentiation. In *The Role of Products of the Histocompatibility Gene Complex in Immune Responses*. Katz, D.H. and Benacerraf, B. (eds.), New York: Academic Press, pp. 355–389.

Kindred, B. and Shreffler, D.C. (1972) H-2 dependence of cooperation between T and B cells *in vivo*. *J. Immunol.* 109:940–943.

Klein, J. (1979) The major histocompatibility complex of the mouse. *Science* 203:516–521.

Kohn, H.I., Klein, J., Melvold, R.W., Nathenson, S.G., Pious, D., and Shreffler, D.C. (1978) The first H-2 mutant workshop. *Immunogenetics* 7:279–294.

Lilly, F., Boyse, E.A., and Old, L.J. (1964) Genetic basis of susceptibility to viral leukemogenesis. *Lancet* ii:1207–129.

McCluskey, R.T., Benacerraf, B., and McCluskey, J.W. (1963) Studies on the specificity of the cellular infiltrate in delayed hypersensitivity reactions.

McKenzie, I.F.C., Morgan, G.M., Sandrin, M.S., Michaelides, M.M., Melvold, R.W., and Kohn, H.I. 1979. B6.C-H-2^{bm12}: a new H-2 mutation in the I region in the mouse. *J. Exp. Med.* 150:1323–1338.

Miller, J.F.A.P. and Vadas, M.A. (1976) Antigen activation of T lymphocytes: influence of major histocompatibility complex. *Cold Spr. Har. Symp. Quant. Biol.* 41:579–588.

Möller, G. and Möller, E. (1965) Plaque-formation by non-immune and x-irradiated lymphoid cells on monolayers of mouse embryo cells. *Nature* 208:260–263.

Najarian, J.S. and Feldman, J.D. (1963) Specificity of passively transferred delayed hypersensitivity. *J. Exp. Med.* 118:341–352.

Oth, D., Oswald, P., and Burg, C. (1969) Restoration of the "hybrid effect" suppressed by whole-body irradiation. *Japan. J. Exp. Med.* 39:649–652.

Sanford, B.H. (1967) Evidence for immunological resistance to a parental line tumor by F_1 hybrid hosts. *Transplantation* 5:557–560.

Snell, G.D. (1958) Histocompatibility genes of the mouse. I. Demonstration of weak histocompatibility differences by immunization. *J. Natl. Cancer Inst.* 20:787–824.

Uhr, J.W., Capra, J.D., Vitteta, E.S., and Cook, R.G. (1979) Organization of the immune response genes. *Science* 206:292–297.

Williams, R.M. (1973) Possible role of the H-2K-*Ir* regions in "allogeneic" inhibition. *Fed. Proc.* 32:880.

Williams, R.M. (1977) Experimental models with possible implications for the role of HLA in malignancy. *Prog. Clin. Biol. Res.* 16:21–28.

Williams, R.M. and Waksman, B.H. (1969) Thymus-derived cells in the early phase of delayed tuberculin reactions. *J. Immunol.* 103:1435–1437.

Williams, R.M., Dorf, M.E., and Benacerraf, B. (1975) H-2 linked genetic control of resistance to histocompatible tumors. *Cancer Res.* 35:1586–1590.

Williams, R.M., Eig, B.M., and Singer, D.E. (1980) Preliminary analysis of hybrid resistance to histocompatible P815 utilizing bone marrow and thymus epithelium radiation chimeras. In *Genetic Control of Natural Resistance to Infection and Malignancy*. Skamene, E., Kongshavn, P., and Landy, M. (eds.), New York: Academic Press, pp. 477–483.

Williams, R.M., Kwak, L.W., and Melvold, R.W. (1981) Evidence for involvement of the H-2K[b] and I-A[b] genes in hybrid resistance to P815-X2. *Immunogen.*, in press.

Zinkernagel, R. and Doherty, P. (1975) H-2 compatibility requirement for T cell mediated lysis of target cells infected with lymphocytic choriomeningitis virus. *J. Exp. Med.* 141:1427–1436.

CHAPTER 21

Role of Accessory Cell *HLA-D* Region Molecules in T Cell Activation by Antigens[1]

E. Thorsby, B. Bergholtz, E. Berle,
L. Braathen, and H. Hirschberg

Tissue Typing Laboratory, Rikshospitalet, The National Hospital, Oslo 1, Norway

Recent studies in mice and guinea pigs have demonstrated that products of the self major histocompatibility complex, MHC, are involved in the cooperative cell events leading to T cell activation by foreign antigen. Most T cell subsets appear to be able to recognize an antigen only when it is presented together with products of the self MHC expressed in the antigen-presenting cells. These constraints on T cell activation, called self MHC restriction, appear to be laid down prior to antigen encounter, during T cell differentiation in the thymus as well as during post-thymic development (see for example Zinkernagel, 1978).

Human T cells are similarly restricted by products of the *HLA* complex, the T helper/amplifier cells by products of the *HLA-D* region, and the cytotoxic T cells by products of the *HLA-A*, *-B* and *-C* regions (for references, see Thorsby et al., 1981; Thorsby, 1981).

Needless to say, these findings are of great relevance to cancer immunology. Several studies have demonstrated that T cell cytotoxicity against target cells expressing tumor specific antigens is restricted by self MHC products (Gomard et al., 1976; Chesebro et al., 1976; Trinchieri et al., 1976). However, other studies, using slightly different assay systems, found less MHC restriction (Holden and Herbermann, 1977; Stutman and Shen, 1978).

Many questions still remain to be answered. The mechanism behind self MHC restriction is not known. One possibility is that T lymphocytes are equipped with one single type of receptors which recognizes an interaction

[1]Supported in part by grants from the Norwegian Council for Science and the Humanities, the Norwegian Cancer Society, the Norwegian Society for Fighting Cancer, and Anders Jahre's Medical Research Fund.

product formed by antigen in complex with self MHC products. Another possibility is that T lymphocytes have two types of receptors (linked or unlinked), one which binds to self MHC products and the other to antigen, and that both must combine for activation to occur.

Another important unresolved question is the nature of the MHC elements which restrict T cell activation. Are these the MHC cell membrane molecules which function as strong histocompatibility antigens in allogeneic combinations, or products of closely linked genes? Closely associated is the question of whether MHC encoded molecules of any cell type can function as restricting elements in T cell activation. For example, can any cell expressing products of the murine *H-2I* or human *HLA-D* region, under appropriate conditions, present antigen in an immunogenic and self MHC restricted way to the T helper/amplifier cell?

Some of our own attempts to answer the last two questions will be briefly summarized in the following, using studies of human accessory cell-dependent T lymphocyte proliferative responses to different foreign antigens as a model. Experimental details are found in the listed references.

HLA-D Restriction of Proliferative T Lymphocyte Responses to Antigen

When T lymphocytes from sensitized donors are mixed with antigen *in vitro*, a proliferative response will usually occur, provided 2–10% peripheral blood-derived autologous monocytes/macrophages (Mø; i.e., adherent cells) are also present. The proliferating cells belong to the helper/amplifier ($T_{h/a}$) subset of human T cells (Reinherz and Schlossman, 1980). This T cell response is restricted by products of the *HLA-D* region of the T cell donor, as has been demonstrated for many different antigens (purified protein derivative of tuberculin: PPD, viral antigens, hapten-conjugated cell membranes, etc.) (Bergholtz and Thorsby, 1977; other references in Thorsby, 1981). An optimal antigen-specific response requires that antigen is presented by macrophages which express the D/DR^2 determinants of the T cell donor.

The results of a typical experiment using purified T cells from a donor with recurrent herpes labialis and herpes simplex virus type 1 (HSV) as antigen, are shown in Fig. 21.1. When T cells from this donor, who is *D/DR* 1/7, were mixed with HSV and Mø, a strong HSV-specific response was seen (compare open and filled columns to the left in Fig. 21.1). When HSV was instead presented with Mø from an allogeneic unrelated donor who shared both *D/DR* determinants with the T cell donor, a response similar to that seen in the autologous combination was obtained (second open and filled columns).

---

[2] The term *D/DR* is used since it is not known whether the T cell activating D determinants and the corresponding *DR* determinants inducing alloantibody production are present on the same or on different *HLA-D* region molecules.

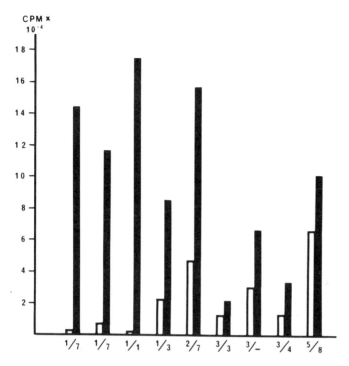

Figure 21.1. *HLA-D/DR* restriction of the T cell herpes simplex virus (HSV) response. 50,000 T cells from a sensitized donor of *HLA-D/DR* type 1/7 were mixed *in vitro* with 5,000 autologous (left column) or allogeneic macrophages and HSV-Ag added (■) or not (□). After 6 days of culture, proliferation was assayed by ³H-thymidine incorporation. The results are given as median cpm of triplicates (ordinate). Along the abscissa, the *D/DR* types of the macrophage donors used are shown.

The sharing of only one *D/DR* determinant between the Mø and T cell donor also resulted in strong or moderate HSV responses. However, when the Mø shared no *D/DR* determinants with the T cell donor, only a slight antigen-specific response was seen when the allogeneic mixed macrophage-T cell response was subtracted (compare the four open and filled columns to the right). Similar data were obtained in other experiments, and macrophages taken from sensitized and non-sensitized donors, for example neonates, functioned equally well (Berle and Thorsby, 1980).

The inability of *D/DR* disparate Mø to induce antigen-specific responses is not due to suppression or cytotoxicity caused by the *HLA* incompatibiltiy between T and Mø, and neither matching nor disparity of *HLA-ABC* determinants has been found to affect these responses (see, for example, Berle and Thorsby, 1980).

The antigen-sensitive T cells are clonally distributed, not only with respect to antigen, but also with respect to the restricting *HLA-D* region elements. Thus, individuals being heterozygous at *HLA-D* have two separable populations of antigen-reactive T cells, each only able to recognize antigen together with products of the one or the other *HLA-D* region expressed in the antigen-presenting Mø membrane (Hirschberg et al., 1979).

The Nature of the Restricting *HLA-D* Region Elements

The elements which restrict the $T_{h/a}$ cells might be the cell membrane molecules expressing the *HLA-D* and *-DR* determinants and which thus function as strong histocompatibility antigens in allogeneic combinations, or other unknown products of the *HLA-D* region. At least two pieces of evidence indicate that the *HLA-D/DR* molecules may themselves function as restricting elements:

1. Our own studies as well as those of others have involved cells from *unrelated* individuals. Thus, in our own studies we found that combinations of macrophages and $T_{h/a}$ cells from unrelated individuals were fully able to cooperate in antigen-specific immune responses, provided they shared both *HLA-D/DR* determinants, based on typing with antisera or cells recognizing allogeneic *D/DR* determinants. In most instances, pronounced antigen-specific responses occurred also when only one *D/DR* determinant was shared (see Fig. 21.1). Although it cannot be entirely excluded that instead products of genes closely linked to and in very high nonrandom association to the *D/DR* genes may be the restricting elements, the rather constant findings in a high number of studies using unrelated combinations make this alternative explanation unlikely.

2. Anti-*DR* antibodies specifically inhibit macrophage-T cell cooperation when reactive with *DR* determinants which may function as restricting elements. We showed this by culturing T cells and Mø from *HLA* homozygous and heterozygous donors in the presense of specific anti-*DR* antibodies without complement (Bergholtz and Thorsby, 1978). Part of the results of four typical experiments are given in Table 21.1. All four experiments demonstrate that antiserum reactive with the *DR* determinant shared between Mø and T cell donors specifically inhibits antigen activation. The first two experiments also show that antiserum only reactive with *DR* of the T cell donor has no effect. More important, as the two last experiments demonstrate, antiserum recognizing only *DR* determinants carried by the macrophages and not the T cell donor, also has no or much less inhibitory effect. Similarly, anti-B27 antiserum which is reactive only with the macrophages does not inhibit, while it does inhibit when only reactive with the T cells.

Our results are in accordance with similar data obtained in studies of mice and guinea pigs (Schwartz et al., 1976; Shevach et al., 1972, 1977), and have later been confirmed by others in man (Geha et al., 1979; Rodey et al., 1979). Antiserum induced cell-mediated killing of the antigen-presenting cells is not a

Table 21.1. Inhibition of Mφ Dependent PPD Activation of T Cells by Anti-*HLA-DR* and *HLA-B* Antibodies.

T cells	Mφ	PPD	NS[a] cpm	αDR2	%RS[b]	αDR3	% RS
DR 2/3	2/2	−	22 ± 14	43 ± 8		36 ± 3	
		+	970 ± 68	564 ± 19		936 ± 222	
			948[c]	521	55%	900	95%
DR 2/3	3/3	−	70 ± 14	70 ± 6		48 ± 16	
		+	1270 ± 61	1469 ± 210		582 ± 99	
			1200[c]	1399	117%	534	45%

T cells	Mφ	PPD	NS cpm	αDR3	%RS	αDR8	%RS	αB27	%RS
DR 3/3	3/8	−	1125 ± 102	963 ± 220		375 ± 26		803 ± 75	
B −/−	27/−	+	2602 ± 181	864 ± 120		1512 ± 189		2206 ± 149	
			1477[c]	0	0%	1137	77%	1403	95%
DR 8/8	3/8	−	393 ± 96	319 ± 110		337 ± 117		422 ± 163	
B 27/27	−/−	+	1982 ± 434	1806 ± 160		816 ± 262		816 ± 212	
			1589[c]	1487	94%	479	30%	394	25%

Note: The anti-*DR* antisera used were free from contaminating anti-*HLA-ABC* antibodies.

[a]Normal serum.

[b]% Relative stimulation = $\dfrac{\Delta \text{ cpm antiserum}}{\Delta \text{ cpm NS}}$.

[c]Incremental cpm = Δ cpm.

likely explanation, since in our studies and those of Rodey et al. (1979), no or much less effect was observed when the antiserum was reactive with determinants carried only by the macrophages, and which thus could not function as restricting elements. The effects of anti *HLA-B*27 antibody on the responding T cells, however, could be explained by Fc receptor dependent T cell killing.

Both the strong correlation between allospecificity and restriction, as well as the antibody inhibition experiments, are strong arguments that it is the *HLA-D/DR* cell membrane molecules responsible for alloimmune reactions which function as restriction elements for $T_{h/a}$ cells. However, the exact relationship between the epitopes responsible for restriction and those inducing allogeneic T cell and antibody production is not known. Furthermore, *HLA* encoded molecules other than the known *D/DR* may also be able to function as restriction elements for $T_{h/a}$ cells.

The Effects of Accessory Cells Other than Blood-Derived Macrophages

Blood-derived monocytes/macrophages are not the only cells expressing the *D/DR* determinants. They are also present on B lymphocytes, Langerhans cells of the skin, endothelial cells, and some others, while they are not detectably expressed on most resting T cells, fibroblasts, etc.

We found that autologous B lymphocytes depleted of monocytes/macrophages were not able to induce a PPD specific response in sensitized T cells. The main reason for this inability might be that an insufficient number of B cells bind the specific antigen. Thus, we repeated the experiments using the hapten trinitrophenyl (TNP), which binds to most cell membranes, and T cells sensitized to TNP *in vitro*. We found that TNP-treated monocyte-deprived B cells were even more effective on a per cell basis than TNP-treated Mø to induce a secondary TNP specific response (Bergholtz and Thorsby, 1979), while TNP treated autologous T cells failed to do so (Thorsby and Nousiainen, 1979).

We then investigated epidermal skin cells, which contained 3–5% *DR* expressing Langerhans cells, with less than 0.1% monocyte-macrophage contamination detectable with peroxidase staining. The results of two experiments are summarized in Table 21.2. It can be seen that epidermal cells are fully able to substitute for macrophages in inducing a virus (HSV) specific response in sensitized T cells, and that this capacity is lost after pretreatment of the epidermal cells with xeno-anti-*DR* antiserum and complement. Other experiments gave similar results (Braathen et al., 1980). In further experiments, we could show that the Langerhans cell dependent antigen activation of T cells was self *D/DR* restricted (to be published). Similar data have been obtained in the guinea pig (Stingl et al., 1978).

Endothelial cells prepared from umbilical cords also express the *D/DR* antigens. Using endothelial cells containing at most 0.5–2% peroxidase positive

Table 21.2. *HLA-DR* Positive Epidermal Cells (Ec) May Replace Macrophages (Mφ) in Herpes Simplex Virus (HSV) Antigen Activation of Autologous T Cells.

	Experiment no. 1 HSV		Experiment no. 2 HSV	
	−	+	−	+
T[a]	116 ± 43	527 ± 23	124 ± 26	293 ± 154
T + Mφ[b]	351 ± 136	6,343 ± 1,368	66 ± 29	5,236 ± 113
T + Ec[c]	533 ± 112	13,336 ± 831	675 ± 105	14,407 ± 780
T + (Ec + NRS)[d]		11,171 ± 987		14,142 ± 472
T + (Ec + αDR)[e]		522 ± 186		415 ± 256

[a] 5×10^4 T cells.

[b] 5×10^3 Mφ.

[c] 5×10^4 Ec (< 0.1% peroxidase positive cells) prepared by a suction blister device.

[d] Ec pretreated with normal serum plus complement.

[e] Ec pretreated with rabbit anti-*DR* antiserum plus complement.

monocytes, we showed that endothelial cells were equally effective as blood-derived macrophages in presenting antigens such as PPD and HSV in an immunogenic way to *D/DR* identical sensitized T cells (Hirschberg et al., 1980). This endothelial cell-T lymphocyte cooperation is restricted by *D/DR* in the same way as is T-Mø cooperation, as will appear in Table 21.3. Endothelial cells from a donor who is *HLA-D/DR* 2/6 could induce a strong PPD specific response in T lymphocytes from a *D/DR* identical sensitized adult donor, to the same extent as when autologous macrophages were used (upper part of Table 21.3). However, the same endothelial cells were much less effective in inducing a PPD specific response in T cells from donors carrying other *D/DR* antigens (lower part of Table 21.3). This finding becomes even more apparent when these data, along with data from two other experiments using other cell donors, are expressed in terms of relative antigen stimulation (to the far right of the table). Thus, endothelial cells can fully substitute for macrophages in these T cell responses, and in other experiments we could demonstrate that the same T cell clones were able to recognize antigen on macrophages and endothelial cells. When fibroblasts were substituted for macrophages, no antigen-specific proliferation was seen.

Taken together, the results strongly suggest that for cells to function as accessory cells in antigen-specific activation of $T_{h/a}$ cells, they must express both the correct *HLA-D/DR* molecules and antigen.

Discussion

The data summarized above demonstrate that the response of the T helper/amplifier sub-set to antigen requires co-recognition of antigen and products of the self-*HLA-D* region expressed in the antigen-presenting cells.

Table 21.3. Endothelial Cells (En) May Replace Macrophages (Mφ) in T Lymphocyte Activation by Antigen.

T^a	Mφ (autol)	En (allog)	Exp. no. 1			% RAgS^c Exp. no.		
			– PPD	+	Δ^b	1	2	3
2/6	–	–	482^d	1062	580			
2/6	2/6	–	270	8342	8072			
2/6	–	2/6	460	7188	6728	83	97	52
7/–	–	–	538	1032	494			
7/–	7/–	–	380	4904	4524			
7/–	–	2/6	778	1988	1210	18	23	15

^{a}5 × 10⁴ T cells mixed with 2.5 × 10³ Mφ or En.

^{b}Incremental cpm (with-without PPD).

^{c}% Relative antigen stimulation: $\dfrac{\Delta \text{ cpm En} - \Delta \text{ cpm T cells alone}}{\Delta \text{ cpm Mφ} - \Delta \text{ cpm T cells alone}} \times 100.$

^{d}Median cpm of triplicates.

Very similar data have been obtained in studies of the cytotoxic T cell subset, the difference being that these cells are restricted by products of the *HLA-A*, *-B* and *-C* regions (for references, see Thorsby et al., 1981; Thorsby, 1981). Both subsets are clonally distributed, both with respect to antigen and the restricting *HLA* element.

Available evidence suggests that the *HLA-D/DR* molecules as such function as restricting elements for the $T_{h/a}$ subset. This does not exclude the possibility that co-recognition of other products of the *HLA-D* region may also permit $T_{h/a}$ cells to respond to antigen. The self *HLA-D/DR* restriction is seldom complete, and there is every reason to believe that additional *HLA-D* region products may exist in man, as they do in the mouse, which may function as restriction elements. For example, Niederhuber and Allen (1980) have provided evidence that in addition to products of the *H-2 I-A* sub-region, products of the *I-J* sub-region may also restrict antigen-specific macrophage-T cell interactions. Another important question to be resolved is whether the epitopes responsible for the alloantigenic specificity are also responsible for the restriction specificity.

One common denominator for cells which may function as antigen-presenting cells appears to be the expression of *HLA-D/DR* molecules. B lymphocytes, Langerhans cells, and endothelial cells may apparently also present antigen in an immunogenic way for the $T_{h/a}$ subset, provided the antigen is also available in the cell membrane. Apparently, strong ability to phagocytose or digest antigen may not be necessary, since B cells, under certain circumstances, can function as accessory cells, and Langerhans cells and endothelial cells are only weakly phagocytic.

The involvement of self MHC molecules in T cell responses to antigen has important implications for MHC linked *Ir* (immune response) gene control, as discussed elsewhere (Benacerraf and Germain, 1978; Thorsby, 1978; Thorsby, 1981). The MHC encoded cell membrane molecules may be important in the generation of T cell receptor diversity, via somatic mutations during anti-self produced proliferation responses in thymic and post-thymic development (Jerne, 1971; von Boehmer et al., 1978). However, they may also influence immunogenicity on the antigen-presenting cell level, for example, by differences in ability to associate with or be modified by antigen. Of particular relevance for cancer immunology are the findings of a close and apparently selective association between some tumor-associated antigens and particular *H-2* allelic products (Gomard et al., 1977; Bubbers et al., 1978). Thus, the *HLA* cell membrane molecules may have a direct immunoregulatory function in T cell immune responses to tumor specific antigens.

References

Benacerraf, B. and Germain, R.N. (1978) The immune response genes of the major histocompatibility complex. *Immunol. Rev.* 38:70–119.

Bergholtz, B. and Thorsby, E. (1977) Macrophage-dependent response of immune human T lymphocytes to PPD *in vitro*. Influence of *HLA-D* compatibility. *Scand. J. Immunol.* 6:679–786.

Bergholtz, B. and Thorsby, E. (1978) *HLA-D* restriction of the macrophage-dependent response of human T lymphocytes to PPD *in vitro*. Inhibition by anti-*HLA-DR* antisera. *Scand. J. Immunol.* 8:63–73.

Bergholtz, B. and Thorsby, E. (1979) *HLA-D* restricted antigen activation of sensitized T lymphocytes. Studies on the ability of *HLA-D/DR* expressing B cells to substitute for macrophages in antigen activation. *Scand. J. Immunol.* 10:267–274.

Berle, E. and Thorsby, E. (1980) The proliferative T cell response to herpes simplex virus (HSV) antigen is restricted by self *HLA-D*. *Clin. Exp. Immunol.* 39:663–676.

Bodmer, J.G. (1978) Summary and conclusions: Ia Serology. In *Histocompatibility Testing 1977*. Bodmer, W.F., Batchelor, J.R., Bodmer, J.G., Festenstein, H., and Morris, P.J. (eds.), Copenhagen: Munksgaard, pp. 351–357.

Braathen, L.R., Berle, E., Mobech-Hanssen, U., and Thorsby, E. (1980) Studies on human epidermal Langerhans cells. II. Activation of human T lymphocytes to herpes simplex virus. *Acta Dermato-Venereologica (Stockholm)* 60:381–387.

Bubbers, J.E., Chen, S., and Lilly, F. (1978) Nonrandom inclusion of H-2K and H-2D antigens in Friend virus. Particles from mice of various strains. *J. Exp. Med.* 147:340–351.

Chesebro, B. and Wehrly, K. (1976) Studies on the role of the host immune response in recovery from Friend virus leukemia. II. Cell-mediated immunity. *J. Exp. Med.* 143:85–95.

Geha, R.S., Milgrom, H., Broff, M., Alpert, S., Martin, S., and Yunis, E.J. (1979) Effect of anti-*HLA* antisera on macrophage T cell interaction. *Immunology* 76:4038–4041.

Gomard, E., Duprez, V., Henin, Y., and Levy, J.P. (1976) H-2 region product as determinant in immune cytolysis of syngeneic tumor cells by anti-MSV T lymphocytes. *Nature* 260:707–709.

Gomard, E., Duprez, V., Reme, T., Colombani, M.J., and Levy, J.P. (1977) Exclusive involvement of H-2D or H-2K product in the interaction between T killer lymphocytes and syngeneic H-2 or H-2 viral lymphomas. *J. Exp. Med.* 146:909–922.

Hirschberg, H. (1981) Presentation of viral antigens by human vascular endothelial cells *in vitro*. *Human Immunology*, (in press).

Hirschberg, H., Bergh, O.J., and Thorsby, E. (1979) Clonal distribution of *HLA* restricted antigen-reactive T cells in man. *J. Exp. Med.* 150:1271–1276.

Hirschberg, H., Bergh, O.J., and Thorsby, E. (1980) Human endothelial cells can present antigen to sensitized T lymphocytes *in vitro*. *J. Exp. Med.* 152s:249–255.

Holden, H.T. and Herberman, R.B. (1977) Cytotoxicity against tumor-associated antigens not H-2 restricted. *Nature* 268:250–253.

Jerne, N.K. (1971) The somatic generation of immune recognition. *Eur. J. Immunol.* 1:1–9.

Niederhuber, J.E. and Allen, P. (1980) Role of I-Region gene products in macrophage induction of an antibody response. II. Restriction at the level of T cell in recognition of I-J-subregion macrophage determinants. *J. Exp. Med.* 151:1103–1113.

Reinherz, E.L. and Schlossman, S.F. (1980) The differentiation and function of human T lymphocytes. *Cell* 19:821–827.

Rodey, G.E., Luehrman, L.K., and Thomas, D.W. (1979) *In vitro* primary immunization of human peripheral blood lymphocytes to KLH: evidence for *HLA-D* region restriction. *J. Immunol.* 123:2250–2254.

Schwartz, R.H., David, C.S., Sachs, D.H., and Paul, W.E. (1976) T lymphocyte-enriched murine peritoneal exudate cells. III. Inhibition of antigen-induced T lymphocyte proliferation with anti-Ia antisera. *J. Immunol.* 117:531–540.

Shevach, E.M., Paul, W.E., and Green, I. (1972) Histocompatibility linked immune response gene function in guinea pigs. Specific inhibition of antigen-induced lymphocyte proliferation by alloantisera. *J. Exp. Med.* 136:1207–1217.

Shevach, E.M., Lundquist, M.L., Geczy, A.F., and Schwartz, B.D. (1977) The guinea pig I region. II. Functional analysis. *J. Exp. Med.* 146:561–570.

Stingl, G., Katz, S.I., Clement, L., Green, I., and Shevach, E.M. (1978) Immunologic function of Ia-bearing epidermal Langerhans cells. *J. Immunol.* 121:2005–2010.

Stutman, O. and Shen, F.-W. (1978) H-2 restriction and non-restriction of T cell-mediated cytotoxicity against mouse mammary tumor targets. *Nature* 276:181–182.

Thorsby, E. and Nousiainen, H. (1979) *In vitro* sensitization of human T lymphocytes to hapten (TNP)-conjugated and non-treated autologous cells is restricted by self-*HLA-D*. *Scand. J. Immunol.* 9:183–192.

Thorsby, E. (1978) Biological function of *HLA*. *Tissue Antigens* 11:321–329.

Thorsby, E. (1981) Involvement of *HLA* cell membrane molecules in T cell activation. In *HLA Typing: Methodological Aspects and Clinical Relevance*. Florida; CRC Press, 1981, in press.

Thorsby, E., Bergholtz, B., Berle, E., Braathen, L., and Hirschberg, H. (1981) Involvement of *HLA* in T cell immune responses. *Transpl. Proc.*, in press.

Trinchieri, G., Aden, D.P., and Knowles, B.B. (1976) Cell-mediated cytotoxicity to SV-40 tumor associated antigens. *Nature* (Lond.) 261:312–314.

Von Boehmer, H., Haas, W., and Jerne, N.K. (1978) Major histocompatibility complex-linked immune-responsiveness is acquired by lymphocytes of low-responder mice differentiating in thymus of high-responder mice. *Proc. Natl. Acad. Sci.* 75:2439–2442.

Zinkernagel, R.M. (1978) Thymus and lymphohemopoietic cells: their role in T cell maturation in selection of T cells H-2 restriction-specificity and in H-2 linked *Ir* gene control. *Immunological Rev.* 42:224–270.

PART III:

Surface Antigens

CHAPTER 22

Possible Clinical Significance of Circulating Immune Complexes in Melanoma Patients[1]

Rishab K. Gupta and Donald L. Morton

Division of Oncology, Department of Surgery, UCLA School of Medicine, University of California, Los Angeles, California and Surgical Service, VA Medical Center, Sepulveda, California

Summary

The incidence of circulating immune complexes (CIC) in serum samples from melanoma patients, non-cancer patients (with immune complex associated diseases) and normal volunteers was analyzed by the complement consumption technique. The incidence of positive CIC was 68% (115/170) in patients suffering from immune complex associated diseases, e.g., systemic lupus erythematosus, rheumatoid arthritis, glomerulonephritis, hepatitis, acute viral infections, etc., compared to only 13% (31/245) in normal volunteers. The positive CIC incidence was 43% (147/341) in melanoma patients. In certain melanoma patients, CIC levels became insignificant when tumor persisted for several months. There were higher incidences of CIC in serum samples from patients with tumor burden of approximately 1–100 g than in those with <1.0 g or >100 g. This finding suggests an antibody excess in sera from patients with low tumor burden (<1.0 g) and an antigen excess in patients with high tumor burden (>100 g). Immune complexes could be generated by admixing a serum sample taken at the time of low tumor burden (early serum sample) with the one taken at the time of high tumor burden (late serum sample). Absorption of the early serum sample with allogeneic melanoma decreased the level of immune complexes. Therefore, CIC in sera of melanoma patients may be due to antigen-antibody complexes related to tumor activity.

[1]These investigations were supported by Grants CA12582 and CB64076, awarded by the National Cancer Institute, DHEW, and grants from Cancer Research Coordinating Committee of the University of California, California Institute for Cancer Research, and Medical Research Service of the Veterans Administration.

Melanoma serum samples with positive CIC activity were significantly more inhibitory to phytohemagglutinin-induced *in vitro* lymphocyte blastogenesis than those with insignificant CIC levels, suggesting that CIC may be one of the several causes of immunosuppression in cancer patients. Twenty-six percent (6/23) of melanoma patients with no evidence of disease but with CIC-positive serum samples had tumor recurrence within 3 months. On the other hand, 92% of patients (34/37) whose sera were negative for CIC had no detectable tumor recurrence for at least 6 months. Thus, assessment of CIC level in melanoma patients may provide relevant information relative to immune status and clinical prognosis of the disease.

Introduction

It is logical to assume that circulating immune complexes *in vivo* should form each time a humoral immune response is made to a free antigen on the cell surface or an antigen released into the circulation. Association between circulating immune complexes and many pathological conditions has been described by various investigators (Zubler and Lambert, 1977). The fact that human malignant melanomas contain tumor-associated antigens that cause the formation of circulating antibodies in patients with this disease has been well documented (Morton et al., 1968; Lewis et al., 1969; Muna et al., 1969; Cornain et al., 1975; Gupta et al., 1979; Gupta, 1980). These circulating anti-tumor antibodies react *in vivo* with antigens present on tumor cells (Phillips and Lewis, 1971; Irie et al., 1974; Gupta and Morton, 1975; Kristensen et al., 1976). In some cases these antibodies have been eluted from biopsied tumor cells and shown to react with melanoma cells (Phillips and Lewis, 1971; Gupta and Morton, 1975). The phenomenon of *in vitro* antigen modulation, capping and shedding after exposing the melanoma cells to antibody has been described by Leong et al. (1977, 1979). A number of possible mechanisms, i.e., cell death, surface bleeding, sublethal autolysis, or secretion that might release tumor antigens into circulation, have been proposed by Price and Robinson (1978). Spontaneous shedding of tumor-associated antigens into the culture medium by melanoma cells is now well documented (Grimm et al., 1976; Bystryn, 1977; Reisfield et al., 1977; Gupta et al., 1978b; Leong et al., 1978), and may represent the mechanism of *in vivo* antigen shedding by tumor cells. Part or all of the antigens shed into circulation may complex with humoral antibodies to form the circulating immune complexes (CIC).

Many serum factors which modify cell-mediated immune reactions have been described (Nelson and Gatti, 1976). However, circulating free antigen and/or immune complexes have received special attention. It can now be postulated that some of the serum factors which block *in vitro* cell-mediated immunity against melanoma cells (Hellstrom et al., 1971; Happner et al., 1973) may be these free tumor-associated antigens and/or antigen-antibody complexes (Sjogren et al., 1971; Baldwin et al., 1973; Currie, 1973; Thomson et al.,

1973; Jose and Seshadri, 1974; Theofilopoulos and Dixon, 1978; Gupta et al., 1979c). Recent developments suggest that an assessment of CIC levels may be useful for monitoring clinical course in patients with malignancy (Mukojima et al., 1973; Heimer and Klein, 1976; Rossen et al., 1977; Samayoa et al., 1977; Theofilopoulos et al., 1977; Gupta et al., 1979b; Eiras et al., 1980; Kristensen et al., 1980; Gropp et al., 1980).

During analyses of sequential serum samples from melanoma patients for anti-tumor antibody by the complement fixation assay, serum samples were frequently positive for anticomplementary activity. In some patients, significant levels of anticomplementary activity were observed prior to or at the time of clinically detectable tumor recurrence (Gupta and Morton, 1978; Gupta et al., 1979e). Many of these anticomplementary serum samples were also capable of inhibiting mitogen-induced lymphocyte blastogenesis (Rangel et al., 1977b). In view of the numerous reports of the association of immune complexes, or similar material, with malignancy in humans, these investigations were designed (a) to compare the incidence of anticomplementary activity in sera from melanoma patients with that in normal sera, (b) to determine the nature of the factors responsible for anticomplementary activity, (c) to determine the correlation between anticomplementary activity and inhibition of mitogen-induced lymphocyte proliferation by melanoma sera, and (d) to determine the clinical significance of the serum anticomplementary activity.

Materials and Methods

Patient Population

Serum samples were selected randomly from 341 melanoma patients seen in the Division of Surgical Oncology at UCLA. All patients had histologically proved malignant melanoma but none had received immunotherapy, chemotherapy, or radiation therapy at the time of serum sampling. The ages of melanoma serum donors ranged for 10–80 years. The melanoma patient population was almost equally distributed among males (175) and females (166).

Control Population

Non-cancer patient sera were procured from the various clinics of the UCLA Center for Health Sciences, and the non-malignant nature of these samples was determined either by consulting with the physician caring for the patient or from the clinical charts. Patients who were likely to have immune complex diseases (hepatitis, acute viral infections, glomerulonephritis, rheumatoid arthritis, systemic lupus erythematosus, etc.) were deliberately selected. The ages of these patients ranged from 17 to 73 years (mean 47 years). Of 170 non-cancer patients, 78 were males and 92 were females.

Blood samples were collected from 245 apparently healthy normal donors, including laboratory personnel and volunteers who had no history of malignancy and who were not receiving any medication that might be immunosuppressive. The normal donors ranged in age from 15–68 years (average 39.8 years).

Serum Samples

Aliquots of whole blood were drawn by peripheral venipuncture, and allowed to clot at room temperature for one hr and then at 4°C for 2 hr. Serum was separated and collected after the sample was centrifuged at 1,000 xg for 15 min. Aliquots of serum in 1–1.5 ml volumes in sterile plastic vials (Costar, Cooke Laboratories, Alexandria, VA) were stored at −35°C. At the time of testing, the serum was thawed at room temperature and heat-treated at 56°C for 30 min to decomplement the sample.

Complement Consumption Assay

The anticomplementary activity of each test serum was determined by the ultramicrocomplement fixation assay described elsewhere (Gupta et al., 1978a). To semi-quantitate the amount of complement consumed, the following procedure was employed: Using a standard technique of complement titration, the complement source was titrated in the absence, and in the presence, of $2\mu l$ of 1 : 4 dilution of the test sera. Two microliters of each dilution (1 : 6, 1 : 8, 1 : 10, 1 : 12 $\cdots$ 1 : 24) of the complement source was used and a reduction in complement titer of greater than 25% in the presence of the test serum was considered to be due to the anticomplementary activity of the serum. The extent of the anticomplementary activity of a test serum was indicated by the magnitude of the complement titer reduction. This anticomplementary activity was calculated as percent complement consumed by the following formula:

$$\% \text{ Complement Consumed} = 1 - \frac{\text{Complement Titer in Presence of Test Serum}}{\text{Complement Titer in Absence of Test Serum}} \times 100$$

The 1 : 4 dilution was chosen after preliminary standardization of the reagents (hemolysin and sheep cells). Dilutions higher than 1 : 4 generally resulted in greatly reduced incidence of anticomplementary activity both for melanoma and non-cancer patients' sera, whereas undiluted or 1 : 2 diluted test sera were consistently anticomplementary. Therefore, anticomplementary activity exhibited by the test sera at dilutions less than 1 : 4 may have been non-specific.

This method of assessing the extent of complement consumption is quite reproducible. We observed that a limited number of freeze-thaw cycles did not influence the results of anticomplementary activity assays.

Melanoma Cell Line

Cultured cells from an established melanoma cell line, UCLA-SO-M14 (M14), were used as target antigen and for absorption of the test sera. This cell line was maintained in serum-free, chemically defined medium (Chee et al., 1976).

Determination of Antibody and Antigen Activities

The microcomplement fixation assay (Gupta and Morton, 1980) was used to assess the antibody titer against extracts of a cultured human melanoma cell line (M14) and autologous and allogeneic biopsy tumor specimens. Extracts of M14 cells were prepared according to the procedure of Eilber and Morton (1970). Veronal buffered saline (VBS), prepared from commercially available Complement Fixation Test Diluent Tablets (Oxoid Ltd., London, England), was used as diluent. Membrane extracts of autologous tumor cells were prepared by hypotonic cell lysis of an autopsied tumor specimen (Oren and Herberman, 1971). Antigen activity in the test serum sample was determined by the complement fixation procedure described by Gupta et al. (1979c).

Absorption of Sera

Serum samples suspect for anti-melanoma antibody were absorbed with cultured melanoma (M14) cells. Aliquots (250 μl) of serum were mixed with two volumes (500 μl) of packed M14 cells, and incubated at 37°C for 1 hr with intermittent agitation on a Vortex Mixer at low speed. The mixtures then were centrifuged at 800 xg for 10 min at 4°C. Supernatants were absorbed once more. After final absorption, supernatants were recentrifuged at 15,000 xg for 30 min. Control samples were not absorbed with M14 cells, but were otherwise processed in the same manner.

Lymphocyte Blastogenesis Inhibition Assay

The blastogenesis inhibition assay was performed as previously described (Rangel et al., 1977a). The ability of the test serum to stimulate or inhibit phytohemagglutinin (PHA)-induced blastogenesis of normal lymphocytes was assessed by the following equation:

$$\Delta CPM = CPM \text{ with reference serum} - CPM \text{ with test serum}$$

A positive ΔCPM value denoted inhibition of lymphocyte blastogenesis and a negative ΔCPM value denoted stimulation by the test serum compared with the reference serum. We arbitrarily considered a serum to be positive for its ability to inhibit PHA-induced blastogenesis when the difference between the incorporation of ^{3}H-thymidine by DNA in the presence of reference (AB) serum and the test serum was greater than +2500 ΔCPM.

Results

Incidence of Positive Anticomplementary Activity

A test serum was considered anticomplementary when 2 μl of its 1:4 dilution consumed greater than 25% complement. Within this constraint, melanoma sera had a significantly higher incidence of anticomplementary activity (43%) than normal sera (13%) (p<0.05). Non-cancer patients with suspected immune complex associated diseases exhibited 68% incidence of positive anticomplementary activity (Figure 22.1).

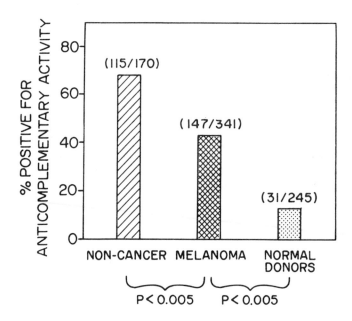

Figure 22.1. Incidence of positive anticomplementary activity in sera from melanoma and non-cancer patients and normal donors. A serum was considered positive when 2 μl of 1:4 dilution consumed greater than 25% complement.

Anticomplementary Activity Correlated with Tumor Burden

Clinical charts of the melanoma patients were reviewed by physicians familiar with their clinical course. Body burden of tumor at the time of serum sampling was roughly approximated in terms of weight. Size and number of palpable tumor masses and tumor nodules seen on radiological films, scans, and tomograms were determined. It was arbitrarily assumed that a 1.0 cm³ nodule weighed about 1.0 g. Based on these estimations, melanoma patients were grouped into categories: No evidence of disease (NED) to <1 g tumor (NED group); 1 to <100 g tumor (medium tumor burden) and ≥100 g tumor (high tumor burden). Patients in the NED group had no detectable disease by physical and radiological examinations. Patients in the 1 to <100 g tumor burden group had from small to fairly large pulmonary or subcutaneous metastases. Patients in the ≥100 g tumor group had grossly large tumor masses.

Results presented in Table 22.1 show that the incidence of positive anticomplementary activity was the highest (71%) for the medium tumor burden group. Anticomplementary activity was significantly lower in the NED and high tumor burden groups (35% and 31%, respectively).

Complement Consumption by Sequential Serum Samples

In some but not all patients who were studied sequentially over a period of at

Table 22.1. Incidence of Positive Anticomplementary Activity in Sera from Melanoma Patients with Reference to Body Burden of Tumor.

Body burden of tumor	No. Positive	No. tested	% Positive	p[b]
NED[a] – < 1	48	136	35	< 0.002
1 – 100	63	89	71	
> 100	16	52	31	< 0.002

Note: A serum was considered positive for anticomplementary activity when 2 μl of 1:4 dilution consumed greater than 25% complement.

[a]No evidence of disease.

[b]Significance was determined by the Chi-square method. NED—<1 group and >100 group compared to 1–100 group.

least one year, the anticomplementary activity in their serum samples decreased below detectable levels as tumor burden increased or persisted over a period of several months. Such a relationship between serum anticomplementary activity and body-burden of tumor is exemplified in Figure 22.2. In some patients, serum samples began to consume complement 2–4 weeks before their tumors were clinically detectable. Antibody levels against autologous and allogeneic melanoma cells also increased. After some fluctuation, the antibodies declined to undetectable levels in serum samples taken shortly before death. Anticomplementary activity of the serum samples also decreased at this time.

Figure 22.2. Correlation between anticomplementary activity and tumor burden during clinical course of a melanoma patient. Tumor burden was assessed by reviewing the clinical chart. Percent complement consumption refers to the amount of complement consumed by 2 μl of 1:4 diluted test serum.

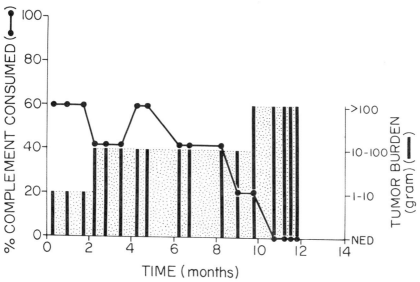

Reactivity Between NED Sera and High Tumor Burden Sera

Since anticomplementary and antibody activities could decrease as a result of excess free antigen in the circulation at the time of high tumor burden, a number of melanoma sera selected from patients with high tumor burden were reacted against antimelanoma antisera by complement fixation. These antisera were raised by immunizing rabbits with human melanoma extracts. Antisera were then absorbed with human normal tissues to remove non-specific antibodies (Gupta et al., 1980). Of 60 melanoma sera from patients with high tumor burden, 15 (25%) showed reactivity against the rabbit antimelanoma antibody. Five of these 15 positive melanoma sera were selected on the basis of their reactivity and were reacted against 12 melanoma sera from patients with no evidence of disease, but whose sera were known to contain complement fixing antibodies to melanoma cells and extracts. As illustrated in Figure 22.3, at least seven sera reacted to all the five high tumor burden sera. Others showed random patterns of reactivity. For example, two serum samples from NED patients were positive against melanoma membrane extracts but were consistently negative against the five sera from high tumor burden patients. These results suggested that the five sera (A, B, C, D, and E) from patients with high tumor burden contained some components, possibly antigens, that reacted with antibody in the serum samples of the NED melanoma patients.

Figure 22.3. Immunologic reactivity between sera from melanoma patients with minimal tumor burden and sera from patients with high tumor burden. All early melanoma sera had a definite reactivity against melanoma tumor cell membrane extract and no reactivity against human normal liver membrane extract by the complement fixation assay. A serum with a titer of $\geq 1:4$ was considered antibody positive.

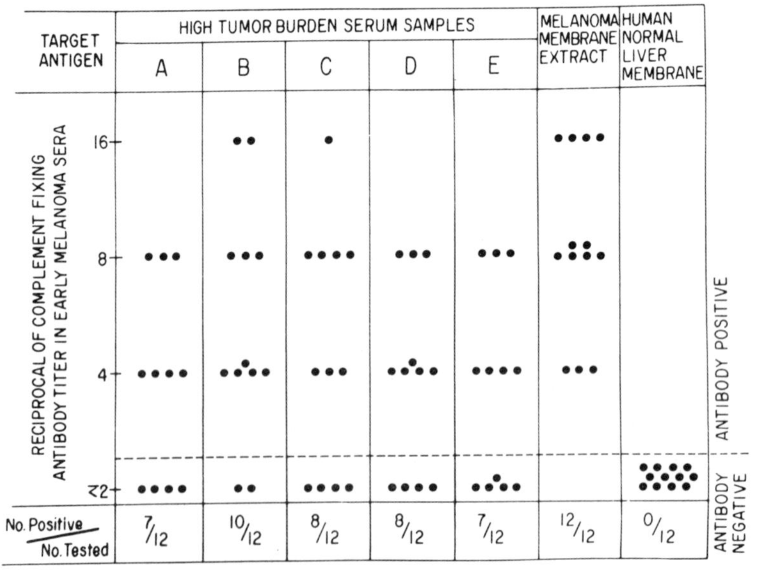

Target Antigen	High Tumor Burden Serum Samples					Melanoma Membrane Extract	Human Normal Liver Membrane
No. Positive / No. Tested	A: 7/12	B: 10/12	C: 8/12	D: 8/12	E: 7/12	12/12	0/12

To rule out the possibility of isoantibodies and histocompatibility antigens as cause for the activity in the above experiment, an early serum sample (taken at the time of no tumor burden) of Patient A was reacted against an autologous and an allogeneic late serum sample (taken at the time of high tumor burden), a melanoma membrane extract, and a human liver membrane extract. Results presented in Table 22.2 show that the early serum sample of melanoma Patient A had detectable complement-fixing antibody levels against his autologous late serum sample, as well as against an allogeneic late serum sample and a melanoma membrane extract. No reactivity was observed against normal liver membrane extract. Absorption of the early serum sample with cultured melanoma (M14) cells decreased the antibody titers below the detectable level.

In Vitro Generation of Immune Complex-Like Activity

Since these experiments suggested the presence of antibody in the early serum sample and antigen-like material in the late serum sample, it was decided to test whether mixture of the two serum samples could generate an immune complex-like activity. Therefore 250 μl aliquots of 1 : 4 dilution of early and late serum samples of melanoma Patient B were mixed, incubated at 37°C for 1 hr and then tested for their complement titer. Neither the early nor the late serum samples alone affected the complement titer significantly. The complement titer in the presence of 1 : 4 dilution of either the early or late serum sample ranged from 1 : 18 to 1 : 20 compared to 1 : 22 in the absence of the test sera. However, when the early and late serum samples were mixed and tested, the complement titer decreased to <1 : 6, indicating that the mixture had become anticomplementary. No such effect on complement titer was observed when the late serum samples were mixed with a normal serum sample that was negative for anti-tumor antibodies.

To determine the specificity of the humoral factors present in early and late sera of the melanoma patients, the samples were absorbed with cultured

Table 22.2. Reactivity of an Early Serum Sample (Taken at the Time of Low Tumor Burden) of Melanoma Patient A Against Autologous and Allogeneic Late Serum Samples (Taken at the Time of High Tumor Burden), Melanoma Membrane Extract, and Human Normal Liver Extract, as Measured by Complement Fixation.

	Reciprocal of antibody titer of early serum sample	
Target antigen	Before absorption with M14 cells	After absorption[a] with M14 cells
Allogeneic melanoma cell membrane	16	< 4
Normal liver cell membrane	< 2	–
Autologous late serum	16	< 4
Allogeneic late serum	8	< 4

[a]One volume of early serum sample was absorbed with 2 volumes of packed M14 cells as described in materials and methods.

melanoma cells. In tests of various combinations, the reduction in complement titer by the autologous mixture of early and late serum samples was affected only when the early serum sample was absorbed with M14 cells. The complement in the presence of a 1:4 dilution of an unabsorbed early or late serum sample was 1:18 compared to 1:22 in the absence of any of these two sera. The complement titer in the presence of an absorbed early serum sample was only slightly reduced (1:14) compared to an unabsorbed sample (1:18). This reduction could have been due to generation of soluble immune complexes during absorption of the serum. However, there was no further reduction in the complement titer (1:16) when the absorbed early serum sample was mixed with the unabsorbed late serum sample. A mixture of unabsorbed early serum and absorbed late serum reduced the complement titer to <1:6, suggesting that the generation of anticomplementary activity was now due to the formation of immune complexes. Antibody of the immune complexes was present in the early serum sample, and combined with the antigenic components in the late serum sample.

Anticomplementary Activity vs Lymphocyte Blastogenesis Inhibition

From the limited number of melanoma sera tested for their ability to inhibit mitogen-induced lymphocyte blastogenesis, 43 sera with positive anticomplementary activity were significantly more inhibitory (ΔCPM$=6,889\pm2,194$) than 55 sera with negative anticomplementary activity (ΔCPM$=-690\pm1,427$). The differences were statistically significant ($p=<0.01$). Eighteen melanoma sera with positive anticomplementary activity and positive reactivity with rabbit antimelanoma antibody (antigen positive) exhibited greater inhibition in the lymphocyte blastogenesis assay (mean $\Delta=10,606\pm3,707$) than 25 samples that were antigen negative but anticomplementary positive (mean ΔCPM$=4,215\pm2,602$). Sera with no antigen and anticomplementary activities or antigen positive but with no anticomplementary activity were not inhibitory in the lymphocyte blastogenesis assay (mean ΔCPM$=-1,098\pm1,572$ and $942\pm3,485$, respectively). These results indicated that the lymphocyte blastogenesis inhibition by melanoma sera with positive anticomplementary activity was potentiated by concurrent antigenic activity.

Prognostic Significance of Sera Anticomplementary Activity in Melanoma

Of 60 melanoma patients who had no evidence of disease at the time of serum sampling and who were followed for at least 6 months, 23 were postitive for anticomplementary activity and 37 were negative. Six of the 23 (26%) positive patients had recurrence within 3 months of follow-up, while only 3/37 (8%) patients with no anticomplementary activity had clinical recurrence of the disease within 3 months. Other patients remained free of disease for greater than 6 months.

Discussion

Several immunological methods have been used to detect immune complexes in human sera from patients with pathological conditions (World Health Organization, 1977). In this investigation, we used the microcomplement consumption technique to assess the anticomplementary activity of melanoma sera as well as to define the cause of the anticomplementary activity. We found that 43% (147/341) meanoma sera were positive for the anticomplementary activity compared to 13% (31/245) of sera from healthy normal donors. Johnson et al. (1975) reported 42% (109/261) of pathological sera as positive for anticomplementary activity compared to 1.4% (1/72) of healthy adult sera. The lower incidence of anticomplementary activity among normal donors in their investigation could have been due to differences in the selection of healthy adults.

Varying amounts of immune complexes or immune complex-like material in sera of patients with malignancy have been reported by other investigators (Rossen et al., 1977; Samayoa et al., 1977; Theofilopoulos et al., 1977). The variations are probably due to the different sensitivities and detection limits of each assay. Samayoa et al. (1977) reported that 29% (42/146) of the sera from cancer patients contained immune complex-like material compared to 5% (2/42) from non-cancer patients and 3% (2/59) from normal donors, as determined by precipitin reaction in gel against monoclonal rheumatoid factor. Bland et al. (1974) reported the presence of immune complexes in 54% (14/26) of sera from patients with advanced gastrointestinal and hepatobiliary carcinoma by detection of "heavy IgG." These investigators suggested that "heavy IgG" was composed of tumor-derived antigen and its corresponding specific antibody.

In our study, melanoma sera were selected from a population manifesting varying degrees of body-burden of tumor. The incidence of positive anticomplementary activity in melanoma sera was lower in patients with no evidence of disease or with high tumor burden than in patients with medium tumor burden. Similar results were observed in other types of malignancies (Gupta et al., 1979b). Assuming that anticomplementary activity is due to immune complexes, then this lower incidence could be the result of antibody excess in sera from patients with low tumor burden (<1 g) and of antigen excess in sera from patients with high (>100 g) tumor burden. Therefore, the quantity or composition of the immune complexes in these extreme groups would be such that neither could consume complement. Theofilopoulos et al. (1977) reported that small immune complexes (about $11-13$ S) fixed complement less effectively and were not detected as efficiently by the Raji cell assay as the large immune complexes. These investigators also reported that melanoma patients with advanced disease had a significantly higher incidence and level of immune complexes than patients with no detectable or only localized disease.

Analysis of anticomplementary activity in sequential serum samples from several melanoma patients revealed that some samples consumed significant amounts of complement in the absence of clinically detectable tumor, whereas some had no anticomplementary activity despite evidence of disease. Some patients who were disease-free had serum samples that were anticomplementary during the disease-free interval. Such patients generally had disease recurrence within 6 months. In some patients, the serum anticomplementary activity decreased as tumor burden increased. Analyses of serial serum samples from these patients for complement fixing antibody levels revealed that the disappearance of antibody was concomitant with or prior to a decrease in anticomplementary activity. These findings suggest that the antigens from tumor released into circulation (Baldwin et al., 1973; Currie, 1973; Thomson et al., 1973) may complex with virtually all the circulating antibody, thus producing an antigen excess in the circulation. These antigen-antibody complexes together with the excess-free antigen could, in turn, directly or indirectly produce immunosuppressive serum factors that could block further production of antibodies.

The results of our investigation show that melanoma sera with anticomplementary activity and free antigen were more inhibitory to PHA-induced blastogenesis than the sera with anticomplementary activity alone. The inhibition caused by sera with positive anticomplementary activity appeared to be abrogated by antibody excess (Gupta et al., 1979c), i.e., the sera that were anticomplementary and that contained detectable levels of antibody were not inhibitory to PHA-induced blastogenesis. This result supports Hellstrom and Hellstrom (1977) in their conclusion that antigen-antibody complexes together with free tumor antigen and possibly other immunosuppressive substances may specifically inhibit *in vitro* cell-mediated immunity.

It is possible that the immune complexes themselves have no inhibitory activity, but that certain pathogenic conditions induce both immune complexes and a higher level of some other serum inhibitory factor. However, in our preliminary studies, we found that absorption with *Staphylococcus aureus* Cowan Strain I of some cancer sera that were inhibitory to PHA-induced lymphocyte blastogenesis but positive for anticomplementary activity resulted in elimination of both activities. Since protein A from this bacterium absorbs immunoglobulin and can remove immune complexes which are inhibitory in other systems (Steel et al., 1974), it is possible that the protein A experiments indicate that the immune complexes themselves are the inhibitory factor. As suggested by Kilburn et al. (1976), immune complexes might interact with other serum components that have inhibitory activity. It is also possible that the immune complexes interact with cells bearing Fc receptors, and that these cells are either directly inhibited or have indirect suppressor functions. Suppressor activity for cells with receptors for the Fc fragment of IgG has been reported in several systems (Moretta et al., 1977).

Since immune complexes are one of the factors that can consume complement, the demonstration of anticomplementary activity in sera might suggest neoplastic activity, provided the possibilities of anticomplementary activity caused by non-tumor-associated immune complexes are eliminated. Even though we have not established that anticomplementary activity is caused by tumor-related immune complexes in each test, our preliminary results do, to some extent, show a correlation with tumor recurrence. Therefore, determination of antibody, anticomplementary activity and tumor-associated antigen(s) in sera of cancer patients and their correlation with *in vitro* cell-mediated immunity reactions may provide an insight into the tumor-host relationship and a better means for predicting the outcome of the clinical course of the patient.

References

Baldwin, R.W., Bowen, J.G., and Price, M.R. (1973) Detection of circulating hepatoma D23 antigen and immune complexes in tumor bearer serum. *Br. J. Cancer* 28:16–24.

Bland, K.I., Ludwig, F.J., Heishman, A.F., Safian, R.D., Pfaft, W.W., and Cusumano, C.L. (1974) Method of detection of circulating immune complexes. *Surg. Forum* 25:111–112.

Bystryn, J.C. (1977) Release of cell-surface tumor-associated antigens by viable melanoma cells from humans. *J. Natl. Cancer Inst.* 59:325–328.

Chee, D.O., Boddie, A.W., Roth, J.A., Holmes, E.C., and Morton, D.L. (1976) Adaptation of human melanoma cell line to grow in chemically defined serum-free medium. *Cancer Res.* 36:1503–1509.

Cornain, S., deVries, J.E., Collard, J., Vennegoor, C., Wingerden, I.V., and Rumke, P. (1975) Antibodies and antigen expression in human melanoma detected by the immune adherence test. *Int. J. Cancer* 16:981–997.

Currie, A. (1973) Circulating antigen as inhibitor of tumor immunity in man. *Br. J. Cancer Suppl. 1* 28:153–161.

Eilber, F.R. and Morton, D.L. (1970) Immunologic studies of human sarcomas: additional evidence suggesting an associated sarcoma virus. *Cancer* 35:588–596.

Eiras, A.S., Robins, R.A., Baldwin, R.W., and Byers, V.S. (1980) Circulating immune complexes in patients with bone tumors. *Int. J. Cancer* 25:735–739.

Grimm, E.A., Silver, H.K.B., Roth, J.A., Chee, D.O., Gupta, R.K., and Morton, D.L. (1976) Detection of tumor-associated antigen in human melanoma cell line supernatants. *Int. J. Cancer* 17:559–564.

Gropp, G., Havemann, K., Scherfe, T., and Ax, W. (1980) Incidence of circulating immune complexes in patients with lung cancer and their effect on antibody-dependent cytotoxicity. *Oncology* 37:71–76.

Gupta, R.K. (1980) Antigenic complexity in human maligant melanoma tumors detected by allogeneic antibody. In *Serologic Analysis of Human Cancer Antigens.* Rosenberg, S.A. (ed.), New York: Academic Press, Inc., pp. 339–380.

Gupta, R.K. and Morton, D.L. (1975) Suggestive evidence for *in vivo* binding of specific anti-tumor antibodies of human melanomas. *Cancer Res.* 35:58–62.

Gupta, R.K. and Morton, D.L. (1978) Tumor-related immune complexes in sera from melanoma patients. *Fed. Proc.* 37:1595.

318

Gupta, R.K. and Morton, D.L. (1980) Detection of tumor antigens by complement fixation using allogeneic antibody. In *Serologic Analysis of Human Cancer Antigens*. Rosenberg, S.A. (ed.), New York: Academic Press, Inc., pp. 611–619.

Gupta, R.K., Irie, R.F., and Morton, D.L. (1978a) Antigens on human tumor cells assayed by complement fixation with allogeneic antisera. *Cancer Res.* 38:2573–2580.

Gupta, R.K., Irie, R.F., Chee, D.O., Kern, D.H., and Morton, D.L. (1978b) Antigens in spent serum-free medium of a human malignant cell line. *Bacteriol. Proc.* 79:54.

Gupta, R.K., Irie, R.F., Chee, D.O., Kern, D.H., and Morton, D.L. (1979a) Demonstration of two distinct antigens in spent tissue culture medium of a human malignant melanoma cell line. *J. Natl. Cancer Inst.* 63:347–356.

Gupta, R.K., Golub, S.H., and Morton, D.L. (1979b) Correlation between tumor burden and anticomplementary activity in sera from cancer patients. *Cancer Immunol. Immunother.* 6:63–71.

Gupta, R.K., Golub, S.H., Rangel, D.M., and Morton, D.L. (1979c) Inhibition of mitogen-induced lymphocyte proliferation correlated to anticomplementary activity in sera from melanoma patients. *Cancer Immunol. Immunother.* 5:221–228.

Gupta, R.K., Silver, H.K.B., Reisfield, R.A., and Morton, D.L. (1979d) Isolation and immunochemical characterization of antibodies from the sera of cancer patients which are reactive against human melanoma cell membranes by affinity chromatography. *Cancer Res.* 39:1683–1695.

Gupta, R.K., Theofilopoulos, A.N., Dixon, F.J., and Morton, D.L. (1979e) Circulating immune complexes as possible cause for anticomplementary activity in humans with malignant melanoma. *Cancer Immunol. Immunother.* 6:211–221.

Gupta, R.D., Silver, H.K.B., and Morton, D.L. (1980) Production and characterization of xenogeneic antisera to tumor-associated antigen(s). *J. Surg. Oncol.* 13:75–89.

Happner, G.H., Stolbach, I., Byrne, M., Cummings, J.J., Donough, E., and Calabresi, P. (1973) Cell-mediated and serum blocking reactivity to tumor antigens in patients with malignant melanoma. *Int. J. Cancer* 11:245–260.

Heimer, R. and Klein, A. (1976) Circulating immune complexes in sera of patients with Burkitt's lymphoma and nasopharyngeal carcinoma. *Int. J. Cancer* 18:310–316.

Hellstrom, I., Sjogren, H.O., Warner, G.A., and Hellstrom, K.E. (1971) Blocking of cell-mediated immunity by sera from patients with growing neoplasms. *Int. J. Cancer* 7:226–237.

Hellstrom, K.E. and Hellstrom, I. (1977) Immunologic enhancement of tumor growth. In *Mechanisms of Tumor Immunity*. Green, I., Cohen, S., and McCluskey, R.T. (eds.), New York: John Wiley and Sons, p. 159.

Irie, K., Irie, R.F., and Morton, D.L. (1974) Evidence for *in vivo* reaction of antibody and complement to surface antigens of human cancer cells. *Science* 186:454–456.

Johnson, A.H., Mowberay, J.F., and Porter, K.A. (1975) Detection of circulating immune complexes in pathological human sera. *Lancet* 1:762–765.

Jose, D.G. and Seshadri, R. (1974) Circulating immune complexes in human neuroblastoma: direct assay and role in blocking specific cellular immunity. *Int. J. Cancer* 13:824–838.

Kilburn, D.G., Fairhurst, M., Levey, J.G., and Whitney, R.B. (1976) Synergism between immune complexes and serum from tumor-bearing mice in the suppression of mitogen responses. *J. Immunol.* 117:1612–1617.

Kristensen, E., Langrad, E., and Reimann, R. (1976) Humoral immunity in malignant skin melanoma. Isolation of melanoma specific IgG from melanoma metastases. *Eur. J. Cancer* 12:945–950.

Kristensen, E., Brandslund, I., Nielsen, H., and Svehag, S.E. (1980) Prognostic value of assays for circulating immune complexes and natural cytotoxicity in malignant skin melanoma (stage I and II). *Cancer Immunol. Immunother.* 9:31–36.

Leong, S.P.L., Sutherland, C.M., and Krementz, E.T. (1977) Changes in distribution of human malignant melanoma membrane antigens in the presence of human antibody by immunofluorescence. *Cancer Res.* 37:293–298.

Leong, S.P.L., Cooperband, S.R., Sutherland, C.M., Krementz, E.T., and Deckers, P.J. (1978) Detection of human melanoma antigens in cell-free supernatants. *J. Surg. Res.* 24:245–252.

Leong, S.P.L., Cooperband, S.R., Deckers, P.J., Sutherland, C.M., Cesane, J.F., and Krementz, E.T. (1979) Antibody-induced movement of common melanoma membrane antigens on the surface of unfixed human melanoma cells. *Cancer Res.* 39:2125–2131.

Lewis, M.G., Ikonopisov, R.L., Nairn, R.C., Phillips, T.M., Hamilton-Fairley, G., Bodenham, D.C., and Alexander, P. (1969) Tumor specific antibodies in human malignant melanoma and their relationship to the extent of the disease. *Br. Med. J.* 3:547–562.

Moretta, L., Webb, S.R., Grossi, C.E., Lydyard, T.M., Cooper, M.D. (1977) Functional analysis of two human T cell subpopulations: help and suppression of B cell responses by T cell bearing receptors for IgM or IgG. *J. Exp. Med.* 146:184.

Morton, D.L., Malmgren, R.A., Holmes, E.C., and Ketcham, A.S. (1968) Demonstration of antibodies against human malignant melanoma by immunofluorescence. *Surgery* 64:233–240.

Mukojima, T., Gunren, P., and Klein, G. (1973) Circulating antigen-antibody complexes associated with Epstein Barr virus in recurrent Burkitt's lymphoma. *J. Natl. Cancer Inst.* 51:1319–1321.

Muna, N.M., Marcus, S., and Smart, C. (1969) Detection by immunofluorescence of antibodies specific for human malignant melanoma cells. *Cancer* 23:88–93.

Nelson, D.S. and Gatti, R.A. (1971) Humoral factors influencing lymphocyte transformation. *Prog. Allergy* 21:261.

Oren, M.E. and Herberman, R.B. (1971) Delayed cutaneous hypersensitivity reactions to membrane extracts of tumor cells. *Clin. Exp. Immunol.* 9:45–56.

Phillips, T.M. and Lewis, M.G. (1971) A method for elution of immunoglobulin from the surface of living cells. *Rev. Europ. Stud. Clin. Biol.* 16:1052–1053.

Price, M.R. and Robinson, R.A. (1978) Circulating factors modifying cell-mediated immunity in experimental neoplasia. In *Immunological Aspects of Cancer.* Castro, J.E. (ed.), Baltimore: University Park Press, pp. 155–181.

Rangel, D.M., Golub, S.H., and Morton, D.L. (1977a) Demonstration of lymphocyte blastogenesis-inhibiting factors in sera of melanoma patients. *Surgery* 82:224–232.

Rangel, D.M., Gupta, R.K., Golub, S.H., and Morton, D.L. (1977b) Demonstration of tumor-associated antigen-IC activity in immunosuppressive melanoma sera. *Proc. Am. Assoc. Cancer Res.* 18:184.

Reisfield, R.A., David, G.S., Pellegrino, M.A., and Holmes, E.C. (1977) Approaches for the isolation of biologically functional tumor-associated antigens. *Cancer Res.* 37:2860–2865.

Rossen, R.D., Reisberg, M.A., Hersch, E.M., and Gutterman, J.U. (1977) The clg binding test for immune complexes: clinical correlations obtained in patients with cancer. *J. Natl. Cancer Inst.* 58:1205–1215.

Samayoa, E.A., McDuffie, F.C., Nelson, A.M., Go, V.L.W., Luthra, S.S., and Brumfield, H.Q. (1977) Immunoglobulin complexes in serum of patients with malignancy. *Int. J. Cancer* 19:12–17.

Sjogren, H.O., Helstrom, I., Bansal, S.C., and Hellstrom, K.E. (1971) Suggestive evidence that the "blocking antibodies" to tumor bearing animals may be antigen-antibody complexes. *Proc. Natl. Acad. Sci. U.S.A.* 68:1372–1375.

Steel, G. Jr., Ankerst, J., and Sjogren, H.O. (1974) Alteration of *in vitro* anti-tumor activity of tumor bearer sera by absorption with *Staphylococcus aureus* Cowan I. *Int. J. Cancer* 14:83.

Theofilopoulos, A.N. and Dixon, F.J. (1978) Immune complexes associated with neoplasia. In *Immunodiagnosis of Cancer*. Herberman, R. (ed.), New York: Marcel Dekker, Inc., pp. 896–937 (Part 2).

Theofilopoulos, A.N., Andrews, B.S., Urist, M.M., Morton, D.L., and Dixon, F.J. (1977) The nature of immune complexes in human cancer serum. *J. Immunol.* 119:657–663.

Thomson, D.M.P., Sellens, V., Eccles, S., and Alexander, P. (1973) Radioimmunoassay of tumor specific transplantation antigen of a chemically induced rat sarcoma: circulating soluble tumor antigen in tumor bearers. *Br. J. Cancer* 28:377–388.

World Health Organization (1977) The role of immune complexes in disease. Report of a WHO scientific group, *WHO Technical Report series 606*.

Zubler, R.H. and Lambert, P.H. (1977) Immune complexes in clinical investigation. In *Recent Advances in Clinical Immunology*. Thomson, R.A. (ed.), New York: Churchill Livingston, pp. 125–147.

Published 1981 by Elsevier North Holland, Inc.
Saunders, Daniels, Serrou, Rosenfeld, and Denney, eds.
FUNDAMENTAL MECHANISMS IN HUMAN CANCER IMMUNOLOGY

CHAPTER 23

Natural and Activated Killer Lymphocytes[1]

Eva Klein and Farkas Vánky

*Department of Tumor Biology and Radiumhemmet, Karolinska Institutet,
S-104 01 Stockholm, Sweden*

Cell-mediated cytotoxicity offers the method of choice in many studies of tumor immunology, because the short-term *in vitro* assays are technically easy and measure anti-tumor effects directly.

The outcome of the short-term assays, performed either with freshly harvested effectors or with lymphocytes kept in culture with various stimuli, depends on several factors, such as the immunological history of the lymphocyte donors, the activation profile of the lymphocyte population, the previous treatment of the effectors (fresh or cultured), the characteristics of the target, and the species or allorelationship of the effectors and target.

Due to the complexity of the immune system, the results obtained under *in vitro* conditions may not accurately reflect *in vivo* events. Absence of lytic effects in a particular system does not rule out the existence of anti-tumor reactivity, since this may be manifested in a less dramatic way than an efficient and prompt direct lytic effect.

On the basis of recent developments in the area of cell-mediated cytotoxicity, a dualistic concept has developed: (1) Killer T cells (CTL) generated upon encounter with antigens present on the tumor cell surfaces are thought to be instrumental in specific resistance; (2) Natural killer (NK) cells, responsible for "non-specific" cytotoxicities, are regarded to represent the "first line of defense," because they have been shown to attack cells with altered surfaces, e.g., virus infected cells or tumors. It has been shown that the NK effect can be promptly boosted by the administration of interferon and other seemingly

[1]Funded in part with funds from the Department of Health, Education, and Welfare under Contract Number N01 CM 74144, Grants awarded by the National Cancer Institute, DHEW, No. 5R01-CA-25250-02A1, and by the Swedish Cancer Society.

"non-specific" measures. This primarily operationally defined distinction has to be modified, however because cytotoxic effects of non-immunized donors, which would thus conform with NK effects when tested against freshly harvested targets, were shown to be due to antigen recognition, and in this respect they were fundamentally similar to CTL.

Natural Killer Effect

Natural killing is an operational designation. It implies the *in vitro* cytotoxicity exerted by lymphocytes derived from donors with no known immunization history against the particular target. Due to the sensitivity of tumor derived lines, in such assays, it was speculated that the NK system plays an important role in the rejection of tumor cells (Haller et al., 1977; Jondal et al., 1978). In the majority of NK studies which led to characterization of the phenomenon, certain culture lines were used as targets. It is likely that membrane properties and not the expression of certain surface antigens defines their sensitivity (Ährlund-Richter et al., 1980).

The lymphocyte is heterogeneous with regard to strength of lytic function. Cells used as targets vary in the lytic threshold that must be surmounted by the lymphocyte in order to bring about lysis. In dose response experiments, the difference in cell sensitivity is reflected by the difference in the size of the effector population containing killer cells needed to kill a fixed number of targets. Increased effectiveness can be achieved by manipulating the assay conditions. If a more prolonged target cell/lymphocyte interaction is permitted to take place, the cytotoxic potential of the effector population is elevated. Interferon projection appears to play a key role in this event (Santoli and Koprowski, 1979).

It was demonstrated by several workers that cultured cells, as compared to directly explanted cells, have relatively higher sensitivities (Becker et al., 1978; de Vries et al., 1975). It is conceivable that NK sensitive variants are eliminated *in vivo* and they arise *de novo* in the growing population when it released from the selective pressure of killer lymphocytes. It is more likely, however, that a change of cell membrane characteristics occurs after explantation. Alternating retransplantation and reexplantation experiments showed that the NK sensitivity changed back and forth, depending on whether the target cells were harvested from the mouse or from the culture.

The majority of human blood lymphocytes which have natural cytotoxic potential belong to the T cell series, although they are heterogeneous with regard to their surface marker characteristics (Bakács et al., 1978; Kall and Koren, 1978; Masucci et al., 1980a; West et al., 1977). The ranking order of different subfractions derived from the nylon nonadherent lymphocyte population with regard to their "specific activity," i.e., their cytotoxic potential on per cell basis, is as follows: (1) Non SRBC rosetting subset (which contains cells reactive with anti-T serum) with and without demonstrated Fc receptors; (2) SRBC rosetting cells with E receptors of relatively low avidity and concomitant expression of Fc receptors; (3) Cells with E receptors of low avidity and without Fc receptors; (4) Cells with E receptors of high avidity and Fc receptors; (5) Cells with E receptors of high avidity without Fc receptors.

Interferon Activates the Cytotoxic Machinery

Short-term exposure of lymphocytes *in vitro* to interferon (IFN) enhances their NK activity, and we denote the resultant action "interferon activated killing" (IAK) (Santoli and Koprowski, 1979; Masucci et al., 1980b; Saksela et al., 1979). IAK was found to be mediated by the same lymphocyte subsets as NK. The cytotoxic ranking of the lymphocyte subsets is similar, but the IAK effects are stronger. In all likelihood, IFN elevates the function of lymphocytes with lytic potential (Masucci et al., 1981). As a result, IAK also affects targets that resist the majority of unmanipulated (NK) killer cells which operate at a lower level of activity.

Short-term assays for NK and IAK differ only operationally, in that IAK involves IFN pretreatment of the effector cells. The results with lymphocytes of individuals with high NK-activity are similar to IFN-activated lymphocytes from donors which function at a lower level of natural (NK) activity. Thus there is an individual difference in the activation profiles of T cell populations. The similarities between the two systems suggest that the rules emerging from IAK experiments are likely to be valid for the NK system as well.

Generation of Killer Cells in Culture

The NK activity of lymphocytes gradually disappears under culture conditions (Masucci et al., 1980a; Poros and Klein, 1978). However, when lymphocytes are activated in culture by specific stimuli (e.g., mixed lymphocyte culture [MLC]), cytotoxicity is generated which affects not only targets related to the stimulus, but also other cells that have no known antigenic relationship to it. This type of cytotoxicity can also be triggered by alloantigens (Callewaert et al., 1978; Seeley and Golub, 1978), calf serum (Zielska and Golub, 1976), some modification that occurs on the surface of cultured tumor cells (Martin-Chandon et al., 1975), EBV infected B cells (Klein et al., 1981), EBV transformed autologous and allogeneic lymphoid lines (Svedmyr et al., 1974), and phytohemagglutinin (PHA) (Stejskal et al., 1973). Activated killing, AK, can also affect certain targets that are NK resistant in short-term tests.

Since there is a correlation between the degree of activation, as reflected by blastogenesis, and the efficiency of AK (Masucci et al., 1980a), the killing potential exerted against sensitive cell lines (K562, Molt-4, etc.) can be used as a sign of activation.

The natural and the cultured activated killer cell populations show slightly different characteristics (Poros and Klein, 1979). A relatively higher proportion of the activated killer cells adhere to nylon wool. The proportion of Fc receptor-carrying killer cells is lower in the AK than in the NK system (Poros and Klein, 1978; Seeley et al., 1979). T cells with high affinity E receptors are the least active, both in the fresh (NK) and cultured (AK) populations.

Neither NK nor AK show the histocompatibility restriction phenomenon. The AK of a lymphocyte culture is not brought about by surviving NK cells, but are triggered *de novo*. Lymphocyte populations depleted of the NK active subsets, i.e., T cells with SRBC receptors of high avidity, became cytotoxic on exposure to appropriate activating stimuli (Masucci, G. et al., 1980c), and lymphocytes kept in autologous plasma *in vitro* for several days, which have lost NK activity, became cytotoxic when cultured further with K562 cells (Poros and Klein, 1978).

In one disease condition, the acute phase of infectious mononucleosis, the properties of the blood lymphocyte population are reminiscent of those of *in vitro* activated lymphocytes. The proportion of T cells with IgG or IgM receptors is decreased, and the lymphocytes exert indiscriminate cytotoxicity which affects a number of cell lines, among them even those which have low NK sensitivity (Klein et al., 1981).

Presentation of antigen to lymphocyte populations *in vitro* triggers the lymphocytes with receptors to divide. After a few days, such mixed cultures develop cytotoxic potential. On the population level, the following cytotoxicity systems can be generated in antigen containing lymphocyte cultures: (1) Enlargement of the specific clone will result in cytotoxicity against cells which carry the stimulating antigens, and cells which carry cross-reactive antigens. (2) Transactivation will recruit lymphocytes with other specificities and thus targets unrelated to the stimulus may be killed if the proportion of lymphocytes with receptors against their antigens is high (Symington and Teh, 1980). (3) Activated lymphocytes kill certain type of targets (cultured lines). This interaction is probably independent of antigen recognition. The simultaneous occurrence of these effects can be detected by using different targets and the overlapping of the various effector subsets by employing the "cold target competition" assay (Landazuri and Herberman, 1972).

From the complexity of the system, it follows that "specificity" on the effector level can only be determined if target cells of similar characteristics are used. As proposed earlier, the detection of reactive cells is perhaps more meaningful at the level of the recognition step (Martin-Chandon et al., 1975).

Allogeneic MLC provides conditions where specific CTL's (directed against the stimulator blast cell as targets, or a corresponding EBV-transformed B cell line of recent origin which is practically nonsensitive to the NK effect) and AK effects (e.g., against autologous B cell line or the HLA negative, K562, and Daudi cell lines) can be studied in parallel. The properties of the two cytotoxic systems can be contrasted as follows: Generation of AK in mixed lymphocyte culture does not require cell division. This implies that AK is not dependent on the enlargement of the specific alloreactive clone(s) (Callewaert et al., 1978). It appears that precursor cells, present at the initiation of the culture, are triggered to AK, as a sequel to the specific recognition step. In accordance, AK which accompanies a specific secondary MLC response, generated by a re-stimulation with the specific target, does not show a similarly strong secondary peak (Seeley et al., 1979).

We have attempted to separate the allospecific CTL from the AK (anti-K562) cells on the basis of E-rosetting and the expression of Fc receptors. E-rosette separation yielded two subsets that damaged both targets, but the anti-allotarget effect was slightly stronger in the sedimented E-rosetting cells, while the anti-K562 (AK) effect was enriched in the interphase (Poros and Klein, 1979). In the second type of experiment, the lymphocyte populations were separated on the basis of Fc receptor expression by absorption to immune complex-coated plastic surfaces. Allospecificity was enriched in the FcR negative fraction, while AK (anti-K562) cytotoxicity was mediated by both the FcR negative and positive subsets, although the latter was more active (Seeley et al., 1979). In the third system, we separated fractions with various affinities to *Helix pomatia* hemagglutinin (a T cell marker). The relative strength of allo- and AK activities of the fractions were similar (Poros et al., to be published). Thus there was a considerable overlapping in the effector populations which killed on the basis of antigen recognition (since the targets were the ones used for generation of cytotoxicity) and affected K562.

Lysis of Allogeneic, Freshly Isolated Tumor Cells by Interferon Treated Blood Lymphocytes

In experiments performed to search for autotumor reactive lymphocytes in blood, we found that freshly harvested tumor cells from human sarcomas and carcinomas lack or possess low NK sensitivity. They were lysed by healthy donor's lymphocytes only when these belonged to the category with very high NK potential as indicated by strong effect on K562 cells, one of the prototypes of NK sensitive lines. However, cytotoxicity could be induced against al-logeneic tumor biopsy cells in 50% of cases by incubation of the lymphocytes for 2–3 hours with Hu-IFN-α prior to the tests (Vánky et al., 1980). Similar results on leukemias were reported by Zarling et al. (1979).

IFN did not induce cytotoxicity against autologous tumor cells. Such activity occurred with untreated lymphocytes in about 25% of cases tested. However, IFN did not elevate its strength, and when it was absent, IFN did not induce it. Our interpretation of the results was that the biopsy cells were killed by alloreactive T cells which were triggered for lytic function by treatment with IFN. Thus, an assay conforming with the operationally classi-fied IFN activated NK effect, detected alloreactive killer cells.

If alloantigens were responsible for the lytic effect, different subsets in the same effector population should function against different targets in the

326

majority of combinations. The cold target competition assay allows the investigation of this question.

In such experiments, tumor cells separated from biopsy specimens from 14 patients were used as targets, and lymphocytes from 6 cancer patients and 14 healthy blood donors were used as effectors. Tumor cells from 23 patients were used as unlabeled competitors. When the competitor was identical with the target, the inhibition was complete in 20/26 experiments at 1:10 ratio of labeled:unlabeled cells and only in 2/35 tests when foreign, unlabeled tumor cells were the competitors. The Daudi and K562 cells were "universal" competitors: their presence abrogated the cytotoxicity as strongly as identical targets (K562 was even more effective) (Table 23.1). Thus we showed that in one lymphocyte population at least, part of the killer cells reactive with various allogeneic biopsy-derived tumors are not identical. These results support the hypothesis that alloreactive lymphocytes were triggered by IFN for the lytic function. Irrespective of their selectivity for the various biopsy cells, these lymphocytes reacted also with K562 and Daudi. Thus the reactivity with the NK reactive cell lines is not clonally distributed. This fact has been proven on clonal lines of mouse natural killer cells (Dennert, 1980).

The lack of IFN effect on autologous cytotoxicity was puzzling. One obvious possibility may be that there were no tumor recognizing lymphocytes, in addition to those which were already functioning in the cases with inherent cytotoxicity. This explanation is unlikely, since in another assay system, in which blood lymphocytes were confronted with autologous biopsy cells and blastogenesis was measured, a high proportion of cases (68%) were positive. We assume that the majority of autoreactive T cells were in a state of differentiation which allowed DNA synthesis in response to antigen presentation, but not in response to IFN. This explanation is likely, since the majority of T cells which express E receptors are not enhanced for cytotoxicity by IFN (Masucci, et al., 1980b).

Table 23.1. Summary of Cold Target Competition Tests in Lytic Systems with IFN Treated Lymphocytes in Allogeneic Effector Target Combinations.

		Ratio labeled : unlabeled target		
	Competitor	2:1	1:1	1:10
Biopsy	Non-identical	5[a]	22	35
	Identical	35	60	95
Daudi		35	63	98
K562		62	82	100

Note: Freshly separated biopsy cells were used as targets, effector target ratio 50:1, 4 hr ^{51}Cr release assay.
[a]Mean % inhibition of cytotoxicity at the indicated ratios.

In the next series of experiments, we attempted to impose a more efficient non-specific stimulus for activation of the autotumor recognizing lymphocytes.

In the experiments of Zarling et al. (1976) and Sharma and Odom (1979), who used freshly harvested leukemia cells, cytotoxicity against autologous leukemia cells was generated *in vitro*, when a strong stimulus was provided by confrontation with a pool of allogeneic lymphocytes from several donors or with bacterial extract. It was also shown that autologous lymphoblastoid cell lines could be killed by lymphocytes activated in MLC (Seeley and Golub, 1978).

In MLC's, in which we used the patients' lymphocytes as responders, 7/19 generated autologous tumor cell killers and 11/13 damaged allogeneic tumor cells (unrelated to the reactants). The results can be interpreted in such a way that in 40% of the cases, autologous tumor recognizing lymphocytes were "transactivated" in the MLC. (It has to be established whether the autotumor and alloreactive subsets were non-identical.) The effects against the allogeneic tumor cells were probably due to cross-reactivities between the allogeneic stimulator lymphocytes and the allogeneic third party target tumor cells. K562 cells were regularly killed by all MLC effectors; thus activation of the lymphocytes occurred in all cultures.

Autoreactivity by specific means, i.e., in the autologous mixed cultures containing lymphocytes and tumor cells, was generated in a higher proportion of tests, 12/19. Even in those cases in which autologous tumor killing was not generated, the lymphocytes killed K562, which indicated that recognition of the autologous tumor cells took place because this interaction provided the stimulus for activation of the lytic effect. In these cases, perhaps the number of autotumor recognizing lymphocytes were low or the tumor cells were relatively resistant to plasma membrane damage.

We can conclude that autologous tumor recognizing cells are present in the blood lymphocyte population of sarcoma and carcinoma patients, and such lymphocytes can be triggered for cytotoxicity, even by non-specific means. Due to stimulation of the relevant clone for proliferation, the autologous lymphocyte-tumor cell cultures provide the most efficient system for generating anti-tumor lytic effects. The occurrence of *in vivo* events related to these *in vitro* observations has been described in experimental systems. Allosensitization was shown to confer protection on mice and rats against the outgrowth of syngeneic tumor cell grafts (Kobayashi et al., 1980).

The strategy of current experimentation concerning autologous tumor reactivity in man aims at generating autoreactive lymphocytes by interaction with the antigenic cells and enrichment of these by cloning and growth stimulation. However, activation by other means may also trigger the autotumor reactive lymphocytes.

The demonstration that the lymphocytes can recognize the autologous tumor biopsy cells and can damage them indicates that immunological recognition of the tumors is a reality and further research on this line is meaningful.

Extrapolation from these experiments to *in vivo* events should be approached with caution, for the immunological interactions are complex, and the anti-autotumor effects were generated and detected under artificial conditions.

If lymphocytes which mediate cytotoxicity are made available for therapeutical administration, some of the dangers encountered in cytotoxic drug or radiotherapy may become operative, i.e., in addition to the anti-tumor effects, the activated lymphocyte population may damage non-malignant cells, too. Such effects may occur in infectious mononucleosis. During the acute phase, a high proportion of the T lymphocytes in the blood are in the activated state, and it is likely that these T cells are instrumental in the elimination or control of EBV infected B cells which are known to have a proliferative capacity *in vitro*. Occasionally, however, autoreactive complications lead to long lasting syndromes (Purtilo et al., 1977).

References

Ährlund-Richter, L., Masucci, G., and Klein, E. (1980) Somatic hybrids between a high NK-sensitive lymphoid (YACIR) and several low sensitive sarcoma or L-cell derived mouse lines exhibit low sensitivity. *Somatic Cell Gen.* 6:89–99.

Bakács, T., Klein, E., Yefenof, E., Gergely, P., and Steinitz, M. (1978) Human blood lymphocyte fractionation with special attention to their cytotoxic potential. *Z. Immun. Forsch. Immunobiol.* 154:121–134.

Becker, S., Kiessling, R., Lee, N., and Klein, G. (1978) Modulation of sensitivity to natural killer cell lysis after *in vitro* explantation of a mouse lymphoma. *J. Natl. Cancer Inst.* 61:1495–1498.

Callewaert, D.M., Lighbody, J.J., Kaplan, J., Joroszowski, J., Petersson, W.D., and Rosenberg, J.C. (1978) Cytotoxicity of human peripheral lymphocytes in cell-mediated lympholysis, antibody dependent cell-mediated lympholysis, and natural cytotoxicity assay after mixed lymphocyte cultures. *J. Immunol.* 121:81–85.

Dennert, G. (1980) Cloned lines of natural killer cells. *Nature* 287:47–49.

Haller, O., Hansson, M., Kiessling, R., and Wigzell, H. (1977) Role of non-conventional natural killer cells in resistance against syngeneic tumor cells *in vivo*. *Nature* 270:609–611.

Jondal, M., Spina, C., and Targan, S. (1978) Human spontaneous killer cells selective for tumor-derived target cells. *Nature* 72:62–64.

Kall, M.A. and Koren, H.S. (1978) Heterogeneity of human natural killer populations. *Cell. Immunol.* 40:58–68.

Kobayashi, H., Hosokawa, M., and Oikawa, T. (1980) Transplantation immunity to syngeneic tumors in WKR rats immunized with allogeneic cells. *Transp. Proc.* 12:156–159.

Klein, E., Ernberg, I., Masucci, M.G., Szigeti, R., Wu, Y.T., Masucci, G., and Svedmyr, E. (1981) *In vivo* control of the proliferative capacity of EBV infected B cells. *Cancer Res.* In press.

Landazuri, O.M. and Herberman, R.B. (1972) Specificity of cellular immune reactivity to virus induced tumors. *Nature New Biology* 238:18–19.

Martin-Chandon, M.R., Vánky, F., Carnaud, C., and Klein, E. (1975) "*In vitro* education" on autologous human sarcoma generates non-specific killer cells. *Int. J. Cancer* 15:342–350.

Masucci, M.G., Klein, E., and Argov, S. (1980a) Disappearance of the NK effect after explantation of lymphocytes and generation of similar non-specific cytotoxicity correlated to the level of blastogenesis in activated cultures. *J. Immunol.* 124:2458–2463.

Masucci, M.G., Masucci, G., Klein, E., and Berthold, W. (1980b) Target selectivity of interferon induced human killer lymphocytes related to their Fc receptor expression. *Proc. Natl. Acad. Sci.* 77:3620–3624.

Masucci, M.G., Masucci, G., Klein, E., and Berthold, W. (1981) Interferon induced cytotoxicity of human lymphocytes. In *New Trends in Human Immunology and Cancer Immunotherapy*. Vol. I. Serrou, B. and Rosenfeld, C. (eds.), Paris-London: Doin-Saunders. In press.

Masucci, G., Poros, A., Seeley, J.K., and Klein, E. (1980c) *In vitro* generation of K562 killers in human T lymphocyte subsets. *Cell. Immunol.* 52:247–254.

Poros, A. and Klein, E. (1978) Cultivation with K562 cells leads to blastogenesis and increased cytotoxicity with changed properties of the active cells when compared to fresh lymphocytes. *Cell Immunol.* 41:240–255.

Poros, A. and Klein, E. (1979) Distinction of anti-K562 and anti-allocytotoxicity in *in vitro* stimulated populations of human lymphocytes. *Cell. Immunol.* 46:57–68.

Poros, A., Ährlund-Richter, L., Klein, E., Hammarström, S., and Koide, N. Inverse correlation between the expression of Helix pomatia hemagglutinin (HP) receptors and cytotoxicity against K562 or alloblasts in lymphocyte populations activated in mixed cultures. Submitted for publication.

Purtilo, D.T., De Floria, D., Hutt, L.M., Bhawan, J., Yang, J.P.S., Otto, R., and Edwards, W. (1977) Variable phenotypic expression of an X-linked recessive lymphoproliferative syndrome. *New Engl. J. Med.* 297:1077–1081.

Saksela, E., Timonen, T., and Cantell, K. (1979) Human natural killer activity is augmented by interferon via recruitment of "pre-NK" cells. *Scand. J. Immunol.* 10:257–266.

Santoli, D. and Koprowski, H. (1979) Mechanism of activation of human natural killer cells against tumor and virus-infected cells. *Immunol. Rev.* 44:125–162.

Seeley, J.K. and Golub, S.H. (1978) Studies on cytotoxicity generated in human mixed lymphocyte cultures. I. Time course and target spectrum of several distinct concomitant cytotoxic activities. *J. Immunol.* 120:1415–1422.

Seeley, J.K., Masucci, G., Poros, A., Klein, E., and Golub, S.H. (1979) Studies on cytotoxicity generated human mixed lymphocyte cultures. II. Anti-K562 effectors are distinct from allospecific CTL and can be generated from NK-depleted T cells. *J. Immunol.* 123:1303–1311.

Sharma, B. and Odom, L.F. (1979) Generation of killer lymphocytes *in vitro* against human autologous leukemia cells with leukemia blasts and BCG extract. *Cancer Immunol. Immunother.* 7:93–98.

Stejskal, V., Lindberg, S., Holm, G., and Perlman, P. (1973) Differential cytotoxicity of activated lymphocytes on allogeneic and xenogeneic target cells. II. Activation by phytohemagglutinin. *Cell. Immunol.* 8:82–92.

Svedmyr, E.A., Deinhardt, F., and Klein, G. (1974) Sensitivity of different target cells to the killing action of peripheral lymphocytes stimulated by autologous lymphoblastoid cell lines. *Int. J. Cancer* 13:891–905.

Symington, F.W. and Teh, H.S. (1980) A two signal mechanism for the induction of cytotoxic T lymphocytes. *Scand. J. Immunol.* 12:1–12.

Vánky, F. and Stjernswärd, J. (1979) Lymphocyte stimulation by autologous tumor biopsy cells. In *Immunodiagnosis of Cancer*. Herberman, R.B. and McIntire, K.R. (eds.), New York: Marcel Dekker Publ., pp. 998–1032.

Vánky, F., Argov, S., Einhorn, S., and Klein, E. (1980) The role of alloantigens in natural killing. Allogeneic but not autologous tumor biopsy cells are sensitive for interferon induced cytotoxicity of human blood lymphocytes. *J. Exp. Med.* 151:1151–1165.

de Vries, J.E., Meyerung, M., Van Dongren, A., and Rümke, P. (1975) The influence of different isolation procedures and the use of target cells from melanoma cell lines and short-term cultures on the non-specific cytotoxic effect of lymphocytes from healthy donors. *Int. J. Cancer* 15:391–400.

West, W.H., Cannon, G.B., Kay, H.D., Bonnard, G.D., and Herberman, R.B. (1977) Natural cytotoxic reactivity of human lymphocytes against a myeloid cell line: characterization of effector cell. *J. Immunol.* 48:355–361.

Zarling, J.M., Raich, P.C., McKeough, M., and Bach, F.H. (1976) Generation of cytotoxic lymphocytes *in vitro* against autologous human leukemia cells. *Nature* 262:691–693.

Zarling, J.M., Eskra, L., Borden, E.C., Horoszewics, J., and Carter, W.A. (1979) Activation of human natural killer cells cytotoxic for human leukemia cells by purified interferon. *J. Immunol.* 132:63–71.

Zielska, J.V. and Golub, S.H. (1976) Fetal calf serum induced blastogenic and cytotoxic response of human lymphocytes. *Cancer Res.* 36:3842–3846.

CHAPTER 24

Monoclonal Antibodies as Probes for Cell Surface Changes in Human Malignancy[1]

Roger H. Kennett, Zdenka L. Jonak, Kathleen B. Bechtol,* and Rebecca Byrd

Department of Human Genetics, University of Pennsylvania School of Medicine, Philadelphia, Pennsylvania and Wistar Institute, Philadelphia, Pennsylvania*

Introduction

It is well accepted that the surface of tumor cells differs from that of corresponding normal adult cells (Ruddon et al., 1978; Sell, 1980). On the other hand, the significance of the molecular changes and their possible genetic basis are not well understood. The observed surface alterations may result from: (1) genetic expression of an oncogenic virus or a somatic mutation, (2) abnormal timing of expression of germ-line genes, (in the case of oncofetal antigens), (3) expression of a differentiation antigen that is not normally detected on normal cells because the cells represented by the differentiated state of the tumor are present in low numbers, (4) perturbations in the arrangement of cell surface molecules resulting from either rapid growth of the tumor cells or loss of expression of a gene product, or (5) any combination of these mechanisms.

As the molecular characteristics of cell surface changes in malignancy become better understood, the relationship of the malignant phenotype to the malignant genotype will have to be analyzed. The phenotype of a tumor which successfully "colonizes" a host could result from a series of events: for example, a primary event might cause loss of growth control, and subsequent events could lead to a generation of clonal variants of the primary tumor which because of selective advantage, overgrow the primary tumor. Such a selection of variant tumors has been shown to play a role in the development of metastatic tumors from non-metastasizing forms (Fidler and Kripke, 1977;

[1]This work was supported by Grants CA 24263, CA 14489, NS 15427, and CA 10815 from the National Institutes of Health and by Grant PCM 79-26757 from the National Science Foundation.

Brunson and Nicolson, 1978). The nature of the initial event is likewise unclear; it remains to be determined whether transformation of a cell from a non-malignant to a malignant form causes (1) the loss of a gene product or function, for example, fibronectin (Ruoslahti et al., 1980), or (2) the production of new gene products. Either possibility may apply in the case of a particular tumor type.

If the molecular basis of malignancy is the loss of a gene product, it will be necessary to carefully characterize the cell surface composition of the tumor cells and compare it to that of corresponding normal cells. For a given tumor cell type, this process may require extensive study and careful analysis of the structure and distribution of its cell surface molecules. If, on the other hand, a new gene product is present, the definition of an antigen as being truly tumor specific requires demonstration that the gene for the antigen is present in the tumor DNA but not in normal human DNA. Analysis of this new genetic structure should then indicate whether it is a new gene of viral origin or a mutant form of a normal germ-line gene.

Before the introduction of monoclonal antibodies by Kohler and Milstein (1975), the possibility of carrying out a discriminating and thorough analysis of the composition of cell surfaces was difficult and impractical. The production of large amounts of very specific monoclonal antibody reagents has made it possible to begin careful analyses of the surface architecture and composition of cell surfaces. Out of such studies should come a more discriminating comparison of tumor cell and normal cell surfaces and a better understanding of both the primary and secondary cell surface changes in malignancy. We will review here the various ways that monoclonal antibodies have already been applied to the study of human tumor cell surface antigens and discuss ways in which these useful new reagents may be applied in the future. We concentrate on human tumor antigens, both because this has been a major interest of ours for some time and because the advent of monoclonal reagents to human antigens make practical a rigorous analysis of human tumor cell surfaces, while earlier investigators working with human tumors were restricted to the use of heterospecific immunizations requiring extensive absorptions to allow detection of the tumor specific response.

Materials and Methods

The immunizations of mice, hybridoma production, and screening of monoclonal antibodies were performed as previously reported (Kennett et al., 1978). The peroxidase-linked antibody assay followed the method of Kennett (1980d). Cells were attached to polystyrene plates (Linbro 76-033-05), and monoclonal antibodies reacting with them were detected with peroxidase-conjugated rabbit anti-mouse immunoglobulin (Cappel), using orthophenyldiamine as a substrate. The optical density at 450 mu of each well was read with a Multiscan Spectrophotometer (Flow). Cytotoxicity assays were performed as described by

Kennett (1980b). The detection of individual cells in bone marrow that express a particular antigen was done with peroxidase-linked anti-immunoglobulin reagents, a procedure described previously (Kennett et al., 1980; Jonak, 1980).

The detection of antibody binding with protein-A conjugated fluorescent Covaspheres (Covalent Technology Corp.) was done to determine whether the antigens detected by two different monoclonal antibodies were expressed in the same cells or different cells. Since PI153/3 is IgM and P3B1-C3 is IgG$_{2a}$, we could use protein-A (coupled to Covaspheres) as a specific reagent for detection of P3B1-C3 binding. The conditions for this assay were the same as for the peroxidase-coupled assay. After the incubation with the monoclonal antibodies, the cells were washed and resuspended in 100 μl of protein A-conjugated Covaspheres. The plates were centrifuged at 1000 xg for 15 minutes to ensure that a monolayer of Covaspheres settled on and around the cells. The plates were then left undisturbed for 20 minutes at room temperature. After this incubation, the mixture was resuspended in 3 ml medium and was transferred to a 15 ml tube with a conical bottom. Unbound covaspheres were removed by underlaying the cell suspension with 1 ml of calf serum, centrifuging at 110 xg for 8 min, and discarding the supernatant. The cells were washed and resuspended in 20 μl of horseradish peroxidase-conjugated rabbit anti-mouse Ig. The procedure was the same as that described above for the peroxidase-coupled antibody assay. The assay was evaluated under a light microscope for peroxidase staining. Fluorescent covaspheres were detected with a Leitz Orthoplan II with Phloem attachment (fluorescence cube N).

Cells which expressed the antigen detected by the IgM antibody PI153/3 were labeled only with peroxidase and thus exhibited a black ring of precipitate. Cells labeled with PI153/3 (IgM) and P3B1-C3 (IgG$_{2a}$) or with P3B1-C3 alone exhibited both a black precipitate and bound fluorescent Covaspheres. Lymphocytes with human immunoglobulin on their surface bound the Covaspheres but did not show a black precipitate resulting from the binding of peroxidase conjugated rabbit anti-mouse immunoglobulin.

Inhibition of cell proliferation with monoclonal antibodies was tested as described previously (Kennett et al., 1980b), except that the antibodies were used directly in hybridoma supernatants without ammonium sulfate precipitation.

Results and Discussion

Monoclonal Antibodies Against Human Tumor Associated Antigens

In the five years since Kohler and Milstein described the first monoclonal antibodies, several investigators have reported isolation of hybridomas making antibodies against human tumor antigens (Table 24.1). In the case of melanomas, individual antibodies have been found which (1) react with antigens present on other cell types as well as melanomas, (2) bind detectably to only some melanomas (Yeh et al., 1979; Carrel et al., 1980), or (3) bind to all

334

Table 24.1. Human Tumor Associated Antigens Detected with Monoclonal Antibodies.

Tumor cell type	Reference
Melanoma	Brown, J. et al., 1980; Carrel et al., 1980
	Koprowski et al., 1978; Steplewski et al., 1979
	Yeh et al., 1979; Imai et al., 1980
Neuroblastoma	Kennett and Gilbert, 1979
Colorectal carcinoma	Koprowski et al., 1979
Thymus-leukemia	Levy et al., 1979
Acute lymphoblastic leukemia (cALL)	Ritz et al., 1980
B Cell lymphoma	Nadler et al., 1980; Brown, S. et al., 1980

melanomas tested (Koprowski et al., 1978; Steplewski et al., 1979; Imai et al., 1980). In the last two cases, the antibodies do not react with other tumor cells or with the normal cells tested. This, of course, does not exclude the possibility that the recognized antigens are present on some small populations of melanocytes or on fetal cells. Nevertheless, these antibodies may be used for the applications listed in Table 24.2, and they certainly represent a major step in the development of tools to decipher the molecular composition of the cell surface of malignant melanocytes. Among the antibodies described by Steplewski, one precipitates an antigen of 84,000 daltons and another precipitates proteins of 116,000, 95,000, 29,000, and 26,000 daltons. Brown et al. (1980) independently described anti-melanoma antibodies, of which 2 of 8 react with melanomas and not fibroblasts. One of these antibodies reacts with an antigen with a molecular weight estimated at 97,000 and the second precipitates

Table 24.2. Potential Uses of Monoclonal Antibodies Against Tumor Associated Antigens.

Application	References reporting initial results
1. Isolation of tumor-associated antigens by immunoprecipitation or affinity chromatography	Momoi, et al., 1980; Steplewski et al., 1979; Brown, J. et al., 1980; Ritz et al., 1980; Levy et al., 1979
2. Tumor identification	
a. Diagnosis	Greaves et al., 1980; Bradstock et al., 1980
b. Detection of metastasis	Kennett et al., 1980; Levine et al., 1980
3. Immunotherapy	
a. Cytolytic antibodies	Bernstein, et al., 1980; Herlyn et al., 1980;
b. Antibodies with attached drugs	Nadler et al., 1980
4. Mapping of genetic locus for antigen to specific chromosome	Barnstable et al., 1978; Kennett et al., 1980a; Solomon and Jones, 1980
5. Isolation of "tumor antigen" genes by combination of monoclonal antibody and recombinant DNA techniques	
6. Detection of cell surface receptors involved in growth regulation	McGrath et al., 1980; Kennett et al., 1980

proteins estimated to be 110,000, 80,000, and 27,000 daltons. The striking similarity of these independent results leads one to believe that we will soon have a better understanding of the antigens present on human melanomas and their significance with regard to the genetic and molecular basis of the neoplasia.

A well-designed and imaginative approach to making tumor-specific antibodies against a human B cell lymphoma has been described by investigators in R. Levy's laboratory (Brown et al., 1980). They have taken advantage of the fact that the B cell lymphoma expresses a human immunoglobulin with a clonally derived idiotype. Antibodies against the immunoglobulin idiotype are then, for all practical purposes, tumor specific. By making mouse human hybrids between the B cell lymphoma and a mouse plasmacytoma (Levy et al., 1979), they derived hybrid clones making significant amounts of this human immunoglobulin. The immunoglobulin was used to immunize mice and to produce monoclonal antibodies against idiotypic determinants. These monoclonal antibodies were useful reagents for identifying and monitoring the specific patient's lymphoma cells.

Although none of the antigens detected by the antibodies listed in Table 24.1 have yet been shown to be truly tumor specific (i.e., produced by a gene not in germ-line DNA), they are nevertheless potentially useful for the applications listed in Table 24.2.

Detection of Metastasized Neuroblastoma with Monoclonal Antibodies

We will describe here the work that was done with a monoclonal antibody made against a human neuroblastoma antigen. The antibody PI153/3 has been used for detection of neuroblastoma cells in bone marrow. Production of the monoclonal antibody PI153/3 was described previously (Kennett and Gilbert, 1979). The antibody was characterized as reacting with human neuroblastomas, retinoblastomas, and glioblastomas; all tumors derived from neuroectoderm. It also reacts with human fetal brain, but not with adult brain (Kennett and Gilbert, 1979). Momoi et al. (1980) have shown that the antigen is a glycoprotein and that the antigenic determinant is present on the carbohydrate portion of the molecule. They estimated that the molecule makes up approximately 1% of the total cell surface glycoprotein. This finding illustrates another advantage of monoclonal antibodies—they can detect and isolate even minor molecular components of the cell surface.

While using PI153/3 to detect neuroblastomas in bone marrow with immunoperoxidase labeling (Kennett et al., 1980a; Jonak, 1980; see Fig. 24.1 for example), we observed that the antibody reacted with tumor cells in an acute lymphoblastic leukemia (ALL) marrow used as a control. We then observed that the PI153/3 antigen is present on B cell ALL and common ALL cells but not on T cell ALL cells (Kennett et al., 1980a). A more extensive analysis of the reactivity of the antibody (Table 24.3), which confirmed our earlier observations, was done with immunofluorescence and fluorescent activated cell sorter analysis (Greaves et al., 1980).

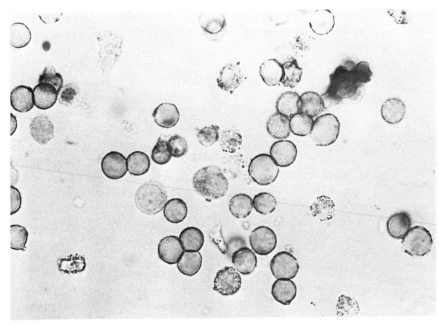

Figure 24.1. Detection of antigen on ALL cells with monoclonal antibody PI153/3. Bone marrow lymphocytes from an ALL patient were incubated with PI153/3 (IgM) and then with protein-A coated fluorescent Covaspheres. The cells were then reacted with peroxidase conjugated anti-mouse Ig, spread on polylysine coated slides and treated with diaminobenzidine and osmium tetroxide. Cells to which PI153/3 binds show a brown precipitate at the cell membrane. The control pictured shows that cells which are positive for PI153/3 do not bind protein-A coated Covaspheres. The spheres can be seen bound to some lymphocytes which presumably have surface Ig to which the protein-A binds. These cells, which do not bind the monoclonal antibody and thus do not show a brown precipitate, are not present in all marrows, but only those in which there is apparently some contamination by peripheral blood lymphocytes. Neuroblastoma marrow with tumor cells present show this pattern of labeling when PI153/3 is used alone and also when PI153/3 and P3B1-C3 are used together. When leukemia cells and immature lymphocytes are treated with both antibodies, all cells labeled show both the precipitate and the fluorescent spheres (Figure 24.2) demonstrating that neither of these cell types express the PI153/3 antigen without also expressing the antigen detected by P3B1-C3.

These data showed that the antibody is certainly useful for classifying certain types of leukemia cells, but its reactivity complicated our attempts to use PI153/3 to detect neuroblastoma cells in bone marrow. What concerned us was that it had been reported by Evans and Hummeler (1973) that bone marrow aspirates of certain children with neuroblastoma, particularly those recently removed from treatment, contained primitive cells with lymphocytic morphology. In the few cases where we identified these cells, they were labeled

Table 24.3. Reactivity of PI153/3 with Leukemic Cells.

Leukemia type	No. tested	No. positive PI153/3	DA2[a]
Acute lymphoblastic leukemia			
cALL[b]	51	51	51
B-ALL[c]	4	4	4
T-ALL[d]	21	0	0
"Unclassified"/"null" ALL[e]	10	6	8
Acute myeloid leukemia			
AML	18	0	13
AMML	1	0	1
AMonL	2	0	2
Ph[1+] CML			
CML	9	0	0
CML-BC "M"[f]	8	0	7
"L"[b]	10	10	10
Acute undifferentiated leukemia			
(a) Ph[1+] AUL in relapse[b]	1	1	1
(b) AUL with "L" phenotype[b]	5	4	5
(c) AUL with "M" phenotype	5	0	3
B cell malignancies[g]			
Hairy cell leukemia	2	2	2
Non-Hodgkin's lymphoma[h]	3	3	3
Myeloma	1	0	0
Plasma cell leukemia	2	0	0
B-CLL	9	9	9
B-PLL	2	2	2
Others			
Megakaryoblastic leukemia	1	0	0
T-CLL	2	0	0
Sezary (T) leukemia	4	0	1
Erythroleukemia	4	0	0

[a] Anti-HLA-DR: reacts with all *DR* types.
[b] Phenotype: cALL[+], TdT[+], SmIg[-], E[-]/T[-].
[c] Phenotype: cALL[-], TdT[-], SmIg[+], E[-]/T[-].
[d] Phenotype: cALL[-], TdT[+], SmIg[-], E and/or T[+].
[e] Phenotype: cALL[-], TdT[+], SmIg[-], E[-]/T[-].
[f] Phenotype: cALL[-], TdT[-].
[g] All malignant cells in this category had monoclonal Ig (or light chains).
[h] Involved marrow studied.
(Source: Greaves et al., 1980.)

lightly with the antibody PI153/3. We therefore postulated that they were expressing the antigenic determinant present on leukemia blast cells. To distinguish these lymphocytes from neuroblastoma cells, we chose a second monoclonal antibody, P3B1-C3, which, as reported previously (Kennett et al., 1980c), reacts with human B cells and with the null cell ALL line Reh derived from a patient with common ALL (Rosenfeld et al., 1975).

Table 24.4 compares the reactivity of the two antibodies PI153/3 and P3B1-C3. Although P3B1-C3 reacts with 20% of peripheral blood lympocytes, there is no reactivity with bone marrow cells from normal transplant donors. As shown in Table 24.5, all leukemia or lymphoma marrows containing cells

338

Table 24.4. Reactivity of Monoclonal Antibodies with Different Human Cell Types, As Determined by Cytotoxicity or Binding Assay.

Monoclonal antibody	IMR6 neuroblastoma	Reh null ALL	B cell line	T cell line	Fibroblasts	Peripheral blood lymphocytes adult	Normal donor marrow
PI153/3	+	+	–	–	–	–	–
P3B1-C3	–	+	+	–	–	20% +	–

that show reaction with PI153/3 also react with P3B1-C3. Five untreated neuroblastoma patients showed a few cells labeled with both antibodies, while 10 patients classified as Type IV, and thus having disseminated neuroblastoma, and one patient classified as Type III, exhibited cells which labeled with only the "anti-neuroblastoma" antibody PI153/3. As we had postulated, nine of the stage IV neuroblastoma patients in remission after treatment showed cells which labeled with both antibodies and were classified as premature lymphocytes. We therefore conclude that we are able to detect neuroblastomas that

Table 24.5. Reaction of Monoclonal Antibodies PI153/3 and P3B1-C3 with Bone Marrow Cells.

Disease	Diagnostic (untreated) (+/+)	(+/−)	(−/+)	(−/−)	Remission (+/+)	(+/−)	(−/+)	(−/−)	Relapse (+/+)	(+/−)	(−/+)	(−/−)
Neuroblastoma stage: I												
II	1											
III	1	1						3	1			
IV	1	10			9		1		1			
IV-S	2				1			1				
Retinoblastoma	1	1										
Non-Hodgkin's lymphoma	1		2					1			1	
ALL	8		3		1		3	3	1		4	
AML			1								1	
Ganglioneuroma			2	1								

Note: Reaction recorded as number of bone marrow samples showing indicated reaction pattern (PI153/3/P3B1-C3) in an immunoperoxidase assay. + indicates that cells showing a ring of precipitation after treatment with diaminobenzidine and osmium tetroxide were found with the specific monoclonal antibody but not with a control antibody.

have metastasized to bone marrow and, by using a combination of antibodies, determine whether or not we are truly labeling neuroblastomas or immature lymphocytes.

To confirm that in the bone marrows, where we could detect cells labeled by both antibodies, the two antigens are expressed by the same cells, we took advantage of the fact that the monoclonal antibodies are of two different heavy chain classes μ (PI153/3) and α_{2a} (P3B1-C3). Both antibodies will react with the peroxidase labeled anti-mouse Ig reagent, but only P3B1-C3 will bind protein-A coated fluorescent Covaspheres. We can thus show that when incubated with both antibodies, neuroblastoma cells are labeled with peroxidase but will not bind the spheres. Reh cells and other leukemia cells positive for PI153/3 and P3B1-C3 label with both peroxidase and the fluorescent spheres. Since there are no leukemia cells labeled with peroxidase that do not bind the spheres, we can conclude that there are no leukemia cells that express the PI153/3 antigen but not the P3B1-C3 antigen. Figure 24.1 shows the labeling of ALL cells with PI153/3 and the peroxidase labeled antibodies and Covaspheres. The only cells that bind the protein-A coated spheres are lymphocytes expressing Ig. Since there is no peroxidase label, we can conclude that no mouse antibody has bound to these cells. Figures 24.2A and 24.2B demonstrate that, when cells from the bone marrow are labeled with both antibodies and both second labels, all cells labeled with peroxidase also bind the spheres. With these labeling procedures, we are confident that we can distinguish neuroblastomas from immature lymphocytes and in fact have in one case detected neuroblastoma cells in a patient's marrow, when standard clinical procedures involving identification of tumor cell clumps did not detect them.

Further analysis of the antigens expressed on leukemia cells and neuroblastomas should allow us to determine if the antigens on the two tumor types are the same antigens, or simply cross-react because they have similar antigenic structures. We are in the process of comparing the antigens isolated from the neuroblastoma line IMR5 and the leukemia line Reh. We are also making more antibodies against the antigen obtained from one cell type to determine if they also react with the second type of tumor cell.

We have shown that the neuroblastoma-leukemia antigen is actually an oncofetal differentiation antigen. It is nevertheless useful, in combination with other antibodies, for both classifying leukemia cells and detecting metastasis of neuroblastoma cells. Other antibodies, which are shown by extensive analysis of normal human adult and fetal cells to detect antigens which appear to be truly tumor specific, should then be used to go to the next, definitive step, which is isolating the gene for the antigen and determining if it is really a "tumor specific gene." It should not be difficult to combine the technologies of monoclonal antibodies and recombinant DNA. An essential step will be to use the first antibody that defines the antigen to isolate the molecule and then make other antibodies against as many determinants on it as possible to

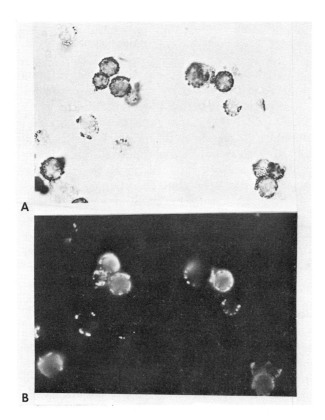

Figure 24.2. Detection of antigens on ALL cells with monoclonal antibodies PI153/3 and P3B1C3. This experiment was performed as described under Figure 24.1, except that the cells were labeled with both PI153/3 (IgM) and P3B1C3 (IgG$_{2a}$). The photographs demonstrate that all cells labeled with PI153/3 also express the antigen detected by P3B1-C3. The PI153/3$^+$/P3B1-C3$^-$ pattern of labeling is seen on neuroblastomas but not on leukemias or immature lymphocytes. A shows cells labeled with peroxidase. B shows the same field under fluorescent illumination.

enhance assay sensitivity. Isolation of the antigen will also allow determination of its molecular weight and estimation of the size of its corresponding messenger RNA. With these facts and immunological tools, it should be possible to use established techniques for isolation and characterization of the "tumor antigen gene."

Recessive Mutations and Cell Surface Receptors

Of course in some and perhaps all tumors, the initial genetic event which produces a malignant cell does not produce new "tumor specific antigens," but causes the loss of a function or gene product. In this case of what would classically be defined as a recessive mutation, one would not find a new antigenic determinant primarily associated with the malignancy. With this model of malignancy, two other applications of monoclonal antibodies could illuminate the molecular basis of malignancy, again concentrating on the cell surface as a likely location for a molecular change that would affect the regulation of cell growth and division.

The first obvious application is to use monoclonal antibodies made against cell surface antigens on normal cells to determine if any antigenic cell surface molecule is missing on the tumor cell, which would normally be expressed on that cell type. Definition of the malignant cell's normal counterpart would of course be difficult, since the differentiated state of a given tumor is in itself often a mystery. On the other hand, we might find it fruitful to concentrate on obtaining monoclonal antibodies that react with cell surface molecules and have an effect on some aspect of cell division and/or differentiation. The rationale for this approach is based upon three observations: (1) several investigators have reported the production of monoclonal antibodies against cell surface receptors for various hormones and growth factors (Table 24.6); (2) antibodies against hormone receptors have been shown in some cases to mimic the effect of the hormones on the cells (Kahn et al., 1977; Kasuga et al., 1978); and (3) tumors in general may be viewed as cells which for some reason do not respond properly to normal signals which would induce the cell to stop dividing and differentiate or to continue its progress down a pathway of differentiation.

The proposed search for missing or non-functional cell surface receptors can be approached in two ways, as diagrammed in Figure 24.3. First, antibodies made against cell surface antigens of normal cells can be tested to see if their reactions with these cells can stop cell division and/or induce cell differentiation. Those antibodies which have such an effect can then be tested against tumor cells to see if the antigen is present and if the antibodies produce the same effect on differentiation and/or division. This approach has the important limitation that the normal human cells necessary for the study may not be as available as tumor cells.

For the second approach (Kennett et al., 1980c), the assumption is made that the tumor cell expresses a mutant form of the cell surface receptor, which

Table 24.6. Monoclonal Antibodies to Cell Surface Receptors.

Receptor specificity	Reference
Estrogen	Greene et al., 1980
Acetylcholine	Gomez et al., 1979
Thyroid stimulating hormone	Tzartos and Lindstrom, 1980
Insulin	Raizada and Fellows, 1980
Epidermal growth factor	Grimm and Fox, 1980
β-adrenergic	Venter and Fraser, 1980

342

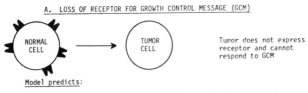

A. LOSS OF RECEPTOR FOR GROWTH CONTROL MESSAGE (GCM)

NORMAL CELL → TUMOR CELL

Tumor does not express receptor and cannot respond to GCM

Model predicts:

Antibodies to receptor on normal cell will not react with tumor cell.

Antibodies to receptors on normal cells may block GCM.

Antibodies may mimic effect of GCM on normal cells.

To test this model:

Find monoclonal antibodies that react with normal cells corresponding to differentiated state of the tumor, but do not react with the tumor cells

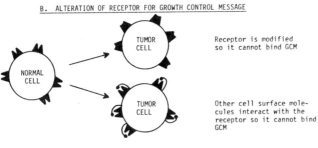

B. ALTERATION OF RECEPTOR FOR GROWTH CONTROL MESSAGE

NORMAL CELL

TUMOR CELL

Receptor is modified so it cannot bind GCM

TUMOR CELL

Other cell surface molecules interact with the receptor so it cannot bind GCM

Model predicts:

Antibodies may bind receptor on normal cells and on tumor cells. Antibodies may mimic the effects of GCM.

To test this model:

Find monoclonal antibodies that react with tumor cells and see if they can mimic the effects of GCM.

Can they stop proliferation and induce differentiation?

Figure 24.3. Two alternative mechanisms by which receptors for growth control messengers (GCM) may be involved in the primary alteration in malignancy. In both models, tumor cells continue to divide and/or fail to differentiate because they lack a functional receptor which would normally receive the message inducing the cell to stop dividing and differentiate. The analysis of both possibilities has been made practical by the availability of monoclonal antibodies, reagents which are directed against single antigenic determinants and are available in large quantities. For the study of most human tumors, it may be more practical to test model B, because tumor cells are more likely to be available for immunization, assays, functional studies, and molecular analyses. Functional studies would also be easier because they could use tumor cells without identification of the GCM by looking for antibodies which by themselves or in combination inhibit cell proliferation and/or induce differentiation.

can no longer receive the molecular signal to stop dividing and differentiate—perhaps because of a mutation, or interaction with an oncogenic viral gene product which alters the normal binding site. It is possible that some of the antibodies made against this receptor molecule may react with the tumor cell receptor and induce that tumor cell to stop dividing and differentiate. Such antibodies would provide insight into the molecular basis of the tumor cell's lack of growth control, and could also be potentially useful for differentiation therapy (Waxman, 1979). Because the molecular changes involved in this type of malignancy-induction mechanism may not produce enough conformational change for the altered receptor to be recognized by the human immune system as a foreign protein, the use of monoclonal antibodies made in mice or rats would have a definite advantage. On the other hand, once such a cell surface molecule or any other type of useful human tumor marker is identified with rat or mouse monoclonal antibodies, it would certainly be useful to attempt to make human monoclonal antibodies. Human lymphocytes sensitized to some form of the molecule could be fused to one of the recently reported human immunoglobulin producing lines form which human hybridomas can be made (Olsson and Kaplan, 1980; Croce, 1980). Using this system as a model, we have recently begun to test our monoclonal antibodies that react with the ALL cell line Reh. We are testing first to see if any of the antibodies inhibit the proliferation of Reh. We have been encouraged by our initial experiments (Kennett et al., 1980c; Figure 24.4) and by a recent report by McGrath et al. (1980) that some of these monoclonal antibodies against a mouse T lymphoma inhibit this tumor's proliferation. Their experiments indicate the antibodies block cell surface viral receptors. This result does not exclude the possibility that the antibodies may be reacting with a cell surface receptor and mimicking the effect of a hormone or other molecule which plays a normal role in the control of cellular differentiation.

The use of the cell line Reh is advantageous because these cells reportedly can differentiate along the B cell-T cell pathway (Lau et al., 1979), and therefore should allow us to see if any of the antibodies which inhibit proliferation also induce the cells to differentiate.

Neurofibromatosis as a Model for the Genetics of Malignancy

Another system with great potential for probing the molecular genetic basis of malignancy is provided by the dominant genetic disease, neurofibromatosis (NF) (Kennett et al., 1980d; Fienman and Yacovac, 1970). This is a common (1/3000 births) genetic disease characterized by various symptoms which appear to result from localized hyperplasia, usually affecting cells of neural crest origin (Bolande, 1974). Individuals with NF manifest symptoms indicating that there may be an abnormality which under certain undefined conditions affects the control of non-malignant cell proliferation, and also show a significant increase in the incidence of certain malignancies. These observations appear to be consistent with Knudsen's (1977) model for the induction of malignancy involving two mutations, in this case a germ-line mutation responsible for NF and a second mutation responsible for the malignant cells which arise in the NF patient. Comparison of the cell surface determinants on cells from NF patients to those on normal cells may define a cell surface change

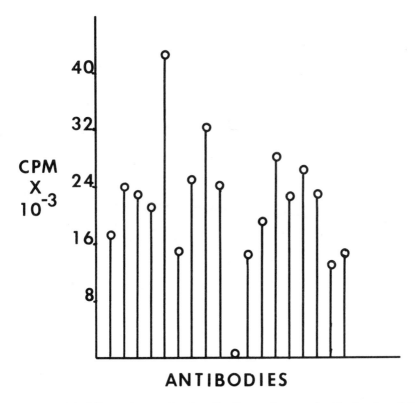

ANTIBODIES

Figure 24.4. Effects of monoclonal antibodies on the growth of leukemia cell line Reh. 10^5 cells in 100 μl of RPMI 1640 with 20% heat inactivated fetal bovine serum were placed in each well of a round-bottomed 96-well microplate. 100 μl of spent hybridoma supernatant containing monoclonal antibodies was added to each well. One day later, 50 μl of ^{3}H-thymidine (1.25 μCi) were added. After incubation overnight, the cultures were harvested and the extent of proliferation measured by the amount of ^{3}H-thymiidine incorporated into TCA precipitable material. Samples were tested in quadruplicate. Results show that some of the hybridoma supernatants appear to inhibit Reh cell proliferation, and further tests of those are in progress.

resulting from the dominant NF mutation. The relatively large number of tumor samples available from NF patients offer the opportunity to use immunochemical and biochemical procedures to define the molecular changes that take place when a tumor is induced by a second mutation. In any case, this dominant genetic disease which appears to affect the control of cell proliferation provides a system from which useful information regarding the role of cell surface molecules in growth control may be obtained.

In our first attempt to produce monoclonal antibodies that react with NF but not normal cells, we obtained antibodies that react with the immunizing NF cells but not normal fibroblasts (Figure 24.5). Whether these antibodies

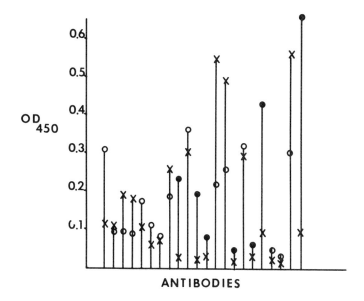

ANTIBODIES

Figure 24.5. Reaction of monoclonal antibodies made against neurofibromatosis fibroblasts MEF against MEF(○,●) and normal fibroblasts MRC-5(X). Monoclonal antibodies were made by fusing spleen cells from a BALB/c mouse immunized with MEF fibroblasts with the plasmacytoma SP2/0 Ag-14 (Shulman et al., 1978). 223 of 596 wells had hybrids. 161 of these made antibodies reacting with MEF fibroblasts. These antibodies were tested for binding to MEF and to a normal fibroblast, MRC-5 using an immunoperoxidase binding assay. The amount of peroxidase conjugated anti-mouse Ig bound was measured by detecting the amount of enzyme activity using orthophenyldiamine as a soluble substrate. This reaction produces a yellow product which is quantitated by reading the OD 450 mu. Data shown is representative of the 161 samples tested. Samples with MRC-5 had twice as many cells as MEF, so most antibodies showed more binding in the MRC-5 samples than in MEF samples. Those which showed significant binding to MEF and not to MRC-5 were considered to be against NF specific or polymorphic determinants, and were selected for further study. These are indicated by the closed circles (●).

really do react with "NF specific antigens" or are simply directed against human polymorphic determinants remains to be defined.

Summary

We have outlined several ways in which monoclonal antibodies have been used to study cell surface changes in malignancy, and suggested other promising applications. Whether the initial events which induce malignancy result in the expression of tumor specific antigens or the loss of a gene product, the technical advances made possible by Kohler and Milstein's introduction of monoclonal antibodies will certainly facilitate exploration of the structure and composition of malignant and normal cell surfaces. These studies will certainly help to elucidate both the changes associated with malignancy and the molecular events involved in normal processes of cellular differentiation.

ACKNOWLEDGMENTS
We want to thank Jeannie B. Hass, Barbara Meyer, Sue Hufnagel, and Marian Butts for their excellent technical assistance.

References

Barnstable, C.J., Bodmer, W.F., Brown, G., Galfre, G., Milstein, C., Williams, A.F., and Ziegler, A. (1978) Production of monoclonal antibodies to group A erythrocytes, HLA, and other human cell surface antigens—new tools for genetic analysis. *Cell* 14:9–20.

Bernstein, I.D., Tam, M.R., and Nowinski, R.C. (1980) Mouse leukemia: therapy with monoclonal antibodies against a thymus differentiation antigen. *Science* 207:68–71.

Bolande, R.P. (1974) The neurocristopathies: a unifying concept of disease arising in neural crest maldevelopment. *Human Pathol.* 5:109–429.

Bradstock, K.F., Janossy, G., Pizzolo, G., Hoffbrand, A.F., McMichael, A., Pilch, J.R., Milstein, C., Beverley, P., and Bollam, F.J. (1980) Subpopulations of normal and leukemia human thymocytes: an analysis with the use of monoclonal antibodies. *J. Natl. Canc. Inst.* 65:33–42.

Brown, J.P., Wright, P.W., Hart, C.E., Woodbury, R.G., Hellstrom, K.E., and Hellstrom, I. (1980) Protein antigens of normal and malignant human cells identified by precipitation with monoclonal antibodies. *J. Biol. Chem.* 255:4980–4983.

Brown, S., Dilley, J., and Levy, R. (1980) Immunoglobulin secretion by mouse x human hybridomas: an approach for the production of anti-idiotype reagents useful in monitoring patients with B cell leukemia. *J. Immunol.* 125:1037–1043.

Brunson, K.W. and Nicholson, G.L. (1978) Selection and biologic properties of malignant variants of a murine lymphosarcoma. *J. Natl. Cancer Inst.* 61:1499–1503.

Carrel, S., Accolla, R.S., Carmagnola, A.L., and Mach, J-P. (1980) Common human melanoma-associated antigen(s) detected by monoclonal antibodies. *Cancer Res.* 40:2523–2528.

Croce, C. (1980) Hybridomas to study viral and tumor antigens and human genetics. In *Monoclonal Antibodies in Endocrine Research*. Fellows, R. and Eisenbarth, G. (eds.), New York: Raven Press. In press.

Evans, A.E. and Hummeler, K. (1973) The significance of primative cells in marrow aspirates of children with neuroblastomas. *Cancer* 4:906–912.

Fidler, I.J. and Kripke, M.L. (1977) Metastasis results from pre-existing variant cells within a malignant tumor. *Science* 197:893–895.

Fienman, N.L. and Yakovac, W.C. (1970) Neurofibromatosis in childhood. *J. Pediatrics* 76:339–346.

Gomez, C.M., Richman, D., Berman, P.W., Burres, S.A., Arnason, B.G.W., and Fitch, F.W. (1979) Monoclonal antibodies against purified nicotinic acetylcholine receptor. *Biochem. and Biophys. Res. Commun.* 88:575–582.

Greaves, M.F., Verbi, N., Kemshed, A., and Kennett, R. (1980) A monoclonal antibody identifying a cell surface antigen shared by common acute lymphoblastic leukemias and B lineage cells. *Blood.* In press.

Greene, G.L., Fitch, F.W., and Jensen, E.V. (1980) Monoclonal antibodies to estrophilin: probes for the study of estrogen receptors. *Proc. Natl. Acad. Sci.* 77:157–161.

Grimm, E. and Fox, C.F. (1980) Precipitation at the EGF receptor using hybridoma antibodies. In *Monoclonal Antibodies in Endocrine Research*. Fellows, R. and Eisenbarth, G. (eds.), New York: Raven Press. In press.

Herlyn, D., Steplewski, Z., Herlyn, M., and Koprowski, H. (1980) Inhibition of growth of colorectal carcinoma in nude mice by monoclonal antibody. *Cancer Res.* 40:717–721.

Imai, K., Molinaro, G.A., and Ferrone, S. (1980) Monoclonal antibodies to melanoma-associated antigens. *Transplant. Proc. XII*:380–383.

Jonak, Z.L. (1980) Peroxidase-conjugated antiglobulin method for visual detection of cell-surface antigens. In *Monoclonal Antibodies: Hybridomas: a New Dimension in Biological Analyses*. Kennett, R.H., McKearn, T.J., and Bechtol, K.B. (eds.), New York: Plenum Press, pp. 378–380.

Kahn, C.R., Baird, K., Flier, J.S., and Jarrett, D.B. (1977) Effects of auto-antibodies to the insulin receptor on isolated adipocytes. *J. Clin. Invest.* 60:1094–1106.

Kasuga, M., Akanoma, Y., Tsushima, T., Suzoki, K., Kosaka, K., and Kebata, M. (1978) Effects of anti-insulin receptor autoantibody on the metabolism of rat adipocytes. *J. Clin. Endocrinol. and Metab.* 47:66–77.

Kennett, R.H. (1980a) Enzyme-linked antibody assay with cells attached to polyvinyl chloride plates. In *Monoclonal Antibodies: Hybridomas: a New Dimension in Biological Analyses*. Kennett, R.H., McKearn, T.J., and Bechtol, K.B. (eds.), New York: Plenum Press, pp. 376–377.

Kennett, R.H. (1980b) Microcytotoxicity assay. In *Monoclonal Antibodies: Hybridomas: a New Dimension in Biological Analyses*. Kennett, R.H., McKearn, T.J., and Bechtol, K.B. (eds.), New York: Plenum Press, pp. 391–392.

Kennett, R.H. and Gilbert, F. (1979) Hybrid myelomas producing antibodies against a human neuroblastoma antigen present on fetal brain. *Science* 203:1120–1121.

Kennett, R.H., Denis, K.A., Tung, A.S., and Klinman, N.R. (1978) Hybrid plasmacytoma production: fusions with adult spleen cells, monoclonal spleen fragments, neonatal spleen cells, and human spleen cells. *Curr. Top. Microbiol. Immunol.* 81:77–91.

Kennett, R.H., Jonak, Z.L., and Bechtol, K.B. (1980a) Monoclonal antibodies against human tumor-associated antigens. In *Monoclonal Antibodies: Hybridomas: a New Dimension in Biological Analyses*. Kennett, R.H., McKearn, T.J., and Bechtol, K.B. (eds.), New York: Plenum Press, pp. 155–168.

Kennett, R.H., Jonak, Z.L., and Eager, K.B. (1980b) Monoclonal antibodies and cell surface differentiation. In *Monoclonal Antibodies in Endocrine Research*. Fellows, R. and Eisenbarth, G. (eds.), New York: Raven Press.

Kennett, R.H., Jonak, Z.L., and Bechtol, K.B. (1980c) Characterization of antigens with monoclonal antibodies. In *Advances in Neuroblastoma Research*. Evans, A. (ed.), New York: Raven Press, pp. 209–219.

Kennett, R.H., Jonak, Z.L., Meyer, B.E., and Bechtol, K.B. (1980d) Monoclonal antibodies as tools for analyzing neurofibromatosis and other genetic diseases. In *Neurofibromatosis*. Mulvihill, J.J. and Riccadi, V. (eds.), New York: Raven Press. In press.

Knudson, A.G. (1977) Genetics and etiology of cancer. *Arch. Hum. Genet.* 8:1–16.

Kohler, G. and Milstein, C. (1975) Continuous cultures of fused cells secreting antibody of predefined specificity. *Nature* 256:495–497.

Koprowski, H., Steplewski, Z., Herlyn, D., and Herlyn, M. (1978) Study of antibodies against human melanoma produced by somatic cell hybrids. *Proc. Natl. Acad. Sci. U.S.A.* 75:3405–3409.

Koprowski, H., Steplewski, Z., Mitchell, K., Herlyn, M., Herlyn, D., and Fuhrer, P. (1979) Colorectal carcinoma antigens detected by hybridoma antibodies. *Som. Cell. Genet.* 5:957–972.

Lau, B., Jager, G., Thiel, E., Rodt, H., Huhn, D., Pachmann, K., Netzel, B., Boning, L., Thierfelder, S., and Dormer, P. (1979) Growth of the Reh cell line in diffusion chamber. *Scand. J. Hematol.* 23:285–292.

Levine, G., Balloo, B., Reiland, J., Solter, D., Gumerman, L., and Hakala, T. (1980) Localization of I-131-labeled tumor-specific monoclonal antibody in the tumor-bearing BALB/c mouse. *J. Nucl. Med.* 21:370–573.

Levy, R., Dilley, J., Fox, R.J., and Warnke, R. (1979) A human thymus leukemia antigen defined by hybridoma monoclonal antibodies. *Proc. Natl. Acad. Sci. U.S.A.* 76:6552–6556.

McGrath, M.S., Pillemer, E., and Weissman, I.L. (1980) Murine leukemogenesis monoclonal antibodies to T cell determinants arrest T lymphoma cell proliferation. *Nature* 285:259–261.

Momoi, M., Kennett, R.H., and Glick, M.C. (1980) A membrane glycoprotein from human neuroblastoma cells isolated with the use of monoclonal antibody. *J. Biol. Chem.* 255:11914–11921.

Nadler, L.M., Staslenko, P., Hardy, R., Kaplan, W.D., Button, L.N., Kufe, D.W., Aritman, K.H., and Schlossman, S.F. (1980) Serotherapy of a patient with a monoclonal antibody directed against a human lymphoma-associated antigen. *Cancer Res.* 40:3147–3154.

Olson, L. and Kaplan, H.S. (1980) Human-human hybridomas producing monoclonal antibodies of predefined antigenic specificity. *Proc. Natl. Acad. Sci. U.S.A.* 77:5429–5431.

Raizada, M. and Fellows, R. (1980) Monoclonal antibodies to insulin receptor. In *Monoclonal Antibodies in Endocrine Research*. Fellows, R. and Eisenbarth, G. (eds.), New York: Raven Press. In press.

Ritz, J., Pesando, J.M., McConarty, J.N., Lazarus, H., and Schlossman, S.F. (1980) A monoclonal antibody to human acute lymphoblastic leukemia antigen. *Nature* 283:583–585.

Rosenfeld, C., Vanuat, A.M., Goutner, A., Guegang, J., Choquet, C., Tron, F., and Pico, J.L. (1975) An exceptional cell line established from a patient with acute lymphoid leukemia. *Proc. Assoc. Canc. Res.* 16:1075.

Ruddon, R.W. (ed.) (1978) *Biological Markers of Neoplasia: Basic and Applied Aspects*. New York: Elsevier/North Holland.

Ruoslahti, E., Hayman, E.G., and Engvall, E. (1980) Fibronectin. In *Cancer Markers*. Sell, S. (ed.), Clifton, New Jersey: Humana Press, pp. 485–505.

Sell, S. (1980) *Cancer Markers, Diagnostic and Developmental Significance*. Clifton, New Jersey: Humana Press.

Shulman, M., Wilde, C.D., and Kohler, G. (1978) A better cell line for making hybridomas secreting specific antibodies. *Nature* 276:269–270.

Solomon, E. and Jones, E.A. (1980) Monoclonal antibodies as tools for human genetic analysis. In *Monoclonal Antibodies: a New Dimension in Biological Analyses*. Kennett, R.H., McKearn, T.J., and Bechtol, K.B. (eds.), New York: Plenum Press, pp. 75–102.

Steplewski, Z. (1980) Monoclonal antibodies to human tumor antigens. *Transplant. Proc. XII*:384–387.

Steplewski, Z., Herlyn, M., Herlyn, D., Clark, W., and Koprowski, H. (1979) Reactivity of monoclonal anti-melanoma antibodies with melanoma cells freshly isolated from primary and metastatic malanoma. *Eur. J. Immunol.* 9:94–96.

Tzartos, S.J. and Lindstrom, J.M. (1980) Monoclonal antibodies used to probe acetylcholine receptor structures; localization of the main immunogenic region and detection of similarities between subunits. *Proc. Natl. Acad. Sci.* 77:755–759.

Venter, J. and Fraser, C. (1980) Monoclonal antibodies to B-adrenegic receptors: use in receptor purification and characterization. In *Monoclonal Antibodies in Endocrine Research*. Fellows, R. and Eisenbarth, G. (eds.), New York: Raven Press. In press.

CHAPTER 25

Immunoglobulin Idiotypes, Allotypes, and Isotypes as Probes for Analysis of B Cell Differentiation[1]

Alexander R. Lawton*, Hiromi Kubagawa, William E. Gathings, and Max D. Cooper

Departments of Pediatrics and Microbiology, Vanderbilt University School of Medicine and Cellular Immunobiology Unit, Lurleen B. Wallace Tumor Institute, Departments of Pediatrics and Microbiology, University of Alabama in Birmingham, Alabama

Introduction

Progress in science and in medicine is always a continuum, with each new observation resting on earlier ones. Nevertheless, it is often possible to identify key observations which initiate quantum leaps in an established area, or open entirely new areas of investigation. In the field of B cell differentiation, the rediscovery by Pernis et al. (1970) and Raff (1970) that a subset of lymphocytes in rabbits and mice bore immunologloglobulins on their cell membranes easily detectable by immunofluorescence represents such a landmark. Möller (1961) had made the same observation 9 years earlier; perhaps its impact was lost because cellular immunology was not yet in vogue. Immunoglobulin spots or caps were reported to mark a population of lymphocytes distinct from those bearing the θ antigen (now Thy 1) in mice (Raff, 1971) or capable of binding sheep erythrocytes at low temperature in humans (Jondal et al., 1972). The terms B cells and T cells were coined to refer to lineages previously known to be distinct only through association of their development with different central lymphoid organs. Within a very short time, these simple techniques were used to identify a subset of acute lymphoblastic leukemia of children as belonging to the T cell lineage (Kersey et al., 1975) and to classify the majority of cases of chronic lymphocytic leukemia in adults as monoclonal proliferations of B lymphocytes (Preud'homme and Seligman, 1972). The central concept emerging from these observations—that cell lineages and differentiation stages within lineages having distinct functions are marked by their expressions of

[1]Research from the authors' laboratories was supported by USPHS-NIH Grants AI 11502, CA 16673, and the March of Dimes 1-608 and 1-625.

sets of cell-membrane "differentiation" antigens (Boyse et al., 1971)—has been singularly important in illuminating the workings of the immune system. It has also made possible development of new and much more precise classifications of human lymphoid malignancies and provided the means for relating malignancies to specific stages of normal lymphoid development.

This review will focus on one system of differentiation antigens—the immunoglobulin molecules expressed by B cells. We will describe how expression of different immunoglobulin gene products has been used to develop information on normal differentiation of this cell line and on the pathogenics of a B cell malignancy which appears to encompass all of the stages of clonal B cell development.

Isotypes, Idiotypes, and Allotypes

The diversity and multichain structure of immunoglobulin molecules have provided an extraordinarily powerful set of tools for analysis of differentiation pathways of the B cells which produce these proteins. Three terms are used to define different facets of immunoglobulin diversity. Isotype refers to the heavy chain class of immunoglobulins; the different isotypes, of which there are 9 in humans, are encoded by a family of closely linked genes (C_H) which determine approximately 3/4 of the carboxy-terminal end of heavy chains, called the constant region. The term idiotype defines unique antigenic determinants associated with the variable regions of immunoglobulin light and heavy chains, which are encoded by separate genes. Anti-idiotypic antibodies are generally produced by heterologous immunization with a monoclonal immunoglobulin, such as a myeloma protein. By absorption with normal immunoglobulin, the antiserum can be made specific for V region determinants of the immunizing protein. Such reagents can then be used to identify the immunoglobulin product of a particular B cell clone, or a family of clones having closely related V region structures. Immunoglobulin genes also exhibit polymorphic variations, or allotypy. Allotypic variants have been identified in heavy and light chain constant regions of man, mouse, and rabbit. In rabbits there are also allotypes associated with the heavy chain V regions.

Early Events of B Cell Differentiation

The significance of the stepwise developmental sequence of B cells can best be appreciated by consideration of the "goals" of this process. The specificity of an antibody depends upon the shape, dimensions, and charge characteristics of a combining site formed by interaction of its V_H and V_L regions. The variety of combining sites which may be formed—thought to number between 10^6 and 10^8—is a function of the genetically encoded diversity of V regions and the possibility that a given V_H may form different combining sites depending upon with which V_L it is associated. The selectivity of the immune response arises from the clonal nature of the lymphoid system. Each clone of lymphocytes expresses only one of all of the possible V_H and V_L combinations, first in the form of a membrane bound receptor, and at later stages of differentiation, as a secreted antibody.

The first "goal" of B cell development is to ensure that most or all of the potential specificity repertoire present in the genome becomes expressed in a clonal fashion on B cells. A second diversification process follows clonal development. By mechanisms which are just beginning to be understood, clonal precursors initially expressing IgM generate progeny which synthesize antibody molecules of each of the other heavy chain classes. This process of isotype switching involves no change in clonal specificity, since the light chain and the heavy chain V region expressed remain constant. This switch is accomplished by translocation of structural genes encoding a V region from a position near the μ chain structural gene to a site close to a new C_H gene (Davis et al., 1980; Sakano et al., 1980).

The first recognizable cell of the B lineage is called the pre-B cell. Pre-B cells were initially identified in mouse fetal liver, where they preceded development of B lymphocytes by several days (Raff et al., 1976). Pre-B cells have several distinguishing characteristics, the most important being that they synthesize intracytoplasmic μ chains but lack detectable cell surface immunoglobulin (Cooper et al., 1977; Burrows et al., 1979; Levitt and Cooper, 1980). This feature permits pre-B cells and B cells to be rather easily distinguished by immunofluorescence. Cell suspensions containing a mixture of the two cell types are first stained in the viable state with fluorescein-labeled anti-μ antibodies, then fixed and stained with rhodamine-labeled anti-μ. The surface immunoglobulin of B lymphocytes is stained both red and green, while pre-B cells are stained only with rhodamine.

Early studies on the ontogeny and tissue distribution of pre-B cells suggested that they play an important role in clonal development. In humans and rabbits, as well as mice, this cell type appeared in fetal liver prior to development of sIg$^+$ lymphocytes (Gathings et al., 1977; Hayward et al., 1978). In adults, pre-B cells were found only in bone marrow, an organ known to be the site of B cell generation. Studies of growth kinetics *in vivo* and *in vitro* indicated an additional important difference between pre-B cells and their B lymphocyte progeny. Large pre-B cells were labeled with ^{3}H-thymidine at a rate consistent with a cell-cycle time of 8–12 hours, while small pre-B cells and sIg$^+$ B lymphocytes rarely incorporated thymidine during a 24-hour labeling period (Owen et al., 1977).

Mice treated from birth with antibodies to μ chains lack B lymphocytes, plasma cells, and the capacity to generate antibody responses (Lawton et al., 1973). We found equal frequencies of pre-B cells in bone marrow of adult anti-μ treated mice and controls, reinforcing the idea that pre-B cells lack surface immunoglobulin receptors. Cultures of bone marrow cells from these animals generated sIg$^+$ B lymphocytes which could be stimulated by bacterial lipopolysaccharide to generate plasma cells of all isotypes. Cultures of spleen cells, which lacked both pre-B cells and sIg$^+$ lymphocytes, did not give rise to sIg$^+$ cells (Burrows et al., 1978). These experiments provide the best evidence available that pre-B cells are the direct progenitors of sIg$^+$ lymphocytes.

Role of Pre-B Cells in Generation of Diversity

B lymphocytes from fetal or neonatal animals are clonally diverse, although not to the same extent as lymphocytes from mature animals. To ascertain the role of pre-B cells in generation of diversity, we did a series of studies to determine which of the various immunoglobulin genes their cells express.

Antibodies to kappa chain constant region allotypes were used to determine whether pre-B cells from allotype-heterozygous rabbits exhibit allelic exclusion. It was found that all of the cells which stained for allotype expressed one or the other, but not both, alleles. In these studies, we failed to appreciate what may be a very important characteristic of the biology of pre-B cells—the fact that the majority of these cells, and in particular the large, rapidly dividing pre-B cells, do not express light chains at all. Burrows et al. (1979) generated a number of pre-B cell hybridomas by fusing mouse fetal liver with a non-producer plasmacytoma. These hybridomas contained cytoplasmic μ chains, but lacked both light chains and cell surface immunoglobulin. Levitt and Cooper (1980) demonstrated by biosynthetic labeling that pre-B cells from normal mouse fetal liver synthesized μ but not light chains. This conclusion has been supported by the recent demonstration that light chain genes from several of the pre-B cell hybridomas are present in embryonic forms; the V-J translocation to form a light chain transcription unit has not occurred (Maki et al., 1980).

Two approaches to the central question of whether pre-B cells express V_H genes have been taken. Gathings et al. (1981) have recently studied the expression of a allotypes in rabbit pre-B cells. These polymorphic determinants are associated with all heavy chain isotypes and serve as general V_H markers. It was found that pre-B cells express a allotypes together with $C\mu$. In $a2a3$ heterozygous animals, bone marrow pre-B cells express one of the other allotypes in a $1:1$ ratio. The latter observation was particularly interesting in light of the consistent $\sim 3:2$ ratio of $a3$ to $a2$ among serum immunoglobulin molecules or on the surface of B lymphocytes. Establishing the "pecking order" of allotypes thus appears to be a selective process acting on a cell beyond the pre-B stage.

The second approach to the question of V_H expression in pre-B cells involved studies of patients with multiple myeloma (Kubagawa et al., 1979), the results of which are summarized in the following section.

Clonal Origin of Multiple Myeloma

In recent years, several groups have observed that a high proportion of circulating lymphocytes from patients with multiple myeloma react with antibodies to idiotypic determinants of the homologous myeloma protein (Mellstedt et al., 1974; Abdou and Abdou, 1975; Preud'homme et al., 1977). It was therefore reasonable to ask whether pre-B cells from patients might also express the myeloma idiotype. Monoclonal proteins, one IgAκ and one IgAλ, were isolated fom the serum of two patients and used for immunization and to prepare solid immunoabsorbent columns. Anti-idiotypic antibodies were prepared by absorption of sera with a variety of myeloma proteins and normal immunoglobulins, and then purified by elution from the homologous immunoabsorbent. The specificity of anti-idiotypic antibodies was confirmed by inhibition radioimmunoassay and by direct hemagglutination. In both assays, end points for homologous binding were on the order of one million-fold greater than those for binding to unrelated proteins, including IgA myelomas having the same light chains and V_H subgroups. Both reagents recognized free homologous α chains with ~100-fold less sensitivity than intact proteins.

Despite their exquisite specificity in serological assays, fluorochrome conjugates of the anti-Ids reacted with 0.5–1% of B lymphocytes, a frequency far in excess of that predicted for a unique B cell clone. Portions of each anti-Id were therefore reabsorbed by several passages over a column containing a large excess of normal gammaglobulin. This procedure yielded two populations of anti-idiotypic antibodies: one recognizing determinants of a family of related clones with cross-reactive idiotypes (IdX), and a second which recognized ⩽0.03% of B lymphocytes from normal donors, called individually-specific anti-idiotype (IdIn).

By using anti-Ids in conjunction with antibodies to heavy chain isotypes labeled with a different fluorochrome, we attempted to define various stages of differentiation of the myelomatous clones. Figure 25.1 shows representative results obtained with peripheral blood and bone marrow cells from one of the patients. The principal observations in the other patient were similar.

Pre-B cells were present in the patient's marrow in about 1/3 normal frequency. Of these, more than 30% were Id$^+$. The proportion of Id$^+$ pre-B cells was approximately the same with either the anti-IdX or anti-IdIn antibodies. The frequency of Id$^+$ pre-B cells in samples of normal bone marrow was <.003%.

In this patient, the frequency of sIg$^+$ cells among total lymphocytes was ~1.5%, or about 15% of normal. In the experiment shown, 22% of these cells stained with anti-IdX, while 7% stained with IdIn. Idiotype was detected by either reagent on each of the major B lymphocyte classes. However, the IdIn idiotype was expressed on a much higher frequency of sIgA$^+$ cells (11%) than of cells bearing other isotypes (1.6–5.4%). As indicated earlier, B lymphocytes from normal individuals stained only with anti-IdX. These determinants were

354

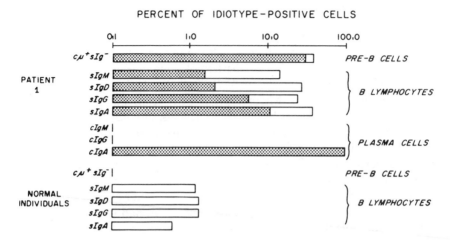

Figure 25.1. Frequency of idiotypic markers among pre-B cells, B lymphocytes, and plasma cells of a patient with IgA myeloma. The open bars indicate percentages of cells with the indicated phenotype which reacted with anti-IdX; closed bars show frequencies obtained with anti-IdIn. Note that a $\log_{10}$ scale is used. Mean frequencies of B lymphocytes from 6 normal individuals reactive with anti-IdX are also shown. Anti-IdIn reacted with <.03% of normal B lymphocytes. The data are representative of several experiments on this patient, performed at different times. Similar results were obtained on another patient. Details of this study are reported elsewhere (Kubagawa et al., Details of this study are reported elsewhere (Kubagawa et al., 1979).

found in approximately equal frequency (0.6–1.3%) on cells bearing each isotype.

All Id$^+$ plasma cells contained IgA, and 99% of IgA$^+$ plasma cells co-stained for idiotype. These results were identical whether idiotype was detected with anti-IdX or anti-IdIn.

Anti-IdX used in these experiments clearly recognizes a family of related B cell clones; anti-IdIn detects a much more restricted population which may be identical to the unique myeloma clone. One of the more interesting results of this study is the observation that among circulating B cells of myeloma patients, there is a greatly expanded population of cells bearing idiotypes related to, but not identical with the specific myeloma idiotype. In the representative experiment shown, 22% of the patient's B lymphocytes were IdX$^+$ and 7% IdIn$^+$. Fifteen percent thus belonged to the related but not identical population. Only this population was seen among normal B lymphocytes, but in 10-fold lower frequency. Furthermore, this population was seen only among B lymphocytes; neither among pre-B cells nor among plasma cells was there a significant difference in the frequency of IdX$^+$ vs IdIn expression. There is evidence in animals that injection of anti-Id can result in expansion of a family of Id$^+$ B cell clones, and that antigen-priming can induce idiotypically related clones which lack specificity for antigen (Cazenave et al., 1974;

Eichmann et al., 1977). A network interaction (Jerne, 1974) based on induction of auto-anti-idiotypic antibodies may be responsible for the phenomenon we have observed.

These data argue strongly that the oncogenic process which culminates in myeloma has its onset at the earliest stage in B cell development. There is clear precedent for this concept in certain myeloproliferative diseases in humans. Polycythemia vera involves a clonal proliferation of erythroid, myeloid, and megakaryocytic lines originating from a common stem cell (Adamson et al., 1976). Chronic myelogenous leukemia apparently results from transformation of an even more primative stem cell, since myeloid, erythroid, megakaryocytic, and B lymphoid cells share a clonal marker (Fialkow et al., 1977, 1978; Janossy et al., 1976; Vogler et al., 1978). Relapse in this disease has involved cells marked by the Ph_1 chromosome but having the phenotypic characteristics of pre-B cells. It will be most interesting to determine whether other clonal proliferations of B cells, such as chronic lymphocytic leukemia, Waldenström's macroglobulinemia, and benign monoclonal gammopathy, also originate at the pre-B stage of development.

Conclusions

We have briefly discussed the implications of the myeloma study on the pathogenesis of this disease. We will conclude by mentioning some of the implications for normal B cell development. First, this data indicates that pre-B cells express V_H determinants, a conclusion recently verified by analysis of μ genes in pre-B cell hybridomas (Maki et al., 1980). Secondly, pre-B cells have been established as a part of a clonal lineage which includes all of the morphologically defined stages of B cell differentiation, and among B lymphocytes, members expressing each of the major isotypes. This information makes it extremely unlikely that pre-B cells represent an aberrant offshoot from the major pathway of B cell development. Finally, the data raise some intriguing questions with regard to the regulation of isotype switching. At what stage of differentiation, and by what mechanism, is commitment of IgA (or IgG) established?

ACKNOWLEDGMENTS
We thank Ms. Carolyn Kosser for preparation of the manuscript.

References

Abdou, N.I. and Abdou, N.L. (1975) The monoclonal nature of lymphocytes in multiple myeloma: effect of therapy. *Am. Intern. Med.* 83:42.

Adamson, J.W., Fialkow, P.J., Murphy, S., Prchal, J.F., and Steinmann, L. (1976) Polycytemia vera: stem cell and probably clonal origin of the disease. *New Engl. J. Med.* 295:913.

Boyse, E.A., Old, L.J., and Scheid, M. (1971) Selective gene action in the specification of cell surface structure. *Amer. J. Path.* 65:439–450.

Burrows, P.D., Kearney, J.F., Lawton, A.R., and Cooper, M.D. (1978) Pre-B cells: bone marrow persistence in anti-μ suppressed mice, conversion to B lymphocytes, and recovery following destruction by cyclophosphamide. *J. Immunol.* 120:1526–1531.

Burrows, P., Lejeune, M., and Kearney, J.F. (1979) Evidence that murine pre-B cells synthesize μ heavy chains but no light chains. *Nature* 280:838.

Cazenave, P-A., Ternynk, T., and Avrameas, S. (1974) Similar idiotypes in antibody-forming cells and in cells synthesizing immunoglobulins without detectable antibody function. *Proc. Natl. Acad. Sci. U.S.A.* 71:4500.

Cooper, M.D., Moretta, L., Webb, S.R., Pearl, E.R., Okos, A.J., and Lawton, A.R. (1977) Studies of generation of B cell diversity in mouse, man, and chicken. *Cold Spring Harbor Symp. Quant. Biol.* 41:139–145.

Davis, M.M., Stuart, K.K., and Hood, L.E. (1980) DNA sequences mediating class switching in α-immunoglobulins. *Science* 209:1360.

Eichmann, K., Coutinho, A., and Melchers, F. (1977) Absolute frequencies of lipopolysaccharide-reactive B cells producing A_5A idiotype in unprimed, streptococcal A-carbohydrate-primed, anti-A_5A idiotype-sensitized, and anti-A_5A idiotype-suppressed A/J mice. *J. Exp. Med.* 146:1436.

Fialkow, P.J., Jacobson, R.J., and Papyannopoulou, T. (1977) Chronic myelocytic leukemia: clonal origin in a stem cell common to the granulocyte, erythrocyte, platelet, and monocyte/macrophage. *Am. J. Med.* 63:125.

Fialkow, P.J., Denman, A.M., Jacobson, R.J., and Lowenthal, M.N. (1978) Chronic myelocytic leukemia: origin of some lymphocytes from leukemic stem cells. *J. Clin. Invest.* 62:815.

Gathings, W.E., Lawton, A.R., and Cooper, M.D. (1977) Immunofluorescent studies on the development of pre-B cells, B lymphocytes, and immunoglobulin isotype diversity in humans. *Eur. J. Immunol.* 7:804–810.

Gathings, W.E., Mage, R.G., Cooper, M.D., Lawton, A.R., and Young-Cooper, G.O. (1981) Immunofluorescent studies on the expression of V_H *a* allotypes by pre-B and B cells in homozygous and heterozygous rabbits. *Eur. J. Immunol.*, in press.

Hayward, A.R., Simons, M.A., Lawton, A.R., Mage, R.G., and Cooper, M.D. (1978) Pre-B and B cells in rabbits: ontogeny and allelic exclusion of kappa light chain genes. *J. Exp. Med.* 148:1367–1377.

Janossy, G., Greaves, M.F., Revesz, T., Lister, T.A., Roberts, M., Durrant, J., Kirk, B., Catovsky, D., and Beard, M.E.J. (1976) Blast crisis of chronic myeloid leukemia (CML). II. Cell surface marker analysis of "lymphoid" and myeloid cases. *Br. J. Haematol.* 34:179.

Jerne, N.K. (1974) Towards a network theory of the immune system. *Ann. Immunol.* (Paris) 125:373.

Jondal, M., Holm, G., and Wigzell, H. (1972) Surface markers on human T and B lymphocytes. I. A large population of lymphocytes forming non-immune rosettes with sheep red blood cells. *J. Exp. Med.* 136:207.

Kersey, J., Nesbit, M., Hallgren, H., Sabad, A., Yunis, E., and Gajl-Peczalska, K. (1975) Evidence for origin of certain childhood acute lymphoblastic leukemias and lymphomas in thymus-derived lymphocytes. *Cancer* 36:1348–1352.

Kubagawa, H., Vogler, L.B., Capra, J.D., Conrad, M.E., Lawton, A.R., and Cooper, M.D. (1979) Studies on the clonal origin of multiple myeloma. Use of individually specific (idiotype) antibodies to trace the oncogenic event to its earliest point of expression in B cell differentiation. *J. Exp. Med.* 150:792–807.

Lawton, A.R., Asofsky, R.M., Davie, J.M., and Hylton, M.B. (1973) Suppression of immunoglobulin synthesis in mice: age dependence of anti-μ suppression and effects of anti (γ1 + γ2) and anti-α. *Fed. Prod.* (Abstract) 32:1012.

Levitt, D. and Cooper, M.D. (1980) Mouse pre-B cells synthesize and secrete μ heavy chains but not light chains. *Cell* 19:617–625.

Maki, R., Kearney, J., Paige, C., and Tonegawa, S. (1980) Immunoglobulin gene rearrangement in immature B cells. *Science* 209:1366.

Mellstedt, H., Hammarström, S., and Holm, G. (1974) Monoclonal lymphocyte population in human plasma cells myeloma. *Clin. Exp. Immunol.* 17:371.

Möller, G. (1961) Demonstration of mouse isoantigens at the cellular level by the fluorescent antibody technique. *J. Exp. Med.* 114:415–432.

Owen, J.J.T., Wright, D.E., Habu, S., Raff, M.C., and Cooper, M.D. (1977) Studies on the generation of B lymphocytes in fetal liver and bone marrow. *J. Immunol.* 118:2067.

Pernis, B., Forni, L., and Amante, L. (1970) Immunoglobulin spots on the surface of rabbit lymphocytes. *J. Exp. Med.* 132:1001–1018.

Preud'homme, J-L. and Seligmann, M. (1972) Surface bound immunoglobulins as a cell marker in human lymphoproliferative diseases. *Blood* 40:777–794.

Preud'homme, J-L., Klein, M. Laboume, S., and Seligmann, M. (1977) Idiotype-bearing and antigen-binding receptors produced by blood T lymphocytes in a case of human myeloma. *Eur. J. Immunol.* 7:840.

Raff, M.C. (1970) Two distinct populations of peripheral lymphocytes in mice distinguishable by immunofluorescence. *Immunology* 19:637–650.

Raff, M.C. (1971) Surface antigenic markers for distinguishing T and B lymphocytes in mice. *Transplant. Rev.* 6:52.

Raff, M.C., Megson, M., Owen, J.J.T., and Cooper, M.D. (1976) Early production of intracellular IgM by B lymphocyte precursors in mice. *Nature* 259:224–226.

Sakano, H., Maki, R., Kurosawa, T., Roeder, W., and Tonegawa, S. (1980) Two types of somatic recombination are necessary for the generation of complete immunoglobulin heavy chain genes. *Nature* 286:676.

Vogler, L.B., Crist, W.M., Vinson, P.C., Brattain, M.G., Sarrif, A.M., and Coleman, M.S. (1978) Philadelphia chromosome-positive pre-B cell leukemia presenting as blastic myelogenous leukemia. *Blood* 52:279.

Published 1981 by Elsevier North Holland, Inc.
Saunders, Daniels, Serrou, Rosenfeld, and Denney, eds.
FUNDAMENTAL MECHANISMS IN HUMAN CANCER IMMUNOLOGY

CHAPTER 26

Quantitation of Isotopic Immunoglobulin Therapy to Tumor Associated Proteins[1]

Stanley E. Order, Jerry L. Klein, David Ettinger,
Moody D. Wharam, Richard Humphrey,
Stanley S. Siegelman, John B. Garrison,
Robert E. Jenkins, John Wallace, and
Peter Leichner
*Divisions of Radiation Oncology, Radiation Immunology, Medical Oncology,
Diagnostic Radiology, Radiation Physics, and Applied Physics Laboratory,
The Johns Hopkins Hospital, Baltimore, Maryland*

Clinical investigators have become increasingly aware that tumor associated proteins, whether they are metabolic products like ferritin (Katz, 1973; Eshhar, 1974), oncofetal antigens like CEA (Gold, 1965), or hormones like HCG (Quinones, 1971), may be exploited for the production of clinically useful antibodies. When radiolabeled (Marchalonis, 1969), these antibodies can be used to scan for tumors containing targeted proteins (Goldenberg, 1978). Therapeutic applications, however, have been restricted by several obstacles, including (1) toxicity, (2) quantitation of dose at tumor sites, in normal tissue, and in the whole body, (3) quantitation of clinical response, (4) integration into conventional therapy, and (5) disciplined protocol development.

This report reviews progress in the use of ^{131}I-labeled antiferritin IgG for cancer therapy. Quantitation of dose distribution and clinical results to date are reported, and future clinical investigations presently under active study are outlined.

Materials and Methods

Antigens

Both ferritin and carcinoembryonic antigen were isolated and purified as previously reported (Katz, 1973; Eshhar, 1974; Gold, 1965; Ettinger, 1979; Order, 1976, 1980).

[1]Supported by National Cancer Institute, National Institute of Health CA-06973-18.

Antibody and Preparation

Production of antisera to ferritin and CEA was accomplished by immunizing New Zealand White rabbits with 100–200 micrograms of ferritin or CEA emulsified in complete Freund's adjuvant. This mixture was injected intradermally at four sites in the thigh, and the injections were repeated two weeks later. Fifty ml of blood were removed by sterile cardiac puncture after an additional two weeks. Samples were allowed to clot at room temperature for one hour, then refrigerated at 4° overnight to allow for clot retraction. The serum was removed under sterile conditions by centrifugation and frozen at $-20°$, after a sample was removed for testing. Additional bleedings were performed two weeks following booster injections.

The reactivity of the antisera was determined by immunoelectrophoresis on commercially prepared agarose plates. Four microliters of purified ferritin or CEA in phosphate buffer (1 mg/ml) were placed in the sample wells, and the agarose plate was activated by electrophoresis with ethylenediaminetetra-acetic acid (EDTA) barbitol buffer pH 8.6 at 15 volts/centimeter for 35 minutes. Forty microliters of antisera were placed in the trough, and the plate was incubated at 25° in a humidified chamber overnight to allow for immunodiffusion and the appearance of bands. The plates were then dialyzed overnight in 1% saline, followed by one hour in deionized water, and then were dried and stained with amido black.

Titration of Antisera

Antisera to CEA or ferritin was titrated by radioimmunoassay against the corresponding radiolabeled antigen. Purified antigen was labeled with ^{125}I using 100 microcuries of Bolton-Hunter reagent (Bolton, 1973) per 100 micrograms of protein. The labeled antigen was separated from free iodine on a prepacked PD-10, G25 column equilibrated with Dextrose Gelatin-Veronal buffer.

The antiserum to be titrated was serially diluted with phosphate buffered saline (PBS) containing 10% normal rabbit serum. Twenty-five microliters of diluted antiserum were added to 25 microliters of diluted labeled antigen in 6 mm×50 mm tubes that were previously coated with fetal calf serum and incubated at 37° for 1 hour. Ten microliters of goat anti-rabbit IgG were added for maximum precipitation. The tubes were incubated at 4° overnight. The precipitates were washed 3 times with PBS and counted in an automatic gamma counting system. The titer of the serum was that dilution of antibody that binds 50% of the labeled antigen when the latter is at a defined concentration. Antibody titers were consistently greater than 1:5,000, using 100 nanograms of ^{125}I-labeled protein per tube.

Preparation and Radiolabeling of IgG

The IgG fraction of the antiserum was isolated by ion exchange chromatography with DEAE cellulose (DE-52, Whatman, Ltd. England). The antiserum was dialyzed against 0.01 M phosphate buffer at 8.0 and incubated with DE-52 equilibrated with the same buffer at a ratio of 1 ml of serum per 5 g of cellulose for 1 hour at 4°C. The IgG was the only serum protein that did not bind to the cellulose at this ionic strength, and it was removed by suctioning through a Buchner funnel or by centrifugation. The IgG solution was dialyzed against phosphate buffered saline and concentrated by ammonium sulfate precipitation or by Amicon Filtration. All samples were sterile-filtered with a 0.22 microfilter (Millipore Corporation, Bedford, Massachusetts) before freezing.

The IgG fraction was labeled with ^{131}I by the lactoperoxidase method (Marchalonis, 1979). For every 5 mg of IgG, 25 micrograms lactoperoxidase, 1 mCi of NaI^{131}, and 10 microliters of 8 mM hydrogen peroxide were added, in that order, in a sterile serum bottle. The mixture was stirred vigorously for 30 minutes at room temperature; the labeled protein was separated from unbound label using a PD-10, G25 column. Sterility and pyrogen testing was carried out before administration to patients.

Affinity Chromatography

Preparation of Ferritin Containing Immunoadsorbent

The purified ferritin was bound to cyanogen-bromide activated Sepharose 4B as described by the manufacturer (Pharmacia Fine Chemicals, Piscataway, New Jersey). In brief, 15 grams (50 ml wet volume) of dried beads were washed and reswelled in 1 mM HCL followed by equilibration with 0.1 M $NaHCO_3$ buffer (pH 8.3)+0.5 M NaCl. Eighty milligrams of purified human tumor ferritin in 100 ml of the same buffer were added and the mixture shaken overnight at 4°C. Remaining active groups were blocked by the addition of 0.5 M Tris buffer pH 8.0 followed by equilibration with 0.1 M sodium phosphate buffer pH 7.0.

Affinity Chromatography Procedure

Adsorption and elution of antibody was accomplished using an automated affinity system (ARK) (Eveleigh, 1978). The ARK was programmed to perform the following steps: (1) 10–15 ml of antiserum were added to an affinity column containing approximately 15 ml of adsorbent, (2) the column was washed with 0.1 M sodium phosphate buffer (pH 7.0) to remove unbound serum proteins, (3) thiocyanate in phosphate buffer was added to elute specific antibody which was bound to the column, and the eluate was dialyzed against running water and then phosphate buffer. The whole procedure was repeated automatically (Eveleigh, 1978). The final preparation was concentrated by Amicon filtration (Amicon Corp., Lexington, Massachusetts) and ammonium sulfate precipitation.

Patient Selection

Patients selected for study have primary non-resectable liver cancers generally replacing 40% of the liver. Some of the patients have had tumors as large as 80 to 85% of the liver with the largest tumor to date being 2,600 grams. Patients must be capable of self care (60% or greater Kainofsky status) in order to be a candidate for isotopic immunoglobulin.

Preparative Regimen for Patients Who Received [131]I

Throughout hospitalization, and at least 2 weeks following treatment, patients received 10 drops of Lugol's solution b.i.d. orally, beginning 7 days prior to radiolabeled antibody administration. Skin testing with radiolabeled antibody and eye testing with unlabeled antibody was carried out 1 day prior to radiolabeled antibody administration. Independent laboratory verification of the sterility and lack of pyrogenicity of the radiolabeled antibody was confirmed before administration. The patients had an intravenous catheter line established with a 3-way stopcock in place for administration of radiolabeled antibody. All patients were taught temperature recording as well as recording of intake and output to minimize contact with the nursing staff while they were radioactive.

Specialized Room Requirements

The patient's room was protected by portable shields designed to reduce the exposure rate to below 2 milliroentgens/hour on the outside of the shields.

Determination of Liver and Tumor Volumes

Computerized axial tomographic scans of the liver, obtained about one week prior to the infusion of radiolabeled antibody, were used to compute liver and tumor volumes. Tomographic slices were 1 cm in thickness with 1 cm between cuts. For the patients studied, 14 to 18 slices bracketed the entire liver. Following a patient's CAT scan, a circular slab of tissue equivalent phantom material, 35 cm in diameter and 2.5 cm in thickness, was imaged employing the same scanner settings used for the patient. The phantom material had two series of holes in the horizontal and vertical directions, 0.20 cm in diameter, with a center-to-center distance of 1.27 cm. The distance between holes in the CAT scan of the phantom material provided a set of spatial calibration points for scaling liver and tumor size in the patient's CAT scan slices.

Normal and tumor bearing regions of the liver were contoured manually in each CAT scan slice. The contours in the entire sequence of each patient's CAT scan slices and the phantom image were then digitized, using a mini-computer controlled electronic digitizing tablet with a spatial resolution of 0.00254 cm. The digitized contours and calibration data were stored on magnetic tape for further processing. For the calculation of liver and tumor volumes, the surface areas in each CAT scan slice were first obtained by numerically integrating around the closed contours representing normal and tumor bearing regions of the liver. The resulting areas for each slice were then numerically integrated using the known sequence, center-to-center distance, and size of each slice, to obtain total liver and tumor volumes. Analogous methods of calculation have been employed in the measurement of normal liver volumes by emission computed tomography. In addition, the computer programs used in the present study permitted three dimensional reconstruction of the liver and tumor and provided anteroposterior and lateral cuts at any level.

To test the reproducibility of manual contouring of the liver and tumor in CAT scan slices, duplicate sets of CAT scans were contoured independently by two investigators. Computed liver and tumor volumes for these CAT scans were in agreement to within 10%. Furthermore, anteroposterior views of the liver and tumor were computer-generated from sequences of manually contoured CAT scan slices and compared with corresponding ^{99m}Tc sulfur-colloid gamma camera images of the liver. The computer generated views satisfactorily reproduced liver shapes and tumor configurations within the liver and provided details that were not observable in radionuclide scans.

Effective Half-Life and Uptake Measurements

The effective half-life of ^{131}I-labeled antibody for total body irradiation was determined from serial measurements of the radioactivity in blood samples by scintillation counting (counts/min/ml of blood) and by monitoring the ^{131}I exposure rate at the bedside, with an unshielded Geiger counter at a distance of not less than 1 meter from the patient. Measurements commenced no later than 1 day post-administration of radiolabeled antibody and were continued daily for the duration of the patient's hospitalization.

Relative measurements of the uptake and decay of ^{131}I-labeled antibody in the liver and tumor were made with a scintillation probe. The probe consisted of a 2×2-in NaI (T1) activated crystal detector coupled to a nuclear spectrometer and time-scaler. A straight-bore collimator, 4 cm in length and 1.9 cm inside diameter, was used to reduce the sensitivity of the probe and to improve its spatial resolution. The 364 keV emissions of ^{131}I were monitored and a 5% energy window selected to reduce scattered radiation effects. When obtaining counts, the scintillation probe was positioned reproducibly on the patient's skin directly over the liver.

In Vivo Quantitation of ^{131}I-Labeled Antibody in the Liver and Tumor

Absolute determination of the ^{131}I activity deposited in the liver and tumor was made by obtaining 180 degree-opposed views with a gamma-ray scintillation camera (Thomas, 1976, 1977). Two to four days prior to the infusion of ^{131}I-labeled antibody, anterior and posterior gamma camera images of the liver were obtained using 3 mCi of ^{99m}Tc sulfur colloid, injected intravenously. These images served to identify normal and tumor bearing regions of the liver in radionuclide scans and to position patients under the gamma camera for optimum views of the liver. Patients were positioned reproducibly, utilizing line lasers and ink marks on the skin. Following the ^{99m}Tc sulfur colloid images, transmission measurements were made for each patient using a flood source that contained about 2 mCi of ^{131}I. A parallel hole 400-keV collimator was employed for the 364 keV gamma emissions of ^{131}I and a 20% energy window selected to reduce scattered radiation effects. The same collimator and energy window were used to measure the 140 keV emissions of ^{99m}Tc sulfur colloid.

Anterior and posterior transmission measurements of the liver and an image of the flood source were obtained. Data were recorded on magnetic tape using a minicomputer interfaced with the large field of view scintillation camera. The computer permitted definitions of regions of interest and provided anterior and posterior count rate information for each region.

Four to eight days post-administration of ^{131}I-labeled antibody, anterior and posterior ^{131}I liver images were recorded using the same gamma camera and computer system. A minimum of 500,000 counts was accumulated for all images, and the system's calibration factor was determined from a standard of known activity. Anterior and posterior count rate information for normal and tumor bearing regions of the liver were obtained from the ^{131}I liver images and for identical regions in the transmission and flood source images. For the patients studied, tumor volumes ranged from about 400 to 900 cm^3, and tumor bearing regions of the liver were clearly demarcated in the radionuclide scans. Mean values of the ^{131}I activity in normal and tumor bearing regions of the liver were computed from the formula

$$A = \left(\frac{I_A I_P}{T} \right)^{1/2} \frac{f}{C}$$

where A is the activity in mCi, I_A and I_p are anterior and posterior count rates, T is the transmission factor, C is the system's calibration factor (counts/mCi/min), and f is a factor which corrects for self-attenuation of the radiation within the organ (Thomas, 1976, 1977). These computations provided quantitative calibrations for the relative uptake measurements made with the scintillation probe.

Distribution of Radiolabeled IgG in the Plasma of Treated Patients

The distribution of ^{131}I-labeled IgG in the plasma of patients treated with either DEAE ion exchange or affinity column purified antibody was analyzed by column chromatography. At various times following initiation of treatment, 1 ml of a patient's plasma was applied to a 3.0×90 cm Sephacryl S-300 chromatography column (Pharmacia Fine Chemicals, Piscataway, New Jersey). Elution in one ml fractions of serum protein was followed by determination of absorbence at 280 nm. Radioactivity was followed with an automatic gamma counting system (Serle Analytic, Inc.).

Rationale for Clinical Trails

The identification of ferritin in neuroblastoma by Hann (1979) and in multiple myeloma by Humphrey in our own laboratories led to scanning trials with radiolabeled antiferritin (Wharam, 1980). More recently a Phase 1 trial of the method was begun in patients with these malignancies who had failed conventional therapy. In lung cancer known to contain ferritin, non-resectable (non-oat cell) tumors will be examined in a Phase 1–2 trial following external irradiation. Ultimately, a Phase 3 randomized trial is anticipated.

The present hepatoma protocol Phase 1–2 trial (without radiosensitizer) was approved for national study through the RTOG (Radiation Therapy Oncology Group, a consortium of radiation centers), with referral to our institution for isotopic antiferritin antibody and maintenance chemotherapy two months later at the referring institution (Sherman, 1978; Freidman, 1979; Order, 1980).

Results

Eight patients have received escalating doses of ^{131}I-labeled antiferritin IgG (hepatoma), two patients affinity chromatography purified antiferritin, and three patients anti-CEA (intrahepatic biliary carcinoma). Three had failed previous treatments which included chemotherapy (adriamycin, 5FU, and mitomycin in one case, and adriamycin, 5FU and bleomycin in the other). One patient had failed partial resection and hepatic artery ligation. Of these 4 patients, three achieved remissions of 6 and 9 months, and one patient continues in remission beyond 15 months. One patient failed to respond and had significant delay prior to radioimmunoglobulin administration. Of 11 patients, 8 have demonstrated clinical remissions as determined by combinations of physical examination, CAT scan, and liver chemistry analysis (Figures 26.1 and 26.2) (Falkson, 1978; Lee, 1979; Malt, 1972; Misra, 1977; Ong, 1976). The median survival of 9 months and mean survival of 11 1/2 months in the Phase 1–2 trial exceeds the published reports for advanced hepatic malignancies (see Figures 26.1 and 26.2). Investigation of the optimum dose of isotopically labeled antiferritin and the best preparation techniques is still in progress.

To date, doses of 50–150 mCi of ^{131}I-labeled antiferritin were given to these patients. The first treatments with 80 mCi and 130 mCi of affinity purified antiferritin have recently been carried out. The comparison of dose rate and total dose achieved has been idealized from quantitating data for a single tumor volume (see Tables 26.1 and 26.2). Affinity chromatography allowed an increase in antibody specificity from 12% antiferritin antibody for polyclonal antisera to 70% for affinity purified antiferritin antibody. Immune complexes were detected in the patients' plasma for the first time in the patients receiving affinity purified ^{131}I antiferritin (Figure 26.3).

Toxicity to date has been limited to clinically important leukopenia and thrombocytopenia in two of the patients previously failing adriamycin-5FU combination therapy at other institutions. In one patient, recovery over a month's time was uncomplicated. The second patient, managed at another institution, experienced a cerebrovascular accident with complete recovery and

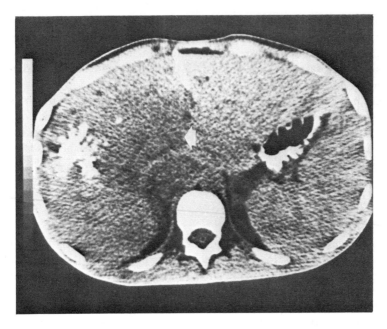

Figure 26.1. Computerized axial tomograph of liver and tumor (dark region—arrow) prior to treatment. White irregularity represents calcific change adjacent to the tumor.

Figure 26.2. Computerized axial tomograph of liver after treatment. White irregularity represents calcific change adjacent to the tumor.

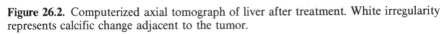

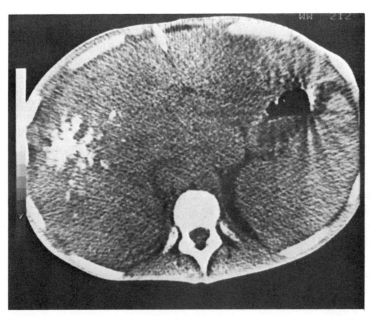

Table 26.1. Comparison of Maximum Dose Rates for Polyclonal and Affinity Chromatographic Purified Antiferritin ^{131}I-IgG.

Antibody	Mean tissue dose (RAD) for 100 mCi of ^{131}I-labeled antiferritin		
	TBI[a]	Liver	Tumor
Polyclonal	150	650	2000
Affinity-purified	28	190	600
Affinity-purified polyclonal	0.20	0.30	0.30

[a]TBI: total body irradiation.

restoration of the white cell and platelet counts, and remains in remission 19 months following treatment, with the CAT scan showing tumor calcification.

Two recent patients received 80 and 130 mCi of affinity chromatography antibody and are being followed through their private physicians presently 1 to 1 1/2 months after isotopic immunoglobulin. Several new observations were noted with affinity chromatography purified antibody: an increased tumor dose rate and decreased total body dose (Tables 26.1 and 26.2), a more immediate uptake of isotopic antibody in the tumor, in contrast to the previous 3–6 day progressive accumulation we reported with polyclonal antiferritin IgG, and the appearance of immune complexes in the blood stream (Order, 1980).

The programs in lung cancer, multiple myeloma, and neuroblastoma are recent developments (Figures 26.4, 26.5, and 26.6). To date, in the non-resectable lung cancer protocol, one patient received ^{131}I antiferritin 100 mCi and progressed with a paraneoplastic hyperparathyroid syndrome, ultimately succumbing to a non-reversible hypercalcemia 5 months after therapy. In that patient, tumor targeting was achieved. A second patient recently received 100 mCi of ^{131}I-labeled affinity purified antiferritin and remains disease-free 3 months after treatment. In addition, in two patients in the pilot feasibility study, lung cancer targeting was achieved. Three neuroblastoma patients' tumors have been visualized with 10 mCi doses of ^{131}I antiferritin. In multiple

Table 26.2. Compairson of the Mean Tissue Dose of Radiolabeled ^{131}I Polyclonal Antiferritin and Affinity Purified Antiferritin IgG.

Antibody	Maximum dose rates (rad/hr) for 100 mCi of ^{131}I-labeled antiferritin		
	TBI[a]	Liver	Tumor
Polyclonal	1.1	2.0	6.0
Affinity-purified	1.0	3.3	11

[a]TBI: total body irradiation.

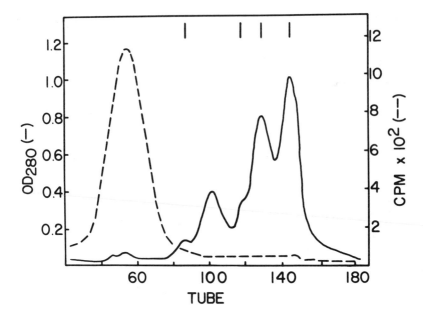

Figure 26.3. The serum profile of a patient as determined by elution after chromatography on Sephacryl S-300, seven days following treatment with ^{131}I antiferritin IgG. The dashed line represents the distribution of radioactivity in heavier immune complexes.

myeloma, the scans with antiferritin ^{131}I-IgG followed 6/6 tissue culture determinations demonstrating ferritin synthesis and secretion by multiple myeloma. Three of three patients have had myeloma tumor localization. One patient received 50 mCi of ^{131}I antiferritin in the Phase 1 study.

Discussion

The present results demonstrate several important relationships:

1. Tumor associated antigen, although not uniquely specific, may be used for tumor localization of radioisotope for scanning and therapy.
2. Tumors known to metabolize and secrete ferritin, i.e., hepatoma, neuroblastoma, and multiple myeloma, could be evaluated for isotopic antiferritin deposition.
3. As specific antibody activity was increased from polyclonal (12%) to affinity chromatographic antiferritin (70%), the kinetics of distribution and dose deposition was altered.

Each of these points requires further amplification. Although ferritin was once thought to be tumor specific, this property has been questioned, because

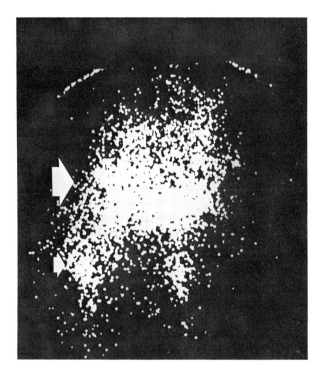

Figure 26.4. Antiferritin [131]I IgG scan of patient with multiple myeloma involving the pelvis (arrow) and right femoral head (smaller arrow).

polyclonal antiferritin has not distinguished significant immunological differences between normal and tumor cells, either *in vivo* or *in vitro*. Cross-reactive ferritin sites in normal spleen, bone marrow, and liver do not demonstrate significant antibody localization.

However, in spleens of patients with Hodgkin's disease, ferritin levels are 10 times greater than in normal spleens (Eshhar et al., 1974), and in our studies of hepatoma, we found that 7% of the tumor protein was ferritin. These findings indicate a large reservior of tumor associated ferritin which is available for antibody deposition. Synthesis and secretion of tumor associated ferritin has been demonstrated in hepatoma (Beck, 1974) and neuroblastoma (Hann, 1979), and recently was found in myeloma by Dr. Humphrey in our group (Order et al., 1981).

Dose rate and total dose are of special significance to isotopic immunoglobin therapy, and our handling of these problems has taken advantage of clinical radiobiologic and radiotherapeutic experience (Shipley, 1979). Conventional mechanical implantation techniques with ^{125}I in prostatic cancer yields dose rates of 5–8 rad/hr and requires higher total doses than conventional isotopic implants with iridium or radium for tumoricidal effectiveness. Dose rates of 10 rad/hr or greater will be cytocidal for tumor cells at total doses of

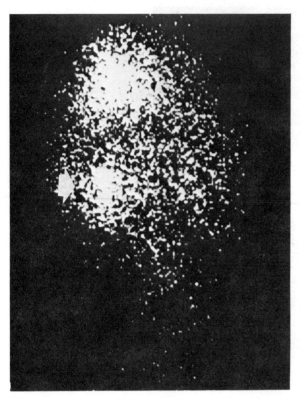

Figure 26.5. Posterior scan after injection of ^{131}I antiferritin IgG of neuroblastoma (arrow) with cardiac image superior (due to free circulating radioimmunoglobulin).

5000–7000 rad. Normal tissue effects, however, also depend upon dose rate; the higher the dose rate to normal tissue, the more extensive the potential normal tissue damage there might be. For example, single doses of total body irradiation of 1000 rad by external beam irradiation exhibit the following dose rate dependencies: at dose rates of 50 rad/minute, there would be significant gastrointestinal toxicity, whereas at 5 rad/minute, no significant gastrointestinal damage occurs. The present dose rate of total body irradiation following ^{131}I antiferritin antibody administration of 1 rad/hr was considerably less toxic than would be expected if dose rates of 5 or 10 rad/hr were administered.

The increase in antibody specificity made possible by affinity chromatography of antibody preparations did not increase the dose rate to the total body nor significantly to the liver (2 to 3 rad/hr) (see Table 26.2). The increased dose rate to the tumor from 6 to 11 rad/hr was, however, significant, and should have enhanced cytotoxic effectiveness. The reduction in total dose of TBI from 150 rad to 28 rad (see Table 26.1) at the same dose rate would allow

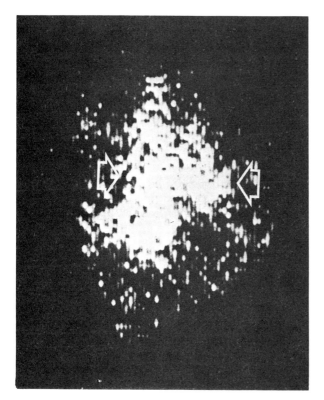

Figure 26.6. Antiferritin ^{131}I-IgG scan of lung cancer between arrows. The patient's neck is superior and part of cardiac silhouette inferior.

a five-fold increase in the dose administered. According to our present experience, this dose increase would lead to an additional 1000 rad (total 3000 rad tumor with 150 rad TBI) with affinity chromatographic purified antiferritin at a higher dose rate. In addition, the increased dose administered would theoretically increase the tumor dose rate further by causing a greater deposition of radiolabeled antibody at the tumor site. Therefore, we anticipate in our continuing studies the further investigation of affinity chromatographic antiferritin in therapeutic trials for patients with hepatoma, myeloma, neuroblastoma, and lung cancer.

Careful and continued monitoring of patients given affinity purified antibody has not revealed toxicity due to the production of immune complexes, but this potential problem will require continual evaluation.

Further attempts to evaluate increased specificity and dose rate and total dose deposition will involve monoclonal hybridoma derived antiferritin antibody, which has been prepared for testing and in preliminary analysis was over 90% immunospecific.

In the hepatoma protocol, external irradiation and chemotherapy have been attempted first, as dose distribution and potential effectiveness of ^{131}I antiferritin was not established (Sherman, 1978; Freidman, 1979). As we near completion of this early phase of clinical investigation, which will allow a maximal single dose of 200 mCi of ^{131}I antiferritin IgG, administration of more than one dose will be considered, since the whole body effective half-life of affinity purified antibody is 1.5 days, while that of polyclonal antibody is 3 days. We have designed a tentative regimen calling for doses distributed at each 1 1/2 day interval during the first week of treatment, with a possible dose of 500 mCi or more of fractionated, radiolabeled antibody. Obviously, careful studies of toxicity, dose distribution, and specific titer of antibody will be required before such an escalation of dose is effected. In addition, pilot studies of combined therapy with radiolabeled antiferritin in conjunction with adriamycin, a chemotherapeutic agent of known activity in hepatoma, and a drug which increases cytotoxicity of low dose rate irradiation, will be considered. Finally, in our most recent hepatoma patients, we have considered maintenance chemotherapy 2 months following isotopic immunoglobulin.

The targeting of more than one ferritin bearing tumor allows for potential investigation of identifying and treating metastasis in lung cancer patients, and for dosimetric evaluation.

The present studies seek to analyze and quantitate specificity and dose deposition. These may well provide a model for more general applications with radiolabeled antibody to varying tumor associated proteins in this rapidly developing field.

Our present data indicate the relative safety of using foreign derived immunospecific antibody to target tumor sites in appropriate malignancies associated with ferritin. The determination of dose distribution and quantitative analysis by a multidisciplinary team representing immunology, nuclear and diagnostic radiology, physics, experimental pharmacology, medical oncology, and radiation therapy represents an initial beginning in the efforts to combine immunological agents, with their special properties of specificity, and radiation, with its established cancerocidal effectiveness, for clinical advancement. Developing the potential of such combined applications in clinical oncology requires quantitation of dose and dose distribution concomitant with investigations of target specificity, in order to establish a rational approach to therapy.

References

Beck, G. and Bollock, C. (1974) Synthesis of ferritin in cultured hepatoma cells. *Fed. Exp. Biol. Soc.* 47:314–317.

Bolton, A.E. and Hunter, W.M. (1973) The labeling of proteins to high specific radioactivity by conjugation to a ^{125}I containing acylating agent. *Biochem. J.* 133:529–539.

Eshhar, T., Order, S.E., and Katz, D. (1974) Ferritin: a Hodgkin's disease associated antigen. *Proc. Natl. Acad. Sci.* 81:3956–3960.

Ettinger, D., Dragon, L., Klein, J.L., Sgagias, M., and Order, S.E. (1979) Isotopic immunoglobulin in an integrated multimodal treatment program for a primary liver cancer: a case report. *Can. Treat. Rep.* 63:131–134.

Eveleigh, J.W. (1978) Techniques and instrumentation for preparative immunabsorbent separations. *J. Chromatog.* 159:129–145.

Falkson, G., Moertel, C.G., Lavin, P., Pretorius, F.J., and Carbone, P.O. (1978) Chemotherapy studies in primary liver cancer. *Cancer* 42:2149–2156.

Friedman, M., Cassidy, M., Levine, M., Phillips, T., Spiwack, S., and Resser, K.J. (1979) Combined modality treatment of hepatic metastases. *Cancer* 44:906–913.

Gold, P. and Friedman, S.E. (1965) Demonstration of tumor specific antigen in human colonic carcinoma by immunologic tolerance and absorption techniques. *J. Exp. Med.* 121:439–462.

Goldenberg, D.M., Deland, F., Kim, E., Bennett, S., Primus, F.J., van Nagell, J.R., Jr., Estes, N., DeSimone, P., and Rayburn, P. (1978) Use of radiolabeled antibodies to carcinoembryonic antigen for the detection and localization of diverse cancers by external photoscanning. *N. Eng. J. Med.* 298:1384–1388.

Hann, H.L., Levy, H.M., Evans, A.E., and Drysdale, J.W. (1979) Serum ferritin and neuroblastoma. *Proc. A.A.C.R. and A.S.C.O.*, no. 126.

Katz, D.H., Order, S.E., Graves, M., and Benacerraf, B. (1973) Purification of Hodgkin's disease tumor associated antigens. *Proc. Natl. Acad. Sci.* 70:369–400.

Lee, Y.T.N. (1979) Hepatic artery ligation and infusion chemotherapy for malignancy of the liver. *J. Amer. Med. Wom. Assoc.* 34:21–26, 31–39.

Mach, J.P., Carrel, S., Merenda, C., Sordat, B., and Cerottini, J.C. (1974) *In vivo* localization of radiolabeled antibodies to carcinoembryonic antigen human colon carcinoma grafted into nude mice. *Nature* 248:704–706.

Malt, R.A., Vroonhaven, T.S.K., and Kakumoto, Y. (1972) Manifestations and prognosis of carcinoma of the liver. *Surg. Gyn. Obst.* 135:361–364.

Marchalonis, J.J. (1979) An enzymatic method for the trace iodination of immunoglobulin and other proteins. *Biochem. J.* 113:299–305.

Misra, N.C., Hiswall, M.S.D., Sangh, R.V., and Das. B. (1977) Infusion of combination of mitomycin-C and 5 fluorouracil in treatment of primary and metastatic liver carcinoma. *Cancer* 39:1425–1429.

Ong, G.B. and Chan, P.K.W. (1976) Primary carcinoma of the liver. *Surg. Gyn. Obst.* 143:31–38.

Order, S.E. (1976) The history and progress of serologic immunotherapy and radiodiagnosis. *Radiol.* 118:219–223.

Order, S.E., Klein, J.L., Ettinger, D., Alderson, P., Siegelman, S., and Leichner, P. (1980) Phase 1–2 study of radiolabeled antibody integrated in the treatment of primary hepatic malignancies. *Int. J. Rad. Onc. Biol. Phys.* 6:703–710.

Order, S.E., Klein, J.L., and Leichner, P. (1981) Antiferritin IgG antibody for isotopic cancer therapy. *Oncol.*, in press.

Quinones, J., Mizejewski, G., and Beierwaltes, W.H. (1971) Choriocarcinoma scanning using radiolabeled antibody to choronic gonadotrophin. *J. Nuc. Med.* 12:69–75.

Sherman, D.M., Weichselbaum, R., Order, S.E., Cloud, L., Trey, C., and Piro, A.J. (1978) Palliation of hepatic metastases. *Cancer* 41:2013–2017.

Shipley, W.W., Ling, C.C., Gerwick, L., and Jennings, W. (1979) Ultra low dose rate radium in Chinese hamster cells. *6th Int. Cong. Rad. Research*, Tokyo.

Singh, B., Sharma, S.M., Patel, M.C., Raghavendran, K.V., and Berman, M. (1974) Kinetics of large therapy doses in patients with thyroid cancer. *J. Nuc. Med.* 15:674–678.

Thomas, S.R., Maxon, H.R., and Kereiakes, J.G. (1976) *In vivo* quantitation of lesion radioactivity using external counting methods. *Med. Phys.* 3:253–255.

374

Thomas, S.R., Maxon, H.R., Kereiakes, J.G., and Saenger, E.L. (1977) Quantitative external counting techniques enabling improved diagnostic and therapeutic decisions in patients with well differentiated thyroid cancer. *Radiol.* 122:731–737.

Wharam, M.D., Order, S.E., Klein, J.L., and Leichner, P. (1980) Radiolabeled antiferritin antibody in Hodgkin's disease and neuroblastoma: tumor localization and potential therapeutic application. *Abst. Int. Soc. Ped. Onc. Budapest.* 98.

CHAPTER 27

Autologous Mixed Lymphocyte Culture Response in Man[1]

Sudhir Gupta and Nitin Damle

Memorial Sloan-Kettering Cancer Center, New York, New York

Introduction

Human T lymphocytes proliferate when exposed *in vitro* to autologous B lymphocytes (Opez et al., 1975; Kuntz et al., 1976; Weksler and Kuntz., 1977; Ilfeld et al., 1977; Tomanari and Aizawa, 1977; Sakane and Green, 1979; Hausman and Stobo, 1979). In this autologous mixed culture reaction (AMLR), the stimulating cells are B cells and serologically distinct antigens appear to stimulate autologous and allogeneic responder T cells (Smith, 1978). The autoreactive T cells demonstrate immunological memory and specificity and contain precursors of Concanavalin A (Con A)-induced suppressor cells (Weksler and Kozak, 1977; Sakane and Green, 1979). Like B cell differentiation into plasma cells, AMLR appears to be part of a highly regulated system.

Functional subpopulations of immunoregulatory T cells (suppressor and helper) have been described for the differentiation of B cells to plasma cells (Gupta and Good, 1980). These functionally distinct subpopulations are characterized by the presence of surface differentiation antigens, as defined by heterologous antisera or monoclonal antibodies, receptors for immunoglobulin isotypes, and by the sensitivity to the inhibitory effect of theophylline on rosette formation between T cells and sheep red blood cells (SRBC's) (Gupta and Good, 1980; Gupta et al., 1980; Shore et al., 1978; Kung et al., 1979).

[1]This work was supported by Grants from the National Institute of Health CA-17404, CA-19267, CA-23766, CA-08748, AI-11843, NS-11457, AG-00541, and Fund for the Advanced Study of Cancer and Judith Harris Selig Memorial Fund. Please send correspondence to Dr. Sudhir Gupta, 1275 York Avenue, New York, N.Y., 10021.

In this study, we have examined the responses of subpopulations of human T cells in AMLR which can be distinguished by monoclonal antibodies and by theophylline sensitivity. Furthermore, we have investigated the regulatory influence of each subpopulation of T cells, as well as the effect of histamine and corticosteroids on autologous and allogeneic mixed lymphocyte reaction.

Methods

Peripheral venous blood from normal healthy donors was used. Mononuclear cells were isolated on Ficoll-Hypaque (FH) density gradients. T cells were separated from non-T cells by rosetting the mononuclear cells with neuraminidase-treated SRBC's and separating on FH gradients. T cells obtained in this way were >96% purified, as determined by their rosette formation with SRBC and their lack of readily demonstrable surface immunoglobin. Non-T cells contained approximately 50% B cells, 20% third population cells, 25% monocyte, and <5% T cells. T and non-T cells were resuspended in RPMI-1640 containing 15% fetal calf serum (FCS), penicillin, streptomycin, and L-glutamine (complete medium), at a concentration 1×10^6/ml. Non-T cells were irradiated at 3000 rads from a Caeseum source and used as stimulator cells.

Theophylline resistant (T_R) and theophylline sensitive (T_S) cells were separated by incubating purified T cells (4×10^6/ml) with 3 mM theophylline for 60 min at 37°C, then mixing with 1% SRBC and heat-inactivated SRBC-absorbed FCS and incubating further for 1 hour on ice. Pellets were gently resuspended and rosetting T cells (T_R) were separated from non-rosetting T cells (T_S) on a FH gradient. T_R and T_S cells were washed and resuspended in complete medium at 1×10^6 cells/ml.

Histamine at various concentrations was either added for the entire period of culture or purified T cells were pretreated with histamine for 24 hours, washed, and then co-cultured with respondent cells.

Monoclonal antibodies for T cell and T cell subsets (OK T_3-PAN T, OK T_4-helper/inducer and OK T_8-suppressor/cytotoxic) were purchased from Ortho Pharmaceutical, Raritan, New Jersey. Anti-Ia antibodies were gifts from Dr. John A. Hansen, Fred Hutchinson Cancer Center, Seattle, Washington. Monoclonal antibodies were present in AMLR and allogeneic MLR for the entire period of culture. No complement was used.

Results

Subpopulation of T cells responding in autologous and allogeneic MLR. One hundred thousand unseparated total T (T_T), T_R, or T_S responder cells were incubated with equal numbers of irradiated autologous or allogeneic stimulator non-T cells at 37°C for a period of 7 days. The proliferative responses were measured on days 5, 6, and 7 of cultures. The peak proliferative response was observed on day 6 in AMLR and on day 5 in allogeneic MLR. Therefore, data are shown at day 6 for AMLR and day 5 for allogeneic MLR. Table 27.1 shows the results of a representative experiment. T_R cells responded with good proliferative response, but T_S failed to exhibit any significant proliferation. The proliferative response of T_R cells in both AMLR and allogeneic MLR was significantly greater than that of unseparated (T_T) T cells.

Regulation of AMLR and allogeneic MLR of unseparated T cells by T_R and T_S cells. Addition of mitomycin-C-treated T_R cells to unseparated T cells in AMLR or allogeneic MLR resulted in a significant augmentation of the peak proliferative response of T_T cells. T_S cells on the other hand suppressed the proliferative response of T_T cells (Table 27.2). On a per cell basis, the suppressor effect of T_S cells in both AMLR and allogeneic MLR of T_T cells was greater than the augmenting effect of T_R cells.

Effect of T_S cells on AMLR and allogeneic MLR of T_R cells. Results from our studies of the effect mitomycin-C-treated T_S cells on AMLR and allogeneic MLR of T_R cells are shown in Table 27.3. T_S cells suppressed the proliferative response of T_R cells in a dose dependent manner. However, the suppressor influence of T_S cells was more profound in autologous than in allogeneic MLR of T_R cells.

In vitro effects of monoclonal antibodies on AMLR and allogeneic MLR. Results of the analysis are shown in Figure 27.1. OK T_3, OK T_4, 7.2, and 17.5 monoclonal antibodies profoundly suppressed both autologous and allogeneic MLR. OK T_8 antibody, which defines suppressor/cytotoxic T cell subpopulations, however, did not influence either AMLR or allogeneic MLR.

In vitro effect of histamine on AMLR and allogeneic MLR. Data from studies of the effect of histamine in culture on AMLR and allogeneic MLR are shown in Table 27.4. Histamine, when present during the entire period of culture,

Table 27.1. Autologous and Allogeneic Mixed Lymphocyte Culture Responses of Human T Cell Subsets.

	^{3}H-thymidine incorporation (Δcpm)	
Cell type	Autologous[d]	Allogeneic[e]
T_T[a]	6458	8152
T_R[b]	11478	11084
T_S[c]	242	377

[a]Unseparated T cells.
[b]Theophylline resistant T cells.
[c]Theophylline sensitive T cells.
[d]Results are expressed for peak proliferative response at day 6 of cultures.
[e]Results are expressed for peak proliferative response at day 5 of cultures.

Table 27.2. Regulatory Influence of T Cell Subsets on Autologus and Allogeneic Response of Unseparated T Cells.

Responder cell type	Regulator cell[a] type			Autologous[b] (Δ cpm)	Allogeneic[c] (Δ cpm)
T_T	−			8964	10538
$T_T + T_S$	+	T_S	(10:1)	5417	8932
$T_T + T_S$	+	T_S	(4:1)	587	4204
$T_T + T_S$	+	T_S	(2:1)	678	1016
$T_T + T_R$	+	T_R	(10:1)	10684	10622
$T_T + T_R$	+	T_R	(4:1)	12675	14494
$T_T + T_R$	+	T_R	(2:1)	15072	14878

[a]Regulator cells were treated with mitomycin C.

[b]Results are expressed for peak proliferative response at day 6 of cultures.

[c]Results are expressed for peak proliferative response at day 5 of cultures.

decreased both AMLR and allogeneic MLR responses. Significant suppression was observed between 10^{-3} to 10^{-7} molar concentration of histamine. When T cells were first treated with histamine for 24 hours, washed, and then co-cultured with irradiated non-T cells, a similar decrease in the proliferative response was observed, as had been found with co-cultures when histamine was present during the entire period of culture (Table 27.5).

In vivo effect of hydrocortisone on AMLR and allogeneic MLR

Following a single intravenous injection of 300 mg of hydrocortisone, both autologous and allogeneic MLR responses decreased significantly at 4-hour periods and the responses returned toward initial levels at 24 hours following administration of hydrocortisone (Figure 27.2).

Table 27.3. Regulatory Influence of Theophylline Sensitive T Cells (T_S) on Autologous and Allogeneic MLC Response of Theophylline Resistant T Cells (T_R).

Responder cells	Regulator cells[a]		Autologous[b] (Δ cpm)	Allogeneic[c] (Δ cpm)
T_R	−		11965	11823
T_R	+	T_S (10:1)	5908	7974
T_R	+	T_S (4:1)	923	5448
T_R	+	T_S (2:1)	ND	803

[a]Regulator cells were mitomycin C-treated.

[b]Results are expressed for peak proliferative response at day 6 of cultures.

[c]Results are expressed for peak proliferative response at day 5 of cultures.

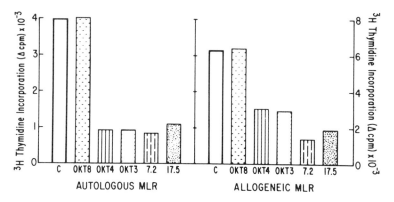

Figure 27.1. Effect of monoclonal antibodies against T cell (OK T_3) and T cell subsets (helper OK T_4, suppressor OK T_8) and Ia antigen (7.2, 17.5) on autologous MLR and allogeneic MLR. (Data from a representative experiment).

Discussion

In autologous MLR, T cells respond with increased DNA synthesis when stimulated *in vitro* by mitomycin-C-treated or irradiated autologous non-T cells (Opez et al., 1975; Kuntz et al., 1976; Weksler and Kuntz, 1977; Ilfeld et al., 1977; Tomonari and Aizawa, 1979; Sakane and Green, 1979; Hausman and Stobo, 1979). The autoreactive T cells have been shown to exhibit immunological memory and specificity (Weksler and Kozak, 1977). Recently, distinct subpopulations of human T cells have been identified by the presence

Table 27.4. Effect of Histamine on Autologous and Allogeneic Mixed Lymphocyte Culture Response.

Histamine (molar/ml)	Autologous[a] (Δ cpm)	% Suppression	Allogeneic[b] (Δ cpm)	% Suppression
0	3732	–	9667	–
10^{-3}	964	74	2746	72
10^{-4}	1298	65	2958	69
10^{-5}	1637	57	5281	45
10^{-6}	2661	28	6467	33
10^{-7}	2625	30	8682	10
10^{-8}	3550	4	9300	4
10^{-9}	3488	6	9816	+2

Note: Histamine was present for the entire period of cultures. +: Augmentation.

[a] Results are expressed for peak proliferative response on day 6 of culture.

[b] Results are expressed for peak proliferative response on day 5 of culture.

Table 27.5. Effect of Histamine Treatment of Responder T Cells on Autologous and Allogeneic Mixed Lymphocyte Culture Response.

Histamine (molar/ml)	Autologous[a] (Δ cpm)	% Suppression	Allogeneic[b] (Δ cpm)	% Suppression
0	2247	–	9193	–
10^{-3}	331	85	2908	68
10^{-4}	390	83	3953	57
10^{-5}	909	59	4749	48
10^{-6}	973	57	4720	48
10^{-7}	1935	14	8012	12
10^{-8}	2289	+2	8811	4

Note: T cells were incubated with various concentrations of histamine for 24 hours, washed × 3 with Hank's balanced salt solution and then cocultured with irradiated autologous or allogeneic non-T cells. +: Augmentation.
[a]Results are expressed for peak proliferative response at day 6 of cultures.
[b]Results are expressed for peak proliferative response at day 5 of culture.

of receptors for immunoglobulin isotypes (Gupta and Good, 1980), the presence of differentiation surface antigens detectable by monoclonal antibodies (Kung et al., 1979), and by their differential sensitivity to theophylline (Shore et al., 1978).

We have analyzed T cell subpopulations identified by the latter two techniques. The inhibitory effect of theophylline on rosette formation between T cells and SRBC can distinguish two subpopulations of T cells, one theophylline resistant, and one theophylline sensitive (Shore et al., 1978). T_R cells exhibit helper activity and T_S cells exhibit suppressor activity in antigen-driven antibody response (Shore et al., 1978). OK T_3 monoclonal antibodies react with the majority of T cells (Pan-T), OK T_4 antibodies react with $50-60\%$ peripheral T cells with inducer/helper activity, and OK T_8 antibodies react with approximately 20% of peripheral T cells that exert suppressor/cytotoxic activity (Kung et al., 1979).

In the present study, we have demonstrated that T_R cells respond vigorously by proliferation in both AMLR and allogeneic MLR. In contrast, T_S cells did not demonstrate any significant proliferative response. Consistent with these results, monoclonal antibodies that are specific for the majority of T cells (OK T_3) and others specific for the helper/inducer T cell (OK T_4) subpopulation, profoundly suppressed the proliferative response in AMLR and allogeneic MLR. In contrast, OK T_8 antibody, which is specific for the suppressor/cytotoxic subpopulation of T cells, had no effect either on AMLR or allogeneic MLR.

These data strongly suggest that the responding cells in AMLR and allogeneic MLR are a subpopulation of T cells with helper activity, while suppressor/cytotoxic T cells are very poor responders. The inhibitory effect of OK T_4 is not due to depletion of a particular cell population, since no

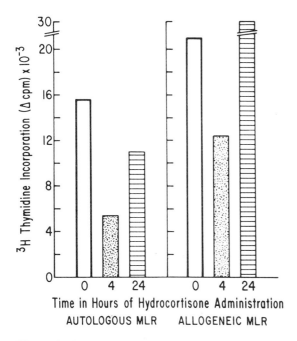

Figure 27.2. Effect of *in vivo* administration of hydrocortisone on autologous and allogeneic MLR. (Data representative of 3 experiments).

complement was used in the cultures and the viability of cells was >94%. Their selective inhibition indicates that these antibodies define the surface antigen through which the responding T cell subsets respond in AMLR and allogeneic MLR. Monoclonal antibodies against Ia determinants markedly suppressed both AMLR and allogeneic MLR, suggesting that the Ia determinant is at least the major stimulator antigen in both AMLR and allogeneic MLR.

Co-cultures of mitomycin C-treated T_S cells with unseparated responder cells in autologous and allogeneic MLR demonstrated a powerful suppression of proliferative response. T_R cells, on the other hand, augmented the proliferative response of unseparated cells. Both suppression by T_S cells and augmentation by T_R cells of the proliferative response of unseparated cells was dose dependent. On a per cell basis, the suppression exerted by T_S cells was more than the augmentation exerted by T_R cells. T_S cells also suppressed the proliferative response of T_R cells in AMLR and allogeneic MLR.

These observations suggest that there is an built-in regulation of AMLR response. Any alteration in helper or suppressor T cells could result in an abnormal AMLR. It has been demonstrated that suppressor cells are generated in AMLR's that are capable of suppressing the MLR and cytotoxic responses (Smith and Knowlton, 1979). Furthermore, it has been observed that autoreactive T cells include precursors for Con A-inducible suppressor cell activity (Sakane and Green, 1979). We believe that AMLR could be at least one if not the only mechanism by which suppressor cells are generated *in vivo*. A deficiency of AMLR responses has been observed in patients with systemic lupus erythematosus and chronic lymphocytic leukemia, which are both associated with a high incidence of serum and tissue autoantibodies (Sakane et al., 1978; Smith et al., 1977).

Hydrocortisone administration *in vivo* results in a marked and transient immunosuppression (Fauci et al., 1980). Haynes and Fauci (1978) have reported a transient decrease in T cells with IgM receptors (Tμ) and an increase in T cells with IgG receptors (Tγ) at 4 hours following a single injection of hydrocortisone. The relative proportions of T cell subsets return to initial levels 24 hours following administration of drug. Tμ cells include cells with helper activity and Tγ cells include cells with suppressor activity (Moretta et al., 1977). We found that *in vivo* administration of hydrocortisone in healthy volunteers brought on marked depression of both AMLR and allogeneic MLR at 4 hours following administration of drug. These responses returned to near initial values 24 hours following administration of hydrocortisone. These functional observations are consistent with the concomitant decrease in Tμ cells at 4 hours following administration, since Tμ cells are included in highly enriched subpopulation of T_R cells.

Histamine, a vasoactive amine, has been demonstrated to exert a number of inhibitory influences on a variety of immune responses (Tomonari and Aizawa, 1979). Recently we have demonstrated that histamine receptors are present on a subpopulation of Tγ cells that suppress B cell differentiation to plasma cells (Gupta et al., 1980). Furthermore, we have been able to produce suppressor factor from histamine activated T cells (Rocklin et al., 1980). Therefore, we have examined the influence of histamine on AMLR and allogeneic MLR. We found that histamine inhibited in a dose dependent manner both autologous and allogeneic MLR, and this inhibition was due to its influence on responder T cells and to its effect on stimulator non-T cells. It remains to be determined whether this decrease in AMLR or allogeneic MLR is attributable to a direct effect of histamine on T_R (helper T) cells, or to activation of T_S (suppressor T) cells.

The analysis of autologous MLR in malignant disorders is currently under investigation.

References

Fauci, A.S., Haynes, B.F., and Katz, P. (1980) Drug-induced T and B lymphocyte and monocyte dysfunction. In *Abnormal Infections in Compromised Host*. M.H. Grieco (ed.), New York: The Year Book Publisher, pp. 163–168.

Gupta, S. and Good, R.A. (1980) Markers of human lymphocyte subpopulations in primary immunodeficiency and lymphoproliferative disorders. *Seminars in Haematol.* 17:1–29.

Gupta, S., Fernandes, G., Rocklin, R., and Good, R.A. (1980) Histamine receptor on human T cell subsets. In *New Trends in Immunology and Cancer Immunotherapy*. B. Serrou and C. Rosenfeld (eds.), Paris: Dion Editieur, pp. 36–47.

Hausman, P.B. and Stobo, J.D. (1979) Specificity and function of a human autologous reaction T cell. *J. Exp. Med.* 149:1537–1542.

Haynes, B.F. and Fauci, A.S. (1978) The differential effect of *in vivo* hydrocortisone on the kinetics of subpopulations of human peripheral blood T lymphocytes. *J. Clin. Invest.* 61:703–707.

Ilfeld, D.N., Krakauer, R. S. and Blaese, R.M. (1977) Suppression of the human autologous mixed lymphocyte reaction by physiologic concentrations of hydrocortisone. *J. Immunol.* 119:428–434.

Kung, P., Goldstein, G., Reinherz, E.L., and Schlossman, S.F. (1979) Monoclonal antibodies defining distinctive human T cell surface antigens. *Science* 206:347.

Kuntz, M.M., Innes, J.B., and Weksler, M.E. (1976) Lymphocyte transformation induced by autologous cells. Human T lymphocyte proliferation induced by autologous or allogeneic non-T lymphocytes. *J. Exp. Med.* 143:1042–1054.

Moretta, L., Webb, S.R., Grossi, C.E., Lydyard, P.M., and Cooper, M.D. (1977) Functional analysis of two human T cell subpopulations. Help and suppression of B cell responses by T cell bearing receptors of IgM (T_M) and IgG (T_G). *J. Exp. Med.* 146:184–200.

Opez, G., Kiuchi, M., Takasugi, M. and Terasaki, P.I. (1975) Autologous stimulation of human lymphocyte subpopulations. *J. Exp. Med.* 142:1327–1333.

Rocklin, R.E., Breard, J., Gupta, S., Good, R.A., and Melmon, K.L. (1980) Characterization of the human blood lymphocytes that produce a histamine-induced suppressor factor (HSF). *Cell. Immunol.* 51:226–237.

Sakane, T. and Green, I. (1979) Specificity and suppressor function of human T cells responsive to autologous non-T cells. *J. Immunol.* 123:584–589.

Sakane, T., Steinberg, A.D., and Green, I. (1978) Failure of autologous mixed lymphocyte reactions between T and non-T cells in patients with systemic lupus erythematosus. *Proc. Natl. Acad. Sci. U.S.A.* 75:3464–3468.

Sakane, T., Steinberg, A.D., Arnett, F.C. et al. (1979) Studies on immune functions in patients with SLE. Characterization of lymphocyte subpopulations responsible for defective AMLR. *Arthritis and Rheumatism* 22:770–776.

Sakane, T., Steinberg, A.D., and Green, I. (1980) Studies on immune functions in patients with SLE. T cell suppressor function and AMLR during active and inactive phase of disease. *Arthritis and Rheumatism* 23:225–231.

Shore, A., Dosch, H.M., and Gelfand, E.W. (1978) Induction and separation of antigen-dependent T helper and T suppressor cells in man. *Nature* (Lond) 274:586.

Smith, J.B. (1978) Stimulation of autologous and allogeneic human T cells by B cells occurs through separate B cell antigen systems. *Cell. Immunol.* 36:203–209.

Smith, J.B. and Knowlton, R.P. (1979) Activation of suppressor T cells in human autologous mixed lymphocyte culture. *I. Immunol.* 123:419–422.

Smith, J.B, Knowlton, R.P., and Koons, L.S. (1977) Immunologic studies in chronic lymphocyte leukemia: defective stimulation of T cell proliferation in autologous mixed lymphocyte culture. *J. Natl. Cancer Inst.* 58:579–585.

Tomonari, K. and Aizawa, M. (1979) Induction of autoreactive cells by the preculture of human peripheral blood mononuclear cells with the autologous fresh plasma. *J. Immunol.* 122:2478–2483.

Weksler, M.W. and Kozak, R. (1977) Lymphocyte transformation induced by autologous cells. V. Generation of immunologic memory and specificity during the autologous mixed lymphocyte reaction. *J. Exp. Med.* 146:1833–1838.

CHAPTER 28

Progress in the Development of Soluble Tumor Antigens for Active Specific Immunotherapy[1]

Barry D. Kahan, Neal R. Pellis, Stephen J. LeGrue, Tsugo Tanaka, and Hisakazu Yamagishi

Division of Immunology and Organ Transplantation, the Department of Surgery, The University of Texas Medical School at Houston, Texas

One approach to the treatment of neoplastic disease is the use of chemically defined, tumor-specific transplantation antigens (TSTA) for active specific immunotherapy to stimulate host resistance. While available therapeutic modes, including surgery, radiotherapy, and chemotherapy may effectively control early neoplasms, local or metastatic recurrence of disease is frequently fatal. The strength of host resistance probably determines disease recurrence and patient survival, by virtue of its capacity to control residual, neoplastic cells. Ineffective resistance may not only fail to destroy residual cells, but may also actually accelerate tumor progression by antagonizing cellular immunity. The studies described here explore the possibility of immunotherapy with purified antigenic materials in a murine model applicable to the human setting: namely, treatment in conditions of supralethal challenge or of residual neoplastic disease.

A variety of studies have demonstrated cell surface, tumor specific markers which elicit host resistance to neoplastic progression: tumor specific transplantation antigens (TSTA; Foley, 1953; Prehn and Main, 1957; Revesz, 1960; Baldwin, 1973). These cell surface membrane antigens, present on tumors induced by exposure to oncogenic hydrocarbons, are individually unique, apparently the result of a distinctive, mutation-like, hereditary event (Basombrio and Prehn, 1972). The TSTA products of the mutated loci appear to be closely associated with (Mondal et al., 1971) but not essential for (Embleton and Heidelberger, 1972) malignant behavior.

[1]Supported by Grant IM62-G from the American Cancer Society.

Sarcomas induced in mice by methylcholanthrene (MCA) are widely employed for studies of TSTA, because of (1) the availability of inbred syngeneic
murine hosts; (2) the high incidence of induction by TSTA of a variety of
neoplasms; (3) the diversity of TSTA; (4) their weak but consistent antigenic
strength in simulating spontaneous neoplasms; (5) ample information on their
tumorigenic behavior; and (6) their amenability to surface membrane extraction techniques.

The TSTA of MCA-induced neoplasms display two important properties:
first, they tend to be unique to each neoplasm. Immunization with one tumor
usually fails to confer protection against challenge with a second tumor, even
though the two neoplasms are not only histologically indistinguishable, but
induced by the same carcinogen in the same host (Basombrio, 1970; Baldwin,
1973). Second, while cells within a primary neoplasm may display antigenic
heterogeneity, due to transformation of a number of parental clones (Embleton
and Heidelberger, 1972, 1975), the cells within most transplantable tumors
keep only a single, or at least a limited number of, antigenic specificities
(Prehn, 1970; Pimm and Baldwin, 1977). These findings suggest that only a
few clones undergo amplification after transformation. A variety of other,
preneoplastic clones are usually not transformed during the life of the host.

The evidence for the existence of tumor antigens in man is indirect: namely,
the capacity of human tumor cells to evoke specific antibody in heterologous
hosts, and the reactivity of human sera or lymphocytes toward neoplastic cells
(for review, see Herberman, 1977).

Tumor Extracts Induce Neoplastic Resistance

In mice, supralethal challenges with some carcinogen-induced neoplasms may
be rejected, following induction of transplantation resistance by prophylactic
treatment with irradiated neoplastic cells (Revesz, 1960) or with tumor extracts
prepared by treatment of cell suspensions with low intensity sonic energy
(Holmes et al., 1971), 3M KCl (Pellis et al., 1974; Meltzer et al., 1975), 0.15M
NaCl (Oettgen et al., 1968), or 2.5% 1-butanol (LeGrue et al., 1980). Extracted
TSTA may be more therapeutically active than intact cells, since they have the
advantages of: (1) potentially definable chemical structure, (2) solubility, (3)
precise quantitation of dosage, (4) focused stimulation of the immune system,
and (5) freedom from adventitious microbes.

Weak Immunogenicity of Tumor Extracts

Resistance against TSTA is weak, even when induced by immunization with
irradiated neoplastic cells: there is unresponsiveness at high antigen doses,
overload by large neoplastic challenges, and decay by two weeks in the absence
of restimulation by tumor challenge (Pellis and Kahan, 1975). In general,
tumor extracts behave as even weaker antigens than irradiated tumor cells,

since they display a higher threshold for the induction of immunity, a narrower dose range of immunoprotective activity, and diminution of immunity following multiple antigen injections.

Several hypotheses may explain the weak antigenicity of tumor extracts. First, the extracted materials may preferentially activate immunomodulatory mechanisms which facilitate rather than retard tumor growth. Although the surveillance hypothesis of Burnett (1970) proposes that the lymphoid system mediates host resistance to malignancy, Prehn (1971) has marshalled evidence that the immune response may actually promote tumor growth. Administration of extracts may result in weak immunoprotection which is not augmented by conventional immunological adjuvants, or even by enhanced tumor growth (Aoki et al., 1968; Fujimoto, 1973; Forni and Comoglio, 1974; Vaage, 1974; Bonavida and Zighelboim, 1974; Milas et al., 1974; Rao and Bonavida, 1976; Paranjpe and Boone, 1975; Bubenik, 1978; Yamauchi et al., 1979). One mechanism which promotes tumor growth is the activation of suppressor T cells, which have been dissected by Nordlund and Gershon (1975), Nelson et al. (1975), Small and Trainin (1976), Manor et al. (1976), Takei et al. (1977), Greene et al., (1979), and Fujimoto et al. (1976). The spleens of hosts sensitized either to allogeneic or syngeneic tumors contain an adherent, Thy 1 positive T cell population which suppresses mixed lymphocyte culture responses and is distinct from cytotoxic T cells (Argyris, 1977, 1978). Embleton (1976) found that administration of 3M KCl extracts of rat MCA sarcomas prevented subsequent immunization with irradiated cells, due to the appearance of inhibitory humoral factors and to the activation of a lymphoid population with suppressor activity. The possibility that suppressor mechanisms are activated by crude 3M KCl extracts of SV40 virus-induced hamster tumors (Coggin, 1979) and of B-77 virus-induced rat tumors (Simkovic et al., 1978) was suggested by the observation that multiple treatments with crude extracts led to no resistance, while single injections induced protection against neoplastic challenge.

A second possible explanation for the weak behavior of tumor extracts is that their antigenic content is so modest that they induce low dose tolerance, similar to that elicited in mice by treating them with sub-immunogenic doses of irradiated mastocytoma cells (Kolsch et al., 1973). This phenomenon may be akin to the growth of small but not large tumor cell inocula, which was denoted "sneaking through" or "dilution escape" (Old et al., 1962; Bonmassar et al., 1971, 1974), and attributed to a nonspecific inhibition of the host response (Bonmassar et al., 1974). This explanation suggests that the potency of antigenic extracts might be augmented by purification of the active component. Enrichment of tumor antigenic activity from crude extracts has been achieved by sieve chromatography (Leonard et al., 1975; Bowen and Baldwin, 1976), ion exchange chromatography (Steele et al., 1975), rate zonal centrifugation (Luborsky et al., 1976), isotachophoresis (Natori et al., 1978) and column isoelectric focusing (Bowen and Baldwin, 1976; Rogers and Law, 1979). Although feasible for the purification of many proteins, these procedures have the common disadvantage of a low antigen yield for *in vivo* tests.

A third explanation for the weak antigenicity of tumor extracts may be their failure to effectively trigger cytotoxic T cells. This defect may be due to separation of the immunogen from critical components in the plasma membrane. Even in the case of histocompatibility antigens, induction of a primary humoral and cellular immune response may demand not only the epitope, but also a "second signal" (Lafferty and Woolnough, 1977), apparently best provided by an intact viable lymphocyte. It has been reported that this signal cannot be provided using a second epitope, such as an extracted Ia antigen or by incorporation of antigens into liposome membranes (Batchelor et al., 1978).

Several workers have suggested that the immunogenicity of TSTA may be enhanced by treatment of the animal with neuraminidase (Rios and Simmons, 1973); dinitrophenylaminocaproate (Martin et al., 1971); dimethyl-diocta-decyl -ammonium bromide, a lipophilic agent (Prager and Gordon, 1978); or derivation with trinitrophenyl (Gillette et al., 1978) or acetoacetyl (Benjamini et al., 1976) groups. Potentiation of the immune response has been achieved by infection of tumor cells with influenza (Boone and Blackman, 1972), Newcastle (Kobayashi et al., 1970), or Friend murine leukemia (Beverly et al., 1973) viruses. However, poor immunogenicity for a primary immune response may not be critical, since in tumor immunotherapy, it is assumed that the neoplasm has *already* afforded a primary antigenic stimulus. The goal of active immunotherapy is to provide an effective secondary stimulus.

The work summarized above demonstrates that many chemically induced murine tumors express membrane structures which can serve as the focus of immune responses. However, the weak immunogenicity of many tumor antigens, coupled with the presence of tumor growth enhancing factors on cells and in extracts, have hampered studies of the biochemical and immunological nature of these molecules.

Extraction of TSTA with 3M KCl

The protocol for the extraction of TSTA from neoplastic cells is adapted from that used for extraction of histocompatibility antigens from lymphoblasts (Reisfeld and Kahan, 1970). Cells enzymatically dissociated from neoplasms are suspended in 0.15 M phosphate buffered saline (PBS, pH 7.2) containing 3M KCl (10 ml PBS/ml packed tumor cell volume). After a 16-hour incubation at 4°C, subcellular particulates are sedimented at 164,000 g. Following concentration by dialysis and removal of precipitated nucleic acids and nucleoproteins, the 164,000 g supernate is designated "crude" KCl extracts. The yield of protein from cultured tumor cells or from animal-propagated cells is about 1 mg/1.3×10^7 tumor cells.

Specific immunoprotection against 100 to 1000-fold the lethal dose of the homologous, but not a second, non-cross-reactive, MCA-induced tumor was elicited in syngeneic hosts by pretreatment with (1) crude 3M KCl extracts

(Pellis et al., 1974; Pellis and Kahan, 1975), (2) fractions sedimented by ammonium sulfate (Pellis et al., 1976), or (3) materials purified by preparative isoelectric focusing (Yamagishi et al., 1979; Pellis et al., 1980). Protective immunity is mediated by T lymphocytes and antagonized by an adherent, phagocytic cell population (Yamagishi et al., 1980). The immunologic character of this response was demonstrated by local adoptive transfer assays (LATA) in which normal syngeneic hosts were endowed with specific tumor resistance, using spleen cells from 3M KCl antigen-treated hosts (Pellis and Kahan, 1978).

Preparative isoelectric focusing (pIEF)

Crude extracts fractionated by preparative isoelectric focusing using a modification of the method of Radola (1973) yield a partially purified TSTA. From 35 to 300 mg crude KCl extract (5 mg/ml) in 1% glycine mixed with carrier ampholyte (40% Ampholine® solution, LKB) are added to a slurry of alcohol-washed, superfine Sephadex G75 (Ultrodex, LKB) and poured into a Multiphor (LKB) preparative isoelectric focusing tray bounded by ampholyte-soaked wicks. The pH gradient is established at 8 watts constant power, maximizing at 1400 volts over a 12 to 16-hour period. Focused slabs are sectioned into 31 zones using a steel cutting grid; 60 to 85% of the protein applied is recovered from the gel bed. The flat bed method of preparative isoelectric focusing has the advantages of (1) a large capacity of crude extract, (2) separation of protective antigens from those facilitating tumor growth, and (3) yield of the active principle by elution not only from, but also within, Sephadex beads (Pellis et al., 1980).

Preparative isoelectric focusing of crude 3M KCl extracts affords a chemical separation of two antigenic principles with antagonistic actions (Figure 28.1): Fraction 1, (pI 2.0–3.5) elicits specific facilitation of tumor outgrowth in primary hosts and upon LATA in naive secondary hosts, in part due to activation of suppressor cells (Yamagishi et al., 1980). On the other hand, Fraction 15 (pI 5.8–6.0) is highly immunoprotective, displaying a 50-fold increased activity over crude 3m KCl extracts. Ten to 45 μg antigen administered ten days prior to challenge halved the mean diameter of tumors resulting from inoculation of 100 minimum tumorigenic dose (MTD) into primary hosts ($p < .0001$) (Table 28.1). The protective effects of the MCA-D and MCA-F (pH 5.9) antigens are specific; there is no cross-protection. Both preparations have the same dose optima (Yamagishi et al., 1979). Figure 28.2 demonstrates that the effect of Fraction 15 is mediated by the immune system: spleen cells derived from hosts treated with this material displayed neutralization in LATA (Pellis et al., 1980). Furthermore, multiple antigen injections of Fraction 15 (Fr 15) at weekly intervals sustain rather than depress host resistance.

Properties of Immunoprotective pIEF Fraction 15

Elicitation of Tumor Specific DTH Relations

Evocation of the delayed type hypersensitivity (DTH) response of footpad

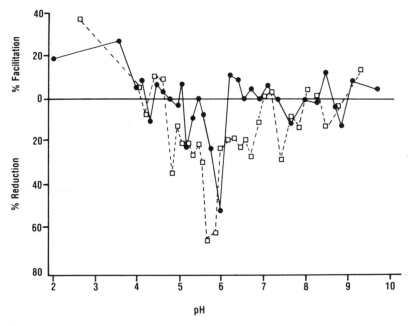

Figure 28.1. *In vivo* activity of isoelectric focusing fractions from crude 3M KCl extracts of MCA-F (●) and MCA-D (□) tumor cells. In individual experiments, crude extracts were fractionated in the PH gradient from 3 to 10. Fractions were eluted from the gel, concentrated, dialyzed, and assessed for immunoprotective activity. Doses of fractions equivalent to 1 mg of the crude extract were administered subcutaneously to groups of 10 mice. Ten days later, control and fraction-treated mice were challenged subcutaneously with 10^4 homotypic tumor cells. Tumor growth was monitored by serial caliper measurements of the mean diameter. Ordinate values were obtained by the formula: (control tumor diameter) − (treated tumor diameter).

swelling in mice previously immunized against a neoplasm affords a rapid alternative to, but correlates with, tumor specific resistance detected by transplantation tests *in vivo* (Takeichi and Boone, 1975). Mice rendered hyperimmune by three to five inoculations of 10^6 irradiated (12,000R) tumor cells at two week intervals were challenged six to ten days later with crude extracts of antigenic fractions (Parish, 1972; Brannen et al., 1974; Kon et al., 1976). Footpad swelling (FPS) in groups of ten immune and control hosts was measured using a dial gauge micrometer caliper and expressed as the difference between the PBS-injected and the antigen-injected footpad of each mouse. Consistent with other manifestations of DTH *in vivo*, there was minimum FPS at 4 hours, maximum at 24 hours, and thereafter a steady decrease to baseline at 48 hours. Antigenic activity was only ascribed to preparations which induced a maximum response at 24 hours.

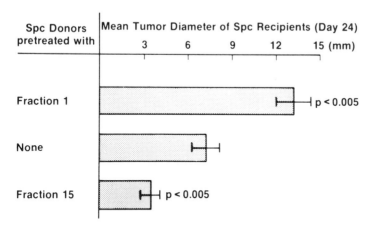

Adoptive Transfer of IEF Fraction Induced
Tumor Facilitation and Neutralization

Figure 28.2. Cell-mediated tumor facilitation and tumor neutralization induced by P2.6 and P6.0, respectively. Spleen cells (10^7) taken 6 days after subcutaneous inoculation of Fr 1 (P2.6) or Fr 15 (P6.0) were admixed with 10^4 MCA-F cells and then inoculated subcutaneously into 10 normal syngeneic recipients. Tumor growth was monitored by caliper measurement.

Hosts immunized with irradiated MCA-F cells displayed positive reactions to MCA-F plasma membranes, to MCA-F spent culture media, and to 10 μg MCA-F Fr 15, but not to these materials prepared from MCA-D cells. On the other hand, after immunization with 10^7 irradiated MCA-D cells, FPS was elicited only by extracts of MCA-D, but not of MCA-F (Macek et al., 1980). Furthermore, immunization with MCA-D 15 induced specific FPS upon challenge with 3M KCl extracts, with purified plasma membranes, and with MCA-F Fr 15, but not with 3M KCl extracts of MCA-D. Thus, Fr 15 induces

Table 28.1. Specificity of Tumor Facilitating Fraction (pI 2.6) and Tumor Protective Fraction (pI 6.0) from MCA-F Extracts.

Host pretreatment	Mean tumor diameter (mm) ± SEM at day 22			
	MCA-F	p	MCA-D	p
None	10.2 ± 0.8	–	7.7 ± 2.1	–
Fr 1 (pI 2.6)	16.8 ± 1.1	< 0.005	8.1 ± 1.6	NS
Fr 15 (pI 6.0)	5.8 ± 0.7	< 0.001	6.8 ± 1.8	NS

T cells which display DTH reactions without a booster stimulus of antigen on the membranes of intact cells.

Dissection of the Lymphoid Populations Sensitized by Fraction 15

The resistance induced by Fr 15 and demonstrated in LATA is mediated by a spleen cell population which is: (a) nonadherent to plastic, (b) radiosensitive to 1000, but not to 500, rads of gamma irradiation, (c) abrogated by anti-Thy 1.2 serum and complement, (d) I-A positive, and (e) non-adherent to nylon wool. The spleen cell activity is sensitive to monoclonal antibodies which individually recognize Lyt 1.1 and Lyt 2.1. The observation that Fr 15-induced tumor neutralization is abrogated by Lyt 1 and Lyt 2 antisera raised the provocative issue of whether Fr 15 induces (1) the Lyt 1, 2, 3 killer cells described by Shiku et al. (1976), or (2) two distinct populations, namely an Lyt 1 helper/delayed hypersensitivity cell, and an Lyt 2, 3 cytotoxic lymphocyte (Stutman, 1977). This question was resolved by demonstrating that it was not possible to reconstitute reactivity by mixing individual cell populations selectively depleted of Lyt 1+ or Lyt 2+ cells. This observation suggests that a single cell (Lyt 1, 2, 3) acts as an effector in Fr 15-induced tumor resistance.

Absence of H-2 Antigenic Activity

While H-2 determinants are present in crude 3M KCl extracts, Fr 15 does not contain H-2 activity in several assays: (a) MCA-F Fr 15 cannot immunize allogeneic BALB/c mice to display second-set rejection of C3H/MCA-F tumor cells. (b) MCA-F Fr 15 cannot elicit DTH responses in FPS assays using DBA/2J mice previously alloimmunized by multiple injections of normal C3H spleen cells. These same mice display FPS upon challenge with crude 3M KCl extracts of MCA-F. (c) Finally, there is a chemical separation of H-2 antigens eliciting FPS with pI values of 5.1–5.5, from TSTA with pI 5.95 (Macek et al., 1980).

Absence of Tumor Growth Facilitating Activity

Spleen cells which were obtained from hosts inoculated 0, 3, 6, 9, 12, or 15 days earlier with 25 μg Fr 15 and were admixed with MCA-F cells at an effector:tumor ratio of 1000:1, never displayed facilitation of neoplastic growth in LATA (Pellis et al., 1980).

Induction of Specific Antibody

Since Thomson et al. (1973, 1976) and Parker and Rosenberg (1977) used sera to demonstrate distinctive tumor antigens on MCA-induced sarcomas, serologic reagents were prepared using the partially purified material. MCA-F Fr 15 (100 μg) emulsified in incomplete Freund's adjuvant (IFA) was administered at three 10-day intervals to New Zealand White rabbits. The resultant sera, which were then heat inactivated and thrice absorbed with C3H spleen cells (10^8/ml serum), displayed "ring"membrane immunofluorescence up to a limiting dilution of 1:8, using an indirect assay with fluorescein isothiocyanate-conjugated, goat-anti-rabbit serum (Baldwin et al., 1971; Zoller et al., 1976).

Antibodies raised against MCA-F Fr 15 did not react with the two antigenically distinct tumors, MCA-D and T. Four lines of evidence suggest that the xenoantisera raised against Fr 15 possess antibodies which specifically recognize tumor specific epitopes: (a) the fluorescence reaction of the rabbit anti-MCA-F serum was only demonstrated on MCA-F, but not on MCA-D, MCA-2A, or MCA-T, target cells, (b) absorption with 10^8 normal C3H spleen cells or 10^8 MCA-D or MCA-T cells did not reduce antibody reactivity or the homotypic MCA-F tumor, (c) the immunofluorescence reaction was competitively inhibited by crude 3M KCl MCA-F extract ($ID_{50} = 3 \times 10^8$ cell equivalents), and (d) there was an inverse correlation between the *in vivo* growth rate of cell strains isolated from the MCA-F tumor, and their degree of reactivity with the rabbit serum (r value = −0.805). This relation is akin to the known correlation between tumor growth rate and antigenic content (Old et al., 1962).

TSTA Extraction with 1-Butanol

The 3M KCl extraction technique has the disadvantages of variable antigen yield, irreversible destruction of cell source and extensive contamination with surface, cytoplasmic, and nuclear proteins. Translation to the clinical setting required a procedure which efficiently and selectively releases TSTA without destruction of the source material, thereby permitting multiple extraction cycles.

The Butanol Technique

Extraction of cell surface or lipid-bound proteins using two phase (greater than 7%) solutions of butanol has been applied to a variety of models: murine erythrocytes (Adachi and Furusawa, 1968), lymphocyte histocompatibility antigens (Kandutsch, 1960; Manson and Palm, 1963), *E. coli* lipopolysaccharide (Morrison and Lieve, 1975; Kanegasaki and Jann, 1979), insoluble particulate enzymes (Morton, 1950; Szewczuk and Baranowski, 1963), proteolipids (Pasquini and Soto, 1972; Godwin and Sneddon, 1975; Ishitani et al., 1978), and blood group antigens (Gardas and Koscielak, 1971; Lambert and Zelinski, 1976, 1978). Recently methods have been developed using single-phase butanol solutions to extract proteins from sarcoplasmic reticulum (Sigrist et al., 1977). Noll et al. (1979) released a specific adhesion protein from sea urchin blastocysts using single-phase butanol extraction without killing the dissociated blastula cells. Extraction of plasma membrane associated moieties with retention of cellular viability is a particularly attractive approach in tumor biology, since yields of antigen tend to be low and source material scarce. Treatment with single-phase, 2.5% (v/v) 1-butanol solution yielded biologically active surface TSTA with retention of viability in 90% of the cells. Following a five-minute exposure of cell suspensions to 2.5% 1-butanol in PBS, cells are immediately sedimented at 500 g. Grossly insoluble material is removed by centrifugation at 10,000 g. The "crude butanol extract" is obtained following dialysis against PBS and ultracentrifugation at 200,000 g for one hour (LeGrue et al., 1980).

Immunoprophylactic Activity of Crude Butanol Extracts

Specific immunoprotection of C3H hosts against a 100 MTD challenge of MCA-F, but not MCA-D, was obtained by pretreatment with 25 μg MCA-F butanol extract. Crude butanol extracts have the same potency as 3M KCl Fr 15 and display exquisite specificity in immunoprophylaxis assays (Figure 28.3). The dose response characteristics of butanol extracts were similar to those of irradiated MCA-F cells, of crude 3M KCl extracts, and of 3M KCl Fr 15. There is a threshold of maximal effect, a plateau, and a supraoptimal level devoid of biological activity (LeGrue et al., 1980).

Preparative isoelectric focusing on a flat bed of Sephadex G75 yielded less than 25% of the pI < 3.0 material observed when 3M KCl extracts were subjected to pIEF. Furthermore, butanol extract Fraction 1 did not enhance tumor growth when administered to syngeneic hosts at doses equivalent to those that facilitated tumor growth by 3M KCl Fr 1. The absence of growth facilitating activity may explain the observation that crude butanol extracts have a similar specific activity to 3M KCl Fr 15.

The immunoprotective activity of MCA-F crude butanol extracts focused at pI 6.4, which in doses of 1–4 μg protein yielded 50–66% reduction of the outgrowth of 100 MTD of MCA-F, but not of MCA-D or MCA-2A (Figure 28.4). The TSTA activity in butanol extracts of the MCA-2A tumor also focused at pI 6.4. The yield from pIEF was excellent: greater than 90% of the applied protein was eluted in the 31 fractions with 3% of the total protein focused at pH 6.4. Of the TSTA units, 90% of the applied activity was recovered in all fractions, with 80% in Fr 16. The pIEF fraction displayed a thirty-fold increase in specific activity compared to the crude butanol extract and a five-fold increase over irradiated cells.

Properties of the Butanol Extract

Noncytolytic Nature of the Extraction Process

Cellular viability after butanol extraction was demonstrated by *in vitro* proliferation and *in vivo* growth. Extracted and untreated MCA-F cells displayed the same *in vitro* plating efficiency and growth rate when assessed five days later by ^{3}H-thymidine uptake (LeGrue et al., 1980). Furthermore, *in vivo* propagated cells extracted with butanol and re-inoculated into groups of syngeneic hosts at doses of 10^2 (MTD), 10^3, and 10^4 cells displayed the same growth rate and tumorigenicity as untreated MCA-F cells.

Relation of TSTA Determinants in 3M KCl and Butanol Extracts

Although many properties of the antigens in the KCl and butanol extracts

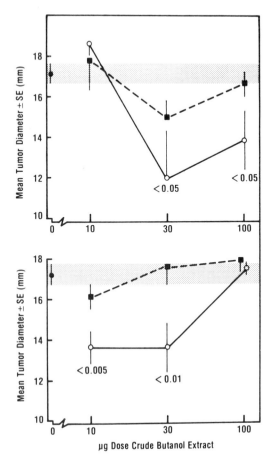

Figure 28.3. Groups of ten mice were immunized with either 10, 30, or 100 μg of butanol extract prepared from MCA-F or from MCA-2A cells, and challenged ten days later with 100 MTD of either MCA-F (upper panel) or MCA-2A (lower panel). The tumor size of hosts receiving homotypic (O—O) annd heterotypic (■--■) extracts were determined 21 days later. Tumor outgrowth (mean±SE) in PBS treated mice is indicated by the shaded areas. Significant differences in the outgrowth of immune and control animals were determined by Student's t-test, and the p-values are indicated.

appeared similar, there was no *a priori* reason to assume that they were crossreactive. In order to ascertain if there were shared antigenic determinants, two assays were utilized which did not require exposure of the host to intact tumor cells. C3H hosts immunized with 3M KCl Fraction 15 responded to footpad challenge with the immunizing antigen or with 7 μg butanol extract from MCA-F, but not to a crude butanol extract from MCA-2A. Secondly, the crude butanol extract specifically inhibited the activity of a rabbit anti-Fr 15 antiserum, demonstrating that xenogeneic hosts recognized an antigenic determinant shared by both antigens.

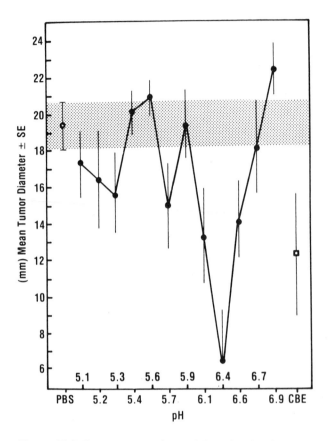

Figure 28.4. Immunoprotective activity of pIEF fractions from an MCA-F butanol extract, which demonstrates the ability of the extract to reduce the outgrowth of MCA-F cells *in vivo*. The mean tumor diameters of PBS-treated animals and animals receiving 2 μg of a pIEF fraction were compared 28 days post-challenge. The range of outgrowth in untreated hosts is indicated. Reduction of mean tumor diameter elicited by the pH 6.4 fraction was significant at a level of p≪0.001.

Antigenic Yield

The yield was calculated by two methods: estimation of relative immunoprotective activity and quantitative absorption of anti-Fr 15 antiserum. About 20% of the total immunoprotective units (one unit reduced tumor outgrowth by half) present on irradiated cells were present in the butanol extract, which comprises 1.8% of the total cell protein. However, this yield may be an underestimate, since numerous critical factors favor the immunogenicity of determinants arrayed on membrane surfaces of viable cells, as compared to antigens in solution. In addition, irradiated cells may synthesize and shed antigen in excess of that expressed at the time of injection, leading to an underestimate of the administered dose. Therefore, the yield was alternatively calculated on the basis of the capacity of putative antigens to absorb a rabbit anti-Fr 15 antiserum, using a method akin to that of Price (1979), who demonstrated a 5% yield with papain extraction. Quantitative absorption experiments show that butanol extraction yields about 60% of the exposed membrane antigen, while the 3M KCl technique yields about 5% (Table 28.2).

Absence of H-2 Alloantigen Activity

The butanol extract was unable to absorb H-2 reactivity from sera produced *in vivo* against K (D23 [b]) or D (D32) private specificities or from monoclonal hybridoma reagents directed against H-2K^k (11–4.1) or Ia^k (10–2.16), whereas whole MCA-F cells have an AD$_{50}$ of 5×10^4 for the H-2K^k reagent but do not absorb the Ia^k monoclonal antibody. The control for specificity was the D33 antiserum directed against H-2K^b, and the positive control was the H-2 antigen present in C3H mouse serum. Furthermore, DBA-2 mice (H-2^d) immunized with 10^7 C3H spleen cells (H-2^k) displayed footpad swelling upon challenge with 3M KCl extracts of either C3H spleen cells or MCA-F, but not with a 3M KCl extract of C57B1/6 (H-2^b) spleen cells, nor with butanol extracts of C3H spleen or of MCA-F cells. These results strongly suggest that butanol extracts do not contain biologically active alloantigens.

Immunotherapeutic Effects of Tumor Extracts

Immunotherapy with 3M KCl Fr 15

Local Disease

Fraction 15 elicited resistance in syngeneic C3H hosts either inoculated with supralethal doses of neoplastic cells or bearing local recurrences after incom-

Table 28.2. Comparison of Protein and Antigenic Yields from Cells and Extracts of MCA-F.

Preparation	Protein yield (mg/10^9 cells)	Antigen yield (TSTA Units/10^9cells)^a	AD$_{50}$ (cell equivalents$\times 10^{-7}$)^b
Irradiated cells	550	1×10^5	1.0 (100%)
Crude 3M KCl extract	25	45	30 (3.3%)
KCl pH 5.9 fraction	0.25	20	15 (6.7%)
Crude butanol extract	7.0	280	1.7 (59%)

^{a}TSTA activity obtained from 10^9 MCA-F cells or extracts of 10^9 cells. One TSTA unit is the mg amount of protein necessary to reduce tumor outgrowth by 50%. The specific activity (U/mg) of preparation is defined as the antigen yield divided by the protein yield.
^{b}The AD$_{50}$ is the cell number or cell number equivalents which reduced the binding of an MCA-F specific rabbit antiserum by 50%. The cell number equivalents for extracts were calculated from the mg amount of extract necessary to reduce surface immunofluorescence by half, divided by the protein yield per 10^7 cells. The percent yield of antigen activity in each preparation is indicated in parentheses.

plete tumor excision. Mice treated, beginning one day after injection of 10^2 (MTD) or 10^3 (10MTD) MCA-F cells, with a course of 3, 4, or 5 weekly injections of 25 μg MCA-F Fr 15 displayed a decreased tumor incidence and rate of neoplastic outgrowth (Kahan et al., 1980). In a second model, animals cured of 1 cm diameter MCA-F tumors by resection were immediately inoculated subcutaneously with a superlethal challenge of 10^3 MCA-F cells to assess immunostimulation by soluble antigen. Mice treated with 3 or 4 injections of 25 μg Fr 15 displayed reduced tumor incidence; indeed, there was abated neoplastic outgrowth in afflicted mice given 4 injections (Kahan et al., 1980). In a third model, about 50% of hosts inoculated with 10^5 MCA-F cells and undergoing resection of 2 cm diameter tumors succumbed to local recurrence by day 19, and died by day 42. On the other hand, treatment with weekly injections of 25 μg Fr 15 decreased the local recurrence rate to 16.7% and the mortality rate to 13.9% by day 19. As shown in Table 28.3, at 60 days 77.8% of Fr 15 treated animals were tumor-free compared to 49.6% of the controls (Kahan et al., 1980). In order to demonstrate that Fr 15 treated hosts were specifically resistant to MCA-F, all surviving animals were challenged with 10 MTD of MCA-D. The MCA-F Fr 15-treated animals succumbed to the antigenically different MCA-D challenge at the same rate as untreated post-resection survivors, and as naive C3H mice not previously inoculated with MCA-F. These findings suggest that the resistance of Fr 15 treated animals was due to specific immunity to MCA-F.

Intravenous Dissemination Model

Although immunogenic TSTA can be isolated from cells derived from a primary tumor, one major obstacle to a therapeutic endeavor might be an

Table 28.3. The Effect of Fr 15 Immunotherapy upon Local Recurrence and Survival Rates after Surgical Resection of 2 cm MCA-F Tumors.

Treatment	No. mice	Operative deaths	Recurrence rate (day 19)[a]	Cure rate (day 60)[b]	Mortality rate (%)[c]
None	40	5	17/35 (48.6)	16/35 (45.7)	18/35 (51.4)
Immunotherapy	40	4	6/36 (16.7)[d]	28/36 (77.8)	8/36 (22.2)[e]

Note: Syngeneic hosts inoculated with 10^5 (1000 MTD) MCA-F and surgically resected when the tumors reached an average diameter of 2 cm; one day later, hosts were divided into two groups: one group was untreated and a second group was treated with weekly doses of 25 μg Fr 15.
[a]Recurrence rate is the proportion of animals displaying a palpable (2 mm) tumor at day 19. Percentage values are in parentheses.
[b]Cure rate is the number of animals with no evident recurrence at day 60. Percentage values are in parentheses.
[c]Mortality rate is the number of animals dead at day 60. All hosts with recurrences by day 60 died.
[d]Statistically significant difference between two groups at the $p < 0.01$ level.
[e]Statistically significant difference between two groups at the $p < 0.05$ level.

antigenic individuality of local recurrences or metastases (Sugarbaker and Cohen, 1972). Diversity in the neoplastic population may occur from an initial or subsequent generation of multiple clones, due to impaired chromosomal replication and/or segregation. Some neoplastic clones display an increased proclivity to metastasis, possibly because of a (1) propensity for migration, (2) affinity for and preferential growth in certain tissues (Fidler and Nicolson, 1976), or (3) deletion of surface markers initially present on the local neoplasm (Fogel et al., 1979). Biologic differences in drug (Trope, 1975) and complement-mediated lytic susceptibility as well as chromosome number (Chu and Malmgren, 1961) may reflect the diversity of clones. Fidler and Kripke (1977) found a difference in the incidence of lung metastases produced by intravenous inoculation of various B16 melanoma clones, suggesting the pre-existence of cells with metastatic propensity in the original tumor population. Pimm and Baldwin (1977) reported antigenically distinct subline pairs derived from surgically excised, primary MCA sarcomas compared to post-surgically recurrent tumors. Baldwin et al. (1979) noted that sublines obtained from pulmonary and gut metastases are in some cases antigenically distinct. Indeed, the immunotherapeutic approach would be of limited value, if the metastases did not bear the surface antigens present on the primary tumor.

Immunotherapy with weekly injections of 25 µg MCA-F Fr 15 decreased the number of pulmonary metastases counted three weeks after intravenous injection via the femoral vein of 10^5 or 10^6 MCA-F cells. These results suggest that at least some of the small fraction of MCA-F cells with metastatic propensity bear the Fr 15 antigen. These findings are consistent with the work of Prehn (1970) showing that antigenic specificity is a stable characteristic of late transplant generations of carcinogen-induced tumors.

Immunotherapeutic Activity of Butanol Extracts

In order to simulate a therapeutic situation in man, mice were treated with weekly subcutaneous injections of 100 µg butanol extract weekly, combined with 25 mg/kg cyclophosphamide injected intraperitoneally, beginning 8 days after inoculation of 10^5 tumor cells. At this time, tumor nodules were 4 mm in diameter. Only the group treated with combined chemoimmunotherapy displayed tumor regression, which was evident by 25 days, and there was little evidence of neoplasms by day 70. While all hosts treated with cyclophosphamide alone were dead at 55 days, 30% of butanol antigen-cyclophosphamide hosts survived over 70 days (Figure 28.5).

Summary

Tumor specific resistance against methylcholanthrene-induced sarcomas was induced by 3M KCl extracts of neoplastic cells. The immunogenic potency of extracts was increased 50-fold by purification upon preparative isoelectric focusing. The partially purified material not only evoked immunoprophylaxis

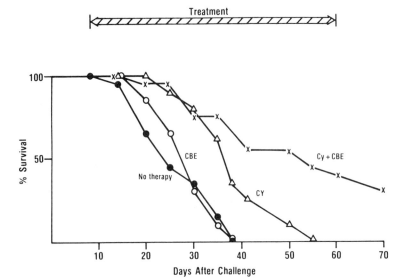

Figure 28.5. Groups of twenty C3H/HeJ mice were inoculated subcutaneously with 10^5 MCA-F cells. At day 8, after challenge, hosts bearing 4 mm established tumors were treated with: (1) Crude butanol extract (CBE), 100 μg weekly, subcutaneously, (O—O); (2) Cyclophosphamide (CY), 25 mg/kg twice a week, intraperitoneally (△—△); (3) CBE plus CY (X—X); or (4) No therapy (●—●). % Survival is shown during 70 days after challenge. Four mice in CBE plus CY group showed complete tumor regression.

against tumor challenge, but also induced specific active immunotherapy against supralethal concomitant or residual neoplastic disease. In order to adapt these methods for future use in the clinical arena, a new method of antigen release was designed. Selective liberation of the active principle from sarcoma cells was obtained with increased yield and with retention of cellular viability by brief exposure to 2.5% (v/v) 1-butanol. The soluble antigen not only was a more potent immunogen than irradiated cells, but also evoked regression of established (4 mm) neoplasms in mice. These findings offer the prospect of intervention with specific active immunotherapy for some neoplasms in man.

References

Adachi, H. and Furusawa, M. (1968) Immunological analysis of the structural molecules of erythrocyte membrane in mice. Analysis of the acqueous phase molecules obtained by butanol fractionation of erythrocyte membrane. *Exp. Cell. Res.* 50:490–496.

Aoki, T., Boyse, E.A., and Old, L.J. (1968) Wild type gross leukemia virus. I. Soluble antigen (GSA) in the plasma and tissues of infected mice. *J. Natl. Cancer Inst.* 41:89–96.

Aoki, T., Herberman, R.B., Johnson, P.A., Lin, M., and Sturm, M.M. (1972) Wild type gross leukemia virus: classification of soluble antigens (GSA). *J. Virol.* 10:1208–1219.

Argyris, B.F. (1978) Activation of suppressor cells by syngeneic tumor transplants in mice. *Cancer Res.* 38:1269–1273.

Argyris, B.F. and DeLustro, F. (1977) Immunologic unresponsiveness of mouse spleen sensitized to allogeneic tumors. *Cellular Immunol.* 28:390–403.

Baldwin, R.W. (1973) Immunological aspects of chemical carcinogenesis. *Advance Cancer Res.* 18:1–75.

Baldwin, R.W., Barker, C.R., Embleton, M.J., Glaves, D., Moore, M., and Pimm, M.V. (1971) Demonstration of cell surface antigens on chemically induced tumors. *Ann. N.Y. Acad. Sci.* 177:268–278.

Baldwin, R.W., Barker, C.R., Embleton, M.J., Glaves, D., Moore, M., and Pimm, M.V. (1979) Neoantigens in chemical carcinogenesis. In *Carcinogens: Identification and Mechanisms of action.* Griffin, A.C. and Shaw, C.R. (ed.), New York: Raven Press, pp. 365–379.

Basombrio, M.A. (1970) Search for common antigenicities among twenty-five sarcomas induced by methylcholanthrene. *Cancer Res.* 30:2458–2462.

Basombrio, M.A. and Prehn, R.T. (1972) Antigenic diversity of tumors chemically induced within the progeny of a single cell. *Int. J. Cancer* 10:1–8.

Batchelor, J.R., Welsh, K.I., and Burgos, H. (1978) Transplantation antigens per se are poor immunogens within a species. *Nature* 273:54–56.

Benjamini, E., Theilen, G.H., Torten, M., Fong, S., Crow, S., and Hennes, A.M. (1976) Tumor vaccines for immunotherapy of canine lymphosarcoma. Part III. Specific active immunotherapy (tumor vaccines) for cancer. *Ann. N.Y. Acad. Sci.* 277:305–312.

Beverly, P.C., Lowenthal, R.M., and Tyrrell, D.A. (1973) Immune responses in mice to tumor challenge after immunization with Newcastle disease virus-infected or x-irradiated tumor cells or cell fractions. *Int. J. Cancer* 11:212–223.

Bonavida, B. and Zighelboim, J. (1974) Modulation of the immune response towards allografts *in vivo*. I. Selective suppression of the development of cell-mediated immunity by soluble alloantigens. *Cell. Immunol.* 13:52–65.

Bonmassar, E., Golding, A., and Cudkowicz, G. (1971) Differential reactivity of mice to alloantigens associated with the D and K end of H-2. *Transplantation* 12:314–318.

Bonmassar, E., Menconi, E., Golding, A., and Cudkowicz, G. (1974) Escape of small numbers of allogeneic lymphoma cells from immune surveillance. *J. Natl. Cancer Inst.* 53:475–479.

Boone, C.W. and Blackman, K. (1972) Augmented immunogenicity of tumor homogenates infected with influenza virus. *Cancer Res.* 32:1018–1022.

Bowen, J.G. and Baldwin, R.W. (1976) Isolation and characterization of tumor-specific antigen from the serum of rats bearing transplanted aminoazo die-induced hepatomas. *Transplant.* 21:213–219.

Brannen, G.E., Adams, J.S., and Santos, G.W. (1974) Tumor-specific immunity in 3-methylcholanthrene-induced murine fibrosarcomas. I. *In vivo* demonstration of immunity with three preparations of soluble antigens. *J. Natl. Cancer Inst.* 53:165–175.

Bubenik, J., Indrova, M., Nemeckova, S., Malkovsky, M., Von Broen, B., Palek, V., and Anderlikova, J. (1978) Solubilized tumor-associated antigens of methylcholanthrene-induced mouse sarcomas. Comparative studies by *in vitro* sensitization of lymph node cells, macrophage electrophoretic mobility assay and transplantation tests. *Int. J. Cancer* 21:348:355.

Burnett, F.M. (1970) The concept of immunological surveillance. *Progr. Exp. Tumor Res.* 13:1–27.

Chu, E. and Malmgren, R. (1961) Microspectrophotometric determination of deoxyribonucleic acid in primary and metastatic mouse mammary tumors. *J. Natl. Cancer Inst.* 27:217–220.

Coggin, J.H. (1979) Induction of transplantation resistance with soluble Simian Virus 40-induced hamster tumor specific transplantation antigen. *Cancer Res.* 39:2952–2959.

Embleton, M.J. (1976) Influence of cell-free tumor-associated antigen preparations on the development of immunity to chemically induced rat tumors. *Int. J. Cancer* 18:622–629.

Embleton, M.J. and Heidelberger, C. (1972) Antigenicity of clones of mouse prostate cells transformed *in vitro. Int. J. Cancer* 9:8–18.

Embleton, M.J. and Heidelberger, C. (1975) Neoantigens on chemically transformed cloned C3H mouse embryo cells. *Cancer Res.* 35:2049–2055.

Fidler, I.J. and Kripke, M. (1977) Metastasis results from preexisting variant cells within a malignant tumor. *Science* 197:893–895.

Fidler, I.J. and Nicholson, G.L. (1976) Organ selectivity for implantation survival and growth of B16 melanoma variant tumor lines. *J. Natl. Cancer Inst.* 57:1199–1202.

Fogel, M., Gorelik, E., Segal, S., and Feldman, M. (1979) Antigenic differences exist between cell surface antigens of the local tumor and its metastases. *Proc. Leukocyte Cult. Conf.* 12:715–723.

Foley, E.J. (1953) Antigenic properties of methylcholanthrene-induced tumors in mice of the strain of origin. *Cancer Res.* 13:835–837.

Forni, G. and Comoglio, P.M. (1974) Effect of solubilized membrane antigens and tumor bearer serum on tumor growth in syngeneic hosts. *Brit. J. Cancer* 30:365–369.

Fujimoto, S., Chen, C.H., Sabbadini, E., and Sehon, A.H. (1973) Association of tumor and histocompatibility antigens in sera of lymphoma-bearing mice. *J. Immunol.* 111:1093–1100.

Fujimoto, S., Green, M.I., and Sehon, A.H. (1976) Regulation of the immune response to tumor antigens. I. Immunosuppressor cells in tumor-bearing hosts. *J. Immunol.* 116:791–799.

Gardas, A. and Koscielak, J. (1971) A, B, and H blood group specificities in glycoprotein and glycolipid fractions of human erythrocyte membrane. Absence of blood group active glycoproteins in the membranes of nonsecretors. *Vox Sang.* 20:137–149.

Gillette, R.W., Berringer, D.C. and Wunderlich, D.A. (1978) Resistance to syngeneic lymphoma cells as a result of immunization with chemically modified allogenic lymphoma cells in mice. *J. Natl. Cancer Inst.* 60:1427–1432.

Godwin, S.F.R. ad Sneddon, J.M. (1975) The binding of 5-hydroxytryptamine to butanol extracts of rat brain stems. *J. Neurochem.* 25:238–288.

Greene, M.I., Perry, L.L., and Benacerraf, B. (1979) Regulation of the immune response to tumor antigen. V. Modulation of suppressor T cell activity *in vivo. Am. J. Pathol.* 95:159–169.

Herberman, R.B. (1977) Existence of tumor immunity in man. In *Mechanisms of Tumor Immunity.* Cohen, S. and Green, I. (eds.), New York: Wiley and Sons, pp. 175–191.

Holmes, E.C., Morton, D.L., Schidlovsky, G., and Trahan, E. (1971) Cross-reacting tumor specific transplantation antigens in methylcholanthrene induced guinea pig sarcomas. *J. Natl. Cancer Inst.* 46:693–700.

Ishitani, R., Miyakawa, A., and Iwamoto, T. (1978) Butanol extracts from myelin fragments. II. Some properties of 5-hydroxytryptamine binding. *Japan. J. Pharmacol.* 28:899–907.

Kahan, B.D. (1972) Solubilization of allospecific and tumor specific cell surface antigens. In *Methods in Cancer Research* Vol. VII. Busch, H. (ed.), New York: Academic Press, pp. 283–338.

Kahan, B.D., Tom, B.H., Mittal, K.K., and Bergan, J.J. (1974) An immunodiagnostic test for transplant rejection. *Lancet* 1:37–42.

Kahan, B.D., Tanaka, T., and Pellis, N.R. (1980) Immunotherapy of a carcinogen-induced murine sarcoma with soluble tumor specific transplantation antigens. *J. Natl. Cancer Inst.* 65:1001–1004.

Kandutsch, A.A. (1960) Intracellular distribution and extraction of tumor homograft-enhancing antigens. *Cancer Res.* 20:264–268.

Kanegasaki, S. and Jann, K. (1979) Demonstration by membrane reconstitution of a butanol-soluble intermediate in the biosynthesis of the 09 antigen of *Escherichia coli. Eur. J. Biochem.* 95:287–293.

Kobayashi, H., Sendo, F., Kaji, H., Shirai, T., Salto, H., Takeichi, N., Hosokawa, M., and Kodama, T. (1970) Inhibition of transplanted rat tumors by immunization with identical tumor cells infected with Friend virus. *J. Natl. Cancer Inst.* 44:11–19.

Kolsch, E., Mengersen, R., and Diller, E. (1973) Low dose tolerance preventing tumor immunity. *Eur. J. Cancer* 9:879–882.

Kon, N.D, Forbes, J.T., and Klein, P.A. (1976) Ability of delayed type hypersensitivity reactions to distinguish tumor associated antigens and histocompatibility antigens in soluble extracts from murine fibrosarcoma. *Int. J. Cancer* 17:613–620.

Lafferty, K.J. and Woolnough, J. (1977) The origin and mechanism of the allograft reaction. *Immunological Rev.* 35:231–262.

Lambert, R.M. and Zelenski, K.R. (1976) The H specificities of butanol extracts of human erythrocytes. *Vox Sang.* suppl. 1, 31:77–83.

Lambert, R.M. and Zelenski, K.R. (1978) Blood group antigens in butanol extracts of animal tissues. *Proc. Soc. Exp. Biol. Med.* 158:220–223.

LeGrue, S.J., Kahan, B.D., and Pellis, N.R. (1980) Butanol extraction of a murine tumor specific transplantation antigen. 1. Partial purification by isoelectric focusing. *J. Natl. Cancer Inst.* 65:191–196.

Leonard, E.J., Richardson, A.K., Hardy, A.S., and Rapp, H.J. (1975) Extraction of tumor specific antigen from cells and plasma membranes of line-10 hepatoma. *J. Natl. Cancer Inst.* 55:73–79.

Luborsky, S.W., Chang, C., Pancake, S.J., and Mora, P.T. (1976) Detergent solubilized and molecular weight estimation of tumor specific surface antigen from SV40 virus transformed cells. *Biochem. Biophys. Res. Commun.* 71:990–996.

Macek, C., Kahan, B.D., and Pellis, N.R. (1980) Delayed hypersensitivity reactions to tumor antigens. *J. Immunol.* 125:1639–1643.

Manor, Y., Treves, A.J., Cohen, I.R., and Feldman, M. (1976) Transition from T cell protection to T cell enhancement during tumor growth in an allogeneic host. *Transplantation* 22:4, 360–366.

Manson, L.A., Foschi, G.V., and Palm, J. (1963) An association of transplantation antigens with microsomal lipoproteins of normal and malignant tissues. *J. Cell. Comp. Physiol.* 61:109–118.

Martin, W.J., Wunderlich, J.R., Fletcher, F., and Inman, J.K. (1971) Enhanced immunogenicity of chemically-coated syngeneic tumor cells. *Proc. Natl. Acad. Sci.* 68:469–472.

Meltzer, M.S., Leonard, E.J., and Rapp, H.J. (1975) Protective tumor immunity induced by potassium chloride extracts of guinea pig hepatomas. *J. Natl. Cancer Inst..* 54:1349–1354.

Milas, L., Hunter, N., Mason, K., and Withers, H.R. (1974) Immunological resistance to pulmonary metastases in C3Hf/Bn mice bearing syngeneic fibrosarcomas of different sizes. *Cancer Res.* 34:61–71.

Mondal, S., Embleton, M.J., Marquardt, H., and Heidelberger, C. (1971) Production of variants of decreased malignancy and antigenicity from clones transformed *in vitro* by methylcholanthrene. *Int. J. Cancer* 8:410–420.

Morrison, D. and Lieve, L. (1975) Fractions of lipopolysaccharide from *Escherichia Coli* 0111:B4 prepared by two extraction procedures. *J. Biol. Chem.* 250:2911–2919.

Morton, R.K. (1950) Separation and purification of enzymes associated with insoluble particles. *Nature* 166:1092–1095.

Natori, T., Law, L.W., and Appella, E. (1978) Immunochemical evidence of a tumor specific surface antigen obtained by detergent solubilization of the membranes of a chemically induced sarcoma, meth-A. *Cancer Res.* 38:359–364.

404

Nelson, K., Pollack, S.B., and Hellstrom, K.E. (1975) Specific anti-tumor responses by cultured immune spleen cells. *Int. J. Cancer* 15:806–814.

Noll, H., Matranga, V., Cascino, D., and Vittorelli, L. (1979) Reconstitution of membranes and embryonic development in dissociated blastula cells of the sea urchin by reinsertion of aggregation-promoting membrane proteins extracted with butanol. *Proc. Natl. Acad. Sci. U.S.A.* 76:288–292.

Nordlund, J.J. and Gershon, R.K. (1975) Splenic regulation of the clinical appearance of small tumors. *J. Immunol.* 114:1486–1490.

Oettgen, H.G., Old, L.J., McLean, E.P., and Carswell, E.A. (1968) Delayed hypersensitivity and transplantation immunity elicited soluble antigens of chemically induced tumors of inbred guinea pigs. *Nature* 220:295–297.

Old, L.J., Boyse, E.A., Clarke, D.A., and Carswell, E.A. (1962a) Part II. Antigens of tumor cells. Antigenic properties of chemically induced tumors. *Ann. N.Y. Acad. Sci.* 101:80–106.

Old, L.J., Clarke, D.A., Benacerraf, B., and Stockart, E. (1962b) Effect of prior splenectomy on the growth of sarcoma 180 in normal and Bacillus Calmette-Guerin infected mice. *Experientia* 18:335–336.

Paranjpe, M.S. and Boone, C.W. (1975) Specific depression of the anti-tumor cellular immune response with autologous tumor homogenate. *Cancer Res.* 35:1205–1209.

Parish, C.R. and Liew, R.Y. (1972) Immune response to chemically modified flagellin. 3. Enhanced cell-mediated immunity during high and low zone antibody tolerance to flagellin. *J. Exp. Med.* 135:298–311.

Parker, G.A. and Rosenberg, S.A. (1977) Serologic identification of multiple tumor-associated antigens on murine sarcomas. *J. Natl. Cancer Inst.* 58:1303–1309.

Pasquini, J.M. and Soto, E.F. (1972) Extraction of proteolipids from nervous tissue with n-butanol-water. *Life Sci.* 11:433–443.

Pellis, N.R. and Kahan, B.D. (1975) Specific tumor immunity induced with soluble materials: restricted range of antigen dose and of challenge tumor load for immunoprotection. *J. Immunol.* 115:1717–1722.

Pellis, N.R. and Kahan, B.D. (1978) Methods to demonstrate the immunogenicity of soluble tumor antigens. II. The local adoptive transfer assay. *Methods in Cancer Res.* 14:29–54.

Pellis, N.R., Tom, B.H., and Kahan, B.D. (1974) Tumor specific and allospecific immunogenicity of soluble extracts from chemically induced murine sarcomas. *J. Immunol.* 113:708–711.

Pellis, N.R., Shulan, D.J., and Kahan, B.D. (1976) Specific tumor immunity induced with soluble materials: purification of antigens inducing tumor resistance. *Biochem. Biophys. Res. Commun.* 71:1251–1258.

Pellis, N.R., Mokyr, M.B. Babcock, J.R., and Kahan, B.D. (1978) Progression of the immune response to solubilized tumor antigens. *Immunol. Commun.* 7:431–440.

Pellis, N.R., Yamagishi, H., Macek, C.M., and Kahan, B.D. (1980) Specificity and biological activity of extracted murine tumor specific transplantation antigens. *Int. J. Cancer* 26:443–449.

Pimm, M.V. and Baldwin, R.W. (1977) Antigenic differences between primary methylcholanthrene-induced rat sarcomas and post-surgical recurrences. *Int. J. Cancer* 20:37–43.

Prager, M.D. and Gordon, W.C. (1978) Enhanced response to chemoimmunotherapy and im-munoprophylaxis with the use of tumor-associated antigens with a lipophilic agent. *Cancer Res.* 38:2052–2057.

Prehn, R.T. (1970) Analysis of antigenic heterogeneity within individual 3-methylcholanthrene-induced mouse sarcomas. *J. Natl. Cancer Inst.* 45:1039–1045.

Prehn, R.T. (1971) Perspectives in oncogenesis: does immunity stimulate or inhibit neoplasia? *J. Reticuloendothel. Soc.* 10:1–6.

Prehn, R.T. and Main, J.M. (1957) Immunity to methylcholanthrene-induced sarcomas. *J. Natl. Cancer Inst.* 18:769–778.

Price, M.R. (1979) I.C.R.E.W. Workshop Report, page 4.

Radola, B.J. (1973) Isoelectric focusing in layers of granulated gels. I. Thin-layer isoelectric focusing of proteins. *Biochim. Biophys. Acta* 295:412–428.

Rao, V.S., Bagai, R., and Bonavida, B. (1976) Specific enhancement of tumor growth and depression of cell-mediated immunity following sensitization to soluble tumor antigens. *Cancer Res.* 36:1384–1391.

Reisfeld, R.A. and Kahan, B.D. (1970) Biological and chemical characterization of human histocompatibility antigens. *Fed. Proc. Fed. Am. Soc. Exp. Biol.* 29:2034–2040.

Revesz, L. (1960) Detection of antigenic differences in isologous host-tumor systems by pretreatment with heavily irradiated tumor cells. *Cancer Res.* 20:443–457.

Rios, A. and Simmons, R.L. (1973) Immunospecific regression of various syngeneic mouse tumors in response to neuraminidase-treated tumor cells. *J. Natl. Cancer Inst.* 51:637–644.

Rogers, M.J. and Law, L.W. (1979) Immunogenic properties of a soluble tumor rejection antigen (TSTA) from a Simian Virus 40-induced sarcoma. *Int. J. Cancer* 23:89–96.

Shiku, H., Takahashi, T., Bean, M.A., Old, J.L., and Oettgen H.F. (1976) Ly phenotype of cytotoxic T cells for syngeneic tumor. *J. Exp. Med.* 144:1116–1120.

Simkovic, D., Chorvath, B., Duraj, J., and Hlubinova, K. (1978) Inhibition and promotion of growth of B77-virus-induced rat tumor with KCl-solubilized tumor cell components. *Neoplasma* 25:647–651.

Small, M. and Trainin, N. (1976) Separation of populations of sensitized lymphoid cells into fractions inhibiting and fractions enhancing syngeneic tumor growth *in vivo*. *J. Immunol.* 117:292–297.

Steele, G., Sjogren, H.O., and Price, M.R. (1975) Tumor-associated and embryonic antigens in soluble fractions of a chemically-induced rat colon carcinoma. *Int. J. Cancer* 16:33–51.

Stutman, O. (1977) Two main features of T-cell development: thymus traffic and postthymic maturation. *Contemp. Top. Immunbiol.* 7:1–46.

Sugarbaker, E.V. and Cohen, A.M. (1972) Altered antigenicity in spontaneous pulmonary metastases from an antigenic murine sarcoma. *Surgery* 72:155–161.

Szewczuk, A. and Baranowski, T. (1963) Purification and properties of γ-glutamyl transpeptidase from beef kidney. *Biochem. Z* 338:317–329.

Takei, F., Levy, J.G., and Kilburn, D.G. (1977) Characterization of suppressor cells in mice bearing syngeneic mastocytoma. *J. Immunol.* 118:412–417.

Takeichi, N. and Boone, C.W. (1975) Local adoptive transfer of the anti-tumor cellular immune response in syngeneic and allogenic mice studied with a rapid radioisotopic footpad assay. *J. Natl. Cancer Inst.* 55:183–187.

Thomson, D.M.P., Sellens, V., Eccles, S., and Alexander, P. (1973) Radioimmunoassay of tumor specific transplantation antigen of a chemically induced rat sarcoma: circulating soluble tumor antigen in tumor bearers. *Brit. J. Cancer* 28:377–388.

Thomson, D.M.P., Gold, P., Freedman, S.O., and Schuster, Y. (1976) The isolation and characterization of tumor specific antigens of rodent and human tumors. *Cancer Res.* 36:3518–3525.

Trope, C. (1975) Different sensitivity to cytostatic drugs of primary tumor and metastasis of the Lewis carcinoma. *Neoplasma* 22:171–180.

Vaage, J. (1974) Circulating tumor antigens versus immune serum factors in depressed concomitant immunity. *Cancer Res.* 34:2979–2983.

Yamigishi, H., Pellis, N.R., and Kahan, B.D. (1979) Tumor protective and facilitating antigens from solubilized tumor extracts. *J. Surg. Res.* 26:392–400.

Yamagishi, H., Pellis, N.R., Mokyr, M.R., and Kahan, B.D. (1980) Specific and non-specific immunologic mechanisms of tumor growth facilitation. *Cancer* 45:1630–1635.

Yamauchi, K., Fujimoto, S., and Tada, T. (1979) Differential activation of cytotoxic and suppressor T cells against syngeneic tumors in the mouse. *J. Immunol.* 123:1653–1658.

Zoller, M., Price, M.R., and Baldwin, R.W. (1976) Inhibition of cell-mediated cytotoxicity to chemically induced rat tumors by soluble tumor and embryo cell extracts. *Int. J. Cancer* 17:129–137.

Published 1981 by Elsevier North Holland, Inc.
Saunders, Daniels, Serrou, Rosenfeld, and Denney, eds.
FUNDAMENTAL MECHANISMS IN HUMAN CANCER IMMUNOLOGY

CHAPTER 29

Carbohydrate Regulated Shedding of Immunochemically Defined Human Melanoma Antigens[1]

A.C. Morgan, Jr., D.R. Galloway,
and R.A. Reisfeld

*Department of Molecular Immunology, Scripps Clinic and Research Foundation,
La Jolla, CA*

Introduction

The search for transformation markers on human and animal tumors has had wide appeal. This interest derives from the potential of these molecules for diagnosis and therapeutic monitoring of neoplastic disease, and from their utility as a tool for exploring the ontogeny and cellular economy of neoplasms.

Many of these studies have employed human melanoma cells as a model system because of the immunogenic nature of this tumor, as detected by assays of both humoral and cell-mediated immunity (Lewis et al., 1969; Skiku et al., 1976; Fass et al., 1970; Fossati et al., 1971; Hellström et al., 1973; Roth et al., 1976; Livingston et al., 1979), and because of the ready availability of long-term cell cultures. The great majority of these studies have focused on human melanoma associated antigens (MAA's) on the surface of melanoma cells. Our laboratory, however, has employed spent culture medium as a source of MAA. The less complex nature of spent culture medium compared to cell surface material has facilitated the identification and purification of two glycoproteins which show specificity for tumor cells.

We have employed indirect immunoprecipitation and sodium dodecyl sulfate polyacrylamide gel electrophoresis (SDS-PAGE) for direct visualization and quantitation of these MAA's, employing both polyclonal and monoclonal antisera. We report on the identification and biochemical characterization of

[1]This is publication No. 2288 from the Department of Molecular Immunology, Scripps Clinic and Research Foundation, La Jolla, CA. This work was supported by USPH Service Grant CA 28420 and Grant IM-218 of the American Cancer Society.

these tumor specific glycoproteins and present evidence for the role of carbohydrates in their shedding from tumor cells.

Identification and Biochemical Characterization of MAA's Shed into Spent Culture Medium

Our approach to identifying tumor specific components in spent culture
medium of intrinsically radiolabeled human melanoma cells involved indirect
immunoprecipitation of such media with polyclonal xenoantisera raised to
human melanoma, carcinoma, and lymphoid cell lines (Galloway et al., 1981a).
Antisera to melanoma cells specifically immunoprecipitated major proteins
with molecular weights of 240K, 220K, and 94K daltons along with non-
specifically absorbed proteins of 45K daltons and small molecules migrating
with the dye front. Figure 29.1A shows a typical profile of immunoprecipitated
components of spent culture medium harvested from melanoma cells following
24 to 72 hours of intrinsic labeling with ^{3}H-amino acids. Antisera to B and T
lymphoid cells did not precipitate either the 240K, 220K, or 94K proteins.
Labeled spent culture medium was previously immunodepleted with anti-
lymphoid cell antiserum absorbed to either formalin-fixed, heat-treated, Pro-
tein-A-bearing *Staphylococcus aureus* Cowan I strain (SACI) or Protein-A-
Sepharose C1-4B. This procedure rendered the subsequent immunoprecipitation by anti-melanoma serum of labeled spent culture medium specific for the
aforementioned 240K, 220K, and 94K proteins. Antiserum to melanoma cells,
human AB erythrocytes, or normal human serum also precipitated a component of 180K daltons. Reactivity to the 180K component was removed by
previous adsorption of anti-melanoma antiserum on normal human plasma
depleted of Ig and coupled to Sepharose 4B (Morgan et al., 1980). In
subsequent experiments, we identified the 220K component present in spent
media as fibronectin, both by specific immunoprecipitation with antiserum to
human plasma fibronectin and by showing its affinity for denatured collagen.
This property of fibronectin allowed us to remove the 220K protein specifically
by absorption of labeled spent medium on gelatin-Sepharose 4B (Ruoslahti
and Engvall, 1977).

In a further series of experiments, we intrinsically labeled a variety of
melanoma and carcinoma cells, fibroblast cell lines of adult and fetal origin,
and cultured human malanocytes derived from fetal uvea (Morgan et al.,
1981b). The 240K component was only shed by melanoma cells of both normal
and uveal origin, whereas the 94K component was shed by both melanoma and
carcinoma cells and, interestingly enough, also by cultured fetal melanocytes,
but not by fibroblasts. Both antigens failed to react with either monoclonal or
monospecific polyclonal antisera to carcinoembryonic antigen (CEA) and
α-fetoprotein, and showed no association with β_2-microglobulin, HLA-A, B or
human Ia-like antigens (Galloway et al., 1981a; McCabe et al., 1980). The
240K and 94K dalton components of spent culture medium were identified as

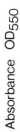

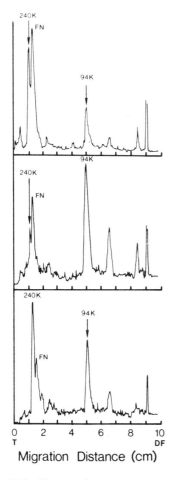

Figure 29.1. Characterization of melanoma associated antigens (MAA's) shed into spent culture medium. Spent culture media of cells, intrinsically labeled with either ^{3}H-3, 4-valine (A), ^{3}H-6 glucosamine (B), or ^{3}H-2-mannose (C), were immunoprecipitated with xenoantiserum to melanoma cells (#6522) and analyzed on 5% acrylamide slab gels.

glycoproteins. Thus, intrinsic labeling of melanoma cells in medium with reduced glucose and pyruvate as an alternative energy source and indirect immune precipitation with antiserum to melanoma cells indicated incorporation of both ^{3}H-6-glucosamine (Figure 29.1B) and ^{3}H-2-mannose (Figure 29.1C) labels into the 240K and 94K molecules. The 240K glycoprotein bound selectively to *Lens culinaris* lectin whereas the 94K glycoprotein had a specific affinity for *Ricinus communis* lectin and did not bind to lentil lectin (McCabe et al., 1979). Similar lectin selectivity was noted for the 94K antigen shed by carcinoma cells.

The similarity of 94K antigen from different sources in lectin affinity and immunological reactivity with polyclonal antisera led us to examine the degree of structural homology in 94K molecules shed by both melanoma and carcinoma cells. Hybridoma antibody, recognizing the 94K protein shed by both M14 melanoma cells and T-24 bladder carcinoma cells (Galloway et al., 1981b), was used for indirect immunoprecipitation of these molecules in the spent culture medium of tumor cells (intrinsically labeled with ^{35}S-methionine). Two-dimensional SDS-PAGE analysis performed by the method of O'Farrell (O'Farrell, 1975) showed that the isolated 94K antigens displayed considerable homogeneity and varied only slightly in pI (e.g., 6.3 for melanoma and 6.2 for carcinoma). This difference could conceivably be due to sialic acid content of the 94K molecules. Evidence for the structural homology of the 94K antigen isolated from either melanoma or carcinoma cells was further strengthened by the results of tryptic peptide analysis of the protein backbone of these molecules. Peptide maps of 94K antigen obtained by high pressure liquid chromatography (Walker et al., 1980) showed nine to ten major peaks, with identical retention times for both 94K antigens isolated either from melanoma or carcinoma cells. This biochemical analysis of 94K antigen suggests that the glycoprotein may serve a similar biological function for different types of human cells, as indicated by its highly conserved structure.

Cytoskeletal Structure and Shedding of MAA's

As a preliminary approach to analysis of the function(s) of shed MAA, we analyzed the role of the cytoskeleton in the shedding process. We made use of cytochalasin B, an inhibitor of microfilament polymerization (Lin et al., 1980), and colchicine, an inhibitor of microtubule polymerization (Margolis and Wilson, 1977). Melanoma cells, as monolayer cultures, were exposed to 0.1–5 μg/ml of cytochalasin B or 0.1–5 μg/ml of colchicine, while they were incorporating either ^{3}H-valine or ^{3}H-glucosamine. After three days, the spent medium was harvested, one aliquot used for determination of triochloroacetic acid (TCA) precipitable radioactivity and another aliquot analyzed by indirect immunoprecipitation with anti-melanoma antiserum and SDS-PAGE. Cytochalasin B, at doses below 1 μg/ml, and colchicine, at doses below 0.5 μg/ml, were not toxic as assayed by trypan blue exclusion of adherent cells and by incorporation of ^{3}H-valine into protein. Shedding of 240K, 94K, and fibronectin was not altered by treatment with colchicine. However, at low, non-toxic doses of cytochalasin B, shedding of all three glycoproteins was markedly enhanced (Figure 29.2). As would be expected, toxic doses of the drug decreased the shedding of these three molecules. Concomitant with the enhanced shedding of 240K, 94K, and fibronectin at non-toxic doses of cytochalasin B, incorporation of ^{3}H-glucosamine label into these glycoproteins was decreased by 80% or more at doses of 0.5–1 μg/ml.

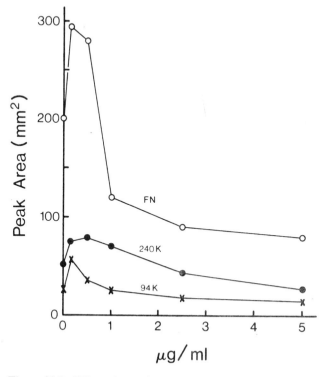

Figure 29.2. Effect of cytochalasin B on shedding of MAA's. 1×10^5 melanoma cells in 16 mm wells were labeled with 10 μCi ^{3}H-3,4-valine during a three-day exposure to cytochalasin B. Spent culture medium was immunoprecipitated with xenoantiserum to melanoma cells, and after SDS-PAGE, peak area of proteins was calculated from scans (at 500 nm) of autoradiographs.

Cytochalasin B, in addition to its effect on the cellular cytoskeleton, is also known to inhibit glucose transport (Mizel and Wilson, 1972). Thus, the decrease in ^{3}H-glucosamine label, observed in the previous experiment, could have been caused by a decrease in glycosylation of these proteins or by a decrease in glucose uptake. To address this issue, melanoma cells were pre-loaded for 24 hours with either ^{3}H-valine or ^{3}H-glucosamine label, the medium changed and cells exposed to non-toxic doses of cytochalasin B for an additional 24 hours. Samples of spent medium were collected at intervals throughout the last 24-hour period and analyzed by indirect immunopreciptia-tion and SDS-PAGE. Under these conditions, no decrease was seen in the association of ^{3}H-glucosamine label with the 240K, 94K, or fibronectin glyco-proteins. Furthermore, there was no evident change in apparent mobility of any shed molecules. These data indicate that the decrease in ^{3}H-glucosamine label associated with shed protein was probably due to an inhibition of glucose transport mediated by cytochalasin B. This also suggests that enhanced shedding at low doses and reduced shedding at high doses of cytochalasin B resulted from its effect on the cytoskeleton rather than on glycosylation. In addition, these data, together with information about the activities of cytochalasin B and colchicine on secretion processes (Hussa, 1979; Chambeau-Guerrin et al., 1978), indicate that shedding of MAA, like fibronectin, is not an active secretion process dependent on microtubule formation, but does require an ordered cytoskeleton structure provided by the microfilament system.

Glucose Regulation of Shedding and Glycosylation of MAA

Numerous descriptions of altered glucose uptake and metabolism in transformed cells have been made since the original description by Warburg of increased anaerobic glycolysis in tumor cells (Warburg, 1926). More recently, glucose was found to be essential for lipid-dependent glycosylation, and it may be necessary for the addition, to N-asparagine residues, of the complex portion of oligosaccharide (Elting et al., 1980). Furthermore, recent investigations indicate a role for glucose in the synthesis and expression of certain glycoproteins. These glycoproteins are induced upon glucose starvation or inhibition of glucose transport (Shiu et al., 1977; Lage-Davila et al., 1979; Olden et al., 1979a) and may represent nonglycosylated precursors of existing glycosylated cell surface molecules (Pouyssegur and Yamada, 1978; McCormick et al., 1979).

These observations on the role of glucose in glycosylation and expression of glycoproteins prompted us to examine its role in glycosylation and shedding of MAA. In preliminary experiments, we found that following an initial adaptation period of one week, melanoma cells would proliferate at rates and reach saturation densities equal to control cells, when grown in minimal essential medium (MEM) supplemented with 1mM glucose, 50mM pyruvate, and undialyzed fetal calf serum. Melanoma cultures in 10mM or 1 mM glucose were subsequently labeled with ^{3}H-valine and spent culture medium and 4 M urea extracts examined by indirect immunoprecipitation and SDS-PAGE. Urea extraction was previously shown to be an effective method for extraction of cell surface MAA's (Galloway et al., 1981b). The 240K and 94K MAA's were markedly inhibited in their shedding in glucose starved cells (Figure 29.3). However, a consistent finding was that residual 240K and 94K continued to be shed. The migration in SDS-PAGE of this residual MAA was unaltered, indicating no apparent change in glycosylation. In contrast, fibronectin was shed in amounts equal to that of cells grown at normal glucose concentration and showed an apparent decrease in mobility indicative of a decrease in glycosylation. Similar changes were noted in these glycoproteins obtained from urea extracts of cells. These results indicated that glucose starvation had a profound effect on shedding and surface expression of MAA's, but did not seem to decrease glycosylation of these molecules. Alternatively, nonglyco-

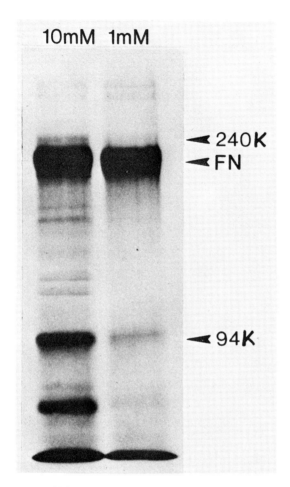

Figure 29.3. Effect of glucose starvation on shedding of MAA. Cultures, adapted to grow in 1 mM glucose (lane 2), were intrinsically labeled with ^{3}H-valine, as were cultures grown in 10 mM glucose (lane 1). After three days, spent culture medium was harvested and analyzed by indirect immunoprecipitation and SDS-PAGE.

sylated MAA's or MAA's reduced in carbohydrate content may have remained in the endoplasmic reticulum due to decreased solubility (Leavitt et al., 1977), thereby allowing only fully glycosylated molecules to reach the surface and be shed.

To study glucose regulation of MAA glycosylation further, we preloaded cells for 24 hours with either ^{3}H-valine or ^{3}H-glucosamine, in medium reduced in valine and glucose. We removed the labeling medium and continued the cultures in medium containing either 10 mM or 100 mM glucose. Samples were removed at intervals up to 24 hours and again analyzed by indirect immunoprecipitation and SDS-PAGE. Shedding of the 240K glycoprotein was unaltered in cells exposed to 100 mM glucose (Figure 29.4B). However, ^{3}H-glucosamine label associated with this glycoprotein was enhanced in cultures exposed to 100 mM glucose when compared to controls (Figure 29.4A). The phenomenon was noted as soon as 2 hours after addition of the increased glucose concentration and continued to increase for the entire 24-hour interval examined. This finding of increased glycosylation was not confined to the

Figure 29.4. Glucose regulation of glycosylation of the 240K glycoprotein. 1×10^5 M10 melanoma cells in 16 mm wells were allowed to incorporate either ^{3}H-6-glucosamine (---) or ^{3}H-valine (—) for 24 hours. The medium was then removed and medium containing 10 mM (O) or 100 mM (●) glucose added. Spent culture medium was harvested at intervals and analyzed by immune precipitation and SDS-PAGE. The quantity of label in the 240K glycoprotein was determined by calculation of peak area from scans of autoradiographs at 550 nm.

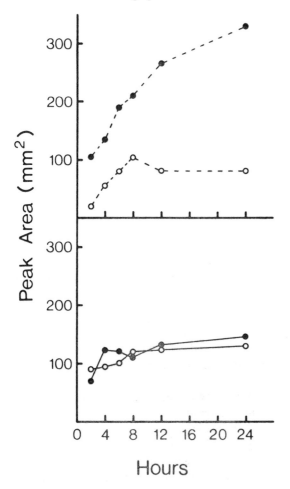

240K molecule but was also apparent in both the 94K and fibronectin glycoproteins.

The results of our experiments stress the fact that MAA sheddings, as well as glycosylation, can be reduced by decreasing glucose in the microenvironment. In contrast, increased extracellular glucose concentrations, though they do not affect the actual amount of MAA shed, enhance the glycosylation of these molecules.

Inhibition of Glycosylation and Shedding of MAA

Experiments detailed previously suggested that carbohydrate plays an essential role in the shedding of glycoprotein MAA. We next undertook experiments with inhibitors of glycosylation, mainly 2-deoxyglucose and tunicamycin, to more rigorously define this requirement. Two-deoxyglucose is a well known inhibitor of lipid-dependent glycosylation (Datema and Schwarz, 1979) and has been used to determine the role of carbohydrate in expression of a number of proteins (Hughes et al., 1977; Nakamura and Compans, 1978). Nevertheless, the agent has other effects on the metabolism of cells in addition to its effect on glycosylation. For this reason, we were careful to choose doses of the drug which resulted in at least two-fold more inhibition of ^{3}H-glucosamine or ^{3}H-2-mannose incorporation than ^{3}H-valine incorporation into shed protein. Under these conditions, the agent showed a selective inhibition of glycosylation at .01 mM. Spent medium from cultures treated with this dose, when analyzed by indirect immunoprecipitation and SDS-PAGE, indicated that, although 2-deoxyglucose did inhibit shedding of MAA's, it was not selective since it also inhibited shedding of other glycoproteins. Fibronectin, which continued to be shed under 2-deoxyglucose treatment, did not show any discernible change in molecular weight and thus was apparently glycosylated. Thus, inhibition of glycosylation with 2-deoxyglucose must result in intracellular retention of most nonglycosylated glycoprotein components of spent medium (Morgan et al., 1981a).

Tunicamycin, an inhibitor of N-asparagine glycosylation, has attracted wide interest because of its specificity for N-acetyl-glucosamine transferase, an enzyme required during the first step in glycosylation of most membrane and secretory glycoproteins (Tkacz and Lampen, 1975; Keller et al., 1979). As with 2-deoxyglucose, this antibiotic can have effects on glucose transport and has recently been shown to be selectively toxic for transformed cells (Duskin and Bornstein, 1977; Olden et al., 1979b). Thus, our first goal was to discern the toxic effects of the drug and if possible, to separate them from the effect on glycosylation. Toxic effects of the drug were reduced by exposure of melanoma cells to 0.5–1 μg/ml of the antibiotic for three days or less. Under these conditions, incorporation of ^{3}H-glucosamine and ^{3}H-2-mannose labels into shed protein was inhibited by 75%, whereas incorporation of ^{3}H-valine was inhibited by 28%. When the major glycoproteins found in spent culture medium were examined by indirect immunoprecipitation and SDS-PAGE, a selective dose-dependent inhibition of 240K and 94K glycoproteins was observed (Figure 29.5). However, some inhibition of fibronectin shedding was observed. Subsequent efforts to remove components of tunicamycin that were toxic to melanoma cells by fractionation of the drug by HPLC proved ineffective. This result contrasted with evidence obtained from experiments with chick embryo fibroblast cultures (Mahoney and Duskin, 1979). However, a fortuitous observation indicated that continued exposure to the antibiotic resulted in adaption of the melanoma cells to the toxicity of the drug without affecting its inhibitory effect on glycosylation. This adaptation was evident from the reduced inhibition of incorporation of ^{3}H-valine into shed protein of adapted versus non-adapted cultures, while no difference in inhibition of incorporation of ^{3}H-glucosamine was observed in the cultures treated with tunicamycin. Further analysis of spent culture medium of adapted melanoma cultures indicated the absence of 240K and 94K MAA but showed the continued presence of other glycoproteins (Figure 29.6). Glycoproteins still

Figure 29.5. Effect of tunicamycin on shedding of MAA. 1×10^5 melanoma cells, seeded into 16 mm wells, were exposed to 0–5 μg/ml of tunicamycin. After 24 hours, 10 μCi of ^{3}H-valine was added and the cultures continued for 48 hours. Spent culture medium was harvested after three days and subjected to indirect immunoprecipitation and SDS-PAGE. The quantity of 240K, 94K, and fibronectin was determined by calculation of peak areas from scans at 550 nm of autoradiographs.

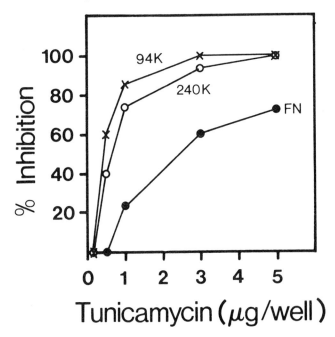

shed into culture medium of drug-adapted cells migrated more rapidly in SDS-PAGE and lacked associated ^{3}H-glucosamine label, which indicated a reduction in or possibly complete absence of carbohydrate.

A second observation enabled us to completely eliminate toxic effects of tunicamycin. We found that when the drug was added to cultures seeded 24 hours in advance, there were no discernible toxic effects of the drug, though glycosylation was still markedly inhibited. In fact, the toxic effects of the antibiotic corresponded with the approximate rate at which the melanoma cells attached and spread after seeding (Figure 29.7). Thus, a gradual reduction in

Figure 29.6. Shedding of MAA cells adapted to grow in tunicamycin. Cultures adapted to continuous growth in 0.5 μg/ml tunicamycin (T) were labeled by the protocol in Figure 29.5 and compared to non-treated cultures (C). Spent culture medium was analyzed by indirect immunoprecipitation and SDS-PAGE.

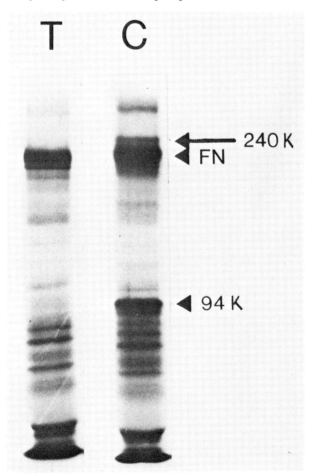

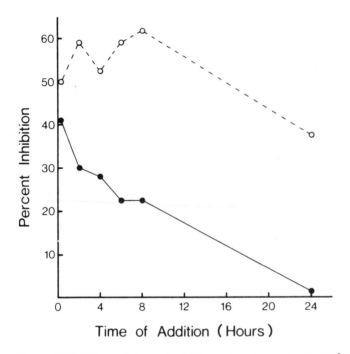

Figure 29.7. Effect of time of addition of tunicamycin. 1×10^5 M10 melanoma cells were seeded in 16 mm wells and incubated at 37°C. Tunicamycin (1 μg/ml) was added to cultures beginning at the time of seeding of the cells to 24 hours after seeding. Twenty-four hours after seeding the melanoma cells, 10 μCi of ^{3}H-valine (●) or ^{3}H-glucosamine (○) was added, and spent culture media were harvested after an additional 48-hour incubation. Radioactivity associated with protein was determined by TCA-precipitation of an aliquot of spent medium.

toxic activity of tunicamycin was apparent with increasing delay in addition of the drug after seeding. These reaction kinetics suggest that the toxic effect, but not the glycosylation effect of tunicamycin, depends at least indirectly on the cytoskeletal structure of the melanoma cell.

These observations with inhibitors of glycosylation and modulation of glucose in the cellular environment serve to emphasize the essential role of carbohydrate in shedding and expression of human melanoma associated antigens.

Conclusions and Speculation

We have described the identification and preliminary biochemical characterization of two glycoproteins shed into spent culture medium of human melanoma cells. Both molecules share a stringent requirement for glycosylation and cytoskeletal organization in order to be shed.

The 94K glycoprotein, shared by tumors of diverse origins, shows remarkable conservation of protein structure, indicative of its essential role in the economy of the neoplastic cell. Since this glycoprotein is also shed by cultured fetal melanocytes, this requirement must also be manifested during embryogenesis and/or differentiation. One common requirement of tumor cells and fetal cells is their mobility and ability to metastasize (Fishman, 1975). It may be relevant to these functions that adult melanocytes will only express the 94K antigen when dividing (P.G. Natali, personal communication). It is at this time that melanocytes may move through the dermis, but while nondividing and in a differentiated state, these cells are immobile (Goerttlar et al., 1980). Similarly, cells in culture become mobile during cell division and only express some differentiated functions while adherent and immobile (Panten, 1975). A similar requirement for movement through other cell populations is required of melanocytes migrating from the neural crest (Du Shane, 1948). Thus, it is interesting to speculate that the 94K glycoprotein may play a role in neoplastic cell mobility and that glycosylation of this molecule may modify or determine its function.

The 240K glycoprotein, on the other hand, though expressed by most melanoma cells, is not common to carcinoma cells and fetal melanocytes. Preliminary evidence, however, suggests that the glycoprotein is shed by SV-40 transformed fetal melanocytes after prolonged culturing. Fetal melanocytes after SV-40 transformation show an absence of desmosomes present before in the non-transformed culture. This loss is indicative of decreased cellular communication and differentiation. Thus, shedding of the 240K component into spent medium may, in a manner similar to LETS protein (Yamada et al., 1978), signal a loss in cellular adhesiveness and a decrease in cell-cell interactions.

We feel that an approach involving both biochemical and biological analysis of specific tumor markers may lead to delineation of the role of these molecules in neoplastic events and to a better understanding of the properties of neoplastic cells.

ACKNOWLEDGMENTS
The authors thank J. Brock and C. Hockman for technical assistance, and J. Bell for preparation of the manuscript.

References

Chambeau-Guerrin, A.-M., Muller, P., and Rossignol, B. (1978) *J. Biol. Chem.* 253:3870–3876.

Datema, R. and Schwarz, R.T. (1979) *Biochem. J.* 184:113–123.

DuShane, G.P. (1948) In *The Biology of Melanomas*. Miner, R.W. (ed.), New York: New York Acad. Sci. Publications, pp. 1–14.

Duskin, D. and Bornstein, P. (1977) *Proc. Natl. Acad. Sci. U.S.A.* 74:3433–3437.

Elting, J.J., Chen, W.W., and Lennarz, W.J. (1980) *J. Biol. Chem.* 255:2325–2331.

Fass, L., Heberman, R.B., Ziegler, J.L., and Kiryabwire, J.W.M. (1970) *Lancet* 1:116–118.

Fishman, W.H. and Singer, R.M. (1975) In *Cancer: A Comprehensive Treatise*. Becker, F.F. (ed.), New York: Plenum Press, pp. 57–80.

Fossati, G., Colnaghi, N.I., Della Porta, G., Cascinelli, N., and Veronesi, V. (1971) *Int. J. Cancer* 8:344–350.

Galloway, D.R., McCabe, R.P., Pellegrino, M.A., Ferrone, S., and Reisfeld, R.A. (1981a) *J. Immunol*. 126:62–66.

Galloway, D.R., Imai, K., Ferrone, S., and Reisfeld, R.A. (1981b) *Fed. Proc*. 40:231–236.

Goerttler, K., Loherke, H., Schweizer, J., and Hesse, B. (1980) *Cancer Res*. 40:155–161.

Hellström, I., Warner, G.A., Hellström, K.E., and Sjogren, H.O. (1973) *Int. J. Cancer* 11:280–292.

Hughes, R.C., Meager, A., and Nairu, R. (1977) *Eur. J. Biochem*. 72:265–273.

Hussa, R.O. (1979) *In Vitro* 15:237–245.

Keller, R.K., Boon, D.Y., and Crum, F.C. (1979) *Biochem*. 18:3946–3952.

Lage-Davila, A., Hoffman-Clerc, F., Torpier, G., and Montagnier, L. (1979) *Exp. Cell. Res*. 120:181–189.

Leavitt, R., Schlesinger, S., and Kornfeld, S. (1977) *J. Biol. Chem*. 252:9018–9023.

Lewis, M.G., Skonopisov, R.L., Nairn, R.C., Phillips, T.M., Hamilton-Fairly, G., Bodenhain, D.C., and Alexander, P. (1969) *Brit. Med. J*. 3:547–562.

Lin, D.C., Tobin, K.D., Grumet, M., and Lin, S. (1980) *J. Cell. Biol*. 84:455–460.

Livingston, P.O., Shiku, H., Bean, M.A., Pinsky, C.M., Oeltgen, H.F., and Old, L.J. (1979) *Int. J. Cancer* 24:34–44.

Mahoney, W.C. and Duskin, D. (1979) *J. Biol. Chem*.254:6572–6576.

Margolis, R.L. and Wilson, L. (1977) *Proc. Natl. Acad. Sci. U.S.A*. 74:3466–3470.

McCabe, R.P., Galloway, D.R., Ferrone, S., and Reisfeld, R.A. (1979) In *Current Trends in Tumor Immunology*. Ferrone, S., Gorini, S., Herberman, R.B., and Reisfeld, R.A. (eds.), New York: Garland STPM Press, pp. 269–286.

McCabe, R.P., Indiveri, F., Ferrone, S., and Reisfeld, R.A. (1980) *J. Nat. Cancer Inst*. 68:703–707.

McCormick, P.J., Keys, B.J., Pucci, C., and Millis, A.J.T. (1979) *Cell* 18:173–182.

Mizel, S. and Wilson, L. (1972) *J. Biol. Chem*. 247:4102–4105.

Morgan, A.C., Galloway, D.R., Wilson, B.S., and Reisfeld, R.A. (1980) *J. Immunol. Meth*. 39:233–246.

Morgan, A.C., Galloway, D.R., Imai, K., and Reisfeld, R.A. (1981a) *J. Immunol*. 126:365–370.

Morgan, A.C., Galloway, D.R., Jensen, F.C., Giovanella, B.L., and Reisfeld, R.A. (1981b) *Proc. Natl. Acad. Sci. U.S.A.*, in press.

Nakamura, K. and Compans, R.W. (1978) *Virol*. 84:303–319.

O'Farrell, P.H. (1975) *J. Biol. Chem*. 250:4007–4021.

Olden, K., Pratt, R.M., Jaworski, C., and Yamada, K.M. (1979a) *Proc. Natl. Acad. Sci. U.S.A*. 76:791–795.

Olden, K., Pratt, R.M., and Yamada, K.M. (1979b) *Int. J. Cancer* 24:60–66.

Panten, J. (1975) In *Cancer: A Comprehensive Treatise*. Becker, F.F. (ed), New York: Plenum Press, pp. 55–100.

Pouyssegur, J. and Yamada, K.M. (1978) *Cell* 13:139–150.

Roth, J.A., Slocum, H.K., Pellegrino, M.A., Holmes, E.C., and Reisfeld, R.A. (1976) *Cancer Res*. 36:2360–2364.

Ruoslahti, E. and Engvell, E. (1978) *Ann. N.Y. Acad. Sci*. 312:178–191.

Shiku, H., Takahashi, T., Oettgen, H.F., and Old, L.J. (1976) *J. Exp. Med*. 144:873–881.

Shiu, R.P., Pouyssegur, J., and Pastan, I. (1977) *Proc. Natl. Acad. Sci. U.S.A.* 74:3840–3844.

Tkacz, J.S. and Lampen, J.O. (1975) *Biol. Biophys. Res. Comm.* 65:248–257.

Walker, L.E., Ferrone, S., Pellegrino, M.A., and Reisfeld, R.A. (1980) *Mol. Immunol.* 17:1443–1448.

Yamada, K.M., Olden, K., and Pastan, I. (1978) *Ann. N.Y. Acad. Sci.* 312:256–277.

PART IV:

Tumor Surveillance

Published 1981 by Elsevier North Holland, Inc.
Saunders, Daniels, Serrou, Rosenfeld, and Denney, eds.
FUNDAMENTAL MECHANISMS IN HUMAN CANCER IMMUNOLOGY

CHAPTER 30

New Approaches to Specific and Non-specific Immunotherapy of Established Cancer Metastases[1]

I.J. Fidler and M.G. Hanna, Jr.

Cancer Metastasis and Treatment Laboratory, National Cancer Institute, Frederick Cancer Research Center, Frederick, Maryland

In this chapter, we address the question of whether augmenting specific and non-specific host immunity might be effective in the treatment of cancer metastasis. Many primary cancers can be treated successfully with surgery and aggressive chemo- and/or radiotherapy, but the metastatic spread of malignant tumors is still responsible for most failures in cancer treatment (Fidler et al., 1978). There are several reasons for this. First, the anatomic location of many metastases may be inaccessible for surgical removal and/or it may prevent an effective dose of therapeutic agents from being delivered. Second, metastases are often too small to be detected at the time the primary tumor is removed, and dissemination of metastases frequently takes place before symptoms of widespread disease are evident. Third, and most serious, metastases can emerge that are resistant to conventional therapy. Recent work (Poste and Fidler, 1979) suggests that metastases arise from the nonrandom spread of specialized subpopulations of cells within the primary tumor (Fidler and Kripke, 1977), and that the responsiveness of these metastatic subpopulations to therapy may differ from that of the non-metastatic tumor cells which constitute the major population of the primary tumor. The process of metastasis is highly selective and represents the end point of several destructive events which few tumor cells survive. Unlike the cells within a solid tumor mass, the progenitors of metastases circulate as small cell clumps and are thereby accessible for interaction with both immunologic and non-immunologic host

[1]Research supported by the National Cancer Institute under Contract N01-CO-75380 with Litton Bionetics, Inc.

factors. Thus, one could speculate that manipulations of the immune system could provide a highly efficient method of controlling metastasis.

The immune response to metastatic tumors involves the interaction of several effector mechanisms. Cell-mediated reactivity against syngeneic tumors can occur in two separate steps. Lymphocytes that are specifically sensitized against tumor surface antigens interact with target cells to lyse them and/or to release soluble mediators. The release of soluble mediators can promote the local accumulation and activation of mononuclear cells to destroy tumor cells. Many studies in experimental tumor systems suggest that the immune system can control metastasis under the appropriate conditions (Fidler and Kripke, 1980). The appropriate conditions, however, appear at present to be very limited. The challenge lies in devising ways to circumvent numerous obstacles to the therapy of disseminated cancer.

We present here the summary of recent work from our laboratory designed to evaluate new approaches to active specific and non-specific immunotherapy in animals bearing metastatic neoplasms.

Active Specific Immunotherapy for Established Metastases with BCG-Tumor Cell Vaccine

Enhancement of host immune reactivity against disseminated neoplasms has been attempted clinically with such microbial vaccines as *Mycobacterium bovis*, strain Bacillus Calmette-Guérin (BCG) (Morton et al., 1974, 1976). The unsuccessful or equivocal results of these clinical studies probably are attributable to the fact that the underlying pathobiology of metastasis, in general, and the optimal conditions for augmenting host immunity, in particular, have not been determined or even thoroughly examined. The L10 hepatocarcinoma syngeneic to strain 2 guinea pigs (Rapp et al., 1968) has several features that make it an interesting model for immunotherapy. It is weakly immunogenic and, following intradermal (i.d.) injection, spontaneously metastasizes to draining lymph nodes and visceral organs. The intratumoral injection of BCG in this experimental guinea pig model not only mediates elimination of regional tumors (skin and regional lymph nodes) but also enhances the induction of systemic tumor immunity, which is obviously required for the control of distant micrometastases (Hanna et al., 1972; Zbar et al., 1972).

Because systemic immunity could be induced by the intratumoral injection of BCG, we then considered whether immunization of animals with vaccines consisting of L10 cells and BCG could be effective against micrometastases. We have demonstrated that, under defined conditions, vaccine preparations consisting of autologous tumor cells and BCG can cure the majority of animals with lethal, established visceral micrometastases. The vaccine therapy is effective over a range of tumor burdens and can be administered after surgery of localized tumor for treatment of lymph node and lung metastases.

Investigations of several variables in vaccine preparations, such as the ratio of viable BCG organisms to viable metabolically active tumor cells, the procedures of cryobiologic preservation, and the x-ray treatment for attenuation of cells, have resulted in the development of an optimal nontumorigenic BCG plus tumor cell vaccine, as well as the most effective regimen for treatment (Table 30.1).

The two variables of adjuvant dose and tumor cell viability were found to profoundly influence the efficacy of the vaccine (Hanna and Peters, 1978; Hanna et al., 1979; Peters and Hanna, 1980). Significant protection against disseminated tumor required a minimum of two vaccinations, administered one week apart, with the initial immunization containing at least 10^7 viable BCG organisms of 70 μg of *C. parvum* admixed with 10^7 tumor cells. Tumor cell viability in the final vaccine preparation was critical. Thus, any manipulation of the tumor cells, such as disaggregation from a solid tumor, cryobiologic preservation or x-irradiation would have to be accomplished while maintaining the requisite cell viability.

To establish disseminated micrometastases in various visceral organs of the strain 2 guinea pigs, freshly harvested L10 ascites cells were washed three times in Hank's balanced salt solution and injected into the dorsal penile vein. Minimum lethal dose (100%) consists of 10^4 viable cells. The time of death from metastasis to the lungs, mediastinal and tracheobronchial lymph nodes, and the viscera varies with the dose of the i.v. inoculum. In this model, as well

Table 30.1. Criteria for Successful Vaccines for Active Specific Immunotherapy.

Adjuvant
  (a) BCG (Phipps, Tice, Connaught): lyophilized, frozen
     (dose-dependence $> 10^6 \neq 10^7 - 10^8$)
  (b) *C. parvum* (Wellcome Labs) (dose-dependence $>7 \mu g \neq 70 \mu g < 700 \mu g$)
Tumor Cells
  (a) Enzymatic dissociation
    (1) Collagenase type I (1.5-2.0 U/ml HBSS)
    (2) DNase (450 K.U./ml HBSS)
    (3) 37° C with stirring
  (b) Cryopreservation
    (1) Controlled-rate freezing (−1° C/min) (7.5% DMSO, 5% FBS, HBSS)
    (2) Viability $\geqslant 80\%$
  (c) x-irradiation
    (1) Rendered nontumorigenic at 12,000-20,000 R.

Components and Administration[a]
  (a) Ratio of adjuvant to tumor cells − 10:1-1:1 (optimum)
  (b) 10^7 tumor cells (optimum)
  (c) 2-3 i.d. vaccinations at weekly intervals.
    3rd vaccination contains tumor cells only.

[a]Isoniazid chemoprophylaxis of BCG infection optional.

as any other, the success of therapy is influenced by tumor burden (number and size of metastases) existing at the time treatment commenced. By 7 days after tumor cell injection (time of second vaccination), pulmonary metastases measured 0.1 mm in diameter. In untreated control animals, a 15-fold increase in volume (2.5-fold increase in diameter) of metastases was noted by day 20. In contrast, metastases were undetected in the vaccine-treated animals by day 20. Thus, at the very least, the BCG plus tumor cell vaccine treatment was effective in preventing the progressive growth of micrometastases.

The preparation of tumor cells for vaccination must meet several criteria (Peters and Hanna, 1980; Peters et al., 1979). The L10 cells are immunogenic when either grown as ascites in the peritoneum or as a solid intramuscular tumor to be enzymatically disaggregated (Table 30.1). Of the various dissociation methods tested, the enzymatic procedure using collagenase type I + DNase in basic salt solution at 37°C was most efficient and produced the highest total viable cell yield per gram of solid tumor without loss of antigenicity. These procedures for the preparation of autologous tumor cell vaccines have been used in the treatment of lung cancer in 19 patients (Maver and McKneally, 1979). Using this technique, we have achieved similar success in preparation of vaccines for human colon cancer and feline mammary cancer. However, the dissociation technique can be applied to clinical solid tumors only when cryopreservation of the resultant tumor cell suspension can be accomplished without reducing the viability and thus the immunogenic potential of the tumor cells. Cells frozen by an optimized cryobiologic procedure were effective in immunization procedures. In contrast, cells frozen by a conventional glycerol method were not effective in immunizing recipient animals (Peters and Hanna, 1980).

Our experimental studies on the morphology of the vaccination induction sites of active specific immunotherapy using BCG-tumor cell vaccines suggested that there is a requirement for persistence of intact tumor cells (and thus presumably tumor antigens) during a critical phase of the development of a chronic inflammatory response (Hanna and Bucana, 1979). This chronic inflammatory response is characterized by a reaction in which the end point is an epithelioid granuloma. Because in this experimental immunotherapy model the injection of L10 cells alone or BCG alone has no therapeutic value, it is clear that the persistence of intact tumor cells in the dermal injection site, while necessary, is not entirely sufficient for induction of effective tumor immunity. Also, the chronic inflammatory response with development of epithelioid granuloma as elicited by the i.d. injection of an optimal dose of viable BCG, in itself, is not immunotherapeutic. The conversion of the BCG-induced acute inflammatory reaction, therefore, to a chronic inflammatory reaction between days 4 and 7, and the destruction and immunologic processing of tumor antigens during this time period by the infiltrating blood-borne monocytes, lymphocytes, and granulocytes are probably all essential factors which contribute to effective induction of specific cell-mediated tumor immunity. From these studies, we conclude that the viability of the tumor cells in the vaccine is important and that some past failures of active specific immunotherapy could have been associated with acute antigenic exposures resulting from suboptimal cryobiologic preservation of tumor cells in the vaccine preparation.

The experimental design for studies of active specific immunotherapy in the guinea pig model is shown in Figure 30.1. Guinea pigs were injected intravenously (i.v.) with 10^6 L10 tumor cells ($100\times$ the minimal lethal dose). Immunizations commenced at either 1, 4, 7, or 10 days after i.v. injection of tumor. Later immunizations were given at weekly intervals. One immunization is not sufficient to bring about eradication of metastases; at least 2 treatments are required. At the time the second vaccine was administered, metastases were large and ranged between 0.1 to 0.25 mm in diameter. The survival of immunized guinea pigs is shown in Figure 30.2. Tumor burden limits therapy, since there was a 25–30% mortality of animals initially immunized on either day 1 or day 4, and a 50–60% mortality of animals initially immunized on day 7 or day 10 after i.v. injection of L10 cells. Significant prolongation of life, however, was achieved in all treatment groups regardless of the tumor burden at the initiation of the immunization procedure.

We conclude the following: The failure of some previous experimental and/or clinical attempts at active specific immunotherapy using BCG or *C. parvum* and autologous tumor cell vaccines could have been due to the non- or low viability of the tumor cells. Such cells disintegrate rapidly and do not provide a chronic antigenic stimulus. Moreover, the immunizing cells need be metabolically active and nontumorigenic. We achieved this goal by exposing

Figure 30.1. Experimental design of active specific immunotherapy in guinea pigs.

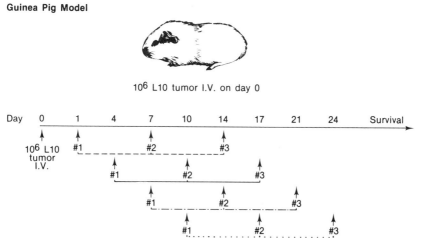

Guinea Pig Model

10^6 L10 tumor I.V. on day 0

Vaccines #1 & #2 = 10^7 BCG plus 10^7 X-irradiated L10 cells.
Vaccine #3 = 10^7 L10 cells only.

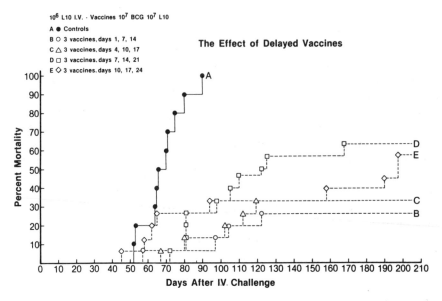

Figure 30.2. Survival of guinea pigs bearing L10 metastases after active specific immunotherapy initiated at various times after tumor cell injection.

the cells to 20,000 R irradiation. Many cells are arrested in the G_1 phase of division, and cells that underwent a limited number of mitotic divisions probably died. Arresting cells in G_1 probably allowed preservation of their metabolic activity.

Stimulation of Macrophage-Mediated Destruction of Metastases by the Systemic Administration of Immunomodulators Encapsulated in Liposomes

Although tumor cell populations are heterogeneous with regard to many characteristics, they are susceptible to destruction by activated, tumoricidal macrophages. Macrophage-mediated destruction of tumor cells, at least *in vitro*, occurs independently of such tumor cell characteristics as antigenicity, invasiveness, metastatic potential, and drug sensitivity (Fidler, 1978). Although tumor cell resistance to a variety of cytotoxic agents, antibodies, cytotoxic lymphocytes, natural killer cells, and/or antibodies has been documented, similar efforts to select tumor cells resistant to lysis mediated by activated macrophages have been unsuccessful (Kerbel, 1979).

Tumoricidal macrophages are effective in the control of metastasis. The i.v. injection of non-specifically activated syngeneic macrophages inhibits both tumor growth at primary sites (Den Otter et al., 1977) and metastasis (Fidler,

1974; Liotta et al., 1977). For clinical use, however, use of these cells as therapeutic agents has several limitations. Foremost is the need to transfuse large numbers of autologous or histocompatible macrophages. It would be preferable if autologous macrophages could be activated *in situ*. Although macrophages isolated from animals bearing progressively growing experimental tumors frequently lack tumoricidal activity, they are still able to respond to exogenous activating stimuli.

One major pathway for macrophage activation *in vivo* is by interaction with the lymphokine, macrophage activation factor (MAF), which is released by sensitized lymphocytes. Therapeutic use of MAF is hindered, however, by the lack of purified preparations of this mediator and because crude lymphokine preparations containing MAF do not activate macrophages *in situ* when injected systemically (Fidler, 1980). We have recently shown that lymphokines encapsulated within liposomes are able to activate macrophages both *in vitro* and *in vivo*, whereas macrophage activation by free (unencapsulated) MAF requires the binding of MAF to a fucoglycolipid receptor on the macrophage surface. Liposome-encapsulated MAF can activate macrophages lacking functional receptors for MAF (Poste et al., 1979; Sone et al., 1980).

Another major pathway for activation of macrophages *in vivo* involves their interaction with microorganisms and/or their product(s). The use of whole microorganisms or their crude products to activate macrophages *in vivo* often has undesirable side effects, such as granuloma formation and allergic reactions (Allison, 1979; Allison and Gregoriadis, 1979). The use of non-toxic compounds that possess immune-potentiating activity would thus be preferable. N-acetyl-muramyl-L-alanyl-D-isoglutamine (muramyl dipeptide, MDP) (mol wt 492) is the minimal structural unit with immune-potentiating activity that can replace *Mycobacteria* in Freund's complete adjuvant (Chedid et al., 1979; Matter, 1979). MDP influences many macrophage functions, including tumoricidal properties. Moreover, like MAF, MDP encapsulated within liposomes rendered mouse and rat alveolar macrophages tumoricidal *in vitro* at concentrations at least 1000 times lower than unencapsulated (free) MDP added to the alveolar macrophage culture medium (Sone and Fidler, 1980).

An attractive feature of liposomes as a carrier vehicle for delivery of activating agents to macrophages *in situ* is that the majority of liposomes injected i.v. are taken up by macrophages, particularly in the reticuloendothelial system of the liver and spleen. Although this is a major obstacle to the targeting of liposomes to other cell types, uptake of liposomes by macrophages offers a means of enhancing uptake of therapeutic agents that stimulate macrophage activity.

In a study of the efficacy of liposome-encapsulated MAF in augmenting host resistance to metastases, C57BL/6 mice were injected in the footpad with 5×10^4 syngeneic B16-BL6 murine melanoma cells (Hart, 1979). Four weeks later, when the implants had reached a size of 10–12 mm, the leg bearing the tumor and the popliteal lymph node were amputated. Three days later, animals were injected i.v. with 5 μmoles of multilamellar vesicles, consisting of phosphatidylserine and phosphatidylcholine (3:7 mole ratio) containing encapsulated MAF suspended in 0.2 ml phosphate-buffered saline. Control animals were injected i.v. with 0.2 ml of supernatants from unstimulated lymphocyte cultures, free MAF (0.2 ml), or liposomes containing saline but suspended in 0.2 ml of free MAF. Both test and control groups were treated twice weekly for 4 weeks. Two weeks after the final treatment, the animals were killed and necropsied. The presence of metastases was determined microscopically. All suspected lesions were confirmed histologically.

Spontaneous pulmonary and lymph node metastases were well established in animals at the time liposome therapy was started, and several individual lung metastases were macroscopically visible (Fidler, 1980). Without therapy, these tumor foci rapidly developed into lesions exceeding 2–3 mm in diameter. As shown in Table 30.2, the majority of mice treated with liposome-encapsulated MAF had no macroscopically or microscopically detectable metastases. Moreover, even in animals with metastasis, the median number of metastases was significantly reduced relative to the other treatment groups. Metastases were consistently present in a high percentage of animals in the various control groups (Table 30.2).

Similar results showing a significant reduction in the incidence of spontaneous lung metastases following i.v. injection of liposome-encapsulated MAF have been obtained using the K-1735 melanoma syngeneic to C3H mice (Fidler, 1980) and the B16-BV8 melanoma in C57BL/6 mice (Poste and Fidler, 1980). In addition to reducing the metastatic burden, therapy with liposome-encapsulated MAF also significantly enhances long-term survival in

Table 30.2. Inhibition of Established B16-BL6 Melanoma Pulmonary Metastases in C57BL/6 Mice Following the Multiple Intravenous Injection of Liposome-Encapsulated Macrophage Activating Agents.

Treatment group	Pulmonary metastasis			
	Negative mice/ total	Median	Range	
PBS control mice	4/48	29	0-107	
Free-MAF	4/20	16	0-38	
Liposome containing HBSS suspended in free MAF	8/26	20	0-65	
Liposome-encapsulated MAF	18/24	0	0-10	< 0.001
Free-MDP (μg/m)	8/10	55	0-94	
Liposomes containing PBS suspended in 2.5 μg MDP	3/26	68	0-308	
Liposomes containing 2.5 μg MDP	20/27	0	0-7	< 0.001

Note: The incidence of metastasis in mice treated with liposome-encapsulated MAF or MDP was significantly decreased (P < 0.001 Chi-square analysis). The data are a summary of 3 separate experiments.

animals injected with the B16-BL6 melanoma. As shown in Figure 30.3, 7 of 10 mice injected i.v. with liposome-encapsulated MAF were still alive when the experiment was terminated after 190 days, whereas virtually all animals in the control groups were dead by 40 days amputation of the primary tumor. Because the median life span of mice injected with the minimum tumorigenic dose (10 B16 cells) is 40-50 days (Griswold, 1972), animals that survive at least 100 days longer than any control mouse can be considered to be essentially disease-free.

Similar experiments were performed in which liposomes containing MDP were administered systemically. C57BL/6 mice bearing spontaneous lung metastases arising from B16-BL6 melanoma cells (implanted 4 weeks earlier in the footpad) were injected i.v. twice weekly for 4 weeks with free MDP (100 μg/mouse), liposomes (5 μmoles phospholipid) containing 2.5 μg MDP, or with a similar dose of liposomes containing PBS and suspended in 2.5 μg free MDP. As in the experiments with liposome-MAF described above, spontaneous lymph node and lung metastases were well established when therapy was initiated 3 days after the removal of the 4-week-old primary tumor implant in the limb. Again, mice were killed 2 weeks after the eighth and final i.v. injection. As shown in Table 30.2 (bottom), control mice injected with PBS and also mice treated with free MDP or "empty" liposomes plus free MDP had extensive metastases. In contrast, 20 of 27 mice injected with liposomes

Figure 30.3. Survival of C57BL/6 mice bearing spontaneous metastases after multiple i.v. injections with liposomes containing macrophage activating factor (MAF).

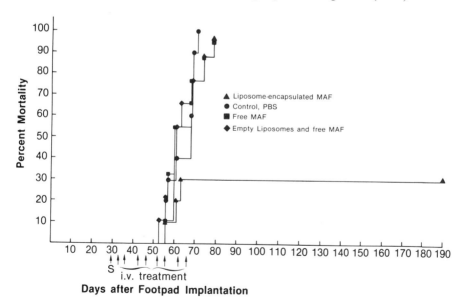

containing MDP were free of detectable disease, and, in the few treated animals with lung metastases, the median number of lesions was significantly lower than in the other treatment groups. Comparison of the same treatment protocols in survival assays revealed that treatment with liposome-encapsulated MDP produced a highly significant increase in survival relative to control mice or mice injected with free MDP or liposomes containing PBS suspended in free MDP (Figure 30.4). On day 190, all the surviving mice were given a subcutaneous (s.c.) challenge of 5×10^4 B16-BL6 cells. Tumors developed in all mice.

In both series of experiments (liposome-MDP and/or liposome-MAF), the regression of lymph node and pulmonary metastases was always associated with the induction of tumoricidal activity in alveolar macrophages (Fidler et al., 1980). In control studies in which systemic administration of liposomes containing control substances failed to activate macrophages, tumor regression also failed to occur (Fidler et al., 1980).

Conclusions

The studies described in this chapter suggest that under the appropriate conditions, the immune system can control cancer metastasis. The challenge now lies in devising ways to expand the conditions necessary to achieve successful immunotherapy of disseminated cancer.

Figure 30.4. Survival of C57BL/6 mice bearing spontaneous metastases after multiple i.v. injections of liposomes containing muramyl dipeptide (MDP).

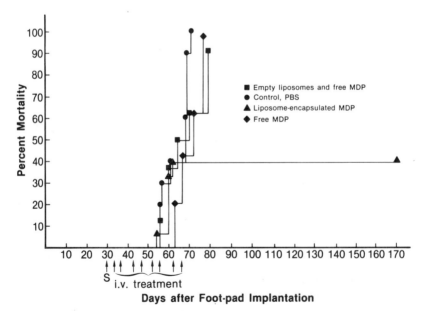

Active specific immunotherapy is a feasible, but demanding, procedure. No longer can we assume that seemingly "unimportant details" do not influence the outcome of the immunization. Perhaps the necessity of adhering to a strict protocol for vaccine preparation (which may differ among different tumors) constitutes the major disadvantage of this procedure. The vaccines must contain viable, nontumorigenic cells prepared from individual tumors. The cells must be admixed with the appropriate dose of the adjuvant (here BCG) and must be administered several times. The major advantage of active specific immunotherapy is that systemic immunity can be generated which could be of immense benefit to a patient harboring dormant tumor cells that may begin to proliferate many months after treatment of the primary neoplasm (Fidler et al., 1978).

The major advantage of activation of tumoricidal properties in macrophages is that these effector cells can destroy tumor cells that are resistant to a variety of cytotoxic agents or other immune cells (Fidler, 1978). The experiments described in this chapter demonstrate that the multiple i.v. injections of immunomodulators encapsulated in multilamellar liposomes activate tumoricidal properties of macrophages and are associated with the regression and/or cytostasis of lymph node and lung metastases arising from s.c. murine melanomas. However, systemic therapy with liposome-encapsulated immunomodulators has a distinct disadvantage inasmuch as it does not lead to generation of systemic immunity.

The establishment and growth of metastases are determined by the rate of tumor cell proliferation and the rate of tumor cell destruction. When tumor cell proliferation exceeds its destruction, metastases will develop. It is important to note that, in both tumor systems used here (L10 in strain 2 guinea pigs and B16 melanoma in C57BL/6 mice), the mass doubling time of metastases is exceedingly short, ranging between 4–7 days. In contrast, the mass doubling time of many human metastases has been calculated to be between 80 and 100 days (Fidler et al., 1978). Because it is reasonable to assume that the rate of target cell killing by murine, guinea pig or human effector cells is similar, immunotherapy directed against metastases with long mass doubling time has more likelihood of success.

The optimal conditions for systemic therapy with either active specific immunotherapy or with liposome-encapsulated immunomodulators, and the efficacy of these modalities alone, or in combination, in treating large metastatic tumor burdens are now being defined. Although the initial results reported here are encouraging, it is unlikely that these therapeutic approaches could serve as a single modality in treating advanced metastatic disease. As with many other anti-tumor therapies, optimal application of these modalities will probably involve their use in combination with other anti-tumor agents. Potential therapeutic regimens designed to stimulate host immunity have to be used in combination with other treatments such as chemotherapy, in order to first reduce the "bulk" tumor burden to a sufficient level at which activated macrophages can kill the surviving or drug-insensitive tumor cells. Moreover, appropriate procedures for active specific immunotherapy should be employed to aid in the destruction of metastases and generate the systemic immunity necessary to control dormant tumor cells.

References

Allison, A.C. (1979) Mode of action of immunological adjuvants. *J. Reticuloendothel. Soc.* 26:619–630.

Allison, A.C. and Gregoriadis, G. (1974) Liposomes as immunological adjuvants. *Nature* 252:252–254.

Chedid, L., Carelli, L., and Audibert, F. (1979) Recent developments concerning muramyl dipeptide, a synthetic immunoregulating molecule. *J. Reticuloendothel. Soc.* 26:631–641.

Den Otter, E., Dullens Hub, F.J., Van Lovern, H., and Pels, E. (1977) Anti-tumor effects of macrophages injected into animals: a review. In *The Macrophage and Cancer.* James, K., McBride, B., and Stuart, A. (eds.), Edinburgh: Econoprint, pp. 119–140.

Fidler, I.J. (1974) Inhibition of pulmonary metastasis by intravenous injection of specifically activated macrophages. *Cancer Res.* 34:1074–1078.

Fidler, I.J. (1978) Recognition and destruction of target cells by tumoricidal macrophages. *Isr. J. Med. Sci.* 14:177–191.

Fidler, I.J. (1980) Therapy of spontaneous metastases by intravenous injection of liposomes containing lymphokines. *Science* 208:1469–1471.

Fidler, I.J. and Kripke, M.L. (1977) Metastasis results from preexisting variant cells within a malignant tumor. *Science* 197:893–895.

Fidler, I.J. and Kripke, M.L. (1980) Tumor cell antigenicity, host immunity, and cancer metastasis. *Cancer Immunol. Immunother.* 7:201–205.

Fidler, I.J., Gersten, D.M., and Hart, I.R. (1978) The biology of cancer invasion and metastasis. *Adv. Cancer Res.* 28:149–250.

Fidler, I.J., Sone, S., Fogler, W.E., and Barnes, Z.L. (1980) Eradication of spontaneous metastases and activation of alveolar macrophages by intravenous injection of liposomes containing muramyl dipeptide. *Proc. Natl. Acad. Sci. U.S.A.*, in press.

Griswold, D.P., Jr. (1972) Consideration of the subcutaneously implanted B16 melanoma as a screening model for potential anticancer agents. *Cancer Chemother. Rep.* 3:315–323.

Hanna, M.G., Jr. and Bucana, C. (1979) Active specific immunotherapy of residual micrometastasis: the acute and chronic inflammatory response in induction of tumor immunity by BCG-tumor cell immunization. *J. Reticuloendothel. Soc.* 26:439–452.

Hanna, M.G., Jr. and Peters, L.C. (1978) Specific immunotherapy of established visceral micrometastases by BCG-tumor cell vaccine alone or as an adjunct to surgery. *Cancer* 42:2613–2625.

Hanna, M.G., Jr., Zbar, B., and Rapp, H.J. (1972) Histopathology of tumor regression following intralesional injection of *Mycobacterium bovis* (BCG). I. Tumor growth and metastasis. *J. Natl. Cancer Inst.* 48:1441–1455.

Hanna, M.G., Jr., Brandhorst, J.S., and Peters, L.C. (1979) Active specific immunotherapy of residual micrometastasis: an evaluation of sources, doses, and ratios of BCG with tumor cells. *Cancer Immunol. Immunother.* 7:165–173.

Hart, I.R. (1979) Selection and characterization of an invasive variant of the B16 melanoma. *Am. J. Pathol.* 97:587–600.

Kerbel, R. S. (1979) Implications of immunological heterogeneity of tumors. *Nature* 280:358–360.

Liotta, L.A., Gattozzi, C., Kleinerman, J., and Saidel, G. (1977) Reduction of tumor cell entry into vessels by BCG-activated macrophages. *Br. J. Cancer* 36:639–641.

Matter, A. (1979) The effects of muramyldipeptide (MDP) in cell-mediated immunity. A comparison between *in vitro* and *in vivo* systems. *Cancer Immunol. Immunother.* 6:201–210.

Maver, C. and McKneally, M. (1979) Preparation of autologous tumor cell vaccine from human lung cancer. *Cancer Res.* 39:3276.

Morton, D.L., Eilber, F.R., Holmes, E.C., Hunt, J.S., Ketcham, A.S., Silverstein, M.J., and Sparks, F.C. (1974) BCG immunotherapy of malignant melanoma: summary of seven-year experience. *Ann. Surg.* 180:635–643.

Morton, D.L., Eilber, F.R., Holmes, E.C., Sparks, F.C., and Ramming, K.P. (1976) Present status of BCG immunotherapy of malignant melanoma. *Cancer Immunol. Immunother.* 1:93–98.

Peters, L.C. and Hanna, M.G., Jr. (1980) Active specific immunotherapy of established micrometastasis: the effect of cryopreservation procedures on tumor cell immunogenicity. *J. Natl. Cancer Inst.* 64:1521–1525.

Peters, L.C., Brandhorst, J.S., and Hanna, M.G., Jr. (1979) Preparation of immunotherapeutic autologous tumor cell vaccines from solid tumors. *Cancer Res.* 39:1353–1360.

Poste, G. and Fidler, I.J. (1979) The pathogenesis of cancer metastasis. *Nature* 283:139–146.

Poste, G. and Fidler, I.J. (1980) Stimulation of macrophage-mediated destruction of lung metastases by administration of immunomodulators encapsulated in liposomes. In *The Study of Drug Activity and Immunocompetent Cell Functions.* Nicolau, C. and Paraf, A. (eds.), New York: Academic Press, in press.

Poste, G., Kirsh, R., Fogler, W.E., and Fidler, I.J. (1979) Activation of tumoricidal properties in mouse macrophages by lymphokines encapsulated in liposomes. *Cancer Res.* 39:881–892.

Rapp, H.J., Churchill, W.H., Jr., Kronman, B.S., Rolley, R.T., Hammond, W.G., and Borsos, T. (1968) Antigenicity of a new diethylnitrosamine-induced transplantable guinea pig hepatoma: pathology and formation of ascites variant. *J. Natl. Cancer Inst.* 41:1–11.

Sone, S. and Fidler, I.J. (1980) *In vitro* activation of tumoricidal properties in rat alveolar macrophages by synthetic muramyl dipeptide encapsulated in liposomes. *Cell Immunol.*, in press.

Sone, S., Poste, G., and Fidler, I.J. (1980) Rat alveolar macrophages are susceptible to activation by free and liposome-encapsulated lymphokines. *J. Immunol.* 124:2197–2202.

Zbar, B., Bernstein, I.D., Bartlett, G.L., Hanna, M.G., Jr., and Rapp, H.J. (1972) Immunotherapy of cancer: regression of intradermal tumors and prevention of growth of lymph node metastases after intralesional injection of living *Mycobacterium bovis* (Bacillus Calmette-Guérin). *J. Natl. Cancer Inst.* 49:119–130.

Published 1981 by Elsevier North Holland, Inc.
Saunders, Daniels, Serrou, Rosenfeld, and Denney, eds.
FUNDAMENTAL MECHANISMS IN HUMAN CANCER IMMUNOLOGY

CHAPTER 31

Immunomodulation by Nutritional Means[1]

J. Wesley Alexander, M.D., Sc.D.

*Professor of Surgery, Director of Transplantation Division and
the Surgical Immunobiology Laboratory, Department of Surgery,
University of Cincinnati Medical Center, and Director of Research,
Cincinnati Shriners Burns Institute*

Introduction

For many centuries, the importance of nutrition to recovery from infection has been recognized. However, only during the last decade has there been significant progress in documenting the powerful influence of nutritional variables on specific immunologic responses. Present knowledge is still quite fragmentary, because nutrient interactions are so numerous and complex, but altered nutritional states are undoubtedly the most common cause of acquired immunologic deficiencies in man. It is also clear that nutritional therapy may not only restore immunologic responses to normal, but in some instances may be used to therapeutic advantage to increase resistance to infection or to control the growth of malignant tumors.

The following review will, of necessity, be brief and incomplete. However, it should become apparent that virtually all studies in fundamental cancer immunology as well as the immunology of resistance to infection must take into consideration the nutritional status of the host.

Effect of Chronic Undernutrition on Immunologic Responses

Protein calorie malnutrition (PCM) or protein energy malnutrition (PEM) are terms frequently used to describe chronic undernutrition. However, patients with chronic undernutrition also have multiple and varying deficiencies of vitamins and minerals, and the clinical states of patients in one area of the

[1]Portions of the research cited herein were supported by USPHS Grant #AI 12936.

world are often different from patients in other geographic regions because of these variables. Marasmus is often used to describe chronic undernutrition in which caloric deficiency predominates, whereas kwashiorkor is used to describe chronic undernutrition in which protein deficiency predominates. Most of the studies of chronic undernutrition have been performed in children, usually in underdeveloped countries where there is the problem of a marked association with chronic infectious diseases such as malaria and parasitism.

Serum Opsonic Proteins

Sirisinha et al. (1976), Chandra (1975), and Olusi et al. (1976) have clearly demonstrated that PEM is associated with low serum levels of nearly all complement components except C4 and C5, and Wunder et al. (1978) have shown a significant reduction in C3 levels in marasmic guinea pigs. There also appears to be an increased consumption of C3, as evidenced by an elevated level of C3 degradation products in the serum. Normal levels of these components may be restored by nutritional repletion (Palmblad, 1977; Dionigi et al., 1977).

B Cell Function

Although germinal centers are often decreased in patients with PEM and there are decreased numbers of peripheral B cells, immunoglobulin levels are usually normal and sometimes elevated. However, there may be depressed reactivity to certain antigens. Chandra (1979) has suggested that the recurrent infections in these children may result in an almost continual immunologic stimulus which may result in hyperimmunoglobulinemia. On the other hand, in very young children with kwashiorkor, there may be a prolonged and profound hypoimmunoglobulinemia (Aref et al., 1970; Chandra, 1979). Primary responsiveness to a variety of antigens has been observed to be somewhat variable but generally depressed (Alexander and Stinnett, in press).

T Cell Function

PEM is associated with marked thymic atrophy and reduction of lymphoid mass, the thymic dependent areas being especially affected. Smythe and his colleagues (1971) demonstrated a marked depression of cell-mediated immunity; only 30% of malnourished children responded to dinitrochlorobenzine (DNCB). Schlesinger and Stekel (1974) also demonstrated that children with kwashiorkor and marasmus failed to respond to DNCB, but isolated lymphocytes from these children had normal blastoid transformation when stimulated with phytohemagglutinin (PHA) *in vitro*. On the other hand, Schopfer and Douglas (1976) found that the lymphocytes from patients with kwashiorkor failed to respond normally to PHA, although pokeweed mitogen caused a better than normal response. Lopez et al. (1972) have shown a marked atrophy of the thymus, decreased responsiveness to DNCB, reduced reactivity to delayed hypersensitivity antigens, and delayed rejection of skin grafts in marasmic guinea pigs. Other reports have both contradicted and confirmed such findings.

Neutrophil Function

A deficiency of the capacity of neutrophils from children with PEM to kill bacteria has been demonstrated repeatedly (Selvaraj and Bhat, 1972; Seth and Chandra, 1972; Schopfer and Douglas, 1976). Phagocytic activity is usually not impaired, but there is a deficient killing of phagocytized bacteria and decreased chemotactic responses. Associated with these defects are metabolic changes showing depression of glycolytic pathway activity.

Response to Bacterial Challenge

Septicemia occurs with high frequency in individuals with kwashiorkor and is often fatal (Scragg, 1978). Bacterial clearance mechanisms in animals with chronic undernutrition are clearly diminished in both the blood and lungs.

Tumor Growth

Moderate degrees of underfeeding may result in depressed B cell function, concurrent with enhanced T cell function and increased resistance to the growth of transplanted tumor cells (Good et al. 1980). This effect on tumor growth results in part from a decreased synthesis of blocking antibody and perhaps also from increased sensitivity of suppressor T cells to moderate protein depletion. Caloric restriction also delays the appearance of spontaneous carcinogen-induced tumors in a variety of animal systems. In the converse situation, overfeeding results in an accelerated growth rate and appearance of induced malignant tumors.

Individual Nutrients and Immunologic Functions

Protein and Amino Acids

Protein deficiency has been shown to alter almost all important immunologic functions. Chronic severe deprivation of protein intake can markedly diminish antibody synthesis, but acute, short-term deprivation can increase antibody synthesis. Moderate degrees of protein restriction with a normal caloric intake will depress B cell function at the same time that T cell function is enhanced, perhaps through a selective effect on suppressor T cells. These conditions result in increased resistance to the growth of transplantable tumors (Jose and Good, 1973; Good et al., 1976). Studies by Malave and Layrisse (1976) suggest that IgG antibody synthesis is restricted more than IgM synthesis during protein deficiency. Kenney et al. (1965, 1968) demonstrated that antibody production on a per cell basis is not diminished in protein depleted animals, but there are fewer cells producing antibody. Law et al. (1974) have demonstrated marked depression of cutaneous hypersensitivity and *in vitro* lymphocyte transformation responses in protein-depleted rats. The clearance of both live and killed bacteria are markedly depressed in protein deficient animals (Ratnakar et al., 1972; Bhuyan and Ramalingaswami, 1972), accompanied by diminished rates of survival. Our own experiments (Wunder et al., 1978) have shown that moderate protein depletion markedly inhibits C3 synthesis and the ability of sera from the affected animals to support opsonization. However, the antibacterial function of neutrophils was not affected nor irregularly depressed.

Our studies have shown that the immunologic defects caused by protein-deficient diets can be reversed by the administration of essential amino acids but not non-essential amino acids, demonstrating that total nitrogen load is not as important as the type of amino acid administered (Wunder et al., 1979). Buzby and his colleagues (1980), using rats with a transplantable mammary adenocarcinoma, showed that total parenteral nutrition with adequate amino acids alone improved host maintenance but also stimulated tumor growth. Adequate amino acids and carbohydrates given together maximized both host maintenance and tumor growth.

Erickson et al. (1979) studied B and T lymphocyte responses in a murine model of malignant melanoma. T cell responses were highly dependent upon dietary protein concentrations, whereas B cell responses were dependent on energy intake and dietary protein. Tyrosine and phenylalanine may have a somewhat selective effect on the growth of melanoma. Pine (1978) showed that murine leukemia was markedly affected by the administration of low phenylalanine diets in mice. Kenney and her colleagues (1970) studied the effect of selected dietary amino acids on the immune response in rats. They showed that tryptophan supplementation in diets increased hemolysin titers of adults and agglutinin titers in young rats after injection of the antigen. Addition of methionine improved weight gain in animals but depressed late primary antibody response. Lysine exerted no significant effect. Petro and Bhattacharjee (1980) studied the effect of selective amino acid deficiency on immunologic responses. Mice fed isoleucine and lysine limited diets had significantly lower levels of C3 than control mice. The animals also had lower levels of transferrin in peritoneal exudates but not in serum. Barbul and her colleagues have shown in a series of articles (1977, 1978, 1980a, 1980b) that dietary arginine supplementation of a diet can minimize post traumatic weight loss, accelerate wound healing, minimize trauma induced thymolysis after injury, increase thymic weight, and increase *in vitro* reactivity of thymic lymphocytes in both animals and man. Milner and Stepanovitch (1979) also showed that tumor growth is inhibited in mice whose diets were supplemented with 5% arginine.

The effects of individual amino acid deficiencies or excesses on immunologic function are just now beginning to be investigated. It may take some time to dissect the precise roles of each individual amino acid in modulating immunologic responses because of the extraordinary complexity and number of possible interactions.

Lipids

Several studies have suggested that the administration of lipids during the course of acute infection may block phagocytosis and potentially worsen the infection. Also, it has been demonstrated that, while intravenous fat emulsions can be a satisfactory energy source in individuals with normal energy expenditure, intravenous fat is not as nitrogen sparing as carbohydrate, calorie per calorie, in injured animals (Freund et al., 1980). Friend and his colleagues (1980) showed that diets containing 20% by weight of fat rich in unsaturated fatty acids reduced the ability of guinea pigs to mount delayed hypersensitivity responses and form antibody. Also, the serum of these animals greatly inhibited the response of mitogens to antigen *in vitro*. On the other hand, Buzby et al. (1980) showed that isocaloric isonitrogenous intravenous diets providing non-nitrogenous calories as fat promoted host maintenance without causing tumor stimulation. Their study suggested that there was a differential utilization of fat calories by normal and malignant cells which could permit normal function of host defense without tumor stimulation. Burns et al. (1978) reported that a diet rich in saturated fat prolonged survival of mice with leukemia better than a diet rich in unsaturated fat.

Carbohydrates

Carbohydrates appear to support nitrogen sparing better than fats when used as an energy source, but no systematic studies have been made of the influence of dietary deficiency of carbohydrates (without caloric deficiency) on immunologic functions. It is well established, however, that carbohydrates usually supply the necessary energy for protein metabolism, and energy deficiency will markedly interfere with immunologic responses.

Vitamins

Isolated vitamin deficiencies are seldom encountered in modern clinical practice. However, animal studies have shown that deficiencies of vitamin intake may affect many of the immunologic processes. Results of these studies are summarized in Table 31.1.

Minerals

Considering the potential importance of several minerals in metaloenzymes, it is surprising that more is not known about the effect of specific mineral deficiencies on immunologic functions. Most of the information currently available concerns iron and zinc, although copper and magnesium have been shown to influence some functions.

Iron

Chandra (1976) has estimated that iron deficiency affects nearly one-third of the population in industrialized countries and nearly two-thirds in developing nations. It has been reported that iron deficient animals have decreased delayed hypersensitivity responsiveness and reduced numbers of circulating T cells. However, others have reported that cell-mediated immune responses in iron deficient subjects are normal (Chandra et al., 1977). It is relatively clear

Table 31.1. Influence of Vitamin Deficiencies on Immunologic Variables.

Vitamin A
    Deficiency impairs epithelial barriers
    Deficiency reduces antibody responses
    Deficiency depresses phagocytic function
        Vitamin A therapy may stimulate mitogenic responses of
            lymphocytes in cancer patients (Micksche et al., 1977) and stimulate cytotoxicity
            in vitro (Lotan, 1979)

Vitamin C
    Deficiency depresses migration of phagocytes
    Marked excesses may impair bactericidal activity of leukocytes (Shilotri and Bhat, 1977)

Pyridoxin (B6)
    Deficiency inhibits both B cell and T cell responses and may induce defective
        phagocytosis and killing of bacteria

Pantothanic acid, theomine, riboflavin
    Deficiency may impair antibody responses

(Source: Alexander and Stinnett, in press.)

that the administration of iron during the course of acute bacterial infection can worsen the infection, since iron acts as a nutrilite for bacteria (Weinberg, 1974).

Zinc

Zinc deficiency has been shown to exert a remarkable effect on specific immunologic functions of the thymus and T cells in both animals and humans (Schloen et al., 1979). The immunologic perturbations that accompany acrodermititis enteropathica dramatically emphasize the role of zinc in immunologic processes. In zinc deficiency, the thymus and thymic dependent regions of second level lymphoid tissues may be severely involuted in zinc deficient animals, and both B cell and T cell functions are inhibited. Primary antibody response is substantially reduced, while secondary responses which require helper T lymphocytes are almost eliminated. Zinc deficient animals also fail to develop cytotoxic T killer cells and natural killer function normally, and they respond poorly to tumor challenges.

Summary and Conclusions

It is obvious from this discussion that nutritional variables may have profound influences on immunologic functions. The potential benefit of immunomodulation by nutritional means on both infection and cancer has not yet been fully appreciated, but it is likely that nutritional approaches will in the future provide an important new dimension in the prevention and treatment of malignant disease.

References

Alexander, J.W. and Stinnett, J.D. Changes in immunologic function. In *Surgical Nutrition*. Fischer, Josef E. (ed.), Boston: Little, Brown & Co., in press.

Aref, G.H., Badr El Din, M.K., Hassan, A.I., and Araby, I.I. (1970) Immunoglobulins in kwashiorkor. *J. Trop. Med. Hyg.* 73:186.

Barbul, A., Rettura, G., Levenson, S.M., and Seifter, E. (1977) Arginine: a thymotropic and wound-healing promoting agent. *Surg. Forum* XXVIII:101–103.

Barbul, A., Rettura, G., Prior, E., Levenson, S.M., and Seifter, E. (1978) Endocrines and Metabolism. Supplemental arginine, wound healing, and thymus: arginine-pituitary interaction. *Surg. Forum* XXIX:93–95.

Barbul, A., Wasserkrug, B.A., and Efron, G. (1980b) Immunostrimulatory action of arginine in humans. *Surg. Forum* XXXI:82–84.

Barbul, A., Wasserkrug, H.L., Sisto, D.A., Seifter, E., Rettura, G., Levenson, S.M., and Efron, G. (1980a) Thymic stimulatory actions of arginine. *J. Par. Ent. Nutr.* 4:446–449.

Bhuyan, U.N. and Ramalingaswami, V. (1972) Responses of the protein deficient rabbit to staphylococcal bacteremia. *Am. J. Pathol.* 69:359.

Burns, C., Luttenegger, D.G., and Spector, A.A. (1978) Effect of dietary fat saturation on survival of mice with L1210 leukemia. *J. Natl. Cancer Inst.* 61:513–515.

Buzby, G.P., Mullen, J.L., Stein, T.P., Miller, E.E., Hobbs, C.L., and Rosato, E.F. (1980) Host-tumor interaction and nutrient supply. *Cancer* 45:2940–2948.

Chandra, R.K. (1975) Serum complement and immunoconglutinin in malnutrition. *Arch. Dis. Childh.* 50:225.

Chandra, R.K. (1976) Iron and immunocompetence. *Nutr. Rev.* 34:129.

Chandra, R.K. (1979) Interactions of nutrition, infection, and immune response. Immunocompetence in nutritional deficiency, methodological considerations, and intervention strategies. *Acta Pediatr. Scand.* 68:137.

Chandra, R.K., Au. B., Woodford, G., and Hyamm, P. (1977) Iron status, immunocompetence, and susceptibility to infection. In *Ciba Foundation Symposium on Iron Metabolism*. Jacob, A. (ed.), Amsterdam: Elsevier, p. 249.

Dionigi, R., Zonta, A., Diminioni, L., Gres, F., and Ballabio, A. (1977) The effects of total parenteral nutrition on immunodepression due to malnutrition. *Ann. Surg.* 185:467.

Erickson, K.L., Fershwin, M.E., Canolty, N.L., and Eckels, D.D. (1979) The influence of dietary protein concentration and energy intake on mitogen response and tumor growth in melanoma-bearing mice. *J. Nutr.* 109:353–359.

Friend, J.V., Lock, S.O., Gurr, M.I., and Parish, W.E. (1980) Effect of different dietary lipids on the immune responses of Hartley strain guinea pigs. *Int. Archs. Allergy Appl. Immun.* 62:292–301.

Freund, H., Yoshimura, N., and Fischer, J.E. (1980) Is intravenous fat nitrogen sparing in the injured rat? *Am. J. Surg.* 140:377–383.

Good, R.A., Fernandes, G., Yunis, E.J., Cooper, W.C., Jose, D.G., Kramer, T., and Hansen, M.A. (1976) Nutrition and immunity under controlled experimental conditions. In *Symposia of the Swedish Nutrition Foundation*. Monograph XIII, Uppsala, Sweden: Almqvist & Wiksell.

Good, R.A., West, A., and Fernandes, G. (1980) Nutritional modulation of immune responses. *FASEB* 39:3098–3104.

Jose, D.G. and Good, R.A. (1973) Quantitative effects of nutritional protein and calorie deficiency upon immune responses to tumors in mice. *Cancer Res.* 33:807.

Kenney, M.A., Arnrich, L., Mar, E., and Roderuck, C.E. (1965) Influence of dietary protein on complement, properdin, and hemolysis in adult protein-depleted rats. *J. Nutr.* 85:213.

Kenney, M.A., Magee, J.L., and Piedad-Pascual, F (1970) Dietary amino acids and immune response in rats. *J. Nutr.* 100:1063.

Kenney, M.A., Roderuck, C.E., Arnrich, L., and Piedad, F. (1968) Effect of protein deficiency on the spleen and antibody formation in rats. *J. Nutr.* 95:173.

Law, D.K., Dudrick, S.J., and Abdou, N.I. (1974) The effect of dietary protein depletion on immunocompetence: the importance of nutritional repletion prior to immunologic induction. *Ann. Surg.* 179:168.

Lopez, V., Davis, S.D., and Smith, N.J. (1972) Studies in infantile marasmus. IV. Impairment of immunologic responses in the marasmic pig. *Pediat. Res.* 6:779.

Lotan, R. and Dennert, G. (1979) Stimulatory effects of vitamin A analogs on induction of cell-mediated cytotoxicity *in vivo*. *Cancer Res.* 39:55–58.

Malave, I. and Layrisse, M. (1976) Immune response in malnutrition. Differential effect of dietary protein restriction on the IgM and IgG response to alloantigens. *Cell. Immunol.* 21:337.

Micksche, M., Cerni, C., Kokron, O., Titscher, R., and Wrba, H. (1977) Stimulation of immune response in lung cancer patients by vitamin A therapy. *Oncology* 34:234–238.

Milner, J.A. and Stepanovich, L.V. (1979) Inhibitory effect of dietary arginine on growth of Ehrlich Ascites tumor cells in mice. *J. Nutr.* 109:489–494.

Olusi, S.O., McFarlane, H., Ade-Serrano, M., Osunkoya, B.O., and Adesina, H. (1976) Complement components in children with protein-calorie malnutrition. *Trop. Geogr. Med.* 28:323.

Palmblad, J., Cantell, K., Holm, G., Narberg, R., Strander, H., and Sunblad, L. (1977) Acute energy deprivation in man: effect on serum immunoglobulins, antibody response, complement factors 3 and 4, acute phase reactants, and interferon-producing capacity of blood lymphocytes. *Clin. Exp. Immunol.* 30:50.

Petro, T.M. and Bhattacharjee, J.K. (1980) Effect of dietary essential amino acid limitations upon native levels of murine serum immunoglobulins, transferrin, and complement. *Infect. Immun.* 27:513–518.

Pine, M.J. (1978) Effect of low phenylalanine diet on murine leukemia L1210, *J. Natl. Cancer Inst.* 60:633–641.

Ratnakar, K.S., Mathus, M., Ramalingaswami, V., and Deo, M.G. (1972) Phagocytic function of reticuloendothelial system in protein deficiency—a study in Rhesus monkeys using ^{32}P-labeled *E. coli. J. Nutr.* 102:1233.

Schlesinger, L. and Stekel, A. (1974) Impaired cellular immunity in marasmic infants. *Am. J. Clin. Nutr.* 27:615.

Schloen, L.H., Fernandes, G., Garofalo, J.A., and Good, R.A. (1979) Nutrition, immunity, and cancer—a review. Part II. Zinc, immune function and cancer. *Clin. Bull.* (Mem. Sloan-Kettering Cancer Ctr.) 9:63–75.

Schopfer, K. and Douglas, S.D. (1976) *In vitro* studies of lymphocytes from children with kwashiorkor. *Clin. Immunol. Immunopathol.* 5:21.

Schopfer, K. and Douglas, S.D. (1976) Neutrophil function in children with kwashiorkor. *J. Lab. Clin. Med.* 88:450.

Scragg, J.N. and Appelbaum, P.C. (1978) Septicemia in kwashiorkor. *S. Afr. Med. J.* 53:358.

Selvaraj, R.J. and Bhat, K.S. (1972) Metabolic and bactericidal activities of leukocytes in protein-calorie malnutrition. *Am. J. Clin. Nutr.* 25:166.

Seth, V. and Chandra, R.K. (1972) Opsonic activity, phagocytosis, and bactericidal capacity of polymorphs in undernutrition. *Arch. Dis. Childh.* 47:282.

Shilotri, P.G. and Bhat, K.S. (1977) Effect of mega doses of vitamin C on bactericidal activity of leukocytes. *am. J. Clin. Nutr.* 30:1077–1081.

Sirisinha, S., Edelman, R., Suskind, R., Charupatana, C., and Olson, R.E. (1976) Complement and C3-proactivator levels in children with protein calorie malnutrition and effect of dietary treatment. *Lancet* 1:1016.

Smythe, P.M., Schonland, M., Brereton-Stiles, G.G., Coovadia, H.M., Grace, H.J., Loening, W.E.K., Mayfoyane, A., Parent, M.A., and Vos, G.H. (1971) Thymolymphatic deficiency and depression of cell-mediated immunity in protein-calorie malnutrition. *Lancet* II:939.

Weinberg, E.D. (1974) Iron and susceptibility to infectious disease. *Science* 184:952.

Wunder, J.A., Stinnett, J.D., and Alexander, J.W. (1978) The effects of malnutrition on variables of host defense in the guinea pig. *Surgery* 84:542–550.

Wunder, J.A., Stinnett, J.D., and Alexander, J.W. (1979) Protein depletion, amino acid repletion, and host defense status in guinea pigs. *Fed. Proc.* (abstract).

Published 1981 by Elsevier North Holland, Inc.
Saunders, Daniels, Serrou, Rosenfeld, and Denney, eds.
FUNDAMENTAL MECHANISMS IN HUMAN CANCER IMMUNOLOGY

CHAPTER 32

Specific Immune Responses to Chemically Induced Tumors: Relation Between Tumor Specific Antigens Recognized by Cloned T Cell Lines and by Antibody Producing Hybridomas, to Tumor Specific Protection in Vivo[1]

Richard T. Smith, Yoshiteru Konaka,
Maron Calderwood, Shiro Shimizu,
Linda Smith, and Paul A. Klein

College of Medicine, Department of Pathology, Tumor Biology Unit, University of Florida, Gainesville, Florida

Introduction and Background

The provocative experiment of Old and colleagues in 1962 first raised the possibility that adoptive immunotherapy might be effective against cancer. Pursuit of this possibility has subsequently challenged, consumed, and frustrated a generation of tumor biologists. Only recently has knowledge regarding the lymphoreticular system been sufficient, and technology for cultivation of all classes of lymphoid cells been adequate, to explore the possibilities meaningfully.

Our efforts have exploited the well established experimental system involving immune responses to chemically induced sarcomas in genetically defined mice. These tumors present to the host immune system a variety of antigenic structures to which it can respond. Each tumor shows in transplantation tests what is widely interpreted as a unique specificity, tumor specific transplantation antigens (TSTA) (Prehn and Main, 1957), as well as specificities, chiefly revealed *in vitro*, which are shared to varying degrees among syngeneic tumors

[1]Supported in part by Grants CA 26882, CA 15334, CA 09126, and HD 00384 from the National Institutes of Health.

(reviewed in Smith and Landy, 1975). As will be discussed in this paper, a rich source of shared antigenic surface structures on these tumors are the products of endogenous murine leukemia virus genomes (DeLeo et al., 1977; Klein, 1980).

Responses to this group of tumors can be elicited from all known elements of the immune system; macrophages, B cells, T cells, and their respective subclasses and various cell products. This chapter reports on experiments which bear upon three questions with which we have been concerned during the past 10 years: (a) Which cell classes or subclasses are responsible for immunologically mediated tumor cell death or inhibition? (b) Toward what tumor antigens are their receptors directed? (c) Can these cells be cultured, cloned, and used to control tumor growth *in vivo*? With due regard for the roles of macrophages, antibody mediated cellular cytotoxicity (ADCC) and natural killer cells in control of tumor growth *in vitro*, the answer to question (a) seems quite clear in studies from our laboratory and those of many other investigators. The T cell is the principle class of lymphoid cells responsible for mediating control of tumor growth *in vivo*. Answers to (b) are now forthcoming with regard to B cell recognition, but are very tentative with respect to T cell recognition. Preliminary experiments relevant to (c) to be reported here suggest potential immunotherapeutic value of lymphoid cells under defined circumstances.

Tumor Borne Antigens Recognized by T Cells

In theory at least, two effector mechanisms are available to T cells which bear receptors for tumor antigen: (a) induction of delayed type inflammatory reactions in which macrophages are instrumental in tumor destruction, and (b) direct T cell-mediated cytotoxicity. Here, we will be concerned exclusively with the latter mechanism, as examined through study of long-term lines of cultured cytotoxic T cells (CTL) both in tests of their effects *in vitro* and *in vivo*, and for purposes of defining the target antigens they attack.

Early studies in our laboratory involved detection of proliferation in lymphoid cell subpopulations in response to solubilized tumor membrane antigen preparations (Forbes et al., 1975). The characteristics and kinetics of the lymphocyte proliferation assay (LPA) which evolved was not different from lymphocyte responses *in vitro* toward bacterial or viral antigens. Distribution of responding cells in blood, lymph nodes, spleen, and tumor, and definition of the cell subclass mixture in these organs, was studied throughout the natural course of tumor bearing. Mixtures of solubilized membrane structures ranging in molecular size between 18,000 and 100,000 D evoked strong proliferative responses in T cells, B cells, and "null" cell classes. Earliest responses were limited to regional lymph node T cells, but by 2–3 weeks all classes were involved (Calderwood et al., 1977, 1980). Cross-stimulation by antigens derived from multiple syngeneic tumors, tested over the natural history of tumor growth, were interpreted as demonstrating polyclonal responses to multiple tumor associated antigens. These antigens were shared among several syngeneic tumors tested. An example of this assay is shown in Figure 32.1.

The *in vivo* behavior of the same lymphoid cell mixtures examined by LPA, were tested for protective effects in a modified adoptive transfer technique (Calderwood et al., 1977). The data confirmed in part the results of Old et al. (1962), in that peritoneal exudate cells (PEC) gave highly significant and specific protection. Our studies showed, however, that unfractionated regional lymph node cells, but not spleen cells, taken 7–12 days after tumor inoculation did give significant specific adoptive protection (Figure 32.2).

The subclasses of lymphoid cells were separated by three different techniques, then tested for LPA reactivity and capacity to provide adoptive protection. LN and spleen sources, as well as the PEC population, were protective in adoptive transfer only when highly enriched for T cells. B cell enriched or null cell subpopulations showed no protective effect despite LPA stimulation equivalent to that of T cells (Table 32.1). These data support the hypothesis that the T cell class contained the principle cells which prevent tumor growth in adoptive transfer. Moreover, this protection was usually specific to the immunizing tumor, despite the fact that B cell or T cell enriched subfractions revealed extensive shared or cross-reactions between syngeneic

Figure 32.1. Lymphocyte proliferation assay in which three soluble tumor antigens (PC1, PC5, PC8) were tested on regional lymph node cells taken after two weeks of bearing either the PC1 (2 left panels) or PC8 (right panel) (●) compared with responses to normal lymph node cells (○). Data are mean cpm±SE of triplicate cultures.

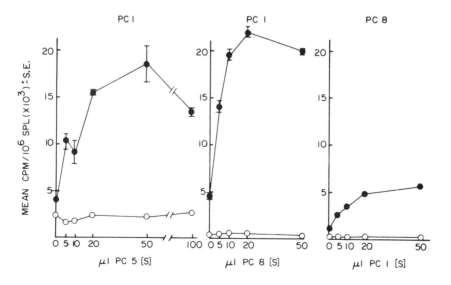

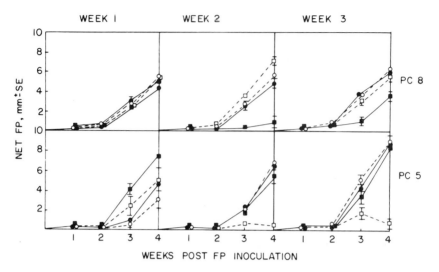

WEEKS POST FP INOCULATION

Figure 32.2. Footpad measurements at intervals following injection of tumor-lymph node cell mixtures into groups of 5 mice in adoptive transfer experiments. Regional lymph node cells taken from C57BL/6 mice bearing the PC1, PC8 or PC5 tumors were mixed at a 1000:1 ratio with either PC8 (upper panel) or PC5 (lower panel) tumor cells, then injected into footpad. (■) PC-8 LNC; (□) PC5 LNC; (●) PC1 LNC; (○) Normal LNC.

tumors *in vitro*. Only when very high ratios of T cells to tumor cells were tested (i.e., >1000:1) was cross protection *in vivo* evident. Despite this, the 4-hour ^{51}Cr release assay gave no evidence of direct cytotoxicity *in vitro* when tested using the same T cell enriched fractions of LN or spleen origin which gave specific protection in the adoptive host. Thus a curious dissociation between *in vitro* and *in vivo* T cell killing propensity and specificity was found.

These data focused our attention upon PEC as the best potential source of tumor specific CTL. PEC taken from tumor hyper-immunized hosts gave significant *in vitro* tumor killing in the short-term ^{51}Cr release assay, at effector to tumor cell ratios between 5:1 and 100:1 (for example, Figure 32.3). T cells appeared to be responsible for cytotoxicity, since killing was abrogated by each preselection technique employed which eliminated T cells. The specificity of killing was examined extensively in this *in vitro* model. As shown in Table 32.2, in 42 separate tests in which significant homologous tumor cytotoxicity occurred, and in which one or more syngeneic tumors were concurrently tested, only 5 instances of significant cross-killing were found. Those PEC found to be generally tumor specific *in vitro* were also tested in the adoptive transfer model and found to provide equally specific protection against the homologous tumor.

It therefore appeared that the T cell class found in PEC was capable of direct *in vitro* killing and *in vivo* protection with a pattern suggestively, but not

Table 32.1. Relationship Between Protection in Adoptive Transfer and Proliferation *in vitro* Among Various Classes of Lymphoid Cells Taken from Tumor Bearing Mice.

Pretreatment of cells	Lymphocyte proliferation assay (^{3}H TdR incorporation mean cpm)	Adoptive transfer assay (Footpad size in mm)
Normal spleen	987	480
Tumor bearing spleen		
Untreated	11,156	283
Anti Ig + C'	17,387	198
Anti Thy-1 + C'	20,017	478

Note: Spleen cells taken 19 days after tumor incubation were tested *in vitro* with solubilized homologous tumor antigen in the LPA, or injected into the footpads of groups of 5 mice after mixing with tumor (E:T-20:1). As indicated, aliquots of these cells were enriched for T or B cells by pretreatment with anti-Ig or anti-Thy-1 plus complement, prior to testing. Footpad measurements were taken at 18 days.

totally, concordant with the unique TSTA pattern revealed by classic transplantation tests. These data led to the use of PEC as the initial cell source from which to culture long-term cytotoxic T cell (CTL) lines. Methods by which this was successfully accomplished differed in no significant way from those which have been used to develop T cell lines carrying other specificities[2] (Gillis and Smith, 1977). Details are given in a separate publication (Konaka et al., manuscript submitted). Briefly, PEC taken from tumor-immunized mice, which had demonstrated specific cytotoxicity, were stimulated twice *in vitro* with irradiated tumor cells and after 5 days were treated with only T cell growth factor (TCGF) derived from Con A treated syngeneic spleen cells. Selection of active lines was based upon *in vitro* tumor cytotoxicity. Long-term T cell lines responsive to six different chemically induced sarcomas and the chemically induced lymphoma EL.4, have been studied in some detail (for example, Figures 32.3, 32.4, 32.5). In addition, short lived (20–35 days) cytotoxic cell lines have been derived from normal spleen cells, stimulated twice or three times *in vitro* with mitomycin C treated tumor cells and cultured in TCGF containing medium (Figure 32.6). None of the latter lines could be extended beyond 35 days.

Each cytotoxic cell line derived from PEC was Lyt-1 negative, Lyt-2 positive, and Thy-1 positive. Each is absolutely TCGF dependent, and antigen independent. The lines retained cytotoxicity for the specific tumor as long as 300 days in continuous culture. Most lines derived from PEC gave greatest cytotoxicity,

[2] The authors are indebted to Drs. Harald von Boehmer and his colleagues at the Basel Institute for Immunology, Basel, Switzerland, and to Drs. Richmond Prehn and Donald Bailey of the Jackson Laboratory, Bar Harbor, Maine, for both the inspiration and the technical education which made this phase of work possible.

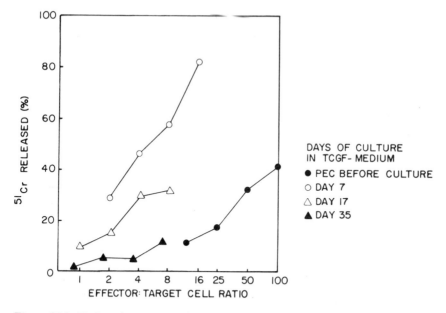

Figure 32.3. Early enhancement of *in vitro* cytolytic activity in cultures containing T cell growth factor of anti-PC-4 immune peritoneal exudate cells toward the PC-4 fibrosarcoma.

as judged by highest percent kill at lowest effector : target (E : T) ratio, between 20 and 60 days. Many lines gradually thereafter lose capacity to kill tumor cells, even though their capacity to divide continues as long as TCGF is supplied in the medium.

Table 32.2. Specificity of Killing by Tumor Immune Peritoneal Exudate Cells *in Vitro*.

Anti-tumor-PEC tested	Incidence of syngeneic cytotoxicity[a]
B6.1	1/11
B6.3	3/10
PC.3	0/2
PC.4	1/6
PC.5	0/3
D2.3	0/2
D2.1	0/4
76.46	0/4

Note: Summary of experiments in which cytotoxicity of PEC elicited by the homologous (immunizing) tumor was concurrently tested with other syngeneic tumors. Out of 42 tests, 5 examples of cross-killing of syngeneic tumors were found.

[a]Significant ^{51}CR release in syngenic tumors/number of syngeneic tumors tested.

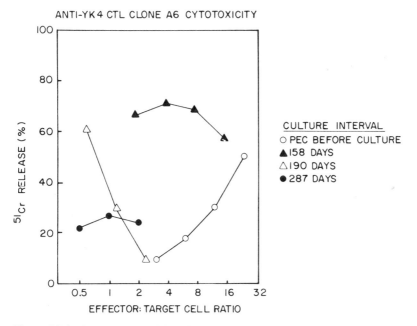

Figure 32.4. *In vitro* cytotoxicity of anti-YK4-clone A6 on YK-4 tumor cells at varying intervals after culture.

Although more difficult to clone than allospecific cells in our hands, two lines (anti-YK 4 and anti-EL.4) have been cloned by limiting dilution on thymus cell feeder layers. The several active clones derived were selected for growth in the cloning medium and for *in vitro* cytotoxicity. Each clone has been characterized individually.

The pattern of *in vitro* cytotoxicity developed by one line during early culture is illustrated in Figures 32.3 and 32.4. Two characteristics of all lines examined are shown: after established growth, the CTL have greater cytotoxicity and E:T ratios which are 20–100 times lower than the original PEC source. Also illustrated is the observation that lines which appear to be established at 30 days frequently enter a "crisis" during which they may die out or lose their killing capacity. All lines successfully cloned survived with significant cytotoxicity longer than 40 days. Two examples are shown in Figures 32.4 and 32.5.

Thus it was possible to derive, sustain, and clone cell lines which have excellent *in vitro* cytotoxicity characteristics toward a class of tumors which are generally resistant to *in vitro* cytotoxicity (Chauvenet and Smith, 1979). Three approaches to the question of *in vivo* functional activity of these CTL against tumors are being made. The modified adoptive transfer technique gives evidence that protection against homologous tumors, both 3-methylcholanthrene (MCA) induced sarcomas and EL-4 lymphomas, is complete at CTL: tumor

456

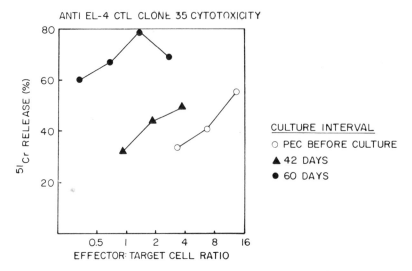

Figure 32.5. *In vitro* cytotoxicity of anti-EL-4 clone 35 on EL-4 tumor cells at varying intervals after initial culture.

ratios in the range of 0.5 : 1 to 5 : 1 (Table 32.3). Sarcomas were mixed with the CTL prior to injection into the footpad, or injected one day before CTL. EL-4 in ascites form was injected i.p. 24 hours before CTL injection. Control cell lines directed against other antigen systems (i.e., BAD-1, an allospecific CTL) failed to protect at any ratio (Figure 32.7).

These techniques clearly show that CTL can function against tumor *in vivo* as well as *in vitro*, and can arrest an established lethal ascites tumor. A more appropriate immunotherapeutic model would, however, pit these lines against more fully established solid tumors. For this to be tested, two unknown elements required resolution: where do CTL home *in vivo* and do they require exogenous TCGF to function *in vivo*? The fate of CTL given intravenously was explored in experiments such as that illustrated in Table 32.4. Although slightly greater concentration of radioactivity was localized in the tumor-bearing area, the overwhelming concentration of CTL was in the liver, not the tumor. Allospecific CTL controls gave a somewhat different homing pattern for reasons that are at present not understood.

The data did not bode well for attempts to affect tumor growth by i.v. injection of specific CTL. This prediction has been borne out in all experiments thus far, which show that no numbers or multiplicity of injections within practical limits of CTL, given i.v., arrested the growth of an established sarcoma in the footpad.

Preliminary experiments suggest that direct injection of specific CTL into an established tumor mass in the footpad results in tumor regression. This type of

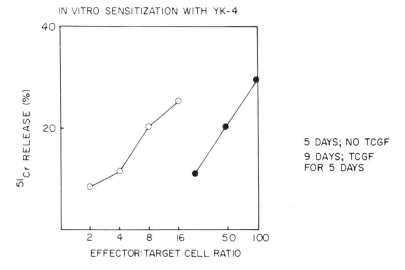

IN VITRO SENSITIZATION WITH YK-4

5 DAYS; NO TCGF
9 DAYS; TCGF
FOR 5 DAYS

Figure 32.6. *In vitro* cytotoxicity of mitomycin treated YK-4 sensitive normal syngeneic spleen cells, against YK-4 tumor cells. *In vitro* sensitization with YK-4 was at a 100:1 ratio of responder to stimulator cells.

Table 32.3. Protection from Lethal Tumor Growth in Adoptive Hosts by Cloned Cytotoxic T Cell Lines (CTL).

Tumor tested	CTL or control cell	Ratio T:CTL	No. with tumor/ no. tested
EL.4 (2 × 10⁵)F.P.			5/5
	EL4. clone 163	1:1	0/5
	EL4. clone 163	1:0.5	0/5
	BAD.1	1:5	5/5
EL.4 (5 × 10⁵)I.P.			
	EL4. clone 163	1:2	0/5
YK-4 (2 × 10⁵)I.P.			4/5
	YK.4.A6	1:0.5	0/5
	YK.4.A6	1:2	0/5
	Normal spleen	1:2	5/5
YK.4 (1 × 10⁵)F.P.			5/5
	YK.4. clone 253	1:2	0/5
	YK.4. clone 341	1:2	0/5
	Normal spleen	1:2	5/5

Note: Three experiments testing anti-tumor effect in adoptive syngeneic hosts of cloned CTL derived from tumor immune syngeneic mice, cultured longer than 40 days in T cell growth factor. EL4 experiments were performed by injecting tumor intraperitoneally, waiting 24 hours, then injecting the indicated CTL. Lethal ascites were scored at 25 days. YK-4 was injected in the footpad after mixing with the indicated proportion of CTL, and progressive tumor growth was scored at 30 days.

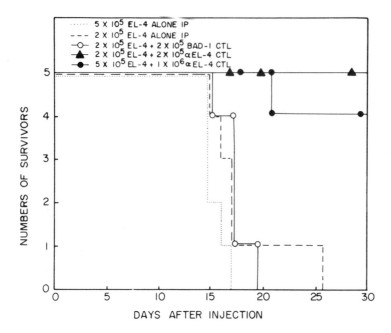

Figure 32.7. Experiment demonstrating *in vivo* protection of groups of 5 syngeneic mice injected i.p. with the indicated numbers of EL-4 ascites adapted tumor cells, by anti-EL-4 CTL injected in the indicated number, 24 hours later.

experiment will require extensive verification with respect to specificity of protection. Experiments will be necessary to separate the direct effects of injected CTL on the tumor mass from that of TCGF injected with CTL on resident host T cells within the tumor mass.

The specificity of CTL derived and/or cloned thus far has shown to a surprising degree that target antigens for killing are shared among some but not all tumors. The extent of cross-killing revealed thus far (Table 32.5) is similar to that found for whole PEC (Table 32.2). Non-cloned CTL killed about 50% of concurrently tested syngeneic tumors, which represents the same or a slightly greater incidence of cross-killing than that produced by the PEC from which the cell lines were derived. The cloned CTL thus far characterized had a higher degree of specific kill, but a significant cross-killing still occurred.

All adoptive transfer tests showed total protection against lethal growth of the homologous combination between CTL and tumor. In combinations of CTL and syngeneic tumor target cells that gave cytotoxicity *in vitro* equivalent to that of the homologous combination, partial protection could be detected *in vivo*.

If it is accepted that cloned CTL bear a single specific receptor, then the target ligand they recognize is probably not unique, but shared by more than one syngeneic tumor. By classic definition, none of the CTL studied thus far

Table 32.4. Distribution of Radioactivity 4 hours after i.v. Injection of YK.4A6 or BAD-1.

| Organ tested | Mean % of ^{51}Cr labeled cytotoxic/ T cell line in organ or tissue | |
	YK 4.A6	BAD-1
Blood	1.2	1.1
L. Foot	0.4	0.5
R. Foot[a]	0.7	0.5
Liver	61.0	38.6
Lung	4.5	42.0
Spleen	5.7	4.0
Kidney	4.2	3.0
Thymus	0.0	0.0
LN	0.1	0.1

Note: 2×10^5 cells each of the cloned T cell lines YK4-A7 (cytotoxic *in vitro* for sarcoma YK.4) or BAD.1 (cytotoxic *in vitro* for cells bearing H-2-D)^d were labeled with ^{51}Cr, then injected intravenously into groups of 5 syngeneic C57BL/6 mice. 8×10^5 YK.4 tumor cells had been injected 4 days previously into the right footpad. Four hours after injection, the various organs were counted. The data are expressed as mean percent of whole body counts.
[a] YK.4 tumor present in footpad resulting from 8×10^5 tumor cells injected 4 days earlier.

can be said to recognize "the" TSTA. The degree to which these CTL clones kill *in vitro* or protect *in vivo* may be a function of the numbers of, or expression of, the ligand recognized by the CTL on the sarcoma cell surface.

Tumor Borne Antigens Recognized by B Cells

Definitive studies on the target antigens for *in vitro* and *in vitro* cytotoxicity by CTL directed against chemically induced sarcomas have been frustrated by the fact that they have not been defined serologically. With the single exception of

Table 32.5. Specificity of Killing by Established Anti-Tumor Cytotoxic T Cell Line.

Line of CTL tested	Incidence of syngeneic killing	
YK.4. Clone.A6	3/10	
EL.4 Clone.163	1/7	4/24
EL.4 Clone.129	0/7	
YK.7 Uncloned	2/4	
YK.5 Uncloned	3/4	7/12
YK.4 Uncloned	2/4	

Note: Summary of *in vitro* cytotoxicity tests on 3 cloned lines and 3 uncloned lines, in which at least one syngeneic tumor was used as a target in addition to that tumor which elicited the CTL. In general, the uncloned lines showed greater cross-killing than the same line after cloning. YK.4 and YK.7 tumor were killed equally *in vitro* by anti-YK.4 clone A6.

the Meth-A and CMS4 BALB/c fibrosarcomas (DeLeo et al., 1977), syngeneic antisera to chemically induced murine sarcomas have shown extensive cross-reactions when tested on apparently identical tumors possessing unique TSTA as determined by transplantation tests (Klein, 1980). Postulated sources of such cross-reacting surface structures on these tumors include fetal or embryonic antigens, differentiation structures, fetal bovine serum components in the case of cultured tumors, and more frequently, murine leukemia virus (MuLV) associated antigens. These are widely but unpredictably expressed on mouse tumor and normal tissues (Old and Stockert, 1977). Furthermore, the natural occurrence of antibodies against MuLV antigens in normal mouse serum as well as in supposedly specific antisera cause apparently anomalous serological reactions on tumor cells (Klein, 1980).

We have applied hybridoma methodology to this problem, using the tumor bearing mouse as the original source of specific anti-tumor B cells (Simrell and Klein, 1979). A series of sixteen monoclonal antibodies derived from C57BL/6 and BALB/c mice bearing syngeneic chemically induced fibrosarcomas have been characterized thus far, in terms of capacity to bind by radioimmunoassay, panels of tumor cells, normal cells, and ecotropic and xenotropic MuLV. By competitive binding, we have also assayed for MuLV on tumor cells using well-characterized anti-MuLV gp70 and p15(E) monoclonal antibodies (Lostrom et al., 1979).

Each hybridoma antibody we have examined shows either MuLV-associated or apparently MuLV-independent cross-reactivity between tumors. Figure 32.8 illustrates these findings. Five syngeneic monoclonal antibodies (L1, 4B1, C5, Q.30, and P4) were derived from tumor-immune mice and the other six (anti-gp70[a,b,c] and anti-p15(E)[a,b,c]) were produced against isolated and purified MuLV (Lostrom et al., 1979). The binding of each antibody to four C57BL/6 sarcomas (M3, PAK-17, PC11, PAK-1) and two BALB/c sarcomas (CS-1 and BH-2) is shown. The positive binding of anti-MuLV antibodies to tumors M3, PC11, and CS-1 identify these tumors as expressing gp70 and p15(E) antigens of ecotropic and/or xenotropic virus on their surfaces.

Two anti-tumor monoclonal antibodies (L1 and 4B1) react only with tumors expressing MuLV antigens. One of these, 4B1, is specific for a determinant identical with, or in close proximity to, the gp70[a] epitope of ecotropic MuLV (Klein and Lennox, manuscript in preparation). In contrast, C5, Q.30, and P4 react with tumor cells independent of their expression of the known MuLV antigens.

The data are consistent with two distinct classes of tumor associated antigens on chemically induced sarcomas. One class includes structures identical with or very closely related to the envelope antigens of MuLV, detected only on tumor cells expressing gp70 and p15(E). The second class is apparently independent of known MuLV gp70 and p15(E) antigens, and are currently of unknown significance.

Antigenic Phenotypes of Selected Tumors As Defined by Monoclonal Antibodies

Antigenic Determinant (original tumor on which detected)

Tumor	gp70[a, b, c]	p15(E)[a, b, c]	LI(M3)	4BI(MC6A)	C5(CS-I)	Q.30(CS-I)	P4(PAK-I)
M3	+	+	+	+	+	-	-
PAK-I7	-	-	-	-	+	+	+
PC II	+	+	+	+	+	-	+
PAK-I	-	-	-	-	+	+	⊕(+)
CS-I	+	+	+	+	△	⊕	+
BH-2	-	-	-	-	+	+	-

Figure 32.8. Binding reactions of monoclonal antibodies (L1, 4B1, C5, Q.30, and P4) raised against 4 tumors (M3, MC6A, CS-1, PAK-1) and against epitopes of murine leukemia virus (gp70[a,b,c] and p15(E)[a,b,c]). Binding was tested against a group of 4 C57BL/6 tumors (M3, PAK-17, PC-11, and PAK-1) and 2 BALb/c tumors (CS-1 and BH-2). Positive binding reactions are indicated by (+). Negative binding reactions are indicated by (−). Reactions enclosed by symbols (rectangle, triangle, circle, and hexagon) refer to independent antigenic determinants on these tumor cells as defined by the monoclonal antibodies. Reactions within rectangles depend on the expression of MuLV determinants on the tumor cells. Positive reactions by C5 antibody (triangle), Q.30 antibody (circle), and P4 antibody (hexagon) are independent of each other and also independent of MuLV expression by the tumor cells. (See text for details).

No epitope recognized by monoclonal antibodies developed thus far in our laboratory is unique to a single tumor. Failure to raise a tumor unique monoclonal antibody may just represent sampling luck, since a TSTA-like structure on a rat carcinoma recognized by a monoclonal antibody has been reported recently (Gunn et al., 1980). On the other hand, it is possible that anti-TSTA B cells are not elicited, and therefore no hybridomas are derived, because recognition of, and effector function against, the postulated TSTA is exclusively a T lymphocyte function. Another possibility is that the shared epitopes simply bind antibody more effectively than putative TSTA structures. The latter would therefore not be selected by current hybridoma methodology. Lastly, it is just possible that TSTA do not actually exist as currently conceived. The appearance of TSTA uniqueness may have other explanations, as discussed below.

Discussion and Conclusions

The concept of a unique TSTA has been attractive partly because it adequately explains *in vivo* tumor transplantation data, and partly because by implication it requires genetic polymorphism, and therefore may be related to expression of the major histocompatibility complex (MHC). In 1975 (Smith and Landy, 1975), we proposed an alternative explanation for TSTA which was not based upon the assumed existence of a unique antigenic ligand as a T cell target for tumor rejection. It depended upon the postulated occurrence of multiple strong and weak tumor associated antigens, including those of MuLV origin, arrayed on the individual sarcoma cell membrane. It was suggested that the apparent uniqueness among individual tumors simply represented the improbability that the pattern of specifically cytotoxic cell clones stimulated by one tumor would be duplicated by the recognition array elicited by another. Effective killing *in vitro* or *in vivo* of chemically induced sarcomas would, by this hypothesis, require "hits" directed against more than one ligand; only the concatenation of "hits" provided by the homologous pattern could provide the effect observed against transplanted tumor. Data presented here affirm that a sufficient variety of MuLV coded and other tumor associated antigens exist on different sarcomas to provide the multiple targets needed, and thereby lend some credence to this idea. However, we can now suggest an additional possibility which would not depend upon a unique TSTA ligand.

If the surface antigens on fibrosarcomas revealed by monoclonal antibodies here are effective targets for T cell killing, as are CTL raised against other MuLV strains, (Levy and LeClerc, 1977; Green et al., 1979) the cytotoxic effect should be restricted by the MHC. The requirement is that virus coded antigens are targets for killing by CTL only in the context of syngeneic MHC products. This factor introduces a major source of potential variability in CTL function and another possible explanation of TSTA.

H2K and H2D structures on MCA induced sarcomas show a highly variable expression in the cell surface membrane, ranging from near absence to twice the concentration expressed on normal cells (Chauvenet and Smith, 1978). Expression of H-2K and H-2D appeared to vary independently in many tumors. Thus the genetic context in which CTL against MuLV or related antigens must function cytolytically may be sufficiently altered in individual tumors, so that killing cannot occur, except in the context of the unique expression of the MHC which stimulated CTL development originally. Thus the shared MuLV coded structures would provide targets for recognition only in the disordered context of the H-2 complex in which it was elicited. Cross-protection toward common, shared virus antigens would not occur when the cell was presented in the context of a syngeneic, but differently disordered MHC. This hypothesis, in effect, also accounts for the observation that MuLV coded structures are shared by MCA induced tumors with respect to T and B cell recognition receptor repertoires, yet act as TSTA *in vivo*.

Either of these possible explanations for TSTA may be as wrong as the unique ligand hypothesis. Each suggests, however, fresh experimental approaches to this intriguing problem, and thus has at least heuristic merit.

References

Calderwood, M.B., Forbes, J.T., and Smith, R.T. (1977) Soluble tumor antigen-induced lymphocyte proliferation: effect of serum from normal and tumor-bearing mice. *Int. J. Cancer* 20:400.

Calderwood, M., Forbes, J., and Smith, R.T. (1980) Immune response to chemically induced tumors: correlation of responding cell class and *in vivo* protection against tumor growth. *Brit. J. Cancer*, in press.

Chauvenet, Ph.H. and Smith, R.T. (1978) Relationship of tumor specific transplantation antigens to the histocompatibility complex: dissociation of *in vitro* alloantigen expression and *in vivo* alloimmunity from tumor specific transplantation antgen strength. *Int. J. Cancer* 22:79.

Chauvenet, P.H., McArthur, C.P., and Smith, R.T. (1979) Demonstration *in vitro* of cytotoxic T cells with apparent specificity toward tumor specific transplantation antigens on chemically induced tumors. *J. Immunol.* 123:2575.

DeLeo, A.B., Shiku, H., Takahashi, T., John, M., and Old, L.J. (1977) Cell surface antigens of chemically induced sarcomas of the mouse. I. Murine leukemia virus-related antigens and alloantigens on cultured fibroblasts and sarcoma cells: description of a unique antigen on BALb/c meth A sarcoma. *J. Exp. Med.* 146:720.

Forbes, J.T., Nakao, Y., and Smith, R.T. (1975) Tumor specific immunity to chemically induced tumors: evidence for immunologic specificity and shared antigenicity in lymphocyte responses to soluble tumor antigens. *J. Exp. Med.* 141:1181.

Gillis, S. and Smith, K. (1977) Long-term culture of tumor specific cytotoxic T cells. *Nature* 268:154.

Green, W.R., Nowinski, R.C., and Henney, C.S. (1979) The generation and specificity of cytotoxic T cells raised against syngeneic tumor cells bearing AKR/gross murine leukemia virus antigens. *J. Exp. Med.* 150:51.

Gunn, B., Embelton, M.J., Middle, J.G., and Baldwin, R.W. (1980) Monoclonal antibody against a naturally occurring rat mammary carcinoma. *Int. J. Cancer* 26:325.

Klein, P.A. (1980) Problems with and approaches to specificity in the serological measurement of histocompatibility and tumor-associated antigens on tumor cell surfaces. *Transpl. Proc.* 12:16.

Levy, J.P. and Leclerc, J.C. (1977) The murine sarcoma virus induced tumor: exception or general model in tumor immunology? *Adv. Cancer Res.* 24:1.

Lostrom, M.E., Stone, M.R., Tam, M., Burnette, W.N., Pinter, A., and Nowinski, R.C. (1979) Monoclonal antibodies against murine leukemia viruses. Identification of six antigenic determinants on the p15(E) and gp70 envelope proteins. *Virology* 98:336.

Old, L.J. and Stockert, E. (1977) Immunogenetics of cell surface antigens of mouse leukemia. *Ann. Rev. Genetics* 17:127.

Old, L.J., Boyse, F.A., Clarke, D.A., and Carswell, F.A. (1962) Antigenic properties of chemically-induced tumors. *Ann. N.Y. Acad. Sci.* 101:80.

Prehn, R.T. and Main, J.M. (1957) Immunity to methylcholanthrene induced sarcomas. *J. Natl. Cancer Inst.* 18:769.

Simrell, C.A. and Klein, P.A. (1979) Antibody responses of tumor-bearing mice to their own tumors captured and perpetuated as hybridomas. *J. Immunol.* 123:2386.

Smith, R.T. and Landy, M. (Eds.) (1975) *Immunobiology and the Tumor-Host Relationship*. New York: Academic Press.

Published 1981 by Elsevier North Holland, Inc.
Saunders, Daniels, Serrou, Rosenfeld, and Denney, eds.
FUNDAMENTAL MECHANISMS IN HUMAN CANCER IMMUNOLOGY

CHAPTER 33

Do Natural Killer Cells Function Through Recognition of Glycoconjugates on Target Cell Membranes?[1]

Christopher S. Henney

Basic Immunology Program, Fred Hutchinson Cancer Research Center, 1124 Columbia Street, Seattle, Washington

Introduction

Natural killer (NK) cells, regardless of the species from which they are derived, are characterized by their ability to lyse a wide variety of cell types, most notably lymphomas and other tumor cell lines. Normal tissues, including fibroblasts, thymocytes, and a portion of bone marrow cells are also lysed, but, in general, normal cells are much less susceptible than tumor cells to NK cell-mediated lysis (Henney et al., 1978; Kiessling and Wigzell, 1979).

There are two principle hypotheses which could account for the unusually wide-range of target cells which are susceptible to NK cell attack. These are: (1) NK cell "specificities" could be clonally distributed. The broad spectrum of target cells lysed would then represent the sum of activity of individual NK cell clones, each of which would have a limited specificity. (2) Cells susceptible to the action of NK cells could share a common feature, which, for the sake of simplicity, one might define as a common target "antigen." (Alternatively, cells susceptible to NK cells might *lack* a surface feature which is displayed on insusceptible cells.)

The experiments presented here were designed to test these hypotheses. No evidence was found to support the concept that NK cell specificity was clonally distributed. On the other hand, several bodies of evidence suggest that NK cells "recognize" configurations of glycoconjugates, possibly glycolipids, on the target cell surface.

[1]This laboratory is supported by Grants A115383 and A115384 and CA24537 from the National Institutes of Health and by Grant IM-274 from the American Cancer Society.

Research Methods and Results

Three sets of related experiments were designed to seek evidence for the possibility that NK cells are clonally distributed. In the first, we asked whether NK cell populations could be adsorbed onto monolayers of susceptible cells, and whether such interactions removed NK reactivity against other susceptible target cells. In one experiment typical of this approach, murine NK cell populations (BCG-induced peritoneal exudate cells of C57BL/6 mice) were incubated (40 min, 37°) on a monolayer of susceptible L5178Y lymphoma cells. Cells non-adherent to the cell monolayer were harvested and their cytotoxic activity against a panel of susceptible target cells was assessed. Incubation on L5178Y cells largely removed cytotoxic activity, not only against this cell but also against Chang cells. Indeed, NK cell adsorption onto L5178Y cells removed cytotoxic activity against all NK susceptible target cells tested. In contrast, parallel adsorption of NK cell populations on NK-insusceptible cell monolayers (e.g., on normal DBA/2 spleen cells), did not remove NK reactivity (Durdik et al., 1980b).

Thus, experiments of this nature established: (a) that NK cells bind to monolayers of NK-susceptible, but not to monolayers of NK-insusceptible cells, and (b) that adsorption on susceptible cell monolayers removed NK reactivity not only to cells of the monolayer phenotype, but also against other NK-susceptible targets.

It proved technically difficult to deplete NK cells totally on cell monolayers, and furthermore, the non-adsorbed cell population was often contaminated with cells that detached from the monolayer. To overcome such difficulties, a different approach was employed which exploited the interaction of effector and target cells in suspension. Susceptible or insusceptible target cells were treated with dichlorotriazinyl amino fluorescein, and the resulting fluoresceinated cells were incubated with NK cell suspensions under conditions allowing target cell-effector cell complexes to form. The resulting mixture was fractionated into fluorescent and non-fluorescent populations using a fluorescence-activated cell sorter (Becton and Dickinson FACS II). The NK reactivity of the non-fluorescent population was then assessed, both against the target cell with which it had been incubated and against a series of other target cells comprising both susceptible and insusceptible phenotypes. It was argued that NK cell interaction with a fluorescent target cell would result in a cell-cell complex which would fractionate with the fluorescent compartment and thus that the non-fluorescent population would be selectively depleted of effector cells capable of binding to the target cell in question. Results of experiments of this type are shown in Table 33.1. As can be seen, incubation with susceptible target cells was associated with a decline in lytic reactivity against all the target cells used. In contrast, incubation with fluorescent but insusceptible target cells (EL4 and cl 27av) was not associated with a decline in NK reactivity (Table 33.1; see also Durdik et al., 1980b).

Table 33.1. Removal of NK Activity Following Binding to Fluoresceinated Target Cells.

NK cells incubated with fluoresceinated target	Phenotype of fluoresceinated cell	% reduction of lytic activity following binding as measured against:		
		Cl 27v	YAC-1	SL-3
L5178Y cl 27v	Susceptible	42	40	42
L5178Y cl 27av	Resistant	< 5	< 2	N.D.[a]
EL4	Resistant	< 2	N.D.[a]	0

Note: Ten million target cells/ml were chemically derivatized with fluorescein (5-10 µg/ml dichlorotriazinyl amino fluorescein di HCl at pH 9, 20°C for 30 min) and then washed three times. Equal numbers of fluorescent target cells and NK cells (BCG induced peritoneal exudates) were mixed, pelleted, and allowed to incubate at 37°C for 30 min and were then separated by fluorescence-activated cell sorter (FACS II) analysis. Criteria for separations were established from independent FACS II analysis of each population. Both low angle scatter and fluorescence parameters were utilized to separate the effector population from the "larger" fluorescent target cell population. After sorting, the non-fluorescent population was tested for its residual NK activity against ^{51}Cr-labeled targets at an E:T of 13:1. NK cells incubated without targets served as controls. The latter had been subjected to conditions identical to those of NK cells mixed with fluorescent targets. Contamination of the fluorescent-negative NK cell populations with fluorescent positive cells was less than 0.3%.
[a] N.D.: not determined.

Results compatible with these binding experiments were also obtained in "cold" target inhibition experiments, in which the lysis of ^{51}Cr-labeled susceptible cells was inhibited by the addition of unlabeled competitor cells. In the series of experiments shown in Table 33.2, one clone of L5178Y cells, cl 27v, which is particularly susceptible to NK cell-mediated attack, was used as the prototype ^{51}Cr-labeled target cell. The number of competitor cells required to inhibit lysis of cl 27v by 50% is reported in Table 33.2. As can be seen, NK susceptible target cells were all effective inhibitors of the lysis of cl 27v. Indeed, the number of such cells required for 50% inhibition was not significantly different from the number of homologous cells required. Cells susceptible to the action of NK cells included: cl 27v; YAC-I, a Moloney virus-induced lymphoma of A/Sn mice; BALB/c 3T3 (clone A31); NSI/I-Ag-4-I of the BALB/c myeloma cell line MOPC 21; Chang cells; a human derived liver cell line; and clone K234 of 3T3 Ki MSV, which were cells from the above 3T3 line infected by a non-productive Kirsten strain of murine sarcoma virus.

In contrast, a series of NK insusceptible target cells were very poor inhibitors. These included: cl 27av, an *in vitro* adapted NK resistant subline of L5178Y lymphoma and three ascites tumors, P815-X2, a methylcholanthrene-induced mastocytoma of DBA/2 mice and EL4, a chemically induced thymoma of C57BL/6 mice. A clear positive correlation was observed between the susceptibility of the cells to NK attack (recorded in Table 33.2 in relation to the susceptibility of cl 27v cells) and their ability to inhibit the NK cell-mediated lysis of cl 27v.

Collectively, these results are incompatible with the concept that distinct subpopulations of NK cells lyse different target cells. We thus found no

Table 33.2. Inhibition Studies Demonstrating Cross-Reactivity of NK Susceptible Target Cells.

Target cell phenotype	Target cell	Relative susceptibility to NK cell lysis	No. cells ($\times 10^{-4}$) required to inhibit lysis of cl 27v by 50%
	cl 27v	100	8
	YAC-1	170	10
NK	3T3	110	9
susceptible	NSI	100	8
	Chang	90	12
	K234	50	9
NK	cl 27av	30	25
insusceptible	P815	20	35
	cl 27a	20	50
	EL4	10	> 100
	Normal spleen cells	0	>> 100

Note: Values shown were compiled from several experiments in which cells were tested for their ability to be directly lysed by BCG-induced NK cells (Wolfe et al., 1977). Relative susceptibility is normalized to that of cl 27v, which is arbitrarily taken as 100. Additionally, 10^4 ^{51}Cr-labeled cl 27v cells were lysed by BCG-induced C57BL/6 NK cells in the presence of increasing numbers of unlabeled competitor cells. The number of such cells required to inhibit lysis by 50% was enumerated. Lysis of cl 27v cells during a 3-hr interval in the absence of competitor cells was 20-40% in various experiments.

evidence that NK "specificities" were clonally distributed. Rather, our findings were consistent with the proposition that susceptibility of target cells to NK attack reflected a shared membrane characteristic. Using yet another approach, that of growing various NK cell populations, and then comparing their specificities, Dennert (1980) has reached the same conclusion.

In light of these observations, we have turned to the proposal that cells susceptible to the action of NK cells might share common surface feature(s). In looking for a potential molecular basis for NK cell-mediated lysis of target cells, one approach we have used has been to seek variants from a given tumor which differ in their susceptibility to NK cell-mediated lysis (Durdik et al., 1980a).

To this end, L5178Y lymphoma cells were cloned by limiting dilutions in RPMI 1640 containing 10% fetal calf serum. Samples from each of the resulting clones, approximately 30 in number, were internally labeled by incubation (30 min, 37°C) with 100 μC sodium ^{51}Chromate (Amersham-Searle, Chicago, Illinois) and tested for sensitivity to BCG-induced NK activity in a 4-hr ^{51}Cr release assay. As a result of this initial screening, one clone, L5178Y clone 27 (cl 27v), was selected as a population particularly susceptible to NK cell-mediated lysis. This cell population has been cultured for a period exceeding 4 years and has retained its susceptibility phenotype throughout this period.

After *in vitro* cloning, a portion of cl 27v cells was transferred to syngeneic (DBA/2) mice and passaged as ascites. In contrast to the *in vitro* line, the ascites cells were very poorly lysed by NK cells. The ascites cells remained as susceptible to anti-H-2^d serum and complement and to alloimmune cytotoxic T cells (C57BL/6 anti-P815 mastocytoma) as were the *in vitro* population from which they were derived. Thus, the ascites cells had not simply become resistant to cell-mediated cytolysis. During the ten months of *in vivo* passage, the ascites cells were adapted *in vitro* and were termed cl 27av (see Table 33.2). These cells have now been cultured for almost two years and have maintained the insusceptible phenotype of the ascites. Cl 27av cells were compared to cl 27v cells by a number of criteria. Serological analysis using anti-H-2^d antisera in the presence of rabbit complement revealed minimal differences. The following antisera were employed in these characterizations: B10 anti-B10.D2; (B10×A)FI anti-B10.D2 (anti-H-2K^d) obtained as NIH serum (D-31(2); (B10.AKM×129)FI anti-B10.A (anti-H-2D^d) obtained as NIH serum D-4(2). With each serum, using dilutions between 1:50 and 1:6400, less than a two-fold difference in surface alloantigen display on the two cell lines was demonstrable. Indeed, quantitative adsorption studies using the same sera revealed no differences between cl 27v and cl 27av cells.

In keeping with the serological analysis, cl 27v and cl 27av were equivalently susceptible to alloimmune cytotoxic T cells and were indistinguishable in their ability to inhibit the T cell-mediated lysis of cl 27v cells (Figure 33.1A). Despite identity as targets for cytotoxic T cells, there was a large and striking difference in the abilities of the two cell lines to serve as targets for NK cell-mediated lysis. This distinction was true not only in direct cytotoxic assays, employing ^{51}Cr-labeled targets, but was also observed when unlabeled cells were used to inhibit the NK cell-mediated lysis of cl 27v cells (Figure 33.1B). As can be seen, cl 27v, the homologous cell type, effectively inhibited NK cell-mediated lysis, whereas cl 27av failed to inhibit lysis at any cell concentration tested. This finding suggests that only the susceptible variant binds to NK cells. Two other points are worthy of emphasis. First, cl 27av has remained insusceptible to NK cells throughout prolonged culture, in contrast to a previous report (Becker et al., 1978) that YAC cells grown as ascites were resistant to NK attack, but reverted to an NK susceptible phenotype when adapted *in vitro*. Second, cl 27 ascites cells have been recloned without finding susceptible cells within the population, which indicates that this population was homogeneous with respect to NK insusceptibility (Durdik et al., 1980a).

The two *in vitro* cell lines derived from L5178Y lymphoma behaved as variants only with respect to their susceptibility to the action of NK cells. The data supporting this conclusion are summarized in Table 33.3. Furthermore, NK cell populations from a variety of sources were all capable of distinguishing between cl 27v and cl 27av. In tests of direct lysis, cl 27v was killed by normal (and BCG-induced) NK cells from CBA spleen, by similar populations of a wide variety of other mouse strains, and by NK cell populations from human and non-human primate (pigtail macaques) peripheral blood. Cl 27av cells were resistant to all of these effector populations (Durdik et al., 1980a).

470

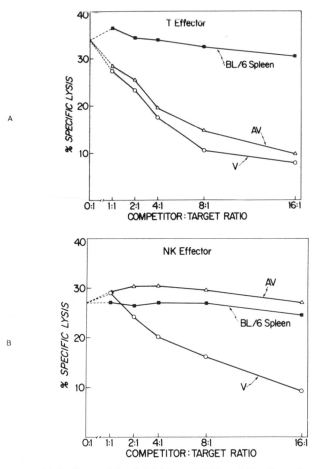

Figure 33.1. Competitive inhibition of NK and T cell-mediated lysis. T (panel A) and NK cell-mediated lysis (panel B) of ^{51}Cr-labeled L5178Y cl 27v cells was followed in the presence of various numbers of unlabeled homologous cells (V, ○), in the presence of cl 27av (AV, △), or in the presence of normal C57BL/6 spleen cells (■). NK cells were obtained from peritoneal exudates of C57BL/6 mice injected with 10^8 BCG, i.p., 5 days previously. Cytotoxic T cells were generated by restimulating for a period of 2 days *in vitro* with x-irradiated P815 cells (responder to stimulator ratio, 50:1) the spleen cells of C57BL/6 mice that had received 10^7 P815 cells 19 days earlier. The effector to ^{51}Cr-target cell ratio was kept constant at 40:1 for NK cells and 10:1 for alloimmune T cells.

SOURCE: *Durdik et al., 1980a with permission of the Williams and Wilkens Co., Ltd.*

Collectively, these findings are most compatible with the proposition that cl 27av cells lack a membrane macromolecule present on cl 27v cells which dictates, or is associated with, susceptibility to NK cells. These observations suggested to us that the variants of L5178Y might serve as useful tools in a

Table 33.3. Characterization of Lymphoma Cell Lines Varying in Susceptibility to NK Cells.

Characteristic	Cell lines derived from L5178Y :	
	cl 27V	cl 27av
Susceptibility to cell-mediated lysis by:		
NK cells	+++	±
"Activated" macrophages	++	++
Cytotoxic T cells	+++	+++
K cells (with anti-H-2^d)	+++	+++
Susceptibility to humoral lysis by:		
Anti-H-2^d + C	++++	+++
Anti-H-2K^d + C	+++	++
Anti-H-2D^d + C	+++	+++
Anti-asialo GM$_2$ + C	+++	–

Note: Both cl 27v and cl 27av cell lines were derived from L5178Y lymphoma. The NK susceptible line cl 27v was derived by cloning at low cell density followed by screening for susceptibility. The cl 27av cell line was derived from cl 27v by ascites passage in DBA/2 mice followed by readaptation *in vitro* (see Durdik et al., 1980a).

search for a molecular basis for NK susceptibility. In collaboration with Drs. W. Young, D. Urdal, and S-I. Hakomori of the Biochemical Oncology Program at the Fred Hutchinson Cancer Research Center, we have begun an extensive and systematic biochemical analysis of membrane extracts from the cl 27v and cl 27av cells (Young et al., 1981).

Following a number of observations that implicated glycoconjugates as cell surface receptor molecules (Fishman and Brady, 1976; Hakomori and Young, 1978), we examined the glycolipids of cl 27 v and cl 27 av cells. Total neutral glycolipid fractions are shown in Figure 33.2. Clone 27 av cells displayed a simple neutral glycolipid and ganglioside pattern with ceramide monohexoside (CMH), ceramide dihexoside (CDH), and hematoside (GM$_3$) as the predominant glycolipids. On the other hand, cl 27v, the NK susceptible cells, showed a strikingly different glycolipid profile. The neutral glycolipid fraction, in addition to CMH and CDH, displayed three prominent glycolipid bands, none of which were detectable on the NK insusceptible variant (Fig. 33.2). Glycolipid chemical analysis indicated that all three bands contained the asialo GM$_2$ carbohydrate moiety and differed only in their lipid portions. Asialo GM$_2$ was not chemically detected on the insusceptible cell line. To demonstrate that asialo GM$_2$ was on the surface of clone 27v cells and available for interaction with specific antibody, the lymphoma cell variants were treated with anti-asialo GM$_2$ followed by a fluoresceinated goat anti-rabbit IgG antiserum. Cell sorter analysis indicated that the majority of the clone 27v cells stained brightly with the antiserum specific for asialo GM$_2$, whereas the clone 27av cells were negative. Furthermore, clone 27av cells were completely resistant to lysis by BALB/c monoclonal IgM anti-asialo GM$_2$ antibody in the presence of complement, whereas cl 27v cells were effectively lysed (Table 33.3; see also Young et al., 1981).

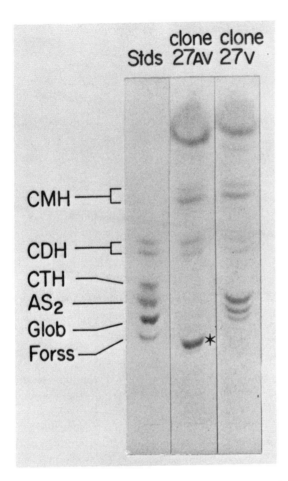

Figure 33.2. Thin-layer chromatography patterns of the neutral glycolipids isolated from L5178Y clone 27av and clone 27v cells. Cells were extracted with chloroform-methanol $(2:1, v/v)$ followed by chloroform-methanol $(1:2, v/v)$. Gangliosides were partitioned by Folch extraction. An equivalent number of cells were chromatographed on Silica gel G plates in the solvent chloroform:methanol:water $(60:35:8, v/v)$. Glycolipids were visualized with orcinol. The star indicates the position of GM_3 ganglioside which remained in the lower phase of the Folch partition. CMH, CDH, and CTH: ceramide monohexoside, dihexoside, and trihexoside respectively; AS2: asialo GM_2; Glob: globoside; and Forss: Forssman antigen.

SOURCE: *Young et al., 1981 with permission of the Williams and Wilkens Co., Ltd.*

There was then, a positive correlation between the display of asialo GM_2 on the two L5178Y variants and their susceptibility to NK attack. Because of this correlation, we directly addressed the possibility that asialo GM_2 might be the substrate, or "trigger," for NK cell-mediated lysis of L5178Y cells. This hypothesis was tested by attempting to inhibit NK cell-mediated lysis with anti-asialo GM_2. Neither BALB/c IgM monoclonal anti-asialo GM_2 antibody, nor an affinity purified rabbit anti-asialo GM_2 antibody preparation could block the NK cell-mediated attack of the clone 27v target cells. This was true of antibody concentrations up to $1:10$, a large antibody excess, considering that the cytotoxic titer of the antisera used was $1:10^6$ to $1:10^7$. Similarly, antiserum directed against MHC products on clone 27v cells also failed to inhibit the NK cell-mediated lysis of these cells, although the same antiserum readily inhibited the T cell-mediated lysis of these cells under the same conditions (Young et al., 1981). Thus, although there was a marked concordance between asialo GM_2 display and susceptibility to NK cells, we could find no direct evidence for a causal relationship between display and susceptibility.

Discussion

The studies presented here do not support the concept that the "specificity" of NK cells is clonally distributed. Indeed, it is clear from the data presented in Tables 33.1 and 33.2, that NK susceptible target cells effectively inhibit the lysis of other susceptible cells and that binding of NK cells to one susceptible target is associated with the removal of activity against all other target cells tested. These observations are, in general, concordant with results obtained from similar experiments by others (Kiessling and Wigzell, 1979; Sendo et al., 1975), although some investigators, using "cold" target inhibition, have interpreted their results to support the hypothesis of restricted specificity (Nunn and Herberman, 1979).

Our findings, and those of several others, are most compatible with the proposition that susceptibility of target cells to NK attack may reflect a shared membrane characteristic which, for want of a better term, we might call an "antigen." (The structure shared would not necessarily have to be antigenic.) Others have argued, from essentially the same premises, that there are several (but a limited number of) subsets of NK cells, each of which is directed against a different "specificity" (Nunn and Herberman, 1979). It is interesting to note that a recent study (Dennert, 1980) in which NK cells were grown as "miniclones," also failed to reveal evidence for a clonal expression of specificity.

It was initially proposed that NK cell activity was directed against either M-MuLV (Kiessling et al., 1975) or some type of endogenous MuLV (Sendo et al., 1975; Zarling et al., 1975), but later studies showed that susceptibility or resistance to NK cells did not correlate with the expression of either serologically defined MuLV antigens or with group-specific antigenic determinants of MuLV (Becker et al., 1976).

In a recent study using an alternative approach, Roder et al. (1979) claim to have isolated target cell structures from NK susceptible cell lines which interact with NK cells. The approach was, however, indirect: detergent-solubilized cell surface proteins of YAC-I lymphoma cells were assessed for their ability to inhibit the binding of mouse spleen cells to YAC targets (a binding assay which the same authors had found to correlate with NK cell activity). Roder et al. found that NK susceptible target cells (but not NK insusceptible targets) possessed glycoproteins of 130,000, 160,000, and 240,000 molecular weight which were capable of preventing NK cell binding to susceptible target cells. No mention was made of the ability of these proteins to inhibit NK mediated lysis, and it remains unclear as to whether the cells measured in the binding assay, while they correlate with the cytotoxic activity of the population, are indeed the killer cells. Nevertheless, the findings are intriguing. They are among the most convincing data to date in support of the hypothesis that there are common cell surface macromolecules on NK susceptible target cells, and are the first to indicate that such common features might be membrane-associated glycoconjugates.

Our data presented above, are, in their broadest sense, compatible with Roder's observations, for we have observed a marked difference in the glycolipid profiles of two cell lines which are variants with respect to their susceptibility to the lytic action of NK cells. Thus, among approximately 20 clones of L5178Y which we have studied, only those bearing asialo GM_2 were susceptible to NK cell-mediated lysis (Young et al., 1981). It should be added however that we have no direct evidence that causally links asialo GM_2 display with NK cell susceptibility and we have thus far been unable to inhibit lysis with anti-asialo GM_2 antibodies. Failure to causally link display with susceptibility should, however, be interpreted in the context of previous studies of this type. Firstly, since no antibody against a target cell structure has yet been shown to inhibit NK cell-mediated lysis, the feasibility of this approach remains to be established. Secondly, it is conceivable that the antibodies employed for the inhibition studies were directed against different structural elements of the glycolipid than those against which NK cells might be directed.

Finally, one other body of evidence suggests that glycoconjugate display may be related to the susceptibility of target tissues to natural cell-mediated cytotoxicity. This is the observation of Stutman et al. (1980) that NK cell mediated lysis is inhibited by a variety of simple sugars, most notably mannose. Two aspects of these observations are noteworthy: (a) inhibition with mannose was observed over a concentration range of 10 mM to 100 mM, and thus could not be attributed to toxic effects and (b) the activity of cytotoxic T cells towards the same target cells was not affected by the presence of mannose, so that the inhibitory effects were selective for NK cell-mediated lysis.

In sum, three pieces of evidence collectively suggest that recognition of cell surface carbohydrates is a salient feature of the action of NK cells: (a) the ability of glycoproteins found exclusively on NK susceptible target cells to inhibit NK cell binding, (b) inhibition of NK mediated lysis by simple sugars, and (c) the display of aberrant glycolipid forms on at least some NK susceptible target cells. It must be acknowledged, however, that to date the evidence is circumstantial, and more definitive evidence causally linking carbohydrate display with NK cell susceptibility is still awaited.

ACKNOWLEDGMENTS
I thank the following colleagues who contributed significantly to various aspects of the work presented here: Barbara North Beck, Jeannine M. Durdik, Sen-itiroh Hakomori, David L. Urdal, and William W. Young.

References

Becker, S., Fenyo, E.M., and Klein, E. (1976) *Eur. J. Immunol.* 6:882–885.

Becker, S., Keissling, R., Lee, N., and Klein, G. (1978) *J. Natl. Cancer Inst.* 61:1495–1498.

Dennert, G. (1980) *Nature* 287:47–49.

Durdik, J.M., Beck, B.N., Clark, E.A., and Henney, C.S. (1980a) *J. Immunol.* 125:683–688.

Durdik, J.M., Beck, B.N., and Henney, C.S. (1980b) In *Natural Cell-Mediated Immunity Against Tumors.* Herberman, R.B. (ed.), New York: Academic Press, Inc., pp. 805–817.

Fishman, P.H. and Brady, O. (1976) *Science* 194:906–915.

Hakomori, S. and Young, W.W. (1978) *Scand. J. Immunol.* 6:97–117.

Henney, C.S., Tracey, D., Durdik, J.M., and Klimpel, G. (1978) *Am. J. Path.* 93:459–468.

Kiessling, R. and Wigzell, H. (1979) *Immunol. Rev.* 44:165–208.

Kiessling, R., Klein, E., and Wigzell, H. (1975) *Eur. J. Immunol.* 5:112–117.

Nunn, M.E. and Herberman, R.B. (1979) *J. Natl. Cancer Inst.* 62:765–771.

Roder, J.D., Rosen, A., Fenyo, E.M., and Troy, F.A. (1979) *Proc. Natl. Acad. Sci.* 76:1405–1409.

Sendo, F., Aoki, T., Boyse, E.A., and Buafo, C.K. (1975) *J. Natl. Cancer Inst.* 55:603–609.

Stutman, O., Dien, P., Wisun, R.E., and Lattime, E.C. (1980) *Proc. Natl. Acad. Sci.* 77:2895–2898.

Wolfe, S.A., Tracey, D.E., and Henney C.S. (1977) *J. Immunol.* 119:1152–1158.

Young, W.W., Durdik, J.M., Urdal, D., Hakomori, S., and Henney, C.S. (1981) *J. Immunol.,* in press.

Zarling, J.M., Nowinski, R.C., and Bach, F.H. (1975) *Proc. Natl. Acad. Sci.* 72:2780–2784.

CHAPTER 34

In Situ, In Vitro, and Systemic Regulation of NK Cytotoxicity[1]

Sidney H. Golub, Ph.D.

Department of Surgery, Division of Oncology, UCLA School of Medicine, Los Angeles, CA 90024

Introduction

Considerable interest recently has focused on natural killer (NK) cells. NK cells have been implicated in natural resistance to tumors, resistance to viral infections, resistance to bone marrow transplants, regulation and maturation of lymphocytes, and resistance to transplanted tumors. However, the actual contribution of NK cells to host resistance against established and growing tumors is not clear. NK activity is apparently depressed in patients with large tumor burdens (Pross and Baines, 1976; Takasugi et al., 1977), and it may well be much more than coincidental that two to the most extensively studied and interesting modes of immunotherapy for cancer, BCG and interferon (IFN), are both associated with augmentation of NK activity. Thus, the observations that NK is apparently depressed in patients with progressively growing tumors and can be augmented by agents known to have both anti-tumor effects and immune modulating effects infer a role for NK cells in resistance to further spread and proliferation of tumor cells. However, direct proof that NK cells can contribute to restriction of clinically apparent tumors is difficult to obtain.

Our studies have focused on possible regulatory mechanisms in NK cytotoxicity. A number of systems have been reported which indicate cellular or humoral mechanisms for regulation of NK cytotoxicity. For example, interferon has been shown to increase NK activity of mouse cells (Djeu et al., 1978a), and this increase is apparently dependent upon the presence of macrophages (Djeu et al., 1978b). Similarly, intraperitoneal administration of

[1] These studies were supported in part by USPHS Grant CA 17013.

BCG in mice results in elevated NK activity of peritoneal exudate cells (Wolfe et al., 1977), and this augmentation of NK activity is apparently dependent upon a macrophage, as administration of silica to mice prevents BCG augmentation of NK (Tracey, 1979). There is limited evidence for the involvement of accessory cells in the development of human NK cytotoxicity, although one *in vitro* model has suggested a T cell control of the development of NK-like cytotoxicity in culture (Ortaldo et al., 1979). Conversely, there is some evidence that cells are able to assert suppressive effects on NK cells. Spleen cells from *Corynebacterium parvum* treated or newborn mice can suppress NK function (Savary and Lotzova, 1978), as can prostaglandin secreting macrophages (Droller et al., 1978). There is also evidence for the existence of suppressors of anti-EL4 NK effectors, but not anti-YAC-1 NK cells, in 89Sr treated mice (Kumar et al., 1979). These findings suggest the presence of regulatory mechanisms which distinguish between heterogeneous NK cells. Thus, a number of model systems have pointed to both positive and negative regulation by non-NK cells of NK cytotoxicity.

We studied the significance of NK activity in the human cancer patient from three approaches. The questions we have addressed are: (a) What are the cellular regulatory events involved in augmentation or suppression of NK activity in patients bring treated with IFN or BCG? Is NK function regulated by interactions with other cell types? (b) What factors regulate NK function at the site of human tumors? Can such factors be manipulated by induction of an inflammatory response at the tumor site with BCG? (c) What are the regulatory events and what lineage of cells is involved in generating NK or NK-like cytotoxicity *in vitro*? We feel that these three approaches may provide us with a broad view of the biological significance of NK activity in the patient with malignant disease.

This report will attempt to provide an overview of these three lines of investigation. I am greatly indebted to my colleagues within the Division of Surgical Oncology, UCLA School of Medicine, for their contributions to these studies. The *in vivo* studies of the effects of IFN and BCG have been assisted by the efforts of Martyn Burk, M.D., Ph.D., and James Goodnight, M.D., Ph.D., in providing clinical information and material. The tumor binding cell data was generated by Paula D'Amore, a graduate student in this laboratory, and the cytotoxicity data and rosette results are the product of the hard work of Dean Hara. The *in situ* studies were initiated upon the suggestion of E. Carmack Holmes, M.D. who has continued to provide excellent clinical collaboration. This work was furthered by the efforts of Richard Edelstein, M.D. and Masayuki Niitsuma, M.D., visiting scientists from France and Japan respectively, with the fine technical assistance of Veronica Routt. I also extend my thanks to Edythe Garvey, R.N., Josephine Shiplacoff, R.N., Jane Stein, R.N., and Robin Bowker, M.T., who have been extremely helpful in providing the clinical material in a remarkably systematic fashion. Two graduate students, Janet Seeley, Ph.D. and Marc Golightly, Ph.D., and a postdoctoral fellow, John Zielske, M.D., contributed greatly to the *in vitro* studies, which benefited from the superb technical assistance of Marcia Rainey. I am indebted to Fred Dorey, Ph.D. and Edward Korn, Ph.D. for their assistance in the biostatistical analysis of the data. Finally, I wish to thank all my colleagues in the UCLA Division of Surgical Oncology, and particularly Donald L. Morton, M.D., Chief of the Division, for their support, advice, and cooperation.

Materials and Methods

Patients

We have analyzed three clinical studies in order to investigate the *in vivo* cells: We have evaluated peripheral blood lymphocytes (PBL) of melanoma patients treated with human leukocyte interferon (IFN-α), PBL from melanoma patients treated with BCG, and tumor infiltrating lymphocytes of lung tumors injected with BCG compared with uninjected tumors.

The UCLA Division of Surgical Oncology is participating in an American Cancer Society sponsored multiinstitutional trial of human leukocyte interferon for the treatment of metastatic malignant melanoma. The patients treated have metastatic disease involving metastases to the subcutaneous tissues and/or lungs. The patients receive daily doses of IFN of 1×10^6 units, 3×10^6 units, or 9×10^6 units for 42 days. This preliminary report includes the evaluation of the first 11 patients treated. We have assessed NK activity against K562 and cell surface markers at daily intervals for the first two days before administration of IFN, for the three days following first administration, and weekly thereafter.

The second study involves the treatment of melanoma patients with either intravenous BCG or intralesional BCG. We have only evaluated three such patients thus far. Two patients with disseminated melanoma received intravenous BCG (1×10^7 organisms of Glaxo strain BCG per treatment) and one patient received 1×10^7 Glaxo strain organisms directly injected into a skin metastasis.

We have also examined NK activity in the tumor infiltrating lymphocytes (TIL) from 20 lung tumors, including both primary lung tumors and metastatic tumors of other sites, and four BCG injected lung tumors. The lung tumors were injected with BCG by percutaneous injection under fluoroscopic control as described previously by Holmes et al. (1979). A larger series of patients has been examined for TIL surface markers and other functional TIL activities. TIL and PBL were obtained from the same patients two weeks following initial BCG injection of the tumor at the time of the surgical resection.

In Vitro Assays

All *in vitro* assays have been previously reported and will only be briefly described here. PBL's were prepared by the standard Ficoll-Hypaque gradient technique. Preparation, cryopreservation, and recovery of cryopreserved cells has been previously described (Golub et al., 1975). T cells were identified by E-rosette formation, Fcγ receptor cells by a rosette formation using ox erythrocytes coated with rabbit IgG, and B cells by EAC rosette formation using sheep erythrocytes, rabbit IgM antibodies, and DBA/2 mouse complement (Golightly and Golub, 1980). NK cytotoxicity tests were performed by standard 4-hr ^{51}Cr release mitrocytotoxicity assay against K562 myeloid leukemia targets. Cold target competition experiments were performed using an assay system previously described (Seeley and Golub, 1978; Seeley et al., 1979). The proportion of target binding cells was determined using the conjugate forming assay of Targan and Dorey (1980). We thank Dr. Targan for his help in establishing this assay in our laboratory. The mixed lymphocyte culture cell-mediated lympholysis (MLC-CML) assay was also performed entirely in microtests, as previously described (Callery et al., 1980). Cell separation procedures employed included E-rosette and nylon fiber column filteration for T cells, EAγ monolayer depletion for removal of Fcγ receptor cells, and enrichment for Fcμ receptor cells by EAμ rosette formation (Golub et al., 1979). The TIL's were prepared by mechanical disaggregation of the tumor. Surgical specimens were first freed of normal tissue and necrotic tissue and then forced through a stainless steel mesh. The resulting single cell suspensions were centrifuged on a standard Ficoll-Hypaque gradient. The cells in the interphase, consisting of lymphocytes, monocytes, and some viable tumor cells, had greater than 90% viability with approximately 20% tumor cell contamination. Subsequently, we have found that the residual tumor cells can be readily removed by filtration through 5 micron or 10 micron nylon monofilament fiber mesh (Niitsuma et al., submitted), although this technique was not employed for the preparations reported here.

Results and Discussion

In Vivo Activation of NK by IFN

Our preliminary results from the analysis of patients receiving human leukocyte IFN have clearly indicated that the systemic administration of this agent results in a consistent increase in NK activity. Thus far, we have evaluated 11 patients who have completed all 42 days of treatment. We have also evaluated 4 healthy control donors, who did not receive IFN, according to the same schedule. The IFN treated patients show a striking, although transient, increase in NK activity. Nine of the eleven patients showed a marked increase in NK activity within the first week of treatment and the remaining two patients started at very high levels of NK cytotoxicity. The most typical pattern is shown in Figure 34.1. This patient showed a marked rise in NK activity at day 7 of treatment, with a subsequent decline to pretreatment levels of activity. The increase at day 7 of treatment was found for this patient group at all effector: target (E:T) ratios. The difference at day 7 compared to day 0 is significant at

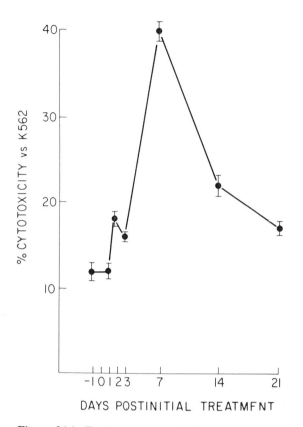

Figure 34.1. Typical pattern of NK cytotoxicity to lymphocytes from an interferon treated patient. Cytotoxicity at E:T of 12.5:1 vs K562 targets by peripheral blood lymphocytes of IFN patient #2. Vertical bars indicate SEM.

$p = <.01$ at E:T ratios of 12.5:1 and 50:1 and at $p = <.025$ at E:T ratios of 25:1 and 100:1, as analyzed by the paired t-test. Since all four doses appear to provide similar time curves, further analysis of the data concentrated on the mean cytotoxicity of the four E:T ratios. Figure 34.2 shows the change in mean cytotoxicity with time for the 11 IFN treated patients and the four control donors. The patients clearly show an increase in cytotoxicity starting at day 2 of treatment and peaking at day 7. The day 7 increase is statistically significant for the mean at $p = <.01$, and this is the only time point that shows a significant rise in NK activity. The normal controls never showed any significant elevation in cytotoxic activity.

Several other time points deserve mention. There is a noticeable decline in activity among the IFN treated patients at day 1 of treatment. Although this decline may be statistically significant ($p = <.10$ for the mean: $p = <.05$ at 12.5:1), it is of doubtful biologic significance, as the healthy control donors

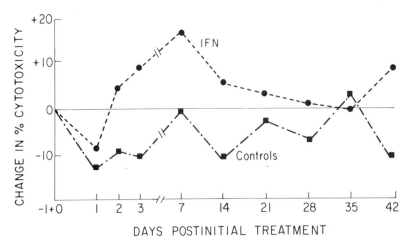

Figure 34.2. Change in mean NK with time. Vertical axis: Change in cytotoxicity =
(mean of four E : T ratios on day of test) − (mean of four E : T ratios of average of day
− 1 and day 0). Horizontal axis: Days following initial IFN treatment. Mean of 11 IFN
treated melanoma patients (●---●) and 4 healthy controls (■---■) are shown.

showed a similar significant decline in day 1 (see Figure 34.2). It seems
probable that this decline is an artifact due to repeated venipuncture of the
same individual. If so, the increases among the IFN patients at day 2 and day
3 are likely to be underestimated. Einhorn et al. (1978) and Huddlestone et al.
(1979) did note more rapid increases in NK activity among their IFN treated
patients than we observed in ours. Differences in dose or purity of IFN used or
type of patient treated probably account for this difference. There is also a
hint of some increase at day 42 and later that may indicate a rebound from
the decline seen after the first week of elevated NK activity. Additional
sampling in this post-treatment period is currently underway to determine if
there is a significant and consistent increase in NK activity once the patient
has completed IFN therapy.

The characteristics of the effector cells stimulated *in vivo* by IFN have been
examined in preliminary experiments. All cytotoxicity, both from the periods
of increased activity and from post-treatment periods, can be abrogated by the
passage of the cells over EAγ monolayers. This indicates that the effectors
appear to be Fcγ receptor bearing cells. Further analysis of the cell surface
markers of the effectors is necessary, but preliminary data do not seem to
indicate any major change during the course of the study in the phenotype of
the cells cytotoxic to K562 targets. We have not found any notable changes in
the proportion of Fcγ receptor cells, T cells, or B cells in the patients treated
with IFN. The results for the first 11 patients show a remarkably stable pattern
for all markers. Thus, there does not appear to be a notable shift in the
proportion of the various lymphocyte populations measured by the relatively
broad assays.

We have examined the number of target binding cells in several patients during the first week of IFN treatment. These results are shown in Figure 34.3. Our preliminary results indicate a notable increase in the proportion of target binding cells shortly after initiation of IFN treatment. Thus, the increased cytotoxicity appears to be associated with a proportion of cells able to bind to targets although we cannot rule out greater cytotoxicity per effector. These target binding cell results contrast with recent reports of increased killing, without increased binding, of human PBL's treated *in vitro* with IFN (Targan and Dorey, 1980). It appears that *in vivo* treatment with IFN affects a different, or additional, stage in the development of mature NK cells than *in vitro* treatment. *In vitro* IFN appears to promote cytotoxicity by directly affecting Fcγ + lymphocytes (Zarling et al., 1979) that are already capable of binding targets (Targan and Dorey, 1980), while *in vivo*, IFN may involve the development of non-binding cells into binding cells.

In summary, treatment of melanoma patients with IFN results in a significant, but transient, increase in cytotoxicity to K562 targets. This increase appears to be associated with an increase in conjugate forming cells, but not with an increase in the proportion of Fcγ receptor cells or in E-rosette or EAC-rosette forming cells. The cytotoxicity generated by *in vivo* treatment by

Figure 34.3. Target binding cells in IFN treated patients. Vertical axis: % of PBL's forming conjugates with K562. Horizontal axis: Days of IFN treatment *in vivo*. Three individual patients are shown with three different symbols. Numbers indicate patient entry number into the study.

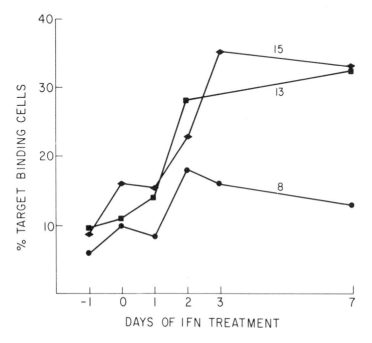

484

IFN peaks approximately one week after initiation of treatment, although there is some evidence for an increase in earlier periods. Following peak cytotoxicity, the activity declines to pretreatment levels, and remains relatively stable throughout the course of the 42 days of treatment.

NK Activity in Patients Treated with BCG

BCG has been shown to augment NK cytotoxicity in mice (Wolfe et al., 1977), in healthy humans (Thatcher and Crowther, 1978), and melanoma patients (Thatcher et al., 1979). In our preliminary results, we have also observed an augmentation of NK activity against K562 target cells in melanoma patients treated with BCG. Thus far, we have evaluated two patients who received intravenous BCG in an experimental protocol for the treatment of disseminated melanoma and an additional patient who received intralesional BCG for a skin metastasis. In all three, NK activity increased following BCG administration. In addition to K562 targets, we have begun to evaluate additional targets for NK susceptibility.

Cytotoxicity was assessed against the NK susceptible K562 cell and against UCLA-SO-M14 cells established from a patient with malignant melanoma. This cell line, henceforth referred to as M14, expresses an oncofetal antigen to which many patients show serologic reactivity (Irie et al., 1976), and is susceptible to natural cytotoxic cells in long-term assays (Golub et al., 1979) but is generally susceptible in standard 4-hour chromium release tests. The second cell line used is the UCLA-SO-L14 cell line (L14), which was established from the peripheral blood lymphocytes of the same melanoma patient who donated the M14 cell line. The L14 cell line was established by infection of peripheral blood lymphocytes from this melanoma patient with Epstein-Barr virus (EBV). The M14 and L14 cells share identical HLA determinants (Pellegrino et al., 1976) and provide an interesting comparison for detection of anti-melanoma activity. The L14 cell line is moderately sensitive to NK activity in the standard 4-hour chromium release test.

Results from a melanoma patient treated with intralesional BCG for a skin metastasis are shown in Table 34.1. Cytotoxic activity against K562 and against L14 targets increased promptly after initiation of treatment and remained high over the course of the following week, although cytotoxic activity was undetectable a month following treatment. Interestingly, cytotoxic activity was never detected in the short-term chromium release assay against M14 targets.

Two other patients who received intravenous BCG have also been sequentially analyzed. Again, both patients showed a transient increase in cytotoxic activity after initiation of therapy, followed by a subsequent decline. This pattern is illustrated in Figure 34.4. These results parallel those obtained in the IFN study, where we also observed a transient increase in NK activity which was not maintained despite repeated administration of the agent.

Table 34.1. NK Activity After Intralesional BCG In a Melanoma Patient.

% Cytotoxicity at E:T[b] of :	Target cells						
	K 562			L14			M14[a]
	50:1	25:1	12.5:1	50:1	25.1	12.5:1	50:1
Day after treatment							
0	13	10	4	8	13	3	0
1	37	27	17	29	23	17	0
2	46	29	21	29	28	20	0
5	33	18	12	22	24	17	0
7	30	14	15	19	19	18	0
33	0	0	0	0	0	0	0

[a]Identical results at E:T of 25:1 and 12.5:1.
[b]E:T = Effector:Target ratio.

Evidence for Regulation of NK in Patients with BCG or IFN

Given the similar results obtained from the BCG and IFN studies, we considered the possibility that the observed cytotoxic increase may involve activation of an accessory cell, while the decline may be associated with activity of a suppressor cell. Removal of adherent cells on Sephadex G10 columns resulted in no change in the pattern of cytotoxicity observed, i.e., the same increase and decline was seen with PBL's from IFN patients in the absence of macrophages. We then examined an alternative approach to studying cell interactions. Since NK-like cytotoxic activity can be induced *in vitro* by stimulation with EBV-transformed lymphoblasts (Svedmyr et al., 1974; Jondal and Targan, 1978), cryopreserved PBL's from one of the i.v. BCG patients were stimulated *in vitro* with an allogeneic lymphoblastoid cell line. After six days of incubation, some samples were tested for incorporation of ^{3}H-thymidine and other samples were tested for cytotoxic activity against the stimulating lymphoblasts. As can be seen in Figure 34.5, cytotoxic activity was augmented in the PBL derived from blood drawn on days 2 and 7 following initiation of BCG treatment as compared to the PBL of the healthy control donor, or the PBL from blood drawn on day 1. This increase is concurrent with the increase in NK cytotoxicity as shown in Figure 34.4. Thus, increased NK cytotoxicity *in vivo* appears to be correlated with increased ability by PBL to generate cytotoxic activity *in vitro*.

It is possible that the increased activity in the cell-mediated lympholysis assay was due to persistence in culture of the increased NK activity. Therefore, we devised the following protocol: PBL's were depleted of active NK cells by passage over EAγ-monolayers; the non-EAγ-adherent, Fcγ receptor negative, NK inactive PBL's were then stimulated with allogeneic lymphoblastoid cells. Cytotoxicity was measured against K562 targets in order to examine only the NK-like cytotoxicity and not allospecific cytotoxic T cell activity. Results of

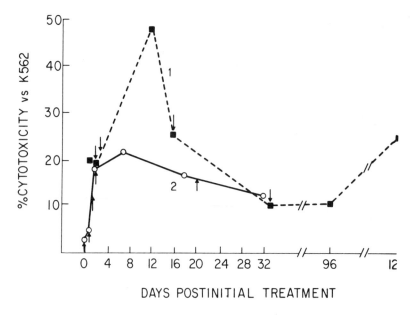

Figure 34.4. NK cytotoxicity of peripheral blood lymphocytes from melanoma patients treated with intravenous BCG. Cytotoxicity vs K562 at E:T of 200:1 with cryopreserved PBL from two melanoma patients. BCG treatments for patient #1 (■--■) shown as downward arrows and for patient #2 (O—O) shown as upward arrows.

one such experiment are shown in Figure 34.6. The cryopreserved PBL's from IFN patient #2 were stimulated with an allogeneic lymphoblastoid cell line and tested for ^{3}H-thymidine incorporation and for cytotoxicity against K562 targets. The cytotoxicity induced *in vitro* against K562 peaked in PBL from day 3 of treatment and progressively declined thereafter, while the NK cytotoxicity detected by directly sampling the patient's PBL's peaked at day 7 and declined thereafter (see Figure 34.1). This finding suggests that IFN treatment is associated with an increase in the number of cells able to generate cytotoxicity and may indicate an increased number of NK precursors. Alternatively, these results could be interpreted to indicate increased activity of accessory or amplifier cells for the generation of NK activity early in IFN treatment. It is interesting to note that the mixed lymphocyte culture results as measured by thymidine incorporation showed no substantial differences over the entire period of treatment. Thus, the increased cytotoxicity was not accompanied by additional lymphocyte proliferative activity. We have obtained similar results with two additional patients which again indicate increased *in vitro* generation of anti-K562 effectors before or at the time of peak *in vivo* NK activity. Cell mixing experiments are being initiated using cells from the peak generation period added to cells of the pretreatment period to determine if increased cell-mediated lympholysis activity against K562 is due to an amplification mechanism.

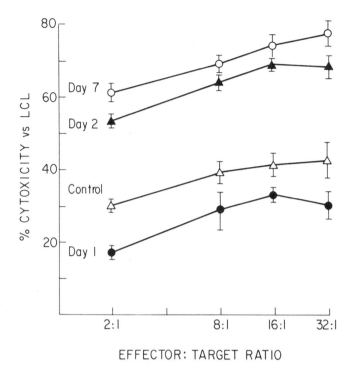

Figure 34.5. Mixed lymphocyte culture-cell-mediated lympholysis with peripheral blood lymphocytes from a melanoma patient treated with intravenous BCG. Cryopreserved PBL's from i.v. BCG patient #2 were stimulated *in vitro* with allogeneic lymphoblastoid cell line cells for 6 days and tested at various E:T ratios (horixontal axis) for cytotoxicity vs LCL targets (vertical axis). Vertical bars indicate standard error. PBL's were obtained one day after BCG treatment (●—●); two days after treatment (▲—▲); seven days after treatment (○—○); and from a healthy control donor (△—△). MLC results (log₁₀ cpm of ³H-thymidine incorporated after stimulation with LCL/log₁₀ cpm incorporated by unstimulated PBL): day 1=4.93/3.43; day 2= 4.94/3.23; day 7=4.91/3.78; control=4.88/3.78. For NK cytotoxicity see Figure 34.4.

These results focused on the possibility that cellular interactions could explain the pattern of increased NK activity followed by decreased NK activity in IFN treated patients. However, one must also consider the possibility of a change in the way cells react to IFN. We have added exogenous IFN *in vitro* to PBL from IFN treated patients. In the experiment shown in Figure 34.7, PBL from an IFN treated patient were preincubated with 100 units of IFN-α for 60 minutes, washed, and tested for cytotoxicity. Samples from the pretreatment period showed cytotoxicity that was increased by additional IFN, as did samples from the early post-treatment period. However, PBL from the period of declining NK activity showed no increased cytotoxicity when preincubated *in vitro* with IFN. Samples from the last day of treatment forward again showed augmented cytotoxicity. It is interesting to note that on day 42,

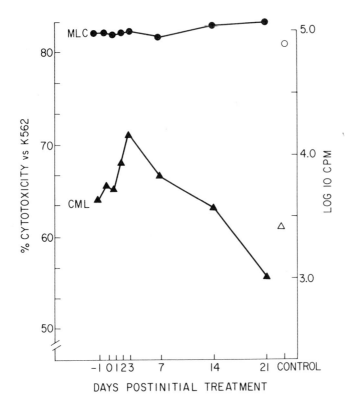

Figure 34.6. Mixed lymphocyte culture-cell-mediated lympholysis with Fcγ-depleted peripheral blood lymphocytes of an IFN treated melanoma patient. Cryopreserved PBL from IFN patient #2, derived from various times during treatment (horizontal axis), were depleted of Fcγ receptor cells by passage over EAγ monolayers. The cells were then stimulated for 6 days *in vitro* with lymphoblastoid cell line cells and tested for cytotoxicity against K562 targets (left vertical axis). Cytotoxicity results (▲—▲) are given as mean of four E:T ratios. MLC results (●—●) are shown as $\log_{10}$ cpm of ^{3}H-thymidine incorporated (right vertical axis). For NK cytotoxicity, see Figure 34.1. Control CML (△) and MLC (○) are results with identically treated PBL from a healthy donor.

after 42 consecutive days with IFN, PBL did show some increased cytotoxicity, and this period is where we are beginning to see some increase in NK activity without the additional *in vitro* IFN. These results have been replicated with two more patients, although two other patients who were treated *in vivo* with low doses of IFN showed consistent *in vitro* augmentation by IFN throughout the course of their treatment. These results suggest that once NK cytotoxicity is enhanced by IFN, the cells may become resistant to further IFN augmentation of NK cytotoxicity.

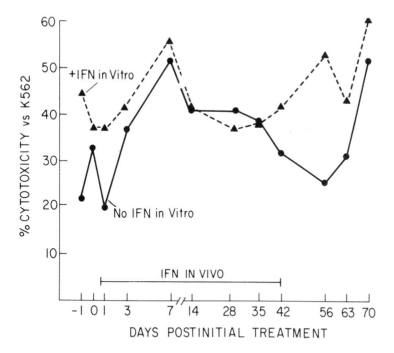

Figure 34.7. Effect of IFN on NK mediated by peripheral blood lymphocytes from an IFN treated patient. Cryopreserved PBL from IFN melanoma patient #3 were obtained at various times during treatment (horizontal axis). PBL were incubated for 60 minutes at 37°C in the presence of 100 units IFN (▲---▲) or in the absence of IFN (●—●) and tested for cytotoxicity against K562 targets at an E:T of 100:1 (vertical axis).

In Situ Cytotoxicity

If NK effectors play a significant role in anti-tumor defenses, one would expect to find active NK cells at the tumor site. We have begun to study the functional activity of tumor infiltrating lymphocytes from human lung tumors, comparing cells from tumors that are and are not injected with BCG (TIL and BCG-TIL). The functional activity and cell populations of the TIL and BCG-TIL have been described elsewhere (Niitsuma et al., submitted) and the data presented here will be confined to NK studies. To briefly summarize our other results, we found that the TIL from human lung tumors had a markedly low proportion of E-rosetting cells and a rather high proportion of Fcγ receptor cells. There was a high proportion of cells ("null cells") with no apparent markers allowing characterization as either T, B, or macrophage. TIL from BCG injected tumors, obtained two weeks following injection, showed a higher proportion of T cells with no notable changes in proportions of Fcγ receptor cells or B cells. Functionally, TIL was found to be severely impaired in MLC-CML assays in both proliferative capacity and ability to generate cytotoxic effectors. In contrast, TIL from BCG injected tumors showed vigorous MLC-CML responses, although these responses were not equivalent to those obtained with lymph node lymphocytes or the peripheral blood lymphocytes from the same patients. Thus, BCG injection of tumors results in an infiltration of functionally reactive T cells while uninjected tumors have a population of functionally anergic cells.

We have obtained similar results in studies of NK function. These results are summarized in Table 34.2. TIL from lung tumors failed to manifest significant levels of NK cytotoxicity against K562 targets. However, TIL from BCG injected tumors showed strong NK cytotoxicity. The BCG-TIL level of cytotoxicity was approximately equivalent to the cytotoxic activity of PBL from the same patients. Three of these patients had more than one lung metastasis detectable at the time of surgical resection. However, only a single metastasis had been BCG injected. Thus, we were able to compare TIL and BCG-TIL from the same patient. The BCG-TIL showed high cytotoxic activity, while the TIL from uninjected tumors from the same patients showed low NK activity. This indicates that the augmentation of the cytotoxicity induced by BCG is confined to the local site and does not result in a noticeable increase in cytotoxic function among cells infiltrating uninjected tumors in the same patient.

We have only begun to study the regulation of cytotoxicity among TIL, but some of our preliminary observations may be of interest. TIL from non-injected lesions which showed low NK activity could not be further augmented with addition of interferon *in vitro*. This suggests a profound state of functional impairment. Addition of TIL to PBL had no effect on PBL mediated NK cytotoxicity. Thus, we have no evidence for suppressor cells such as pros-

Table 34.2. NK Cytotoxicity of Tumor Infiltrating Lymphocytes (TIL) and BCG-TIL.

Cell source	Number tested	% cytotoxicity vs K562 (E:T=50:1) (Mean)	Standard error
BCG uninjected patients:			
TIL	20	7.7	4.8
PBL[a]	19	28.6	4.0
BCG-injected patients:			
BCG-TIL	4	24.8	8.3
TIL	3	5.7	4.7
PBL	4	36.5	7.9
Healthy controls			
PBL[b]	20	20.6	2.4
PBL[c]	4	24.3	5.1

[a]PBL vs TIL, P = < .0005 by t-test.
[b]Controls tested simultaneously with TIL.
[c]Controls tested simultaneously with BCG-TIL.

taglandin secreting macrophages or other types of suppressors which might impair NK activity. This does not mean that TIL does not contain suppressor cells, as Vose and Moore (1979) have demonstrated cells among human TIL that can suppress mitogen-induced responses. However, such suppressor cells do not appear to affect NK effector function. Furthermore, the failure of TIL to inhibit PBL mediated NK suggests that residual tumor cell contamination is not blocking NK cytotoxicity by cold target competition. Thus, there appears to be a local microenvironment within a tumor which is not conductive to functional activity of lymphocytes, including NK activity. Our findings on the lack of activity in human TIL confirm the observations of other investigators (Vose et al., 1977; Totterman et al., 1978). Our data also indicate that the immunosuppressive microenvironment of the tumor can be changed by the introduction of an immunotherapeutic agent such as BCG. Under those conditions, the tumor infiltrating cells can be shown to have strong functional activity, including NK activity.

In Vitro Regulation of NK Cytotoxicity

We have previously described two systems for generating NK-like cytotoxicity *in vitro*. The first system required only *in vitro* culture of normal human peripheral blood lymphoid cells in the presence of a xenogeneic serum source such as fetal bovine serum (Zielske and Golub, 1976). Fetal bovine serum incubated PBL showed increased proliferation and induction of non-specific cytotoxic function. The development of this cytotoxic activity was shown to require T cells, although the cytotoxic activity was mediated at least in part by Fcγ receptor bearing NK-like cells (Golub et al., 1979). We have examined in greater detail a similar system for the induction of NK-like cytotoxicity. This system involves the activation of cytotoxic effectors by standard mixed lymphocyte culture (MLC). Our results with MLC induction have been reported (Seeley and Golub, 1978; Seeley et al., 1979; Golightly and Golub, submitted), and will only be summarized here. We found that MLC induces two very distinct cytotoxic effectors. The first is the usual allospecific cytotoxic T lymphocytes. Cytotoxic T lymphocytes were detected with targets of mitogen induced blasts of the appropriate target type and peak cytotoxicity was found at day 6 of culture. The second type of cytotoxicity was detectable against NK-sensitive targets such as K562 and against lymphoblastic cell lines derived from PBL of the MLC responder. This "anomalous killing" or "NK-like" killing showed peak activity at day 3 in culture and could be further distinguished from T lymphocyte cytotoxicity by the target spectrum of susceptible cells and by cold target competition analysis. The NK-like effectors could be inhibited by NK sensitive targets but not by the specific alloantigen to which the cells were sensitized. In contrast, allospecific cytotoxic T lymphocytes were inhibitable only by cells bearing the appropriate alloantigens.

We have examined the surface phenotypes of the cells mediating cytotoxicity against K562 after alloantigen stimulation. We have also examined the surface markers of the cell types necessary to generate such activity. These results are summarized in Table 34.3. NK cytotoxicity against K562 targets is always associated with cells bearing the Fc receptor for IgG (Fcγ) and we have found no activity associated with cells bearing the Fc receptor for IgM (Fcμ). In agreement with many other laboratories, we find NK activity associated with both the cells forming E-rosettes and cells that fail to form high affinity E-rosettes.

The pattern is quite different with the cells mediating cytotoxicity against K562 after MLC stimulation. In this case, only low levels of cytotoxicity have been found associated with cells bearing the Fcγ receptor. Passage of MLC stimulated cells over EAγ-monolayers fails to reduce cytotoxicity. Since both Fcγ positive and Fcγ negative cells may contribute to the total cytotoxicity, removal of one subpopulation would necessarily result in enrichment of the other one; therefore, failure to change this cytotoxicity by Fcγ depletion does not indicate that the Fcγ cells are inactive or absent. Direct enrichment of such cells on immobilized immune complexes resulted in a low yield of cytotoxic cells. However, the evidence for increased antibody dependent cellular cytoxicity (ADCC) following MLC (Callewaert et al., 1978; Evans et al., 1978) indicates that MLC does induce active Fcγ receptor bearing cells. In the fetal bovine serum cytotoxicity system, we have seen a more marked depletion of cytotoxic activity by the passage of activated cells over EAγ-monolayers.

The situation is more straightforward with regard to the Fc receptor for IgM. We regularly detected strong anti-K562 cytotoxicity induced in MLC among cells bearing this receptor. Peak activity was found after 3 days of MLC which coincided with peak total cytotoxic activity. These cells are uniformly positive for the E receptor but do not bear the Fcγ receptor. Although considerable cytotoxicity was associated with the Fcμ+ fraction, cytotoxicity was also detectable with cells that lacked the ability to form rosettes with IgM coated erythrocytes. Designation of cells as Fcμ- must be interpreted with some caution, as PBL depleted of Fcμ+ can generate additional positive cells within 24 hours (Golightly and Golub, 1980). Furthermore, detection of Fcμ

Table 34.3. Summary: Mixed Lymphocyte Culture (MLC)-Induced Natural Killing.

	Marker						
	E+	E−	Fcγ+	Fcγ−	Fcμ+	Fcμ−	Fcγ-μ-
Standard PBL NK[a]	+	+	+	−	−	+	−
MLC-induced NK	+	±	±	+	+	+	+
Precursors of MLC-induced NK	+	−	±	+	+	+	+

[a]PBL: Peripheral blood lymphocyte natural killing.

receptors appears to be quite sensitive to the IgM concentration on the erythrocytes (Itoh and Kumagai, 1980). Thus, cells described as Fcμ− in this review may have receptors at surface densities or with affinities not detectable by our standard rosetting reagent. In summary, the cytotoxic effectors induced in MLC appear to be quite heterogeneous with regard to the three receptors we have examined: The E-receptor, the Fcγ receptor, and the Fcμ receptor.

In order to generate this cytotoxicity, there is an absolute requirement for E-rosette forming cells. This is true both in the MLC and fetal bovine serum systems. This NK-like cytotoxicity can clearly be generated from cells depleted of active NK cells by passage over EAγ-monolayers. The cytotoxicity can also be generated from cells enriched for Fcμ receptor cells, but it is not exclusively a property of such cells. We have had some conflicting results in attempting to generate cytotoxicity with cells enriched on the basis of the Fcγ receptor. Cells enriched by adherence to immobilized soluble immune complexes were ineffective at generating cytotoxicity in MLC, while cells enriched by EAγ-rosette formation were able to generate cytotoxic cells which bore the Fcγ receptor. The reasons for these differences are not readily apparent.

In summary, we have found considerable heterogeneity among the NK-like MLC induced cytotoxic cells and also among the cells able to generate such activity. One possible interpretation is that a variety of cell types can be activated by alloantigen. These cells might then secrete interferon which in turn would activate NK function from either NK inactive precursors or more mature active NK cells. Thus, the appearance of NK-like activity would simply reflect the production of interferon during the MLC. Evidence for such a model has been reported by Saksela et al. (1979). An attempt to explain our data on the basis of this model encounters several problems. First of all, secondary stimulation in MLC, which would be expected to also produce IFN, fails to augment NK-like cytotoxicity to the same extent that primary sensitization does. More directly, the MLC induced anti-K562 effectors contain a population with strong expression of the Fcμ receptor. These cells have been shown to be inactive in cytotoxicity or cold target competition assays with alloantigen bearing cells, but are quite cytotoxic for K562 or MOLT 4 targets, both of which are very NK-sensitive. However, IFN has been shown to diminish the expression of the Fcμ receptor while enhancing the expression of the Fcγ receptor (Itoh et al., 1980).

An alternative explanation would assume that the Fc receptors, and the E receptor, are not stable markers of subsets of lymphocytes but are instead event markers indicating some stage in the activation of cells. Thus, the different phenotypes of cells we have seen mediating MLC induced cytotoxicity, and the different phenotypes which can serve as precursors of this type of cytotoxicity, may all reflect a single cell type in various stages of activation or maturation. We have proposed that the standard NK activity seen in peripheral blood lymphocytes may be an intermediate stage in T cell activation (Golightly and Golub, submitted). One can visualize a pathway whereby normal T cells, bearing the E receptor, are occasionally activated by antigenic stimulation and in consequence gain expression of the Fcγ receptor, with a concomitant partial loss of expression of the E receptor. Further stimulation of such cells may result in subsequent loss of the Fcγ receptor and gain of the Fcμ receptor, followed by loss of both receptors. The fact that many of the cultured T cell lines maintained in T cell growth factor supplemented medium demonstrated NK-like cytotoxicity (Masucci et al., 1980) would be consistent with this model. In this sense, there may be no such thing as a distinct NK-cell but instead there may be NK activity associated with certain activation events of T cells or perhaps other cell populations.

Regulation of MLC-Induced NK Cytotoxicity

The *in vitro* generation of NK activity bears a notable temporal similarity to the *in vivo* induction of NK cytotoxicity by interferon or BCG. In both *in vitro* and *in vivo* studies, we have seen an early rise in NK cytotoxicity followed by a subsequent decline. In both cases, subsequent decline could not be reversed by additional *in vitro* activation. We have begun studies on the *in vitro* model to determine if suppressor cells prevent restimulation of NK cytotoxicity. To address this question, we have taken cells from later periods in MLC and added them to fresh PBL along with a fresh source of alloantigen. The addition of cells from late MLC (8 to 12 days post-stimulation) suppressed the induction of new NK cytotoxicity by alloantigen stimulation. The nature of the suppressor cells and the mechanism of suppression are currently under study, but these preliminary results indicate that NK cytotoxicity may be under cellular regulation as well as regulation by soluble factors such as interferon.

Summary

We have investigated three models for studying the regulation of NK cytotoxicity in humans. *In vivo* studies of patients treated with IFN or BCG indicates that both agents elevate NK cytotoxicity in a consistent, but transient, fashion. Augmentation of cytotoxicity appears to be correlated with increased numbers of target binding cells and may also be associated with increased ability to generate NK-like cytotoxicity *in vitro* by stimulation with allogenic lymphoblasts. The reasons for the subsequent decline in cytotoxicity are not well established, but this decline does correlate with an inability to augment cytotoxicity *in vitro* with exogenous IFN. Studies of NK cytotoxicity at the tumor site indicate very low levels of NK function despite the presence of considerable numbers of cells bearing the Fcγ receptor. However, intralesional injection of tumors with BCG results in an infiltration of functionally active NK cells. *In vitro* models have indicated that NK-like cytotoxicity can be developed by alloantigen stimulation. The effectors of such cytotoxicity are quite heterogeneous and may bear surface markers, such as the

Fc receptor for IgM, not usually associated with standard NK activity. All three systems point to possible regulatory events in the development and effector function of NK cells.

References

Callery, C.D., Golightly, M., Sidell, N., and Golub, S.H. (1980) Lymphosurface markers and cytotoxicity following cryopreservation. *J. Immunol. Meth.* 35:213–223.

Callewaert, D.M., Lightbody, J.J., Kaplan, J., Jaroszerski, J., Peterson Jr., W.D., and Rosenberg, J.C. (1978) Cytotoxicity of human peripheral lymphocytes in cell-mediated lympholysis; antibody dependent cell-mediated lympholysis and natural cytoxicity assays after mixed lymphocyte cultures. *J. Immunol.* 121:81–85.

Djeu, J.Y., Heinbaugh, J.A., Holden, H.T., and Herberman, R.B. (1978a) Augmentation of mouse natural killer cell activity by interferon and interferon inducers. *J. Immunol.* 122:175–181.

Djeu, J.Y., Heinbaugh, J.A., Holden, H.T., and Herberman, R.B. (1978b) Role of macrophages in the augmentation of mouse natural killer cell activity by poly I:C and interferon. *J. Immunol.* 122:182–188.

Droller, M.J., Schneider, M.V., and Perlmann, P. (1978) A possible role of prostaglandins in the inhibition of natural and antibody-dependent cell-mediated cytotoxicity against tumor cells. *Cellular Immunol.* 39:165–177.

Einhorn, S., Blomgren, H., and Strander, H. (1978) Interferon and spontaneous cytotoxicity in man. II. Studies in patients receiving exogenous leukocyte interferon. *Acta Med. Scand.* 204:477–483.

Evans, R.L., Chess, L., Levine, H., and Schlossman, S.F. (1978) Antibody-dependent cellular cytotoxicity by allosensitized human T cells. *J. Exp. Med.* 147:605–610.

Golightly, M.G. and Golub, S.H. (1980) The *in vitro* culture characteristics and requirements for expression of receptors for IgM on human peripheral blood lymphocytes. *Clin. Exp. Immunol.* 39:222–232.

Golightly, M.G. and Golub, S.H. Natural killer cytotoxicity mediated by human lymphocytes with receptors for IgM: implications for the lineage of NK cells. Submitted for publication.

Golub, S.H., Sulit, H.L., and Morton, D.L. (1975) The use of viable frozen lymphocytes for studies in human tumor immunology. *Transplant.* 19:195–202.

Golub, S.H., Golightly, M.G., and Zielske, J.V. (1979) "NK-like" cytotoxicity of human lymphocytes cultured in media containing fetal bovine serum. *Int. J. Cancer* 24:273–283.

Holmes, E.C., Ramming, K.P., Bein, M.E., Coulson, W.F., and Callery, C.D. (1979) Intralesional BCG immunotherapy of pulmonary tumors. *J. Thorac. Cardiovasc. Surg.* 77:362–368.

Huddlestone, J.R., Merigan Jr., T.O., and Oldstone, M.B. (1979) Induction and kinetics of natural killer cells in humans following interferon theory. *Nature* 282:417–420.

Irie, R.F., Irie, K., and Morton, D.L. (1976) A membrane antigen common to human cancer and fetal brain tissues. *Cancer Res.* 36:3510–3517.

Itoh, K. and Kumagai, K. (1980) Effect of tunicamycin and neuraminidase on the expression of Fc-IgM and -IgG receptors on human lymphocytes. *J. Immunol.* 124:1830–1836.

Itoh, K., Inoue, M., Kataoka, S., and Kumagai, K. (1980) Differential effect of interferon on expression of IgG- and IgM-Fc receptors on human lymphocytes. *J. Immunol.* 124:2589–2595.

Jondal, M. and Targan, S. (1978) *In vitro* induction of cytotoxic effector cells with spontaneous killer cell specificity. *J. Exp. Med.* 147:1621–1636.

Kumar, V., Ben-Ezra, J., Bennett, M., and Sonnenfeld, G. (1979) Natural killers in mice treated with 89 Strontium: normal target-binding cell numbers but inability to kill even after interferon administration. *J. Immunol.* 123:1832–1838.

Masucci, M.G., Klein, E., and Argov, S. (1980) Disappearance of the NK effect after explanation of lymphocytes and generation of similar non-specific cytotoxicity correlated to the level of blastogenesis in activated cultures. *J. Immunol.* 124:2458–2463.

Niitsuma, M., Golub, S.H., Edelstein, R., and Holmes, E.C. Lymphoid cells infiltrating BCG injected lung tumors. Submitted for publication.

Ortaldo, J.R., MacDermott, R.P., Bonnard, G.D., Kind, P.D., and Herberman, R.B. (1979) Cytotoxicity from cultured cells: analysis of precursors involved in generation of human cells mediating natural and antibody-dependent cell-mediated cytotoxicity. *Cell. Immunol.* 48:356–368.

Pellegrino, M.A., Perrone, S., Reisfeld, R.A., Irie, R.F., and Golub, S.H. (1976) Expression of histocompatability (HLA) antigens on tumor cells and normal cells from patients with melanoma. *Cancer* 40:85–86.

Pross, H.F. and Baines, M.G. (1976) Spontaneous human lymphocyte-mediated cytotoxicity against tumor target cells. I. The effect of malignant disease. *Int. J. Cancer* 18:593–604.

Saksela, E., Timonen, T. and Cantell, K. (1979) Human natural killer cell activity is augmented by interferon via recruitment of "Pre-NK" cells. *Scand. J. Immunol.* 10:257–266.

Savary, L.A. and Lotzova, E. (1978) Suppression of natural killer cell cytotoxicity by splenocytes from *Corynebacterium parvum* injected, bone marrow-tolerant, and infant mice. *J. Immunol.* 120:239–243.

Seeley, J.K. and S.H. Golub. (1978) Studies on cytotoxicity generated in human mixed lymphocyte cultures. I. Time course and target spectrum of several distinct concomitant cytotoxic activities. *J. Immunol.* 120:1415–1422.

Seeley, J.K., Masucci, G., Poros, A., Klein, E., and Golub, S.H. (1979) Studies on cytotoxicity in human mixed lymphocyte cultures. II. Anti-K562 effectors are distinct from the allospecific CTL and can be generated from NK-depleted T cells. *J. Immunol.* 123:1303–1311.

Svedmyr, E.A., Deinhardt, F., and Klein, E. (1974) Sensitivity of different target cells to the killing action of peripheral lymphocytes stimulated by autologous lymphoblastoid cell lines. *Int. J. Cancer* 13:891–903.

Tagasugi, M., Ramseyer, A., and Takasugi, J. (1977) Decline of natural nonselective cell-mediated cytotoxicity in patients with tumor progression. *Cancer Research* 37:413–418.

Targan, S. and Dorey, F. (1980) Interferon activation of "PRE-spontaneous killer" (PRE-SK) cells and alteration in kinetics of lysis of both "PRE-SK" and active SK cells. *J. Immunol.* 124:2157–2161.

Thatcher, N. and Crowther, D. (1978) Changes in non-specific lymphoid (NK, K, T cell) cytotoxicity following BCG immunization of healthy subjects. *Cancer Immunol. Immunother.* 5:105–107.

Thatcher, N., Swindell, R., and Crowthor, D. (1979) Effects of repeated *Corynebacterium parvum* and BCG therapy on immune parameters. A weekly sequential study of melanoma patients. *Clin. Exp. Immunol.* 36:227–233.

Totterman, T.H., Hayry, P., Saksela, P., Timonen, T., and Eklund, B. (1978) Cytological and functional analysis of inflammatory infiltrates in human malignant tumors. II. Functional investigations of the infiltrating inflammatory cells. *Eur. J. Immunol.* 8:872–875.

Tracey, D.E. (1979) The requirement for macrophages in the augmentation of natural killer cell activity by BCG. *J. Immunol.* 123:840–845.

Vose, B.M. and Moore, M. (1979) Suppressor cell activity of lymphocytes infiltrating human lung and breast tumors. *Int. J. Cancer* 24:579–585.

Vose, B.M., Vanky, F., Argov, S., and Klein, E. (1977) Natural cytotoxicity in man: activity of lymph node and tumor infiltrating lymphocytes. *Eur. J. Immunol.* 7:753–757.

Wolfe, S.A., Tracey, D.E., and Henney C.S. (1977) BCG-induced murine effector cells II. Characterization of NK cells in peritoneal exudates. *J. Immunol.* 119:1152–1158.

Zarling, J.M., Eskara, L., Borden, E.C., Horoszewcz, J., and Carter, J.M. (1979) Activation of human natural killer cells cytotoxic for human leukemia cells by purified interferon. *J. Immunol.* 123:63–70.

Zielske, J.V. and Golub, S.H. (1976) Fetal calf serum-induced blastogenic and cytotoxic responses of human lymphocytes. *Cancer Research* 6:3842–3846.

Published 1981 by Elsevier North Holland, Inc.
Saunders, Daniels, Serrou, Rosenfeld, and Denney, eds.
FUNDAMENTAL MECHANISMS IN HUMAN CANCER IMMUNOLOGY

CHAPTER 35

Characteristics of NK Cells and Their Possible Role in Resistance Against Tumor Growth

Ronald B. Herberman, Tuomo Timonen,
John R. Ortaldo, Guy D. Bonnard,
Eli Kedar, and Eliezer Gorelik

Laboratory of Immunodiagnosis, National Cancer Institute, Bethesda, Maryland

Introduction

The phenomenon of cytotoxicity toward tumor cells and cultured cell lines derived from tumors by lymphocytes of many normal individuals was first recognized during the course of studies attempting to examine specific cytotoxic activity of lymphocytes of tumor-bearing individuals against their own tumors or against tumors of the same histologic or etiologic type. It gradually became apparent that lymphocytes of some normal controls were actually more cytotoxic against some target cells than were those of the tumor-bearing individuals under study. These findings have necessitated a reevaluation of supposed disease-related cytotoxic reactivity of cancer patients, with a need to discriminate clearly between the activity of natural effector cells and of more specific immune effector cells (Herberman and Oldham, 1975).

The most extensively studied and characterized natural effector cell in man and rodents has come to be called a natural killer (NK) cell. This chapter will summarize what is known about NK cells, emphasizing recent findings from our laboratory. It should be noted, however, that other types of natural effector cells have been found and these may also have important *in vivo* roles. For more details on NK cells and information on other aspects of natural cell-mediated immunity, the reader might consult recent reviews (e.g., Herberman et al., 1979a) and a new comprehensive book on this subject (Herberman, 1980).

Characteristics of NK Cells

NK cells have generally been found to be non-adherent and non-phagocytic and therefore are considered to be a subpopulation of lymphocytes, not macrophages or monocytes. On the basis of initial cell separation studies, NK cells appeared to be null cells, i.e., they lack characteristic markers of either T cells or B cells. They clearly appear to be distinct from mature T cells, since high levels of NK activity have been found in nude or neonatally thymectomized mice. However, through use of more sensitive techniques, evidence has accumulated for some association of NK cells with the T cell lineage. There have also been some suggestions that NK cells may be promonocytes (for detailed discussion, see Herberman, 1980).

Expression of T Cell Associated Markers

In mice and humans, NK cells have been found to have several markers that suggest some relationship to T cells, perhaps indicating them to be early prethymic cells of the T cell lineage (summarized in Herberman, 1980). Each of these markers has been detected on at least a portion of NK cells and appears to be strongly associated with peripheral T cells. In experiments using optimal conditions for formation of rosettes with sheep erythrocytes (E rosette), 50–80% of human NK cells were found to have low affinity receptors for E (West et al., 1977). As a further recent indication that human NK cells belong to the T cell lineage, treatment with specific anti-T cell sera plus complement caused virtual elimination of cytotoxic activity (Kaplan and Callewaert, 1978). In mice, treatment with high concentrations of anti-Thy 1 plus complement, or repeated treatments, eliminated most NK activity (Mattes et al., 1979). In addition, it has been possible to positively select for a portion of NK cells from nude or conventional mice, using a monoclonal anti-Thy 1 antibody and the fluorescence activated cell sorter (Mattes et al., 1979). Similarly, Koo and Hatzfeld (1980) have reported that monoclonal antibodies to Ly 1 can react with about one-fourth of mouse NK cells. Thus, it appears that at least some human and mouse NK cells have characteristic markers of the T cell lineage.

Expression of Fc_γ Receptors and Relationship of NK to K Cells

Another surface marker on NK cells is the $Fc_\gamma R$ (receptor for Fc portion of IgG). $Fc_\gamma R$ are readily detected on human NK cells and methods which deplete $Fc_\gamma R^+$ cells result in virtual elimination of NK activity. In mice and rats, NK cells initially appeared to lack $Fc_\gamma R$. However, when more sensitive depletion procedures were used, more than half of the NK lytic units were removed (Herberman et al., 1977a; Oehler et al., 1978a). The finding of $Fc_\gamma R$ on NK cells of each of the species studied raised questions about the relationship between NK cells and K cells mediating antibody-dependent cell-mediated cytotoxicity (ADCC). However, extensive studies in our laboratory and in some others have failed to confirm that IgG is involved in natural cell-mediated cytotoxicity (Herberman, 1980). Despite this, the NK and K cells appear to be in the same subpopulation of lymphocytes and share many characteristics. On the basis of experiments in which some target cells sensitive to NK activity were able to inhibit ADCC, it appears that NK and ADCC activities may be mediated by the same cells. It may be that the same cell can produce cytotoxic effects either by interaction with antibody-coated target cells via its $Fc_\gamma R$ or with some target cells via separate "NK receptors."

Large Granular Lymphocytes

Although several markers on mouse NK cells appear quite promising for selective depletion of cytotoxic activity (see Herberman, 1980), none has yet been shown to provide the basis for purification of NK cells. In contrast, some recent findings with human and rat NK cells have indicated that isolation of this effector cell population can be achieved. Timonen et al. (1979) found that the majority of human lymphocytes binding to NK-sensitive target cells and thereby forming conjugates were large lymphocytes with an indented nucleus and prominent azurophilic granules in the cytoplasm.

It has been possible to enrich for these large granular lymphocytes (LGL) on discontinuous Percoll density gradients (Saksela and Timonen, 1980; Timonen and Saksela, 1980) and we have recently used this procedure to better characterize human NK cells (Timonen et al., 1980). Most of the NK and also ADCC activity has been found in the fractions with 75–85% LGL, whereas these fractions contained only 10–20% of the input peripheral blood lymphocytes. In contrast, the fractions containing most of the small-to-medium lymphocytes have been virtually devoid of NK or ADCC activity. Thus this procedure consistently results in at least 5-fold enrichment of NK and ADCC activities. The possibility that the LGL are responsible for the cytotoxic activity has been supported by observations that about 50% of the LGL can form conjugates with K562 (a highly NK-sensitive target) or antibody-coated target cells and that most of these conjugate-forming LGL have the capacity to kill the attached target cells. Furthermore, almost all LGL were found to contain $Fc_\gamma R$, as measured by adherence to monolayers of immune complexes. The combination of Percoll gradient centrifugation and monolayer adsorption procedures has yielded fractions containing 90% LGL and most of the NK activity of the input population.

LGL could also be discriminated from other lymphocytes by rosetting with E. About one-half of the LGL had low affinity E receptors, forming rosettes at 4° but not at 29°, and the remainder lacked detectable receptors. In contrast, most other nylon-non-adherent lymphocytes had high affinity E receptors, rosetting at 29° as well as at 4°. This finding has provided the basis for an alternative procedure for further purification of NK cells (Timonen et al., 1980). Removal of high affinity E-rosette forming cells from the LGL-containing Percoll fractions resulted in a subpopulation highly enriched for LGL and NK activity.

Because of reports that the natural effector cells in mice that react against monolayer target cells differ somewhat from NK cells (Stutman et al., 1980; Burton, 1980), it was of interest to determine whether LGL were the effector cells for cytotoxicity against human monolayer target cells as well as against the K562 cell line, that grows in suspension. We have found that only LGL-enriched Percoll fractions were reactive against the whole range of targets tested (Landazuri et al., 1980), indicating that, in man, LGL appear to account for natural cytotoxicity against both suspension and monolayer targets.

These studies on separation of lymphocytes also have defined two morphologically distinct subpopulations of cells with $Fc_\gamma R$ and E receptors (i.e., T_G cells). A functional division was also possible: only the T_G cells with LGL morphology had NK and ADCC activities. Studies are now in progress to determine the distribution between the two cell types of other immune functions that have been associated with T_G cells, particularly suppressor activity.

Rat NK cells in spleen and peripheral blood also appear to be LGL and can be enriched by a procedure similar to that used for human cells (Reynolds et al., 1980). In contrast, LGL have not been detectable in mouse spleens or peripheral blood and the mouse NK cell has not yet been found to have any special morphological features that would distinguish it from other lymphocytes.

The strong association between human NK cells and LGL has allowed us to perform more detailed studies on the phenotype of these effector cells and to compare it with small lymphocytic T cells. We have tested these subpopulations by fluorescence activated cell sorter, using a series of monoclonal antibodies (Ortaldo et al., 1980a), including those recently reported to react selectively with T cells or other cell types (Hoffman et al., 1980). The T cell fraction gave the expected pattern of results, whereas a considerable portion of the LGL reacted with OKM1 and anti-Ia antibodies and about 25% reacted with OKT8 (like the T cells). In contrast, very few LGL reacted with OKT3, which reacts with a high proportion of T cells. The explanation for this pattern of reactivity is not clear, but this phenotype is clearly distinct from that of typical T cells. The reactivity with OKM1 raises the question of some relationship of LGL to monocytes, but this antigen may be a differentiation antigen shared by cells of various lineages.

Augmentation of NK Activity by Interferon (IFN)

A variety of IFN-inducers has been found to augment NK activity in mice and inoculation of IFN itself led to boosting of activity within 3 hours (Djeu et al., 1979; Gidlund et al., 1978). Incubation of mouse spleen cells with poly I:C or with IFN has also resulted in appreciable increases in NK activity. Similar observations have been made with human NK and K cells (Trinchieri and Santoli, 1978; Herberman et al., 1978, 1979a,b). Administration of poly I:C to some patients resulted in increased levels of cytotoxicity after 2 days. Incubation of human peripheral blood lymphocytes with three different IFN preparations for 1 hour or 18 hours caused increased NK and K cell activities with most donors.

During the course of the above studies, there remained some concern as to whether IFN was indeed the molecule responsible for augmenting cytotoxic activity, since the antiviral substance in all of the preparations was actually less than 1-10% of the total protein. To more definitively determine the role of IFN, we have recently had the opportunity to perform experiments with pure human leukocyte IFN (Rubinstein et al., 1979). Incubation of human lympho-cytes with this homogeneous protein for 1 hour at 37°C resulted in substantial augmentation of NK activity, thus confirming the role of IFN in positive regulation of NK activity (Herberman et al., 1980).

The ability to separate LGL from conventional lymphocytes on Percoll gradients and to measure binding of lymphoid cells to NK-susceptible targets has allowed detailed examination of the interactions between effector cells and targets and the mechanisms for augmentation of NK activity by IFN. Two issues examined were whether only LGL formed conjugates with K562 and whether only this subpopulation could be activated for NK activity by IFN. There have been several previous indications for pre-NK cells that can be induced by IFN (e.g., Oehler et al., 1978b; Bloom et al., 1980) and these precursors may have some characteristics that differ from those associated with spontaneously active NK cells. Therefore, Percoll separated fractions of LGL and of conventional lymphocytes, with or without pretreatment by IFN, were tested for conjugate formation with K562 (Timonen et al., 1980). In addition to considerable conjugate formation by LGL, some conventional lymphocytes also formed conjugates. However, this was not accompanied by any detectable cytotoxic activity, even after pretreatment with IFN. These data indicate that both active NK cells and IFN-inducible precursors are LGL and that the conventional lymphocytes forming conjugates with K562 cells are not directly related to NK cells.

Another important question investigated has been the mechanism for aug-mentation of NK activity by IFN. IFN was found to substantially increase the reactivity of LGL as well as unseparated lymphoid cells (Timonen et al., 1980), indicating that IFN can act directly on NK cells and cause augmentation of activity, without the need for accessory cells. Measurements of the kinetics of cytotoxicity also indicated that augmentation by IFN could be detected during the first hour of the assay. However, such cytotoxicity experiments failed to provide insight into which step or steps in the cytotoxic process were affected by IFN. Three main possibilities were considered: (a) induction on pre-NK cells of receptors for recognition of NK-susceptible targets; (b) triggering of the lytic machinery of conjugate-forming inactive NK cells; and (c) augmenta-tion of the activity of already active NK cells.

Measurement of conjugate formation by LGL provided a means to directly examine the first possibility. The treatment of LGL with IFN did not increase the proportion of cells forming conjugates with K562, indicating that the augmenting effects of IFN are beyond the induction of recognition receptors on LGL. To examine which of the other possibilities for IFN action were involved, we have performed experiments with the single cell agarose assay, developed by Grimm and Bonavida (1979). This method allows one to directly determine the proportion of conjugate-forming cells that produce lysis of their attached targets. During the first four hours of the interaction between LGL and K562, both the rate of lysis and the proportion of active conjugate-forming cells were higher for the IFN-treated cells. However, with further incubation, the proportion of targets lysed by the untreated effectors approached or sometimes equalled that affected by the IFN-treated LGL.

These data imply that IFN acts mainly to accelerate the rate of lysis by already active NK cells. However, since contact with target cells can induce LGL to produce IFN (Saksela et al., 1980), the possibility remains that the late rise in the proportion of active NK cells in the control group was due to activation by the endogenously produced IFN. Another important result from these studies was that a high proportion of conjugate-forming LGL, often greater than 90%, were shown to have the ability to act as NK cells. Thus, not only are virtually all NK cells in the LGL population, but a substantial proportion of LGL (about 50%) can act as NK cells against one sensitive target cell. It remains to be determined whether many of the LGL that fail to bind and lyse K562 have reactivity against other NK-sensitive target cells.

Cytotoxicity by Cultured T Cells

A major factor which limits detailed analysis of the characteristics and specificity of NK cells is that these cells only represent a small portion of the lymphoid cells in the blood or spleen (probably less than 5%). Even with the development of satisfactory isolation procedures, like the methods for enrichment of LGL, the low yield of cells imposes serious restrictions on the studies that can be performed. It would therefore be highly desirable to be able to propagate NK cells and expand them to large numbers. Culture of NK cells would also allow direct testing of our hypothesis that NK cells are polyclonal, with differing specificities.

During the past few years, it has become possible to propagate human or mouse T cells in the presence of T cell growth factor (Morgan et al., 1976). Cultured T cells (CTC) from normal human donors were found to have considerable cytotoxic activity against a wide array of target cells (Alvarez et al., 1978; Bonnard et al., 1978; Schendel et al., 1980a,b). Since K562 was one of the target cells that were susceptible to lysis by CTC, we have investigated the possibility that at least some of the cytotoxicity was due to propagation of NK cells. In detailed studies on the nature of cytotoxicity by human CTC, we have obtained evidence for four separate types of activity (Ortaldo et al., 1980b; Ortaldo, 1980): (a) cytotoxicity against K562 target cells; (b) cytotoxicity against allogeneic but not autologous or histocompatible mitogen-induced lymphoblasts; (c) ADCC against antibody-coated mouse lymphoma cells; and (d) lectin-induced cytotoxicity against the mouse lymphoma cells. The cytotoxicity against K562 and the alloblasts was distinguishable by the augmentation of only the former activity by pretreatment of CTC with IFN. Furthermore, in cold target inhibition experiments, unlabeled K562 could strongly inhibit lysis of ^{51}Cr-labeled K562 but did not appreciably affect lysis of labeled alloblasts. Conversely, unlabeled alloblasts only inhibited the lysis of labeled alloblasts. It seems likely that the activity against alloblasts was due to polyclonally activated cytotoxic T cells (Schendel et al., 1980a,b) and that the effectors for K562 were of a different nature and specificity. The possibility that the anti-K562 activity was due to NK cells was supported by the parallel finding of CTC reactivity against antibody-coated targets. This appeared to be true ADCC by K cells, since addition of protein-A selectively blocked this reaction, as was previously demonstrated for ADCC (Kay et al., 1979). The fourth type of cytotoxicity, tested in the presence of phytohemagglutinin (PHA), resulted in substantial cytotoxicity against the ordinarily resistant mouse lymphoma target cell.

The finding of apparent NK activity in CTC was encouraging and was consistent with our hypothesis of the T cell lineage of NK cells. However, the heterogeneity of effector cells in CTC interfered with the possible use of such cells for detailed studies of NK cells. To circumvent this heterogeneity, we have attempted to initiate cultures from Percoll-separated fractions of lymphocytes from normal human donors. The LGL-containing fractions, as well as the fractions with conventional lymphocytes, have proliferated in the presence of T cell growth factor. The CTC from LGL fractions maintained substantial levels of IFN-augmentable cytotoxic activity against K562 and antibody-coated target cells. In contrast, the CTC from the fractions containing conventional lymphocytes had little or no activity against these targets, even after pretreatment with IFN. Thus it appears promising that selected effector cell populations can be expanded by this procedure. We have recently initiated cultures from LGL-enriched fractions, further purified by removal of high affinity E-rosette forming cells. After 7–14 days, almost all of the cells in the cultures had the morphology of LGL, and high levels of cytotoxic activity were seen.

In other laboratories, a few clones of mouse CTC, with cell surface characteristics of NK cells, have already been obtained (Dennert et al., 1980; H. Cantor, personal communication). The clones from the two laboratories differed in specificity, supporting the concept of heterogeneity of NK cells. Clones of mouse and human CTC have also been obtained and studied in our laboratory (E. Kedar, B. Sredni, and N. Navarro, unpublished observations). Three clones of human CTC have been found to have appreciable levels of cytotoxicity against K562 and other NK-susceptible target cells. A large number of clones of mouse CTC have been obtained and most of these have had high levels of cytotoxic activity. Some of these clones have shown a broad range of cytotoxic activity against mouse lymphoma and monolayer target cells and also against some heterologous target cells, whereas other clones have been more restricted in their pattern of reactivity. Characterization of the phenotype of these clones is still in progress, but some have been found to contain abundant azurophilic granules (and thus resemble human and rat LGL) and markers that have been associated with mouse NK cells (asialo GM1 and Ly 5). Thus, it seems likely that some clones of CTC are derived from NK cells and that these cells will be very useful for more detailed characterization of NK cells, their specificity, and the nature of their interaction with target cells.

In Vivo Role of NK Cells

The most important practical issue to be settled is the role of NK cells *in vivo*. There is increasing evidence that NK cells may play an important role in resistance against tumor growth and also in rejection of bone marrow transplants (summarized in Herberman, 1980).

Rapid In Vivo Clearance of Radiolabeled Tumor Cells

To obtain more direct information about the role of NK cells in rapid *in vivo* elimination of tumor cells, we have recently examined the correlation between levels of NK activity and the ability of mice to destroy intravenously inoculated tumors that were prelabeled with ^{125}I-iododeoxyuridine (Riccardi et al., 1979, 1980b,c). In young mice of strains with high NK activity, there was a greater decrease in recovery of radioactivity when measured in various organs at 2–4 hours after inoculation than was seen in strains with low NK activity. In parallel with the decline of NK activity in mice after 10–12 weeks of age, *in vivo* clearance of intravenously inoculated tumor cells was also found to decrease (Riccardi et al., 1979, 1980b,d). Furthermore, a variety of treatments of mice that produced augmented or decreased *in vitro* reactivity also resulted in similar shifts in *in vivo* reactivity. Thus, this *in vivo* assay has correlated very well with NK cell reactivity against a variety of established tumor cell lines.

As further confirmation of the role of NK cells in resistance to growth of NK-susceptible transplantable tumors, transfer of NK cells into mice with cyclophosphamide-induced depression of NK activity was shown to significantly restore both *in vivo* and NK reactivities (Riccardi et al., 1980a). The effectiveness of the transfer correlated with the levels of NK activity of donor cells in a variety of situations: (a) NK-reactive spleen cells were able to transfer reactivity, whereas NK-unreactive thymus cells were ineffective; (b) spleen cells from young mice of high NK strains were considerably more effective than cells from older mice or from strains with low NK activity; (c) the cells responsible for transfer had the characteristics of NK cells, being non-adherent, non-phagocytic, expressing asialo GM1 and lacking easily detectable Thy 1 antigen; and (d) cells from donors with drug-induced depression of NK activity were unable to transfer reactivity. These results extend the recent findings of Hanna and Fidler (1980), who showed that the transfer of NK-reactive spleen cells to cyclophosphamide-treated mice could decrease the number of metastases developing in the lungs after challenge with NK-susceptible solid tumor cells.

A similar pattern of results was obtained when radiolabeled cells were inoculated subcutaneously into the footpads of mice (Gorelik and Herberman, 1980). Clearance correlated in several ways with the levels of NK activity in the recipients, and cells with the characteristics of NK cells were effective in local adoptive transfer. However, in contrast to NK activity and the results with intravenously inoculated tumor cells, no decrease in clearance was observed in older or beige mice. Those results suggest that other effector cells may also be involved in reactivity in subcutaneous tissues [e.g., the natural cytotoxic cell described by Stutman et al. (1980)] or that in some situations, local factors may augment the NK cell activity.

In Vivo Reactivity Against Normal Cells

It has been shown that NK cells can also lyse some normal cells such as subpopulations of bone marrow and thymus cells (Nunn et al., 1977; Welsh et al., 1979; Hansson et al., 1979). To determine whether natural reactivity against normal cells could also occur *in vivo*, we have tested both *in vivo* and *in vitro* reactivities of normal mice against bone marrow cells and fetal fibroblasts (Riccardi et al., 1980c). As with tumor targets, young mice of high NK strains rapidly eliminated a higher proportion of these normal cells than did older mice or those of a low NK strain. Furthermore, both *in vivo* and *in vitro* reactivities against these targets were modulated in parallel by NK-augmenting or depressing treatments.

Role of NK Cells Against Primary Tumors

It will be particularly important now to obtain information about the possible *in vivo* role of NK cells in resistance against primary tumors. The original formulations of the theory of immune surveillance focused on the central role of the immune response as a natural defense against neoplasia. Although most attention has been focused on the relationship of thymus-dependent immunity to immune surveillance, NK activity now has to be considered as an alternative mechanism.

One prediction of the immune surveillance hypothesis is that chemical carcinogens would cause depressed immune function, thereby impairing the ability of the host to reject the transformed cells. This postulate has been examined by many investigators in regard to the possible role of mature T cells and humoral immunity, and conflicting results have been obtained. In contrast, there is little information available on the effects of chemical carcinogens on NK cells. We have recently performed studies to determine the effects of urethane on NK activity (Gorelik and Herberman, 1980). A/J mice, which are sensitive to the carcinogenic effects of urethane, showed depressed NK and *in vivo* reactivity at 7 days after treatment and later developed multiple lung adenomas. In contrast, the *in vitro* NK and *in vivo* reactivities of C57BL/6 mice, which are resistant to urethane carcinogenesis, were virtually unaffected by this treatment. Thus, the carcinogenicity of urethane correlated with its ability to depress NK activity and this effect on host resistance may contribute to the development of neoplastic lesions.

References

Alvarez, J.M., de Landazuri, M.O., Bonnard, G.D., and Herberman, R.B. (1978) Cytotoxic activities of normal cultured human T cells. *J. Immunol.* 121:1270–1275.

Bloom, B.R., Minato, N., Neighbour, A., Reid, L., and Marcus, D. (1980) Interferon and NK cells in resistance to virus persistently infected cells and tumors. In *Natural Cell-Mediated Immunity Against Tumors*. Herberman, R.B. (ed.), New York: Academic Press, pp. 505–524.

Bonnard, G.D., Schendel, D.J., West, W.H., Alvarez, J.M., Maca, R.D., Yasaka, K., Fine, R.L., Herberman, R.B., de Landazuri, M.O., and Morgan, D.A. (1978) Continued growth of normal human T lymphocytes in culture with retention of important functions. In *Human Lymphocyte Differentiation: Its Application to Human Cancer*. Serrou, B. and Rosenfeld, C. (eds.), Amsterdam: Elsevier/North-Holland Biomedical Press, pp. 319–326.

Burton, R.C. (1980) Alloantisera selectively reactive with NK cells: characterization and use in defining NK cell classes. In *Natural Cell-Mediated Immunity Against Tumors*. Herberman, R.B. (ed.), New York: Academic Press, pp. 19–35.

Dennert, G. (1980) Cloned lines of natural killer cells. *Nature* 287:47–49.

Djeu, J.Y., Heinbaugh, J.A., Holden, H.T., and Herberman, R.B. (1979) Augmentation of mouse natural killer cell activity by interferon and interferon inducers. *J. Immunol.* 122:175–181.

Gidlund, M., Örn, A., Wigzell, H., Senik, A., and Gresser, I. (1978) Enhanced NK cell activity in mice injected with interferon and interferon inducers. *Nature* 223:259–261.

Gorelik, E. and Herberman, R.B. (1980) Radioisotope assay for evaluation of *in vivo* natural cell-mediated resistance of mice to local transplantation of tumor cells. *J. Natl. Cancer Inst.*, in press.

Grimm, E. and Bonavida, B. (1979) Mechanism of cell-mediated cytotoxicity studied at the single cell level. I. Determination of cytotoxic T lymphocyte frequency and relative lytic efficiency of individual effector cell populations. *J. Immunol.* 123:2861–2869.

Hanna, N. and Fidler, I.J. (1980) The role of natural killer cells in the destruction of circulatory tumor emboli. *J. Natl. Cancer Inst.*, in press.

Hansson, M., Kärre, K., Kiessling, R., Roder, J., Anderson, B., and Häyry, P. (1979) Natural NK cell targets in the mouse thymus: characteristics of the sensitive cell population. *J. Immunol.* 123:765–771.

Herberman, R.B. (ed.) (1980) *Natural Cell-Mediated Immunity Against Tumors*. New York: Academic Press.

Herberman, R.B. and Oldham, R.K. (1975) Problems associated with study of cell-mediated immunity to human tumors by microcytotoxicity assays. *J. Natl. Cancer Inst.* 55:749–753.

Herberman, R.B., Bartram, S., Haskill, J.S., Nunn, M., Holden, H.T., and West, W.H. (1977) Fc receptors on mouse effector cells mediating natural cytotoxicity against tumor cells. *J. Immunol.* 119:322–326.

Herberman, R.B., Djeu, J.Y., Ortaldo, J.R., Holden, H.T., West, W.H., and Bonnard, G.D. (1978) Role of interferon in augmentation of natural and antibody-dependent cell-mediated cytotoxicity. *Cancer Treat. Rep.* 62:1893–1896.

Herberman, R.B., Djeu, J.Y., Kay, H.D., Ortaldo, J.R., Riccardi, C., Bonnard, G.D., Holden, H.T., Fagnani, R., Santoni, A., and Puccetti, P. (1979a) Natural killer cells: characteristics and regulation of activity. *Immunol. Rev.* 44:43–70.

Herberman, R.B., Ortaldo, J.R., and Bonnard, G.D. (1979b) Augmentation by interferon of human natural and antibody-dependent cell-mediated cytotoxicity. *Nature* 227:221–223.

Herberman, R.B., Ortaldo, J.R., Djeu, J.Y., Holden, H.T., Jett, J., Lang, N.P., and Pestka, S. (1980) Role of interferon in regulation of cytotoxicity by natural killer cells and macrophages. *Ann. N.Y. Acad. Sci.*, in press.

Hoffman, R.A., Kung, P.C., Hansen, W.P., and Goldstein, G. (1980) Simple and rapid measurement of human T lymphocytes and their subclasses in peripheral blood. *Proc. Natl. Acad. Sci. U.S.A.* 77:4914–4917.

Kaplan, J. and Callewaert, D.M. (1978) Expression of human T lymphocyte antigens by natural killer cells. *J. Natl. Cancer Inst.* 60:961–964.

Kay, H.D., Bonnard, G.D., and Herberman, R.B. (1979) Evaluation of the role of IgG antibodies in human natural cell-mediated cytotoxicity against the myeloid cell line K562. *J. Immunol.* 122:675–685.

Koo, G.C. and Hatzfeld, A. (1980) Antigenic phenotype of mouse natural killer cells. In *Natural Cell-Mediated Immunity Against Tumors.* Herberman, R.B. (ed.), New York: Academic Press, pp. 105–116.

Landazuri, M.O., Lopez-Botet, M., Ortaldo, J.R., and Herberman, R.B. (1980) Role of large granular lymphocytes in human natural cytotoxicity against monolayer target cells. Submitted for publication.

Mattes, M.J., Sharrow, S.O., Herberman, R.B., and Holden, H.T. (1979) Identification and separation of Thy-1 positive mouse spleen cells active in natural cytotoxicity and antibody-dependent cell-mediated cytotoxicity. *J. Immunol.* 123:2851–2860.

Morgan, D.A., Ruscetti, F.W., and Gallo, R.C. (1976) Selective *in vitro* growth of T lymphocytes from normal human bone marrows. *Science* 193:1007–1008.

Nunn, M.E., Herberman, R.B., and Holden, H.T. (1977) Natural cell-mediated cytotoxicity in mice against non-lymphoid tumor cells and some normal cells. *Int. J. Cancer* 20:381–387.

Oehler, J.R., Lindsay, L.R., Nunn, M.E., and Herberman, R.B. (1978a) Natural cell-mediated cytotoxicity in rats. I. Tissue and strain distribution, and demonstration of a membrane receptor for the Fc portion of IgG. *Int. J. Cancer* 21:204–209.

Oehler, J.R., Lindsay, L.R., Nunn, M.E. Holden, H.T., and Herberman, R.B. (1978b) Natural cell-mediated cytotoxicity in rats. II. *In vivo* augmentation of NK cell activity. *Int. J. Cancer* 21:210–220.

Ortaldo, J.R. (1980) Cytotoxicity by human cultured T cells. Submitted for publication.

Ortaldo, J.R., Sharrow, S.O., Timonen, T., and Herberman, R.B. (1980a) Analysis of surface antigens on highly purified human NK cells by flow cytometry with monoclonal antibodies. Submitted for publication.

Ortaldo, J.R., Timonen, T., and Bonnard, G.D. (1980b) Natural killing and antibody-dependent cell-mediated cytotoxicity by human cultured T cells. *Behring Inst. Mitt.*, in press.

Reynolds, C.W., Timonen, T., and Herberman, R.B. (1980) Natural killer (NK) cell activity in the rat. I. Isolation and characterization of the effector cells. Submitted for publication.

Riccardi, C., Puccetti, P., Santoni, A., and Herberman, R.B. (1979) Rapid *in vivo* assay of mouse NK cell activity. *J. Natl. Cancer Inst.* 63:1041–1045.

Riccardi, C., Barlozzari, T., Santoni, A., Herberman, R.B., and Cesarini, C. (1980a) Transfer to cyclophosphamide-treated mice of natural killer (NK) cells and *in vivo* natural reactivity against tumors. Submitted for publication.

510

Riccardi, C., Santoni, A., Barlozzari, T., and Herberman, R B, (1980b) Role of NK cells in rapid *in vivo* clearance of radiolabeled tumor cells. In *Natural Cell-Mediated Immunity Against Tumors*. Herberman, R.B. (ed.), New York: Academic Press, pp. 1121–1139.

Riccardi, C., Santoni, A., Barlozzari, T., and Herberman, R.B. (1980c) *In vivo* reactivity of mouse natural killer (NK) cells against normal bone marrow cells. *Cell Immunol.*, in press.

Riccardi, C., Santoni, A., Barlozzari, T., Puccetti, P., and Herberman, R.B. (1980d) *In vivo* natural reactivity of mice against tumor cells. *Int. J. Cancer* 25:475–486.

Rubinstein, M., Rubinstein, S., Familletti, P.C., Miller, R.S., Waldman, A.A., and Pestka, S. (1979) Human leukocyte interferon: production, purification to homogeneity, and initial characterization. *Proc. natl. Acad. Sci. U.S.A.* 76:640–644.

Saksela, E. and Timonen, T. (1980) Morphology and surface properties of human NK cells. In *Natural Cell-Mediated Immunity Against Tumors*. Herberman, R.B. (ed.), New York: Academic Press, pp. 173–185.

Saksela, E., Timonen, T., Virtanen, I., and Cantell, K. (1980) Regulation of human natural killer activity by interferon. In *Natural Cell-Mediated Immunity Against Tumors*. Herberman, R.B. (ed.), New York: Academic Press, pp. 645–653.

Schendel, D.J., Wank, R., and Bonnard, G.D. (1980a) Genetic specificity of primary and secondary proliferative and cytotoxic responses of human lymphocytes grown in conditioned culture. *Scand. J. Immunol.*, in press.

Schendel, D.J., Wank, R., and Bonnard, G.D. (1980b) Generation of proliferative and cytotoxic human cultured T cell lines specific for major histocompatibility complex (HLA) antigens. *Behring Inst. Mitt.*, in press.

Stutman, O., Figarella, E.F., Paige, C.J., and Lattime, E.C. (1980) Natural cytotoxic (NC) cells against solid tumors in mice: general characteristics and comparison to natural killer (NK) cells. In *Natural Cell-Mediated Immunity Against Tumors*. Herberman, R.B. (ed.), New York: Academic Press, pp. 187–229.

Timonen, T. and Saksela, E. (1980) Isolation of human NK cells by density gradient centrifugation. *J. Immunol. Methods* 36:285–291.

Timonen, T., Saksela, E., Ranki, A., and Hayry, P. (1979) Fractionation, morphological and functional characterization of effector cells responsible for human natural killer activity against cell-line targets. *Cell. Immunol.* 48:133–148.

Timonen, T., Ortaldo, J.R., and Herberman, R.B. (1980) Characteristics of human large granular lymphocytes and relationship to natural killer and K cells. Submitted for publication.

Trinchieri, G. and Santoli, D. (1978) Antiviral activity induced by culturing lymphocytes with tumor-derived or virus-transformed cells. Enhancement of human natural killer cell activity by interferon and antagonistic inhibition of susceptibility of target cells to lysis. *J. Exp. Med.* 147:1314–1333.

Welsh, R.M., Zinkernagel, R.M., and Hallenbeck, L. (1979) Cytotoxic cells induced during lymphocytic choriomeningitis virus infection of mice. II. "Specificities" of the natural killer cells. *J. Immunol.* 122:475–481.

West, W.H., Cannon, G.B., Kay, H.D., Bonnard, G.D., and Herberman, R.B. (1977) Natural cytotoxic reactivity of human lymphocytes against a myeloid cell line: characterization of effector cells. *J. Immunol.* 118:355–361.

PART V:

Perspectives and Prospects

Published 1981 by Elsevier North Holland, Inc.
Saunders, Daniels, Serrou, Rosenfeld, and Denney, eds.
FUNDAMENTAL MECHANISMS IN HUMAN CANCER IMMUNOLOGY

CHAPTER 36

Basic Studies

J.C. Daniels, M.D., Ph.D.

Associate Professor of Medicine and Microbiology, Director, Division of Clinical Immunology, Department of Internal Medicine, University of Texas Medical Branch, Galveston, Texas

Diverse approaches to the study of human immunology, and tumor immunology in particular, have in recent years suggested many new ways to attack the problem of malignant disease. The contributions included in this volume demonstrate the multidisciplinary nature of current approaches to human cancer, which are gradually uncovering the interwoven network of relationships underlying the complex processes of tumor formation and immunologic response. These basic studies in cancer immunology are only beginning to generate new therapeutic protocols which promise to significantly enhance the methods of treatment currently in use. Future clinical developments depend upon continued exploration of the basic mechanisms of the immune system at the genetic, biochemical, and cellular levels.

Cell Surface Studies

Monoclonal Antibodies and Tumor Associated Antigens

Dr. Roger Kennett (Chapter 24) presented new information on the sources of tumor associated antigens produced by viral mutation, differentiation, and cellular interaction processes. He emphasized the usefulness of monoclonal antibodies specific for tumor antigens for the identification of tumors, the localization of metastases, the delivery of drugs, and the characterization of specific antigen. Neuroblastoma antibodies have been applied to bone marrow with a peroxidase labeled second antibody for the typing of leukemias and classification of their morphologic types. Dr. Kennett reviewed the use of fluorescent beads as a second detection antibody and described how monoclonal antibody techniques are used for the detection of genetic predisposition to malignancy, as in the case of neurofibromatosis, through monitoring surface changes on premalignant cells.

Dr. Ralph Reisfeld (Chapter 29) reported that SDS-polyacrylamide gel electrophoresis of antigens shed from melanoma cells have a prominent amount of fibronectin. Monoclonal antibodies to biochemically separated components demonstrated that one 94,000 dalton molecular weight moiety is identical between melanoma and carcinoma cells, based upon tryptic peptide mapping. Reisfeld suggested that mechanisms of shedding may include the proteolytic cleavage of surface material into a vesicle. He further demonstrated that carbohydrate is essential in the shedding process. It was also shown that 2-deoxyglucose inhibits the shedding of all material except fibronectin. Other inhibitors of glycosylation of lipids, such as tunicamycin, prevent shedding. Non-carbohydrate surface protein is still recognizable by monoclonal antibody, but cannot be shed.

Dr. Richard Smith (Chapter 32) also applied monoclonal antibodies to a basic cell system. He was able to demonstrate that tumor specific antigens are intricately related to cell surface products of the major histocompatibility complex in murine cell lines. Antibody-dependent T cell cytotoxicity for target tumor cells was studied by experiments using monoclonal antibodies from tumor-bearing mice. Specific cytotoxic cells have been cultured, cloned, and used to control tumor growth.

Dr. Stanley Order (Chapter 26) has utilized polyclonal antiferritin antibodies to carry localized radiation for treatment of hepatoma and intrahepatic biliary carcinoma. Ferritin is preferentially deposited in the spleen and is produced actively by lymphocytes in Hodgkin's disease. Dr. Order left open the question of whether monoclonal antibodies, now under development, will improve the specificity over the polyclonal antibodies used in his initial clinical trials. He underlined his concern that monoclonal antibodies may complex and alter the kinetics of antigen-antibody reactions documented with polyclonal antiferritin antibodies carrying I^{131}. In theory, however, the heightened specificity of monoclonal antibodies should allow favorable adjustments of relative dose rate, total dose, and total body irradiation.

Dr. Barry Kahan (Chapter 28) reported that 3M KCl tumor extracts are protective in a murine system. Irradiated tumor cells are also protective. Kahan suggested that soluble antigens probably activate T suppressor cells. By isoelectric focusing, both potentiating and protective tumor antigens could be shown in the system. Tumor-modulating soluble antigens appeared not to be H-2-restricted. Multiple injections of protective antigen led to a decreased protective effect. However, butanol extraction allowed improved preparation of protective material.

Cell Surface Biochemistry

Dr. Garth Nicolson (Chapter 3) reported studies of the metastatic behavior of tumor cells, in which he observed an inverse relationship between metastatic potential and Gp70 content. These findings led to the hypothesis that the loss of cell surface antigen may promote metastasis by removing the target for the immune system. Specifically, in animals inoculated with progressively colonized cell lines of murine lymphosarcoma, a linear increase in liver or lung nodules and decreased survival time concomitant with sequential selection of the tumor colony have been observed. These colonization steps are accompanied by measurable decreases in cellular Gp70 content and by increases in metastatic potential. Characterization of cells with differing metastatic potential has also been accomplished by sequential selection of cells bearing lectin receptors using NH_2-derivatized lectin, such as Concanavalin A, on a plastic Petri dish. This line of research appears to be particularly promising for illuminating the relationship between cell surface properties and metastatic behavior.

Dr. Max Burger (Chapter 8) reported on a model, using a lectin-removal system for surface carbohydrates such as that presented by Nicolson, which permitted the selection for non-lectin binding cells. Burger was able to devise a melanoma system with clear discrimination between the properties of tumorigenicity and metastability. He found that adhesion did not correlate with metastasis but that actin filaments which increase in the microtubules did correlate. In his system, T cell immunity did not seem to be important in rejection of tumors, as shown by experiments in nude mice. He emphasized that biochemical surface changes, which may be compared with biological properties, exist at the level of glycopeptide differences. Defined oligosaccharide deletions account for both altered biochemistry and modified biologic potential with respect to metastasis.

Dr. Leonard Warren (Chapter 7) pointed out that glycoprotein differences between normal and neoplastic cells appear to be quantitative, gross-dependent features of the cell surface, as opposed to qualitative features. Since carbohydrate accounts for 80% of the glycoprotein changes associated with malignant transformation, these molecules appear to be most vulnerable as a point trigger for malignancy. Carbohydrates and glycoproteins have been noted to be primitive, ubiquitous, extremely heterogenous, and capable of delivering very complex signals to the cell. The immunologic inertia of carbohydrates may relate to their evolutionary stability and ubiquity.

Membrane Composition and Properties

Dr. Michael Inbar (Chapter 2) emphasized that the cell surface is an area of important interaction between cholesterol and phospholipid, which normally exists in an intermediate fluid state optimal for membrane function. As doubling time of cells increases, surface microviscosity decreases accordingly. This change appears to be controlled largely by the addition of cholestene derivatives to the membrane. Fluorescence polarization data show that cholesterol has a brief half-life and is increased with membranes of relatively high viscosity. Leukemia cells show a marked increase in total cholesterol, reflecting both *de novo* synthesis by lymphocytes and degradation of low density lipoprotein in the serum. The cholesterol-to-phospholipid ratio in leukemia cells approaches normality with control of the leukemic process. Total cellular content of cholesterol appears to be lower in leukemic cells, despite the increased cholesterol input. The paradox of an increased input of cholesterol and a decreased cholesterol-to-phospholipid ratio in these cells has proved intriguing. Possible explanations for this discrepancy include the release of membrane into the supernatant, concentration by leukemic antigens of cholesterol into vesicles which are then shed from the surface, or formation of antibodies to cell-detached vesicles resulting in circulating immune complexes. Triggering of increased cell proliferation with an escape from immune rejection may result from shedding of membrane vesicles during malignant transformation. The relationship between detached membrane vesicles and the residual cell surface appears to be a fertile area for further investigation.

Receptor Studies

Dr. Raymond Frade (Chapter 1) reported the availability of long-term cultured cell lines expressing malignant potential which have led to a detailed exploration of the cell surface. For example, from 40–100% of B lymphocytes have been shown to express the C3b receptor. Changes in receptor expression parallel numerous manipulations of such cells, which have suggested that C3b receptors may be cellular differentiation markers.

   Dr. Darrell Carney (Chapter 4) observed that transformed cells lose high affinity thrombin binding. Thrombin initiates division of virtually all kinds of mammalian cells in serum-free, chemically defined medium. Recently, thrombin receptors have been identified on certain cells and appear to increase markedly during cell division. Cell surface action of thrombin, which appears to involve cleavage of the receptor molecule, may be sufficient to trigger cell division. A cell's mitogenic response to various thrombin doses is directly related to receptor occupancy. Stoichiometry suggests a causal relationship between thrombin receptor binding and mitogenicity. Since transformed cells are not capable of high affinity thrombin binding, one must consider that the receptor may be released from the membrane, an abnormal receptor may be present, or the receptor may be occupied by competitive molecules. One can speculate that these transformed cells subvert the thrombin receptor mechanism to potentiate uncontrolled proliferation.

Specific Cell Population Studies

Natural Killer Cells

Dr. Ronald Herberman (Chapter 35) has reported that natural killer (NK) cells carry various surface receptors, prominently Fcγ receptors, and reviewed the relationships between NK activity and antibody dependent cell-mediated cytoxicity (ADCC). The evidence was discussed for participation of NK cells in the *in vivo* clearance of tumor cells, reactivity against normal cells, and their recently investigated role against primary tumors. He emphasized the general biologic role of NK activity in host protection from malignancy.

Dr. Eva Klein (Chapter 23) reported on cytotoxic targets for natural killer (NK) cells. These included the Daudi cell line, with an Fc receptor, and the K562 cell line, without an Fc receptor. She suggested that all cytotoxic cells are of T cell lineage as indicated by surface markers. In her system, interferon did not recruit new NK cells but did increase the cytotoxic activity of the existing NK cells. This result is consonant with the idea that interferon triggers lymphocytes for increased natural killer activity. When tumor cells were used as a target, increased NK activity in cytotoxicity cultures after interferon exposure *in vitro* was observed with allogeneic lymphocytes but not with autologous lymphocytes. Allogeneic NK activity was always lower than autologous activity against biopsied tumor material, raising a question of genetic restriction of the cytotoxic lymphocyte. Dr. Klein emphasized that differential target sensitivities may account for apparent cytotoxic lymphocyte differences in many experiments. She thought a more relevant question than natural killer activity is whether T cell specificity for tumor antigen is present and whether cells expressing such specificity can be activated to kill tumor non-specifically.

Dr. Christopher Henney (Chapter 33) reported three lines of evidence to suggest that recognition of cell surface carbohydrates is an important feature of NK cell activity. Glycoproteins exclusive to NK susceptible target cells inhibit NK cell binding. Simple sugars inhibit NK-mediated lysis. Aberrant glycolipids are displayed on some NK susceptible target cells, and these carbohydrates may be linked with these cells' vulnerability.

Dr. Sidney Golub (Chapter 34) reported on several models for studying the regulation of human NK cytotoxicity. Interferon and BCG transiently increase *in vivo* NK cytotoxicity. Such NK augmentation is associated with *in vitro* cytotoxicity in mixed lymphocyte cultures. NK activity at tumor sites occurs at low levels which can be augmented by intralesional injection of BCG. Regulatory events appear critical to the development and effector function of NK cells.

Dr. Hans Wigzell (Chapter 12) focused attention on NK cells in the human and reported that they appear to be in part null cells. Hypothetically, the NK cells cause rapid contactual lysis of target cells. The surface markers on NK cells are quite diverse, indicating that NK cells are not synonymous with null cells. Surface markers reported on the NK-active cells include receptors for the Fc portion of IgG, H-2, Lyt-5 and other markers. Target associated structures for NK activity include viral, tumor-associated, hematopoietic-differentiation, and general membrane features. Genetically high and low responders appear to be particularly relevant to NK activity. Interferon appears to be responsible for the enhancement of NK activity. Estrogens tend to increase NK activity and hydrocarbon interferon-inducers such as tilirone have recently been shown to increase NK activity. It is certainly hoped that the current fervor for characterization and understanding of the NK system will prove of therapeutic potential in human malignancy.

B Cells

Dr. Sandy Lawton (Chapter 25) reported on the use of monoclonal antibodies for understanding B cell differentiation. Pre-B cells have both cytoplasmic IgM and *DR*-antigen. The immature B lymphocyte then develops surface immunoglobulin and expresses *DR*-antigen at the surface. Upon maturity, B lymphocytes have been shown to carry at their surface receptors for the Ebstein-Barr virus, a C3 receptor, surface immunoglobulin, *DR* antigen and Fc receptors. Lawton also reported that in childhood acute lymphoblastic leukemia, about 25% of circulating peripheral blood lymphocytes are of the pre-B type. He has developed anti-idiotypic antibody against myeloma M-protein. This antiserum cross reacts only slightly (1%) with other nonmyelomatous B lymphocytes and is therefore apparently "myeloma specific." It detects no T cells. Its idiotypic specificity appears to be distributed across isotypes. It is different from the non-cross-reacting "individual specific" anti-idiotype which is specific for B cells, but is different from the myeloma specific antisera for plasma cells. Presumably, these tools for studying the maturation and differentiation sequence of B cells will add to our knowledge of the biology of that system. Additionally, this technique for investigating cellular differentiation may be applicable to other cell lines.

Macrophages

Dr. Richard Niemtzow (Chapter 5) described the application of single-cell intracellular measurement of transmembrane electrical potentials as a tool for illuminating the physicochemical events in macrophage populations. He utilized a murine tumor model to demonstrate differing electrokinetic properties between macrophages of animals harboring malignancy and those of normal animals. Furthermore, there appeared to be a linear increase in macrophage electronegativity with progressive tumor growth. This was interpreted as a correlation between electronegativity and macrophage activation, triggered by malignant transformation of adjacent cells. Similar measurements were undertaken in human lymphoid subpopulations. Distinct electrokinetic differences were found between human T lymphocytes, B lymphocytes, and null cell populations. It is hoped that this tool will help to shed light on macrophage and lymphoid cell subpopulations as well as different differentiation states of the macrophage.

Dr. Thomas Stossel (Chapter 18) reviewed the current biology of the monocyte-macrophage system as well as the interaction with polymorphonuclear leukocytes. Phagocytosis, the common denominator between these two cell lines, has been explored in considerable depth. Possible parallels between the properties of mobile phagocytes and certain transformed cells deserve further investigation.

Dr. Malcolm Mitchell (Chapter 17) reported on experiments probing the *in vivo* effects of immune complexes formed from antigens of murine lymphoblastoid cells and antibodies against them. Such complexes inhibited peritoneal macrophage activity, mediated by suppressor T lymphocyte activation and subsequent suppressor T cell-macrophage interaction. The latter process probably involves soluble mediators. This chain of events appears relevant to host protection against tumors.

T Cells

Dr. Michael Williams (Chapter 20) discussed studies of the immunogenetics of T cells, emphasizing the immunoregulatory role of the histocompatibility genes in hybrid murine models which demonstrate the allogeneic effect. Stimulation of helper and cytotoxic/suppressor lymphocyte subpopulations was found to occur. Genetic control of tumor resistance appears from these studies to be critical to host defense against malignancy.

Dr. Fritz Bach (Chapter 10) addressed himself to activation mechanisms of T cells. Cloned T cells have added measurably to our knowledge of this process. He reported that administration of cyclophosphamide with specific immune T cells is much more effective in promoting murine tumor survival than cyclophosphamide alone or cyclophosphamide combined with non-immune or indifferently immune cells. Cultured T suppressor cells are radioresistant and release interleukin-2, which appears to be a T cell growth factor which increases the proliferation of activated lymphocytes only. Further investigation of these discriminations between activated and nonactivated lymphocytes should illuminate the differences between these differentiation states of the T cell.

Dr. Erik Thorsby (Chapter 21) demonstrated that the interaction of antigen with human T cells is intimately involved with the HLA system. For activation, there must be simultaneous corecognition by the human T cell of foreign antigen and determinants within the HLA structure of the antigen-presenting cell. Thorsby contrasted a single receptor model, in which antigen recognition with an HLA difference at the cell surface occurs, with the double receptor model in which there is dual recognition of the antigen and the HLA structures at the cell surface. His interpretation of available data was that the double receptor model is the more likely to occur in the human. Genetic restriction elements are almost certainly present within the HLA cell membrane molecules. Thorsby confirmed other work suggesting that human T cell-macrophage interactions are probably *DR* restricted. Interestingly, he also showed that Langerhans cells of the skin are *D/DR* positive and can substitute for macrophages in models of such interactions.

Dr. Ethan Shevach (Chapter 6) reported interesting work on the macrophage Ia cell system which appears to be important in the mixed lymphocyte culture, in aldehyde induced mitogenesis and in antigen-specific immune responses. He demonstrated histocompatibility restriction of T macrophage interaction in inbred guinea pigs. He then discussed models of T cell-macrophage interactions based upon cellular interaction structures and complex antigenic determinants. His data suggested that cells are brought closer together by either Ia, aldehyde, or specific antigen in order to permit critical cell-to-cell interactions. These studies promise to help reveal the relationship of immunogenetics to subsequent immunobiologic consequences.

Conclusions

Studies of cell-to-cell interactions, cellular differentiation, and immunogenetic mechanisms have demonstrated that the cell surface is critical to the formation and maintenance of malignant cell lines. Newer tools, discussed above, are permitting the more detailed study of differentiation of the various cellular components of the immune system, particularly as it relates to host protection against malignancy. Intensive investigation of the cell surface and of cytotoxic mechanisms, and employment of new tools for understanding basic cell biology, such as monoclonal antibodies, are steadily developing our potential for understanding the malignant condition. It is hoped that the reports of this symposium will result in effective clinical applications in the near future.

Published 1981 by Elsevier North Holland, Inc.
Saunders, Daniels, Serrou, Rosenfeld, and Denney, eds.
FUNDAMENTAL MECHANISMS IN HUMAN CANCER IMMUNOLOGY

CHAPTER 37

Therapeutic Advances: Immunomodulation

B. Serrou, M.D.

Department of Immuno-Chemotherapy and Laboratoire d'Immunopharmacologie des Tumers, Centre Paul Lamarque, Hôpital St. Eloi, B.P. 5054, 34033 Montpellier Cedex, France

Immunotherapy, mainly in the form of immunostimulation, was introduced some years ago in cancer treatment with the use of agents such as BCG and *Corynebacterium parvum*. However, it was rapidly clear that (1) under optimal conditions, these agents can improve the prognosis of treated cancer patients only to a maximum of 10% (immunosensitive tumor), and (2) these agents can increase but also modulate the immune response. Depending on the time of injection and the drug employed, the same agents can either increase or, when suppressor cells are induced, decrease the immune response. Immunotherapeutic agents were a sort of immunological soup, composed of a very complex aggregate of many undefined antigens capable of stimulating the immune response. These problems, linked with the limited clinical effect of these controversial stimulators, brought about the search for very well characterized and biochemically defined immunomodulating agents, such as Mdp, isoprinosine and NPT, retinoic acid derivatives, thymic factors, cyclomunine, interferon and many others. These drugs, the products of a rapidly developing field, form a very long list which has only evolved during the last 2 or 3 years (Serrou et al., 1981d). This research has also been stimulated by the fact that we do not possess any substances able to significantly control the common viral infections, nor some bacterial infections. Even outside the cancer field, many clinical diseases demand careful management involving correction of immune imbalance, such as autoimmune diseases, which are becoming more and more common, and immune deficiencies.

I would like to emphasize a few points concerning this rapidly expanding field, remarks suggested partly by some of the papers included in this volume. These remarks will deal with (1) tumor specificity; (2) monoclonal antibodies as a means of defining lymphocyte subsets (in particular, T lymphocytes, NK cells, and suppressor cells); (3) neoplastic disease as a tool for characterizing lymphocyte subsets and cell interactions; and (4) modulating agents. Each of these areas offers new possibilities (interferon, cloning of T cytotoxic cells, monoclonal antibodies) for manipulation of the immune system for cancer therapy. Finally I shall make a few brief comments on the definition of the phase 1 and 2 trials of biological response modifiers.

Tumor Associated Antigen Specificity

For many years now, specific tumor antigenicity, particularly against solid tumors, has been the object of much discussion. This point is raised and defended by R.W. Baldwin (Chapter 13), who advocates specific immune resistance. Production of monoclonal antibodies can help to define very limited, minute specificities which could be expressed on many spontaneously arising tumors. If Baldwin's results are confirmed and can be elaborated, this research may open the way to specific immunotherapy. The greatest anti-tumor effect is observed when the vaccine containing viable tumor cells is in contact with adjuvant like BCG.

However, for the non-immunogenic, so-called "spontaneous tumors," neither the role of the specific immune response nor that of the non-specific immune response, particularly that involving NK cells and macrophages, has yet to be defined. In man, little has been known until recently concerning the host-tumor relationship. The role of the immune system in the control of tumor expression and growth has yet to be elucidated. However, if we consider the fact that spontaneous tumors arise from autologous normal cells and that tumor cells do not express strong tumor associated antigens, an investigation into autologous immune reactions may help to elucidate how tumors develop and might be controlled by the immune system. This kind of approach is developed by S. Gupta (Chapter 27), who suggests that autologous reactions could be involved in stimulating the production of suppressor cells, which is characteristic of cancer. We advocate the same kind of approach, and developed the auto-rosette forming cell assay for this purpose. This test characterizes a T cell subset that responds principally in allogeneic and autologous mixed lymphocyte reaction and whose numbers drop very significantly in the relapsed cancer patient (B. Serrou, Chapter 16).

Characterization and Functions of Lymphocyte Subsets

Another area of investigation which has elucidated host-tumor relationships and improved our appreciation of the potential of immunomodulation is the characterization of lymphocyte subsets. During the two last years, this approach advanced significantly with experiments using monoclonal antibodies directed against one cell subset expressing a precise function. Among these cells, I would like to focus on T lymphocytes (cytotoxic, helper, and suppressor) and NK cells, which may prove to be very closely related cells, as suggested by E. Klein (Chapter 23).

T Lymphocytes (Cytotoxic, Helper, and Suppressor T Lymphocytes)
The field of cytotoxic T lymphocytes is covered by F. Bach (Chapter 10). Although T helper cells respond primarily to *HLA-D* region encoded LD antigens, T cytotoxic cells primarily recognize *HLA-B* and C region encoded CD antigens. The precursor cytotoxic T cells express Lyt 1-2 antigens, whereas effector cytotoxic T cells could be of two types: one expressing the Lyt 1-2 antigens and the other expressing only the Lyt-2 antigens. Interestingly, Dr. Bach has proposed new markers to differentiate different cell types and to characterize cytotoxic antigen specific cells based on biochemical characterization of a 200,000 molecular weight molecule which appears in three bands. Furthermore, he has shown that cytotoxic cells generated in mixed lymphocyte culture are *DR* negative, whereas cells active on the K562 target cell are *DR* positive. The last point which he emphasizes is the possibility of cloning T lymphocytes expressing different functions.

Results such as these pave the way for potential immunomodulation by clarifying the role of each functional subset, and providing more precise and biochemically defined markers which could be very useful for evaluating the immune imbalance of the cancer patient. Furthermore, the cloning of functional T cells, if efficient and practical, could make possible autologous adoptive immunotherapy (see M.A. Cheever, Chapter 11), offering the possibility of a patient-adapted treatment. If *in vitro* growth of very specialized cells is possible, we probably should also be able to modulate or increase *in vitro* functional expression of these subsets. In other respects, the potential value of the Tumor Cell Growth Factor (TCGF) should be defined in the near future.

To explore such problems more deeply, we need a perfect human model. In this particular case, diseases could provide an appropriate tool, as pointed out by S. Broder (Chapter 15), who has defined helper diseases (like Sézary syndrome) and suppressor cell diseases (like some leukemias). Along the same lines, we demonstrated that the null ALL leukemia Reh cell line possesses suppressor cell activity which depends on the production of a suppressor factor (Serrou et al., 1981d). These facts could be of major importance in illuminating the pathophysiology of leukemias and other diseases. Furthermore, manipulation and modulation using monoclonal antibodies, either as cytotoxic agents or as drug carriers, is not far from being applicable to cancer treatment.

NK Cells and Interferon
E. Klein (Chapter 23) has suggested that cytotoxic T cells and NK cells could be closely related. However, the biological significance of NK cells remains obscure. Nevertheless, they are becoming better characterized and we know they could play a major role in regulation of autologous immune reactions. In

addition, we now have a very long list of phenotypic markers, as noted by H. Wigzell (Chapter 12). *In vivo*, there is a clear correlation with survival if mice are injected with NK sensitive tumor cells. These results are further improved by previous thymectomy, as previous studies in nude mice have suggested. These mice express a high NK activity. Thymocytes, which do not express any NK activity, are very susceptible to NK cells, as are certain stem cells, particularly embryonic cells. This kind of susceptibility is diminished by retinoic acid, which suggests a modulation and/or differentiating effect at the target level.

Many research teams have demonstrated that this particular type of cell is susceptible to interferon and interferon inducers, which can give rise to a significant increase in NK activity. This effect is independent of the type of interferon used, as reported by S. Baron (Chapter 9), who describes in detail the different types of interferon and the possible mechanisms of action of this fascinating natural antiviral agent. Interferon appears to be an immunomodulatory drug acting on cell multiplication. Also it appears to have opposite effects: (1) it can increase NK activity. The *in vivo* significance of this observation has yet to be defined, but may be crucial in regulating normal cells. (2) It can significantly improve *in vivo* delayed hypersensitivity reactions and the level of non-suppressor T cell subsets. (3) Depending on the schedule and dose employed, it can increase Con A-induced suppressor cell activity, while, preventing antigen sensitization, and produce a smaller effect on memory cells and no effect at all on mature plasma cells. A major problem is the degree of purity of interferon preparations, which if impure can give non-comparable and sometimes conflicting results. These results emphasize the fact that we must be cautious in using this kind of drug for treating patients and not claim too quickly the value of such agents without well-conducted and carefully evaluated studies. Premature optimism can not only be very detrimental for the study itself, but can also delay progress in the field of immunotherapy.

Potential Application in Man

Several potentially significant applications of these studies to human therapy emerge.

First, there is urgent need for tests permitting a precise evaluation of immune imbalance in the cancer patient. For example, as noted by A.F. LoBuglio (Chapter 14), ADCC does not seem to add any complementary information, since monocyte ADCC is not impaired at all in the cancer patient. We need new tests not only to evaluate the immune status of cancer patients but to also screen new immunomodulating or stimulating agents. For the moment, we do not have at our disposal any very simple, reproducible, and reliable tests. From experience in our own laboratories, we proposed using the auto-rosette forming cell assay as a screening test, but up to now we have not found any convincing relationship between our *in vitro* and *in vivo* data. However, progress in subset characterization, mainly from studies using monoclonal antibodies, is beginning to appear encouraging.

Effective screening and precise evaluation of the immune status of the cancer patient during therapy are the keys to immunomodulation, a term which I propose to use in place of immunotherapy because it suggests self-control of tumor development.

This is a rapidly growing field. For the last three years, many new agents which can modulate very specific functions, including natural or biochemically purified or synthesized substances, have appeared in research laboratories and in clinics. It must be remembered that the effects of many of these agents are dose- and time-dependent, and these conditions must be taken into account for the immunomodulation potential of the agents to be maximized. Some of these drugs, such as interferon, numerous thymic factors, bestatin, azimexon, isoprinosine and its derivative NPT, vitamin A and retinoic acid derivatives, cyclomunine, a thymic factor inducer, DTC, and MDP seem to be of great interest. To this long and very incomplete list, I would like to add two interesting agents: first cimetidine (Serrou et al., 1981b), which is widely used in the treatment of gastric ulcer lesions and which very significantly increases mitogen and mixed leukocyte culture responses and the production of plaque forming cells *in vitro* and *in vivo*; second, an RNA extracted from *Klebsiella pneumoniae* (Serrou et al., 1981c), which has no effect on the NK cell activity but which, *in vivo*, very markedly decreases local tumor growth and the number of lung metastases. This drug has no known side-effects, and we are in the process of initiating a phase 1 clinical trial. The greater the number of well-characterized drugs, the better we shall be able to manipulate and normalize an immune imbalance in cancer patients. This possibility becomes even more likely as cell subsets are more and more precisely defined, particularly from a functional point of view.

Need for Definition of Phase 1 and 2 Clinical Studies for Immunomodulating Agents

There is a distinct danger in applying all these new immunomodulatory techniques (immunomodulating agents, monoclonal antibodies used either as cytotoxic antibodies or as drug carriers, autologous adoptive *in vitro* immunomodulation, TCGF, autologous "specific" *in vivo* immunomodulation, etc.), without precisely defined protocols, as was previously done in early chemotherapeutic trials. There is a pressing need not only to adopt phases 1 and 2 chemotherapy trials to immunomodulating agents, but to redefine well-adapted protocols. As Secretary of two EORTC Groups (Cancer Immunology and Immunotherapy Group, CI2G, and Tumor Immunology Project Group, TIPG), I believe development of new protocols to be a major goal today. Indeed, many basic discoveries are now in the process of being applied to the human situation, as elegantly demonstrated by this Symposium, which has been a perfect meeting place for the basic scientists and clinicians.

References

Serrou, B., Rucheton, M., Rey, A., Caraux, J., Estève, C., and Thierry, C. (1981a) Auto-rosette forming cells: Further characterization and immunopharmacology. *Clinical Immunology News Letter*, In press.

Serrou, B., Rey, A., Cupissol, D., Thierry, C., Estève, C., and Rosenfeld, C. (1981b) Modulation of the immune response by cimetidine. In *Human Cancer Immunology. Vol. 4. New Immunomodulating Agents*. Serrou, B. and Rosenfeld, C. (eds.), Guest Editors: Wybran, J. and Meyer, G. Amsterdam New-York: North-Holland, In press.

Serrou, B., Rey, A., Cupissol, D., Estève, C., Dussourd-d'Hinterland, L., Normier, G., Pinèle, A.M., and Rosenfeld, C. (1981c) Efficacy of *Klebsiella pneumoniae* RNA on tumor growth in mice. In *Human Cancer Immunology. Vol. 4. New Immunomodulating Agents*. Serrou, B. and Rosenfeld, C. (eds.) Guest editors: Wybran, J. and Meyer, G. Amsterdam-New-York: North-Holland, In press.

Serrou, B., Rosenfeld, C., Rucheton, M., Thierry, C., and Cupissol, D. (1981d) Suppressor activity of the human ALL null cell line Reh. A tool for the study of suppressor cell mechanisms. *Cancer Immunol. Immunoth.*, In press.

Author Index

Subject Index

retinoic acid derivatives, 225-226

S

Sézary syndrome, 200-205
shedding of MAA, 407-419
SMLR (*See* syngeneic mixed leukocyte reaction)
suppressor cell assays, 277
syngeneic mixed leukocyte reaction (SMLR), 92-97
syngeneic preference (*See* hybrid effect on tumor resistance)

T

T cells (*See* cells: T cells)
T cell growth factor (TCGF) or IL-2, 138-139, 148-157, 453-462, 504
theophylline resistant and sensitive T cells, 376-382
therapy, isotopic immunoglobulin, 359-372
thioglycollate, 74-75
thrombin receptors, 41-53
thymidine, 9-11
thymocytes, 243-256
thymosin, 218-222
transformation, effects on thrombin receptor, 44

tumor-host interaction, 167-178, 196-200, 275-282
tumor resistance, genetic studies in experimental, 283-289
tumor specific immunity, 168-178
tumor-specific transplantation antigens (TSTA), 385-400, 449-462
troponin, 261
TSTA (*See* tumor-specific transplantation antigens)
tumor, chemically induced, 449-462
immunotherapeutic effects, 397-400
tumor volume, measurement of, 362-367
tunicamycin, 416-419

V

vitamins, as nutrients, 443
vitamin A, 225

W

WGA (*See* wheat germ agglutinin)
wheat germ agglutinin (WGA), 110-118

Z

zinc, as nutrient, 444